Obstetrics, Gynaecology and Women's Health

This is the essential textbook for students of obstetrics and gynaecology as well as women's health more generally. Thoroughly modern in approach, it covers clinical topics and surgical procedures as well as providing detailed commentary on the contemporary social, psychological and economic issues that affect women's health.

Many authors who are the acknowledged leaders in their respective research fields have contributed succinct chapters. In this way both students and health professionals are able to benefit from their expertise in a lively and accessible text. It will be a valuable resource for health professionals, including general practitioners, nurses, physiotherapists and health workers. Specific sections address women's mental health, genetics, prescribing for women, health promotion, hormones throughout the life cycle, and psychological and behavioural issues. The text is fully illustrated with many useful guides, tables, photographs and diagrams.

Vivienne O'Connor is a Senior Lecturer in Obstetrics and Gynaecology at the University of Queensland. She is acknowledged as a leading innovator in teaching techniques in the field.

Gabor Kovacs is Professor of Obstetrics and Gynaecology at Monash University in Melbourne. He is a reproductive gynaecologist, the Medical Director of Monash IVF and one of the world's leading IVF clinicians and researchers. He has written five books on reproductive health topics, is the editor of three textbooks, and the author of over 30 book chapters.

Obstetrics, Gynaecology and Women's Health

Edited by
Vivienne O'Connor
University of Queensland

Gabor Kovacs
Monash University

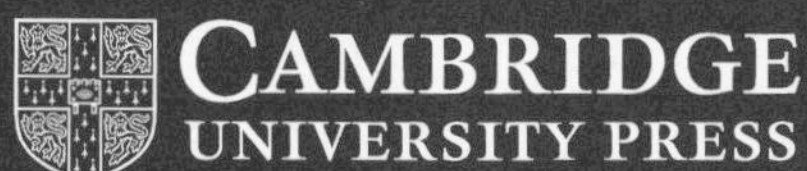

PUBLISHED BY THE PRESS SYNDICATE OF THE UNIVERSITY OF CAMBRIDGE
The Pitt Building, Trumpington Street, Cambridge, United Kingdom

CAMBRIDGE UNIVERSITY PRESS
The Edinburgh Building, Cambridge CB2 2RU, UK
40 West 20th Street, New York, NY 10011-4211, USA
477 Williamstown Road, Port Melbourne, VIC 3207, Australia
Ruiz de Alarcón 13, 28014 Madrid, Spain
Dock House, The Waterfront, Cape Town 8001, South Africa

http://www.cambridge.org

First published 2003

Printed in Australia by BPA Print Group

Typeface New Caledonia (*Adobe*) 10/13 pt. *System* QuarkXPress® [BC]

A catalogue record for this book is available from the British Library

National Library of Australia Cataloguing in Publication data
Obstetrics, gynaecology and women's health.
Includes index.
ISBN 0 521 81893 1.
1. Obstetrics. 2. Gynecology. 3. Women – Health and
hygiene. I. O'Connor, Vivienne. II. Kovacs, Gabor, 1947– .

ISBN 0 521 81893 1 hardback

Contents summary

Contents

List of colour photos

List of contributors

Lisa Amir MBBS, MMed, IBCLC
General Practitioner and Lactation Consultant, Women's Clinic on Richmond Hill, Melbourne and Lecturer, Key Centre for Women's Health, University of Melbourne
Lactation, breastfeeding, breastfeeding difficulties

Richard Anderson MD, PhD, MRCOG
Clinical Scientist and Consultant in Reproductive Medicine, MRC Human Reproductive Sciences Unit and Royal Infirmary, Edinburgh
Conception and implantation

Agnes Bankier MBBS(Hon), FRACP(Paed), HGSA
Certified Clinical Geneticist, Associate Professor, Director, Genetic Health Services Victoria
Genetics

Bryanne Barnett MD, FRANZCP
Professor of Perinatal and Infant Psychiatry, University of New South Wales; Director, Paediatric Mental Health Services, SWSAHS
Mood changes in pregnancy and post partum

Lisa Begg MBBS, FRANZCOG, MPH, DDU
Maternal-Fetal Medicine Specialist, Melbourne
Premature labour, prelabour premature rupture of membranes

Michael J Bennett MB, ChB, MD (UCT) FCOG(SA), FRCOG, FRANZCOG, DDU
Professor and Head of Obstetrics and Gynaecology, School of Women's and Children's Health UNSW; President of The Australian Society of Paediatric and Adolescent Gynaecology
The adolescent: puberty and its disorders

Dr Ruth Best MBBS
General Practitioner and Research Assistant in Department of Obstetrics and Gynaecology, University of Queensland
Breast screening: breast problems

Kirsten Black MMed, MRANZCOG
Fellow in Clinical Effectiveness, Royal Women's Hospital, Melbourne
The adolescent: pregnancy, STIs, Pap tests

Clare Boothroyd MBBS (Hons), MMed Sci, FRACP, FRANZCOG, CREI
Reproductive Endocrinologist and Gynaecologist, Greenslopes Private Hospital, Brisbane
Amenorrhoea, irregular bleeding, PCOS, hirsutism

Henry Burger AO, FAA, MD, BS, FRCP, FRACP, FCP(SA), FRCOG, FRANZCOG
Emeritus Director, Prince Henry's Institute of Medical Research, Monash Medical Centre, Clayton
Hormones through the life cycle

Sharon Cameron MB ChB, MD, MRCOG
Lecturer in Reproductive Medicine, Department of Obstetrics and Gynaecology, Centre for Reproductive Biology, University of Edinburgh
Conception and implantation

Susan V Carr MD
Consultant in Family Planning and Reproductive Health and Honorary Senior Lecturer at the University of Glasgow, Scotland
Sexual health: sexual problems

Michael Carr-Gregg BA(Hons), MA, PhD
Consultant Adolescent Psychologist, Albert Road Centre for Health, South Melbourne
The adolescent: normal development and risk taking

Colleen Cartwright BSocWk (Hons), MPH
Senior Research Fellow, Australasian Centre on Ageing, and Lecturer in Healthy Ageing, School of Population Health, University of Queensland
Ageing: normal common complaints, prescribing for the elderly

Fung Yee Chan FRANZCOG, FRCOG, DDU, CMFM, MD
Professor of Maternal Fetal Medicine, University of Queensland, Mater Misericordiae Health Services, Brisbane
Small for dates, large for dates, fetal well-being

Michael Chapman MD, MBBS, FRCOG, FRANZCOG, CREI
Professor of Obstetrics and Gynaecology, School of Women's and Children's Health, University of New South Wales; St George Hospital, Kogarah, NSW; Unit Manager, IVF Australia, Southern Sydney; St George Private Hospital Kogarah, NSW
Subfertility

Chris Del Mar BSc, MA, MB BChir, FRACGP, FAFPHM, MD
Professor of General Practice at the University of Queensland.
Asking a clinical query

Graeme Dennerstein RFD, MBBS, FRCOG, FRANZCOG
Obstetrician and Gynaecologist, Melbourne
Benign vulvar diseases

James A Dickinson MBBS, PhD, FRACGP, FAFPHM
Professor of Family Medicine, Department of Family Medicine, University of Calgary, Alberta, Canada
Screening

Hans Peter Dietz MD, FRANZCOG, DDU
Fellow in Urogynaecology, Royal Prince Alfred Hospital, Sydney; Visiting Medical Officer, Royal Hospital for Women and Conjoint Lecturer, University of NSW
Urinary and bowel incontinence

Lesley Doyal BA/MSc
Professor of Health and Social Care, School for Policy Studies, University of Bristol
Gender and health

Michael P Dunne BA(Hons), PhD
Senior Lecturer in Epidemiology, Queensland University of Technology School of Public Health, Brisbane, Australia
Sexual behaviour

Kevin Forbes MD BS, FRANZCOG, CREI
Deputy Head of School, School of Medicine, The University of Queensland
Endometriosis

Colin Furnival MBChB, PhD, FRCS, FRACS
Specialist Breast Surgeon, Wesley Medical Centre; Clinical Director of the Centre for Breast Health, Royal Women's Hospital, Brisbane
Breast cancer

Janice L Goerzen BSc, MSc, MD, FRCSC, FRCOG, FACOG, FRANZCOG
Associate Professor of Obstetrics and Gynaecology, University of Tasmania; Director Women's and Children's Services, Launceston, Tasmania
Embryology: ambiguous genitalia at birth, development of the female child, vulvovaginitis in the female child

Jane Gunn PhD, MBBS, FRACGP, DRANZCOG
Associate Professor, Research Director, Department of General Practice, University of Melbourne, Melbourne, Australia
Normal postnatal period

Louise Gyler MA, BSoc Stud
Psychoanalyst in private practice, Sydney
Mood changes in pregnancy and post partum

Kelsey Hegarty MBBS, DipRACOG, FRACGP, PhD
Senior Lecturer, Department of General Practice, University of Melbourne
Abuse against women including minority groups, in pregnancy and the elderly, female genital mutilation

Mary Hepburn BSc, MD, MRCGP, FRCOG
Senior Lecturer in Women's Reproductive Health and Consultant Obstetrician and Gynaecologist, University of Glasgow and Princess Royal Maternity Glasgow
Smoking, alcohol and drugs

Cherrell Hirst AO, MBBS, BedSt DUniv(Hon)
Director of Wesley Breast Clinic 1984–2001, Chancellor of Queensland University of Technology since 1994
Breast screening, breast problems

Michael Humphrey MBBS, PhD, FRANZCOG, FRCOG
Professor of Obstetrics and Gynaecology, James Cook University School of Medicine; Director, Obstetrics and Gynaecology, Women's and Children's Health Service, King Edward Memorial Hospital, WA
Abnormal labour, assisted delivery, induction of labour

Ian SC Jones MB ChM, Dip Obst, Grad Cert Ed, MHA, FRCOG, FRANZCOG, FACS
Head, Department of Obstetrics and Gynaecology, University of Queensland; Head School of Medicine, Southern Division, University of Queensland
Bleeding in pregnancy

Gavin Kemball MBBS, MRCOG
Clinical Research Fellow, IVF Australia, Southern Sydney, St George Private Hospital, Kogarah, NSW
Subfertility

Soo Keat Khoo MBBS, MD, FRCOG, FRANZCOG
Professor/Director, Division of Gynaecology, University of Queensland and Royal

Women's Hospital, Brisbane
Hydatidiform mole, chorionic carcinoma
Gab Kovacs MD, FRCOG, FRANZCOG, CREI
Professor Director of Obstetrics and Gynaecology, Eastern Health, Box Hill Medical School, Monash University
Antenatal care, common presentations in the first trimester
Nicole McCarthy MBBS(Hons), FRACP
Medical Oncologist, Royal Brisbane Hospital, Brisbane
Chemotherapy for breast cancer
Treasure McGuire BPharm, BSC, PostGradDipClinHospPharm
Assistant Director of Pharmacy (Education and Information), Conjoint Lecturer Mater Pharmacy Services, Mater Misericordiae Health Services, Brisbane, School of Pharmacy, University of Queensland, Brisbane
Prescribing for women
Ruth McNair MBBS DRACOG, DA(UK), FRACGP, FACRRM
Senior Lecturer and Director of Undergraduate Education, Department of General Practice, University of Melbourne
Sexuality: sexual history taking; lesbian health: STIs, Pap tests, fertility
Karen McNeil MBBS, MPH, TM
Advanced Trainee in Endocrinology, Austin and Repatriation Medical Centre, Heidelberg, Victoria
Hormones through the life cycle
Geoffrey Mitchell MBBS, FRACGP FAChPM
Associate Professor in General Practice, University of Queensland and Director of the Centre for Palliative Care Research and Education
Death and dying
Adam Morton FRACP
Physician, Mater Misericordiae Hospital, Brisbane
Medical problems in pregnancy
Judith Murray BA(Hons), DipEd, BedSt, PhD
Senior Lecturer and Director of the Loss and Grief Unit, School of Population Health, University of Queensland
Loss and grief
Jonathan Morris MB, ChB, MM, PhD, FRANZCOG
Senior Lecturer and Maternal-Fetal Medicine Specialist, University of Sydney, Royal North Shore Hospital, Sydney
Infections in pregnancy
Balakrishnan R Nair FRCP (Glasgow), FRCP (Edinburgh), FRCP (Ireland), FRACP, GradDipEpi (Clin Epid)
Professor and Director, Geriatric Medicine, John Hunter Hospital, Newcastle
Ageing: normal events, common complaints, prescribing for the elderly
Jeremy Oats MBBS, DM, FRCOG, FRANZCOG
Clinical Director of Obstetrics and Gynaecology, Royal Women's Hospital, Victoria
Diabetes in pregnancy

Vivienne O'Connor MB ChB, FRANZCOG, FRCOG
Senior Lecturer, Department of Obstetrics and Gynaecology, The University of Queensland
Interpersonal skills, prepregnancy counselling, normal labour stages, abortion, normal sexual response, STIs, menorrhagia, vaginal discharge, menopause, pre-cancer and screening, premenstrual syndrome, labour and childbirth, postmenopausal bleeding, medical and surgical issues

Rhian Parker BSc(Econ) Hons, MSc
Lecturer, Department of General Practice, The University of Melbourne
Obesity, body image, health of women from minority groups

Michael Permezel MD, MRCP(UK), MRCOG, FRANZCOG
Professor and Deputy Head, Department of Obstetrics and Gynaecology, University of Melbourne
Iso-immunisation, hypertension, pre-eclampsia, eclampsia

Rodney Petersen MBBS, MBA, FRANZCOG
Senior Lecturer, Department of Obstetrics and Gynaecology, University of Melbourne
Gynaecological cancer

Julie A Quinlivan PhD, FRANZCOG
Senior Lecturer in Obstetrics and Gynaecology, The University of Melbourne
The adolescent: pregnancy, STIs, Pap tests

Michael Quinn MB ChB, MGO, MRCP(UK), FRANZCOG, FRCOG, CGO
Director of Oncology, Royal Women's Hospital; Associate Professor, Dept of Obstetrics and Gynaecology, University of Melbourne
Gynaecological cancer

Chris Riddoch CertEd, BA MEd, PhD
Senior Lecturer in Exercise and Health Science, University of Bristol
Physical activity

Wendy Rogers MBBS, BA, PhD, MRCGP, FRACGP
NHMRC Sidney Sax Fellow, Department of General Practice, Flinders University, South Australia
Ethics and women's health

Alexis Shub FRANZCOG
Fellow Maternal Fetal Medicine, Mater Mothers' Hospital, Brisbane
Small for dates, large for dates, fetal well-being

Suruchi Thapar-Bjorkert BA (Delhi), MA (Delhi), MPhil (Cam), PhD (Warwick)
Lecturer in Sociology, University of Bristol
Physical activity

Mark Thompson-Fawcett FRACS
Senior Lecturer and Colorectal Surgeon, University of Otago and Dunedin Hospital, New Zealand
Urinary and bowel incontinence

David Tudehope AM, MBBS, MRACP, FRACP
Director of Neonatology, Mater Mothers' Hospital, South Brisbane, Queensland; Professor of Paediatrics and Child Health, University of Queensland
The newborn infant

Derek Tuffnell MB, ChB, FRCOG
Consultant in Obstetrics and Gynaecology, Bradford Hospitals NHS Trust, Bradford UK
Obstetric emergencies

Jane Turner MBBS, FRANZCP
Senior Lecturer in Psychiatry, The University of Queensland
Depression and anxiety; puberty: psychological development; psychological effects of cancer

Edith Weisberg MBBS, MM (Syd), FACSHP, FRANZCOG ad eundem
Director of Research, Sydney Centre for Reproductive Health Research, Research Division of FPA Health; Senior Clinical Lecturer, Department of Obstetrics and Gynaecology, University of Sydney
Contraception

Alexandra Welborn MBBS (WA), FRACGP, DMJ (Clin)
Formerly Forensic Physician, Victorian Institute of Forensic Medicine and Honorary Senior Lecturer in Forensic Medicine, Monash University. Currently Psychiatry Registrar c/o WA Postgraduate Training in Psychiatry
Sexual assault

Christine West MD, DCH, FRCOG
Consultant Obstetrician and Gynaecologist, Simpson Centre for Reproductive Health, Royal Infirmary of Edinburgh
Pelvic pain and pelvic mass

Don Wilson MD, FRCS, FRANZCOG, FRCOG, CU
Professor of Obstetrics and Gynaecology and Head of the Department of Women's and Children's Health, Dunedin School of Medicine, University of Otago, Dunedin, New Zealand
Urinary and bowel incontinence

Preface

The traditional obstetrics and gynaecology curriculum in many medical schools around the world has been superseded by 'women's health'. This includes core obstetrics and gynaecology in a broader context that is more relevant for women and those who care for them. At the same time many schools are taking a problem-based learning or case-based approach to health. This text is designed to provide a resource that incorporates both of these developments.

Asking the right questions in clinical practice

Health is more than just the absence of disease or infirmity. It also involves the context of people's lives, their well-being and their dignity. Certainly the issues for women are broader than those of reproduction alone.

This book has a biomedical focus. It is intended for students and practising clinicians caring for women in health and illness. The importance of the psycho-social–cultural aspects of women's lives is emphasised early in the book. We encourage the reader to use it to think of the whole woman and her interaction with her environment as each 'clinical' problem is encountered. Hopefully this approach will provide the reader with an introduction to a comprehensive picture of health and illness.

Although this text is not intended to cover every disease affecting women, it should stimulate the reader to consider the impact of health and disease on the whole person by asking such questions as:

> *If this patient were of a different gender, would the presentation, management and outcomes be different?*
>
> *If this patient lived in a different location, belonged to a different ethnic group, or belonged to a different socio-economic group, what would be the implications for health maintenance or illness?*

Using this book

The structure of this book reflects the fact that a clinical problem may vary in presentation and management depending on the stage of the person's life cycle. Therefore, while the main section on a topic (such as breast disease) might be included in the reproductive years section, for example, cross-references to relevant information in other sections of the book are provided where appropriate. The index can also be used to find appropriate cross-references across the life cycle, as well as to identify specific topics.

Some topics, such as screening and evidence-based medicine, are not confined to women's health, but are included as they form the foundation of current clinical practice. Similarly, a reference list is provided at the end of this book because the information in the text is based on current evidence from the literature. Pregnancy and childbirth issues are at the forefront of this approach, with the large collection of evidence in the Cochrane Library.

The section on the clinical interview is general, and highlights the need for sensitivity and respect that applies to any interaction with patients.

Vivienne O'Connor
Gabor Kovacs

Acknowledgements

We are grateful to the many people who have contributed to this book by providing comment and support during its development. Among the many thanks due are those to: Professor Ross Young, Head, School of Psychiatry and Counselling, Queensland University of Technology; Dr Ian Scott, Medicine Department, The University of Queensland; and Dr Katherine Robertson, Senior Lecturer in Department of General Practice, University of Melbourne, for their comments on the communication skills section; Dr Vanita Parekh, specialist in Sexual Health and Assault Medicine at Canberra Hospital, for comments on the STI section; Dr Gary Pritchard, Obstetric Sonologist, for providing ultrasound photos; Professor Bruce Ward, for providing clinical slides; and Sister Janelle Laws, Mater Mothers' Hospital, for assistance with the clinical photos.

Special thanks to Professor Ian Jones, Head of Southern Clinical Division, Head of Department of Obstetrics and Gynaecology, School of Medicine, The University of Queensland, for providing clinical slides and continued support during this project.

Thanks also to Dr Ruth Best for editorial support, and Ms Julie Buchan, Personal Assistant to Vivienne O'Connor, who has overseen and coordinated the development of this book at all stages.

This book has been developed under the guidance of the skilled team at Cambridge University Press: Peter Debus, Amanda Pinches and Kay Waters.

SECTION 1

Part 1 Women's health

The health professional role

Interpersonal and clinical skills

The interpersonal skills required to work with and for women include an empathic approach to the socio-cultural context of the individual woman's life and a desire to provide quality, equitable health care for women. This involves the ability to sensitively explore all the issues relevant to the woman's health needs, skill and sensitivity in the clinical examination, requesting appropriate investigations to support or refute the differential diagnoses, applying clinical reasoning to reach a diagnosis, and management of the problem. Sound communication skills and a collaborative approach to decision making with the woman are essential.

A thorough grounding in the core skills of consultation and examination is essential during training. Experience in performing intimate examinations may be more difficult for male students, even those trained by special teaching programs.[1] A good clinician will recognise the limitations in their practice and knowledge and be prepared to acknowledge and improve these. Lifelong learning and an ability to search and critically evaluate the relevant literature to obtain answers and apply research to clinical practice are essential for the health professional in the twenty-first century.

Safety in practice is of increasing concern to the public and the profession alike. This major concern covers four main areas: diagnosis, prescribing, communication and organisational change.

Diagnosis

Good clinical reasoning should avoid misdiagnosis. It is, however, not always possible to provide a certain diagnosis. It is essential to be honest about what is known and what is not known. It is possible for the doctor to acknowledge uncertainty about a diagnosis or prognosis while giving the patient a clear, positive message about what they can expect to happen, or what options might be suggested for the problem and what to do if things do not go according to expectation. It is also useful to give an indication, if possible, of the likely time that will elapse before the situation becomes clearer, either through the provision of diagnostic results or further symptom changes. This safety net is likely to be perceived positively by the patient, who may feel even more empowered as the doctor has clearly planned for the uncertainty that all patients know exists. Pretending to know the exact diagnosis or prognosis is likely to lessen satisfaction and cause patients to lose faith in your honesty. Helping patients to cope with uncertainty effectively is an important part of empowerment and a core clinical task. It is also important to acknowledge that you may not have all the answers immediately to hand, but are skilled and willing to obtain the most recent and best available evidence. Most patients are grateful for this approach and will willingly return to discuss your findings. Patients require their doctor to be humane and competent, to give them time, to include them in decision making, and to be honest and trustworthy.[2,3]

Prescribing

Prescribing errors may occur by under-use (failure to use proven treatments in appropriate dosage or duration), over-use (using treatments when they are not needed) and misuse (actually making an error or mistake, such as not responding to an abnormal test, or not checking interaction with the woman's current medications).[4] Errors will become more likely as more complex drugs are available, polypharmacy increases and consultation time is at a premium (Box 1.1).

BOX 1.1 **Errors with pharmaceuticals**

- Poor adherence caused by failure to:
  - explore and integrate patients' preference and beliefs about medicines
  - explain why a drug is being prescribed
  - explain how the drug is supposed to work
  - explain clearly and check the patient's understanding of the regimen
  - recognise a lack of explicit agreement between the woman and her doctor on this course of action
- Inappropriate drugs, dosages or drug combinations
- Common side effects not discussed and anticipated by patients
- Transcribing errors from transfer of information between documents

Adapted from Coulter 2002.[3]

Organisation and change

In order to practise safely, health professionals must be able to work in a team, practise ethically, and be aware of medico-legal issues and the need to deliver optimal care within available resources. Patients must be at the centre of a health care service and must be treated as partners by health professionals. Regular, systematic feedback from patients is essential to improve quality of care and for public accountability. For instance, in recent times there has been a move to reduce the time spent in hospital. For women in particular who form the major carers for a family, it is essential that this early discharge be backed up with appropriate community resources that support the woman's recovery. Prompt and comprehensive communication between services and health care professionals is required to provide follow-up and continuity of care.

Organisation of time is important. Health care professionals (HCPs) who have established a relationship with a patient can make good use of both telephone and email consultations.[5] This would provide HCPs with the added benefit of being able to vary the consultation time, allowing minor issues to be dealt with quickly and providing longer times for those patients who would benefit from this.[6]

Communication

The health professional with well-developed communication skills will have better diagnostic accuracy and clinical satisfaction. Communication skills can be learned and improved on, and can benefit from practice and self-reflection.[7]

1 Woman-centredness

Outcomes for patients can be improved by sound communication and integrating both the health care professional's and patient's agendas, based on their knowledge, understanding, expectations, beliefs and concerns—the patient-centred approach.[8,9] Woman-centred health care involves shared problem definition and decision making in the management of each problem.[10] The main partners in this process are the health professional and the woman—both contribute different areas of expertise. The woman brings to the clinical encounter her own experiences and attitudes (Box 1.2).

BOX 1.2 Woman's contribution to the clinical encounter

- Individual preferences
- Attitude to risk
- Personal and cultural values
- Experience of illness
- Social circumstances
- Habits and behaviour

The health professional can provide appropriate clinical information for discussion, remembering that this may be influenced by doctors' attitudes and values. Health professionals need to support women in making decisions by turning raw data into information that is digestible and therefore helpful to the discussion. This information should include relevant clinical findings, the results of investigations and management options. It should be as complete and balanced as possible and based on the best available evidence (Box 1.3).

BOX 1.3 Information from the health professional

- Causes of the complaint
- Diagnostic tests and their limitations
- Results of investigations and their interpretation
- Treatment options, including:
  - side effects
  - complications: short- and long-term
- Prognosis/outcomes/follow-up
- Preventive strategies

Women provided with this information can be assisted in making their own choice. It must be accepted that this may be different from the one that the clinician might make for him/herself. It should also not be assumed that decisions are always made on a rational basis, and the HCP must be clear about his or her own boundaries. Taking a woman-centred approach to the exploration and management of clinical problems will improve communication and patient satisfaction, and minimise problems if an adverse event should occur (Box 1.4).

The quality of clinical communication is related to positive health outcomes.[11] Patients who are well informed are more likely to maintain treatments and have better health outcomes. The time taken to reach a meaningful shared decision will

BOX 1.4 Improving communication

- Health professionals should aim to:
  - Involve women in making decisions about health
  - Keep women informed
  - Provide women with counselling and support
  - Gain informed consent for all procedures and processes
  - Elicit feedback from women
  - Listen to women's views and experiences
  - Be open and candid when adverse events occur.

depend on the background of the patient, their level of education and the condition under discussion. At all times during a consultation it is important to show the woman respect, allow time for the clinical relationship to develop with trust and honesty, listen to her, provide clear explanations, give the opportunity to ask questions and allow her to be in control—during history taking, examination and discussions of management.

KEY POINT

Women must be treated as partners by health professionals—as 'equals with different expertise'.

2 Providing information

Most women would like more information in the consultation. Doctors typically overestimate how much information has been provided. However, it may be difficult for an individual woman to retain all the information provided, so care must be taken not to provide too much information—it may be necessary to provide information over several consultations. Providing information is not always easy. The usefulness of information is affected by how the HCP presents it. It may be helpful to use pictures and diagrams to show the normal state and the change that the woman's body has undergone. These, together with easily understandable written information, can be taken home by the woman for discussion with friends and family. Generic information should be personalised and made specific to the individual woman. In some situations, where the situation is complex (such as deciding about options for cancer treatment) or sensitive (where there has been a loss), a clinician may choose to record the interview on audiotape for the woman to review later under less stressful circumstances.

Some areas are easier to explain than others. Management options address treatments that may involve a variety of choices, each with different benefits and risks. Risk communication is a particular challenge.[12] It is defined as the open, two-way exchange of information and opinion about risk, leading to better decisions about clinical management. Information on risk must be presented in a balanced manner.

There is no uniform method that has been shown to be the ideal way of presenting this information. It will vary with the issue involved, the amount of relevant information available, the areas that are unknown, and the doctor's level of communication skills. Women can make good use of information that is presented clearly and effectively. The visual presentation of risk information in the form of bar graphs, scales and pie charts can also sometimes be helpful, depending on the individual woman. Providing patients with evidence-based information and being able to explain information accessed by the patient is a current challenge to the health professions.[13]

3 Reducing complaints and litigation

Poor communication and failure to take account of the patient's perspective are at the heart of most formal complaints and legal actions.[14] The patient-centred approach will reduce error rates and influence the patient's reaction to errors when they do occur.

4 Informed consent

Consent should be obtained for any sensitive enquiry or examination, but it only applies if the woman has both heard and understood what is going to happen. Always include an explanation of what you are going to do and why it is necessary, and provide opportunities for the woman to ask questions or stop the procedure. Consent is required before any intimate examination can proceed.

It is also essential that a true informed consent be obtained before any decision is made about treatment. This involves discussion with full and balanced information about the risks and uncertainties of procedures and treatments, the options and alternatives, and the possible outcomes of each. A variety of decision aids using both written, visual and computer-generated material are being developed to assist patients in making decisions.[15,16]

Interviewing

The medical interview is ultimately the most powerful diagnostic tool. When used correctly it is a combination of cognitive and technical skills of the clinician and his/her feelings, beliefs and personality together with those of the woman. Although the interview is structured, the experienced interviewer is able to be flexible and appear spontaneous while putting the woman at ease. Relevant facts should be elicited to provide information to assist the woman in resolving her health concern.

1 Opening the consultation

Always welcome the woman and introduce yourself. If she is accompanied by someone, ask if she would like that person to attend the interview (and ask again before any examination). Offer her a seat nearby rather than across the desk. Be aware of your body language and the body language of the patient throughout the consultation (Box 1.5).

BOX 1.5 Body language to establish good rapport

- An interpretation of body language depends on the context, culture and congruity. In general:
  - Be friendly but professional in your manner.
  - Be open and welcoming.
  - Establish eye contact.
  - Listen and show interest.
  - Encourage and make appropriate responses (facial and verbal).
  - Appear unhurried.

2 Open-ended questions

Open-ended questions are useful to gain information and avoid presuming answers. For example, ask 'Tell me more about …' or 'Can you describe …' or 'How do you feel about that?'

This needs to be balanced with not allowing the patient to diverge too much. Politely keeping the patient on track but allowing the story to unfold is one of the skills of good interviewing and effective communication (Box 1.6).

BOX 1.6 Effective communication

- Use words the woman understands.
- Be unambiguous.
- Let the patient talk.
- Talk less yourself.
- Be non-judgemental.
- Ask 'open-ended' questions.
- Offer encouragement to continue.
- Ask 'Is there anything else you want to tell me or I should know?'

3 Direct questions

Direct questions clarify and add to the information already received. Care must be taken to ask the question in a way that will not bias the response. Establishing the sequence of events in the patient's history is important, and it may assist your understanding to start back at a time when there were no problems and then move forward in time, noting the events as they occurred. Each symptom can be clarified en route or after the sequence of events has been established (Box 1.7).

4 Closing the interview

It is useful to make a brief summary at the end of the consultation to check that both parties have reached agreement on defining the problem(s) and an approach to management and follow-up. Thank the woman for attending and reiterate the next

BOX 1.7 Clarifying symptoms

1 When did it start and how often does it occur? (onset and frequency)
2 Can you show me where you feel it? (location)
3 When it is there, how long does it last? (duration)
4 Do you feel it anywhere else? (radiation)
5 How bad is it? (severity)
6 How would you describe it? (nature)
7 Does anything seem to bring it on? (precipitating factors)
8 Does anything seem to lessen or improve it? (relieving factors)
9 What are/were you doing when it started? (setting)
10 Did you notice any other problems at this time? (associated factors)

event (make another appointment, arrange a test, contact for a result etc). Check the woman's knowledge and understanding of the interview by asking, for example, that she repeat key information in her own words (Box 1.8).

BOX 1.8 Check knowledge and understanding

1 Ensure the correct information has been obtained. ('Let me see if I have understood the problem.')
2 Prioritise the information given (patients recall best what they are told first and last).
3 Provide information that is simple and backed up with written/diagrammatic material.
4 Repeat the problem and the agreed plan of action.
5 Check understanding and consent to the plan.
6 Ask for any questions, queries or concerns.

5 Using an interpreter

Most metropolitan hospitals have interpreter services. It is essential to arrange an interpreter who is not a relative. It is also important to be aware of sensitivities about differences between ethnic groups from the same part of the world and to arrange for the correct language/dialect if appropriate. A female interpreter must be booked, and be trained in medical terminology. Always speak to and watch the patient and keep the questions brief.

KEY POINT

Make careful use of:

- ***reflection*** **(a response that echoes the information just provided)**
- ***silence*** **(to support the woman expressing emotion)**
- ***support*** **(to indicate reassurance and empathy).**

The gynaecological history

The consultation often follows a standard format (Box 1.9), although there are occasions when this format is inappropriate. The additional information that should be covered from a female patient relates partly to her gender (Box 1.10), but also addresses the particular issues important in women's lives (Box 1.11).

The sexual history

Interviewing regarding sexual history is one of the most sensitive components of a health care interview. Health care professionals may tend to avoid broaching the subject, assuming that patients will ask specific questions if relevant. Most patients, however, will not raise the subject unless invited to do so, despite having relevant issues they wish to discuss. It is therefore useful to ask one or two sexual health screening questions during most consultations. The health care professional is in a unique position to assist patients with questions and concerns about sexual function. The interview is private and bound by rules of confidentiality, and the professional should have knowledge or be able to access reliable information regarding sexual health.

Adequate preparation of the interviewer for taking an effective sexual history includes understanding his or her own attitudes, developing skills through reflective practice, gaining adequate knowledge of key issues, and lack of embarrassment. Attitude formation in this area involves developing a non-judgemental approach toward the diverse range of ways in which women choose to express their sexuality. In particular, avoid making assumptions about the nature of a patient's sexual practices. Lesbian women, for example, are constantly aware of the assumption of heterosexuality that pervades social interactions, including interactions with health care providers. Practitioners can assist by developing skills including effective introduction of the subject, facilitation of disclosure of sensitive issues, the use of gender-neutral language, avoiding jargon and clarifying the meaning of language that the patient uses. Knowledge of the range of sexual behaviour and identities and the common sexual problems with which patients present is essential (Section 12). It is important to be able to recognise when to refer the patient for expert advice. This includes having a referral network of knowledgeable and accessible specialists.

BOX 1.9 General history

- Presenting complaint
- History of presenting complaint
- Associated factors
- General system history that is relevant
- Past medical and surgical history
- Social history
- Family history

BOX 1.10 Specific history

1 Menarche
- Age of onset, initial cycle

2 Menses
- Current cycle: frequency, duration, amount of bleeding, last menstrual period
- Abnormal bleeding: intermenstrual bleeding, postcoital bleeding, postmenopausal bleeding
- Premenstrual problems

3 Pain
- Dysmenorrhoea, dyspareunia, pelvic pain

4 Menopause
- Age, symptoms

5 Pregnancies
- Number, outcome, complications

6 Contraception
- Current, past, problems

7 Sexual history
- Current partner, sexual orientation
- Change of partner in previous six months
- Vaginal discharge, sexually transmitted infections
- Sexual concerns
- Sexual abuse

8 Pap test history
- Last one, frequency, any abnormalities, management

9 Breast problems
- Nature, outcomes

10 Investigations
- Ultrasound, mammography, X-ray, blood tests

11 Urinary and bowel symptoms

12 Previous gynaecological complaints (investigation, diagnosis, treatment)

BOX 1.11 Social history

- Marital status
- Partner preference
- Family: children/siblings/parents (carer role)
- Work/study
- Drugs: alcohol, nicotine, cannabis, medications, OTC, complementary medicines and other recreational drugs
- Diet/physical activity/exercise
- Relationship functioning
- Current stressors

How to ask

Rapport building prior to discussing sexuality assists in developing trust and will improve the chance of open and full disclosure of sexual issues. This should be followed by an explanation of the reason for sexual history questions for this particular person and reassurance that many patients feel somewhat embarrassed discussing these matters.

It is important to then seek permission to proceed, and to emphasise confidentiality. Effective communication skills include using open questions, avoiding leading questions initially, observing cues from the patient, and being willing to probe to encourage further discussion. Ensure that you give the patient permission to discontinue the discussion or not answer particular questions if she wishes.

Examples of questions for consultations

- ☐ Signpost and permission
  'It is helpful for your health care for me to understand you as a person more fully. Do you mind if I ask about your sexual and relationship history?'
- ☐ Screening questions
  'Are you or have you been sexually active?' (Section 2 for definition)
  or
  'Do you have a current sexual partner?'
  If no: *'How do you feel about that?'* (if there is a cue from the patient that there may be a problem)
  If yes: *'Are you sexually active with men, women or both?'*
  'Is there anything you would like to discuss regarding your sexual life?'
- ☐ Establishing relevance
  'You mentioned that you would like to have a Pap smear. This can also be a good chance to take tests for infection if needed. Can I ask about your sexual practices to understand whether you may have had any risks for infection?'
  Or
  'Your pain could be due to an infection that could be sexually transmitted. Do you currently have a sexual partner? Have you had any other sexual partners before him/her (and since you have been with your current partner)? How long ago? What types of sexual activity do you do? Do you use any protection during these activities?'
- ☐ Probing following a cue
  'You looked uncomfortable when you mentioned your last boyfriend.'
  The use of reflection can be enough to prompt disclosure of lack of control, unprotected sexual activity or abuse issues. If not, a further probe may be necessary:
  'Would you like to talk about that relationship?'
- ☐ Normalising and broadening sexuality and clarifying sexual orientation
  'Many women are sexually or emotionally attracted to people of either or both sexes.'
  'Many women may be concerned about their sexual response/sexual activities.'

Physical examination

The woman needs to understand the reason for undertaking an examination and what information this may provide to explain her symptoms or exclude particular problems. It is essential to explain what the examination will involve (the use of a diagram or model may be useful) and any discomfort that she may expect (Figures 1.1–1.3).

Check whether she has had a similar examination/procedure before and whether there were any problems experienced. It is not unusual for patients to find the examination distressing or embarrassing. Provide reassurance that the patient can exercise control over the examination and ask for her consent to proceed with the examination. She should be asked if she would like a support person present (a friend,

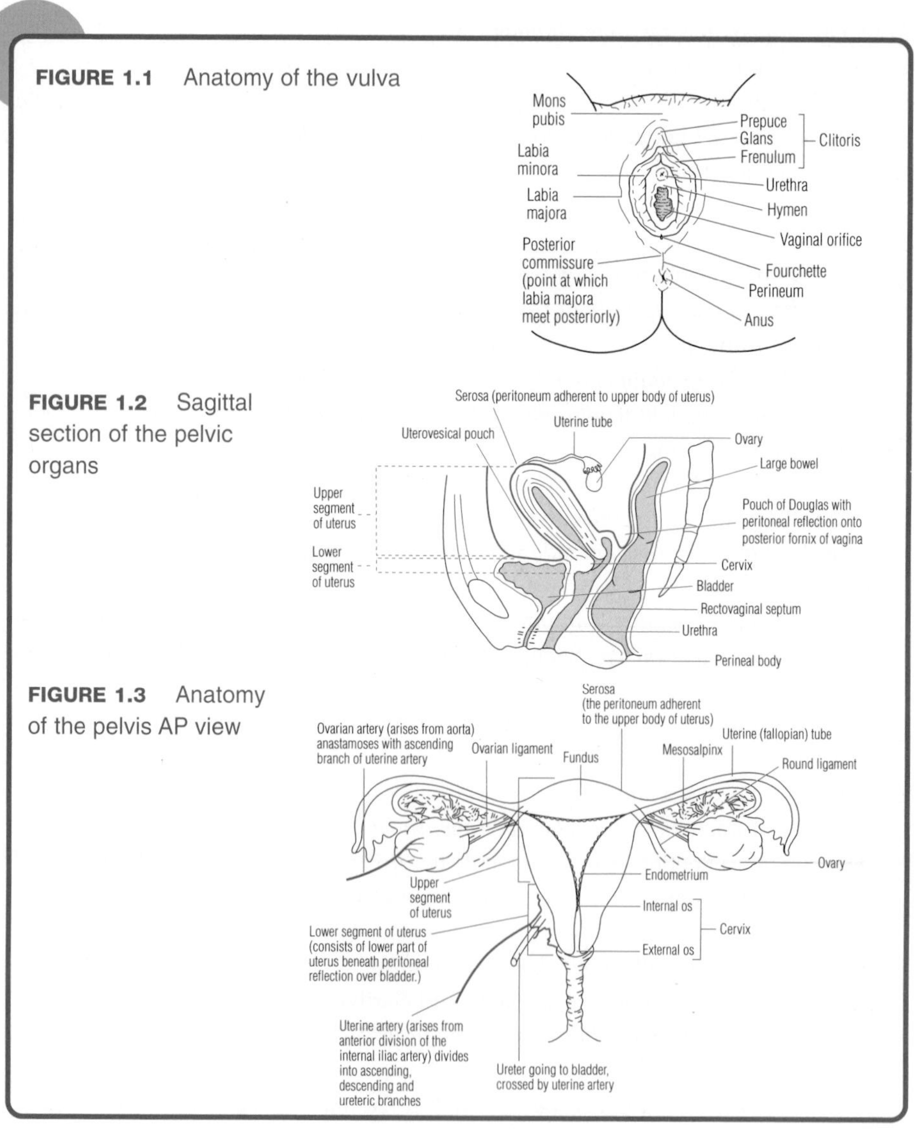

FIGURE 1.1 Anatomy of the vulva

FIGURE 1.2 Sagittal section of the pelvic organs

FIGURE 1.3 Anatomy of the pelvis AP view

relative or nurse) and the health professional should decide if a chaperone would be appropriate for their own support.

The woman may wish to empty her bladder before this examination. Explain which clothes to remove, where to put them and where to sit, and provide a sheet or gown large enough for her to comfortably cover herself in privacy. The room should be a comfortable temperature and well lit. While the woman is preparing for the examination, check that the appropriate equipment is available.

Preparation of equipment

Organise the equipment and ensure that the clinical examination area is prepared (Box 1.12).

BOX 1.12 Examination equipment

- Specula: small, medium, large (metal/disposable)
- Spatulas, brush, cervibroom
- Slide: labelled with woman's name and date of birth
- Thin prep container
- Fixative sprays
- Swabs for culture (suspected/screening sexually transmitted infections)
- Gloves
- Water for warming speculum
- Mirror to offer woman

Examination

There are different approaches to the physical examination that are equally valid. It is important that the clinician is systematic, thorough and skilled, but also flexible to the particular requirements of the woman and the clinical situation. For example, a woman with large breasts may require a different technique for breast examination.

During the examination, provide ongoing details of what is being examined and why. This helps to maintain an atmosphere of safety, perceived control and trust. When examining any part of the body it is also important to observe the woman's response by her facial expression, as discomfort or pain may not be communicated verbally.

The examination may include:

- general (blood pressure, pulse rate, mucous membranes)
- systems if indicated from the history
- specific to the woman: breast, abdominal and pelvic examination.

Breast examination

Inspection

The aim of inspection is to identify specific changes in the breasts (Box 1.13).

BOX 1.13 Changes observed in the breasts

- Asymmetry of breasts
- Skin changes:
  - Dimpling, 'Peau d'orange'
  - Rash (rawness of nipple suggests Paget's disease)
  - Ulceration
  - Discoloration
- Nipple changes:
  - Discharge (amount, spontaneous or with pressure, colour: clear, blood-stained
  - Inversion or retraction
- Lump
  - Size, position, consistency, mobility

The woman should sit facing you with her arms relaxed by her sides (Figure 1.4). Ask her to move to allow observation of the breasts in relation to the chest wall by:

1 Placing her arms above and behind her head (Figure 1.5)
2 Leaning forward so that the breasts move off the chest wall
3 Sitting upright with her hands on her hips to contract the pectoralis major muscle to which the suspensory ligaments of the breast are attached (Figure 1.6).

If a change is noticed, ask the woman whether or not she has observed this and, if she has, how long it has been present.

Palpation

If the woman has a specific breast complaint, examine the asymptomatic side first. Ask the woman to lie on her back with a small pillow under the shoulder of the side of the breast to be examined first. This allows the breast to sit evenly on the chest wall. The arm on the side to be examined should be raised, bent and the hand placed under the head. Palpate the breast with the hand flat and with the pulps of the outstretched fingers, not pinching with the tips of the fingers (Figure 1.7). The breast should be examined to include all quadrants including retro-areolar regions and axillary tail (Figures 1.8, 1.9). The method used should be systematic and may include a circling, vertical lines or quadrant method (Figure 1.10). Examine the axilla for lymph nodes (pectoral, posterior, lateral, central, apical) and examine for the supraclavicular and infraclavicular lymph nodes and check the upper chest wall (Figures 1.11 and 1.12). Now ask the woman to reverse the position of her arms and repeat the examination with the other breast.

Abdominal examination

The abdominal examination (Box 1.14, Figure 1.13) should always be performed prior to a pelvic examination. Ask the woman to adjust the sheet to uncover the abdomen from xiphisternum to the pubic hairline. Abdominal wall relaxation is maximised by

FIGURE 1.4 Breast examination: arms relaxed by side

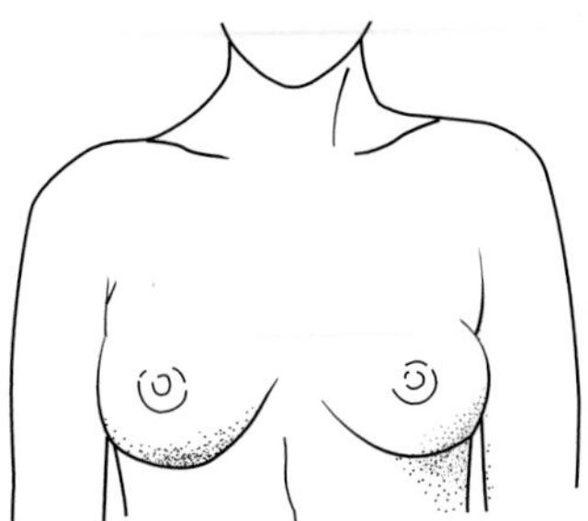

FIGURE 1.5 Breast examination: arms raised and hands behind head

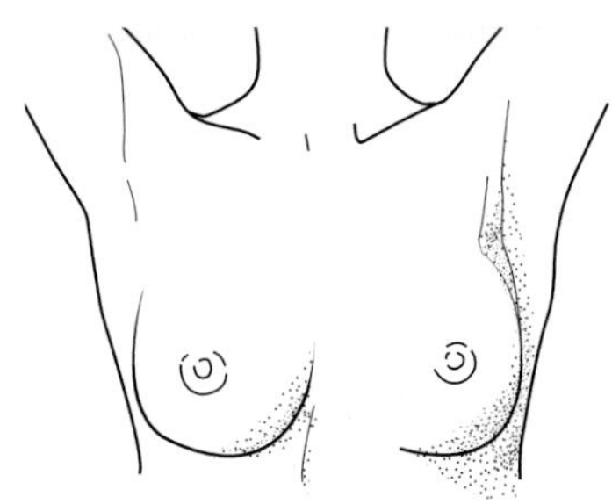

FIGURE 1.6 Breast examination: leaning forward and flexing the pectoral muscles by pushing hands into hips

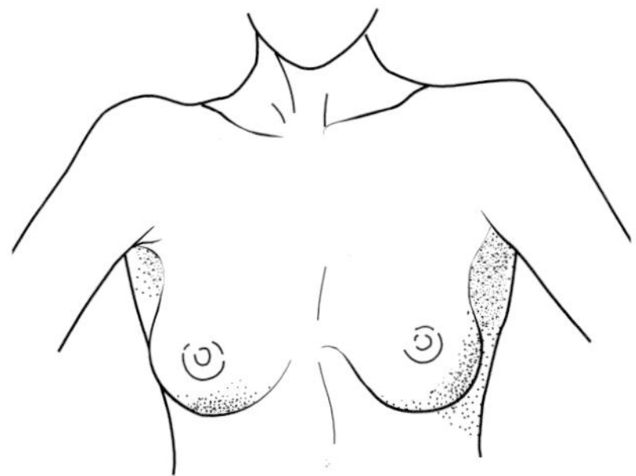

FIGURE 1.7 Breast examination: place a small pillow under the shoulder of the side to be examined so that the breast lies more evenly on the chest wall. Palpate the entire breast using the flattened aspect of the fingers.

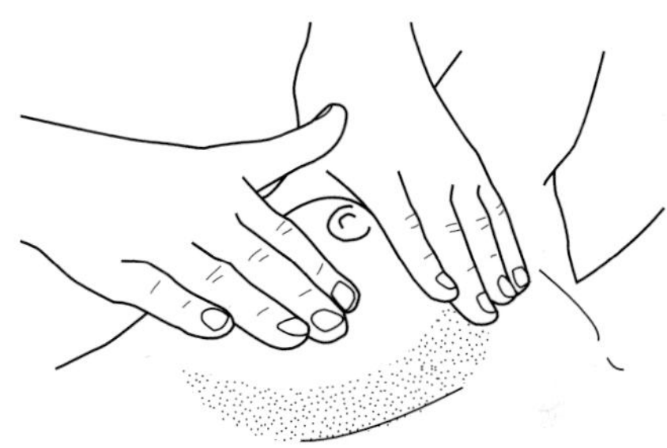

FIGURE 1.8 Breast examination: carefully palpate the tissue beneath the nipple and areola. Visually inspect the nipple for any abnormalities.

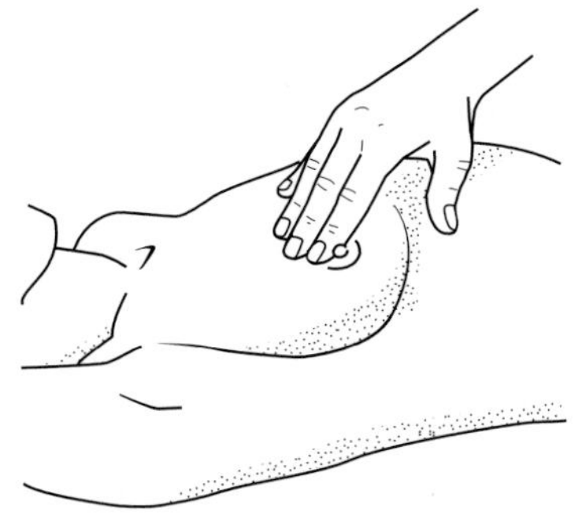

FIGURE 1.9 Breast examination: palpate the axilla by resting the woman's arm on the arm of the examining hand. This may be performed either with the patient seated or with her

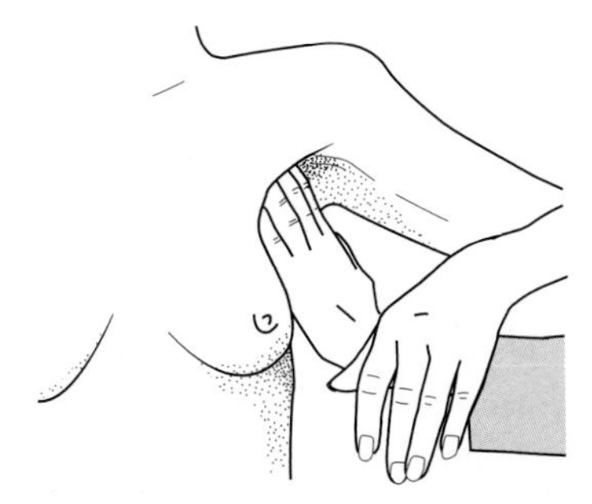

FIGURE 1.10 Methods of breast palpation (a) Spokes of a wheel (b) Concentric circles (c) Quadrant method. Any method can be used provided the examination is thorough.

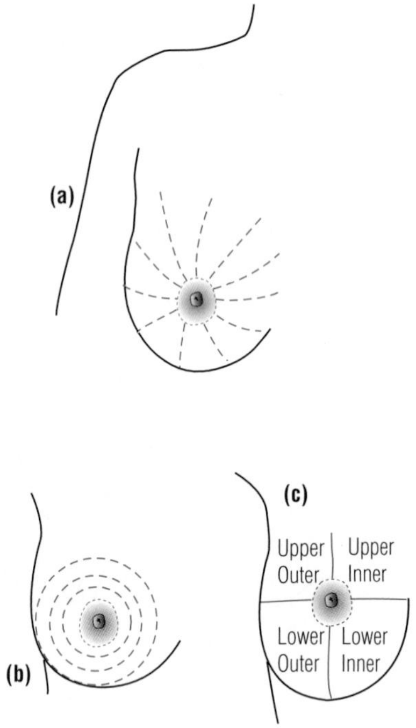

FIGURE 1.11 Breast examination. Check for the presence of enlarged supraclavicular nodes.

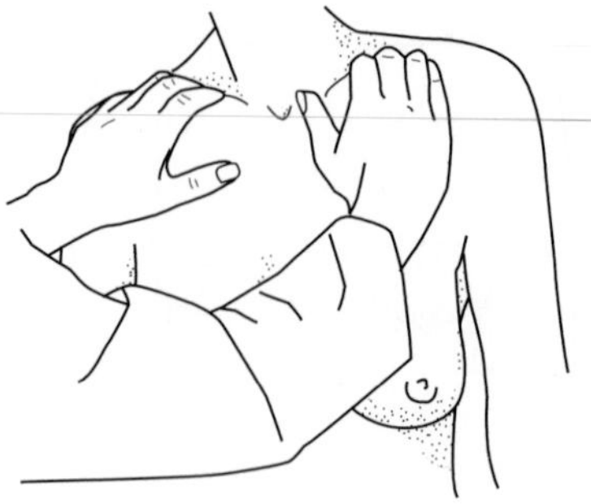

FIGURE 1.12 Breast examination. Palpate the chest wall above the breast mound.

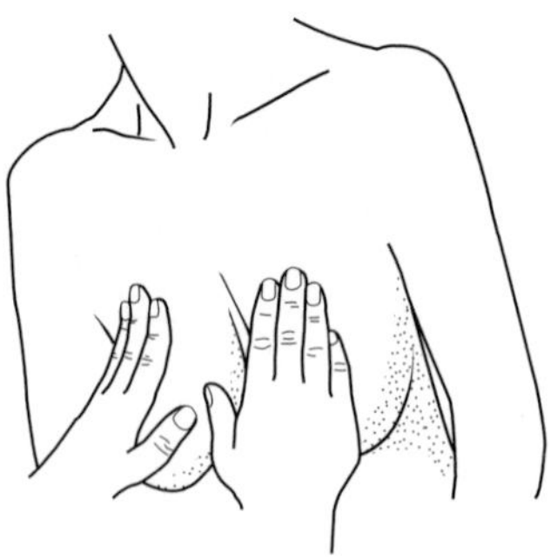

the patient resting her arms alongside her abdomen. Once this part of the examination has been completed, cover the woman with the sheet and explain that the pelvic examination is next.

Vaginal and pelvic examination

After washing and drying your hands, put on disposable gloves. Ask the woman to lift the covering sheet to the knees, bend the knees, rest the feet in a comfortable position and let the legs fall apart. First inspect the vulva and perianal region. Note any skin lesions: erythema, leucoplakia, discoloration, ulcers, lumps or condylomata (Sections 12 and 16). Warm the speculum with water. This should also provide sufficient lubrication (the use of gel interferes with the interpretation of the Pap test). Part the labia minora with the index finger and thumb of the left hand. Continue to explain to

BOX 1.14 Abdominal examination

- Position
  - Lying flat on back, arms at sides
- Observation
  - Skin (colour, rash, lesions)
  - Scars
  - Moving freely with respiration (compromised by pain or peritoneal irritation)
  - Visible peristalsis
  - Abdominal distension
    - Generalised: fat, fluid, fetus, flatus
    - Localised: specific organ, hernia
- Palpation (superficial and deep) all regions of the abdomen (Figure 1.13)
  - Rebound tenderness and guarding (peritonism)
  - Pulsation
  - Presence of a mass. Note:
    - Size, mobility, shape, tenderness, consistency, pulsatile nature, indentability, position
- Percussion
- Auscultation
  - Bowel sounds
    - Increased: increased peristalsis (bowel obstruction, diarrhoea, blood in bowel)
    - Reduced/absent: intestinal paralysis (ileus), perforation, generalised peritonitis
    - Vascular sounds
    - Bruit: systolic arterial—aortic, femoral, renal (stenosed, aneurysmal)

FIGURE 1.13 Abdominal examination: the specific regions of the abdomen used to describe the position of a normal or abnormal change

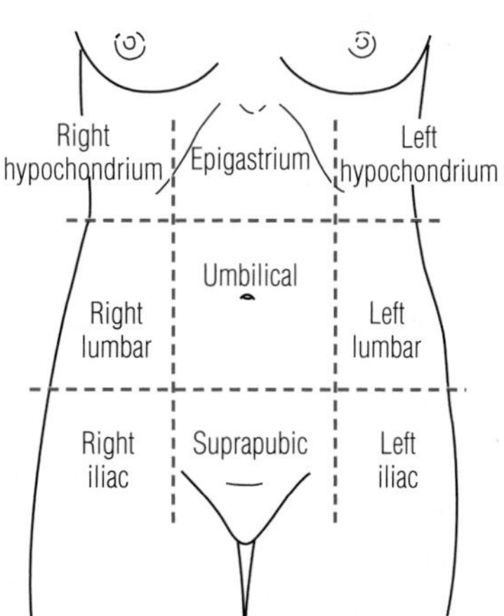

the woman each step of the procedure. Introduce the speculum at the introitus according to its anatomical appearance (the bills horizontal, vertical or at an angle). The opening to the vagina will vary according to the woman's age, size, whether she has had a vaginal delivery, and her degree of relaxation. Occasionally the patient may be too tense to allow the examination to proceed. This may be a conditioned reflexive reaction indicating the presence of sexual pain disorder such as dyspareunia or vaginismus. Gradually insert the speculum to its full length into the vagina, running it along the posterior vaginal wall (Figure 1.14). Once completely inserted, open the bills of the speculum. The handle of the speculum may point either downwards or upwards according to the examiner's preference and experience. A clear view of the cervix should be obtained. Should the cervix not be visualised the speculum may be withdrawn a little and directed anteriorly to locate the cervix of a retroverted uterus. If the cervix still cannot be located, a gentle vaginal examination should be performed to locate its position before attempting to look again with the speculum. Once adequately visualised, lock the speculum in this open position. The cervix is examined for the presence of any discharge, colour, erosion, polyps, ulcers or growths suggestive of neoplasia (Section 16). Cervical swabs, if required, may be taken at this stage from the endocervix and vagina.

FIGURE 1.14 Vaginal speculum examination (a) Parting the labia: it is important to be able to view the introitus. (b) Inserting the speculum. (c) Opening the speculum.

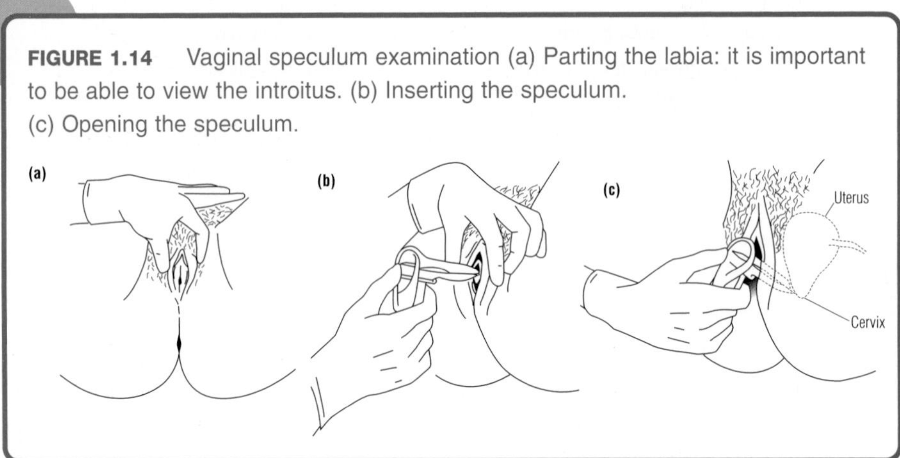

The Pap test

Insert one end of the spatula into the endocervix and rotate through 360 degrees, sampling the squamo-columnar junction under direct vision. The long narrow end is mostly suited to the nulliparous or postmenopausal cervix, the broader end to the parous cervix. Remove the spatula and spread the smear thinly over two-thirds of the glass slide. Place the endocervical brush in the endocervical canal and rotate through 90 degrees (Figure 1.15). Smear this thinly on the remaining one-third of the glass slide. Spray the glass slide with fixative and allow to air dry, in the slide holder. If a thin prep test is to be sent, swirl the endocervical brush and spatula into the fluid in the special bottle.

FIGURE 1.15 Sampling the cervix (a) Taking a cervical and vaginal swab (b) Ectocervical sample of squamocolumnar junction using a cervibroom under direct vision. (c) Endocervical sample using an endocervical brush. (d) Equipment for taking a Pap test. 1. Cervibroom: this can be used for an ecto- or endo-cervical sample. 2. Cytobrush for endocervical canal sample. 3. Spatula for ectocervical sample

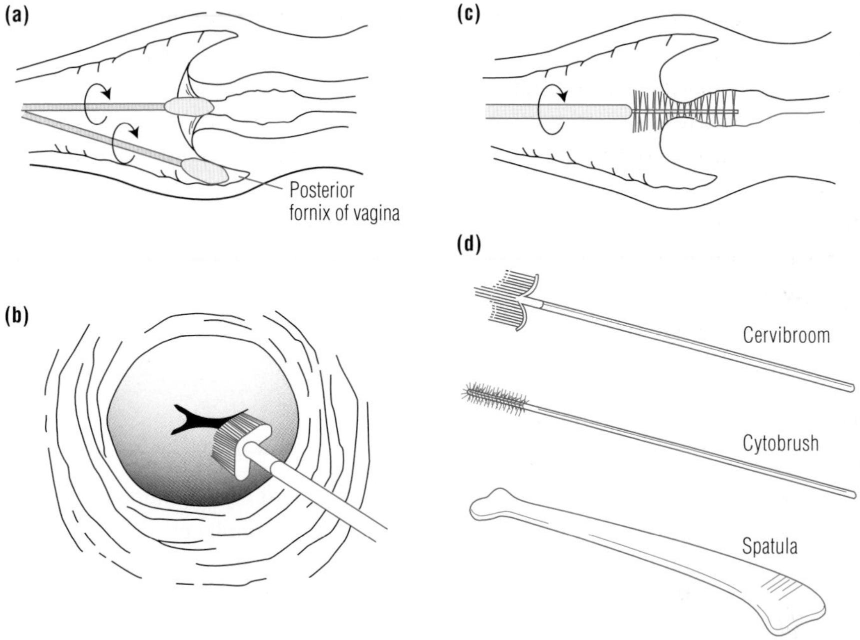

Unlock the speculum while holding the bills apart and then carefully lift the speculum away from the cervix and remove it, gently allowing the bills to come together in the vagina after the cervix has been cleared. As you remove the speculum inspect the walls of the vagina.

Bimanual examination

A bimanual examination of the pelvic organs is usually performed *after* the smear test, to minimise interference with the cervical cytology. However, some HCPs choose to perform a digital examination before the speculum examination to assess the position of the uterus and cervix. The introitus is opened with the fingers of the left hand, avoiding the sensitive clitoral area. The index and middle fingers of the right hand are lubricated with jelly and gently inserted into the vagina and the cervix identified. The cervix of an anteverted uterus is directed posteriorly and that of a retroverted uterus anteriorly (Figure 1.16). Feel the cervix for the shape of the internal os, and the presence of any polyps or cervical growths. With your non-dominant hand on the lower abdomen, gently rock the cervix forwards and backwards to assess uterine mobility. Assess the size, shape, consistency and regularity of the uterus. By moving the cervix from side to side, thus disturbing the adnexal organs and overlying peritoneum, tenderness of the pelvis is elicited (termed 'cervical excitation'). The fingers in the vagina stabilise the pelvic organs while the other hand palpates the organs with pressure through the abdominal wall. Place your non-dominant hand in the right lower abdominal quadrant and the vaginal examining fingers in the right lateral vaginal fornix. The non-dominant hand is gradually brought down to the right inguinal region to meet the other hand. The normal ovary might be felt as an almond-sized mobile structure slipping between the examining hands as they are approximated and is tender if squeezed. The size of the woman's abdomen and the depth of the pelvis influence how much can be felt and it is common not to be able to feel a normal ovary. It is important to place the examining hand initially high in the abdomen, in order to avoid displacing upwards a mobile ovarian cyst. Any identified abnormal adnexal masses should be described in terms of size, shape, consistency, tenderness, mobility and separation from the uterus. The patient's left adnexal area is similarly examined. Finally, the pouch of Douglas and uterosacral ligaments are examined for masses and the uterosacral ligaments palpated. Note any tenderness and nodularity of these ligaments.

FIGURE 1.16 Bimanual examination. (a) Anteverted uterus: the fundus of the uterus is easily palpated by the abdominal hand, which gently pushes it towards the internal hand resting on the cervix. (b) Retroverted uterus: the uterine fundus is difficult or not able to be felt abdominally. The internal examining fingers can feel the posterior wall of the uterus and can gently lift the uterus towards the abdominal hand.

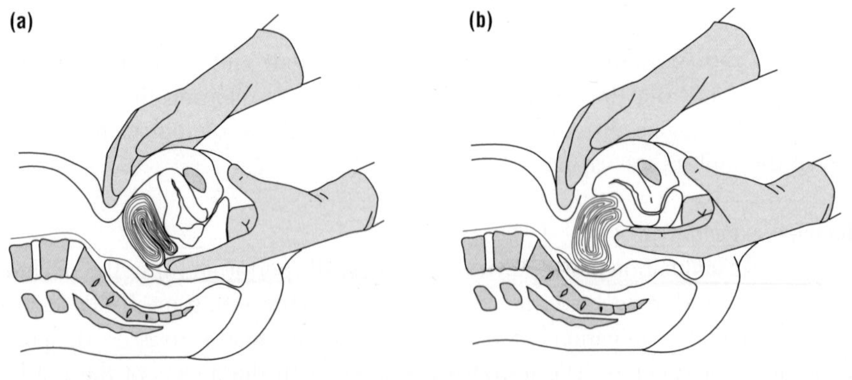

Vaginal examination to identify uterovaginal prolapse

The patient should be asked to lie on her left side with her knees bent. A Sims' speculum is gently introduced into the vagina. Pressure on the posterior vaginal wall exposes the anterior vaginal wall. Note the presence and size of any urethrocele or cystocele. The cervix may also be inspected in this position. Should uterine descent be sought, warn the patient that she may experience momentary discomfort as an instrument (tenaculum) is placed on the cervix to exert gentle traction. The degree of uterine descent is noted and the tenaculum is then removed. The speculum is withdrawn and reinserted, this time placing gentle pressure on the anterior vaginal wall to expose the posterior vaginal wall. Note the presence and size of any rectocoele or enterocoele.

After the examination

It is important on conclusion of the examination that you state that the examination is finished and that the patient can get dressed in privacy. Ask her to return to the consultation setting before explaining the findings of the examination. Next discuss the options for management, arrange appropriate follow-up and complete the appropriate forms (Box 1.15).

BOX 1.15 Pathology request for cervical cytology

- Woman's full name
- Identifying health record number
- Date of birth
- Date of last menstrual period
- Pap smear history
- Hormone therapy
- Relevant symptoms
- Appearance of the cervix

Investigations

In some countries the number of investigations undertaken for each patient has been increasing with seemingly little improvement in their health care. There may be a number of reasons for this (Box 1.16). Investigations should be performed to support or refute a diagnosis and should only be undertaken if it affects the management. It is appropriate to try to achieve a more rational and lower use of investigations, thereby reducing costs or achieving a better cost–benefit ratio. Reducing unnecessary and inappropriate tests is not likely to have any ill effects on the patient.

BOX 1.16 Reasons for the increasing number of investigations

- Patient:
  - Considers tests important for management and understanding
  - Offers concrete evidence for and against a diagnosis
  - More reliable than an opinion
- Doctor:
  - Back up opinion by positive test
  - Insecure/uncertain about diagnosis
  - Fear of missing significant disease
  - Satisfy patient expectations
  - Patient pressure
  - New technology available
  - Litigation concerns

Clinical reasoning

The major task of clinical reasoning is to sort out the symptoms and signs associated with a specific illness. This involves knowledge of the epidemiology and pathophysiology of a disease and the symptoms and signs that tend to cluster together for that particular condition. Hypotheses tend to be generated quite early in the consultation and are tested, rejected or retained as new information is added using focused, hypothesis-driven verbal enquiries and physical examination. This method is termed hypothetico-deductive (or 'guess-and-test') reasoning. This interactive process of hypothesis testing aims to provide a diagnostic formulation (which need not be a specific diagnosis), to account for all the key clinical findings elicited to date. Further testing and final verification of the diagnosis may entail the performance of laboratory investigations and/or observing the patient over time to see whether his/her clinical course, including response to administered treatments, corresponds to that expected on the basis of the original diagnosis.

A useful tool for reflecting on the symptoms and compiling a differential diagnosis is Murtagh's diagnostic principles:[17]

- Probable diagnosis
- Serious disorders not to be missed
- Conditions often missed (pitfalls)
- Masquerades: depression, diabetes, drugs, anaemia, thyroid diseases, spinal dysfunction, urinary tract infections
- Is the patient trying to tell me something else?

Over time, clinical knowledge becomes better organised in terms of the diagnostic (or predictive) value of various clinical findings for different conditions, hypothesis generation and testing become easier, and, as clinical experience and expertise increase, rapid reasoning in the form of pattern recognition is used more frequently in diagnosing commonly occurring presentations. However, unfamiliar clinical problems will continue to require application of the 'guess-and-test' method, as well as skills in searching the literature for well-conducted diagnostic studies that have identified useful heuristics (or 'rules of thumb') for particular clinical scenarios.

Obstetric history: first antenatal visit

The goals of the first antenatal visit are to:

- Determine the health of the mother and fetus
- Identify any factors that will affect the pregnancy
- Identify conditions that the pregnancy will affect
- Determine the model of care
- Establish rapport between woman and health care personnel.

Pregnancy is a highly emotional time for many women. There may be positive responses to a much wanted pregnancy, or negative emotions associated with an unplanned pregnancy. Women may be experiencing doubt, ambivalence, fear and uncertainty. There may also be issues involving partners, friends and family and their response to the pregnancy.

History of this pregnancy

The first antenatal visit should include a history to establish the expected date of delivery (EDD) and look for specific risk factors. Most health professionals would use a standardised chart to include all the important information and a management plan (see Figure 6.10). It is important not to forget psychological factors. There are few events that will be encountered clinically that generate such extreme and polar emotions as pregnancy. Unexpected conception can generate significant stress, and conception after a long period of attempting to conceive can be elating. The first antenatal visit provides an opportunity to initiate discussion about any concerns that can have a significant impact on the woman's mental health, such as the partner's attitude to pregnancy (Section 3).

Calculating the EDD

Use the date of the last menstrual period to calculate the EDD. Pregnancy lasts 9 months or 280 days. An example of one method of calculation is as follows:

Establish the LMP	23/4/03
Go back 3 months	23/1/03
Add 1 year	23/1/04
Add 7 days	30/1/04

The EDD may be modified by taking into account cycle regularity (the calculation above is based on a 28-day cycle) and history of recent contraceptive pill use. Bleeding in early pregnancy (eg bleeding at the time of implantation, threatened abortion at 4 weeks) can cause confusion with the dates for the woman. Most women will have an early ultrasound to assess the gestational age.

Obstetric risk factors

Obstetric risk factors include:

- *Age:* women over 35 years have an increased risk of having a child with a chromosomal abnormality.
- *Parity:* women having a first baby (primigravida) are an unknown quantity with regards to child-bearing. Women with three or more children are at increased risk for a number of problems including haemorrhage and abnormal implantation of the placenta.
- *Height:* women less than five feet (132 cm) are at increased risk of cephalo-pelvic disproportion.
- *Pregnancy weight:* an increased perinatal mortality occurs in women with low prepregnancy weight (< 54 kg/120 lb) or poor pregnancy weight gain (< 5 kg/11 lb).
- *Drug use* (alcohol, tobacco, other drugs): the fetus is at risk for intrauterine growth retardation and developmental problems with high drug usage. If use is significant, preterm birth is more likely, as is the possibility of the neonate undergoing drug withdrawal.

- *Medical history:* women with diabetes, hypertension, renal disease or heart disease have an increased risk for intrauterine growth retardation, premature labour, pregnancy-induced hypertension and other problems.
- *Previous pregnancy/birthing problems:* some pregnancy complications can increase the risk of a problem next time, such as postpartum haemorrhage or premature delivery. The previous pregnancy is the most useful predictor for the current pregnancy and its outcome.
- *Evidence of previous postpartum psychiatric problems* including depression or psychosis may be associated with significant fear as the pregnancy advances. Psychiatric referral early in the pregnancy is prudent.
- *Infections* (sexually transmitted and others): HIV infection treated during pregnancy can reduce the chance of transmission to the fetus by two-thirds; treatment of syphilis can avert developmental problems.

A general history should also be included:

- past medical and surgical history: in particular enquire about diabetes, hypertension, cardiovascular, renal or thyroid disease
- Papanicolaou smear history, date and results of last smear
- medications
- allergies
- social history
- psychological history
- family history.

The booking examination

A full general examination is undertaken to include:

- general inspection (demeanour, pallor, scars, tattoos or rashes)
- observations: blood pressure—take with the woman sitting down and using the same arm each visit
- thyroid examination
- CVS examination: check for heart murmurs
- respiratory system examination if indicated
- breast examination (pigment changes and inversion of the nipples, other breast problems).

Abdominal examination in pregnancy

As the pregnancy advances some women feel weak or nauseous as a consequence of lying supine, as the enlarging uterus may compress the inferior vena cava and compromise venous return; this can be averted by using a small pillow under one side to tilt the woman slightly. The examination should cover all areas of inspection, palpation and auscultation.

Inspection

- Scars
- Colour changes: pigmentation (linea nigra), moles

- Striae gravidarum
- Skin rashes
- Contour. As the pregnancy advances the outline of the fetus is seen.
- Fetal movements can be observed later in pregnancy.

Palpation

See Figures 1.17–1.20.

- Uterine size may be more reliable to estimate gestation when < 18 weeks rather than later.
- Fundal height later (relating the fundal height to the pubic symphysis, the umbilicus or the xiphisternum in centimetres or finger breadths)
- Fetal lie (longitudinal, transverse or oblique)
- Fetal presentation (palpation of the fetal part—most often the head—suprapubically)
- Fetal position: the fetal occiput/sacrum in relation to the mother's pelvis
- Engagement of the fetal head. This is determined by evaluating the extent of the head palpable per abdomen, described in terms of fifths of the fetal head. It may simply be described as being free, fixed or engaged (only two-fifths palpable above the pelvic brim).

FIGURE 1.17 Palpation of pregnant abdomen (a) Determining height of fundus (b) Determining fetal lie: the length of the fetus in relation to the mother's spine (c) Determining fetal presentation: that part of the fetus that addresses the mother's pelvic inlet (d) Determining engagement of the fetal head.

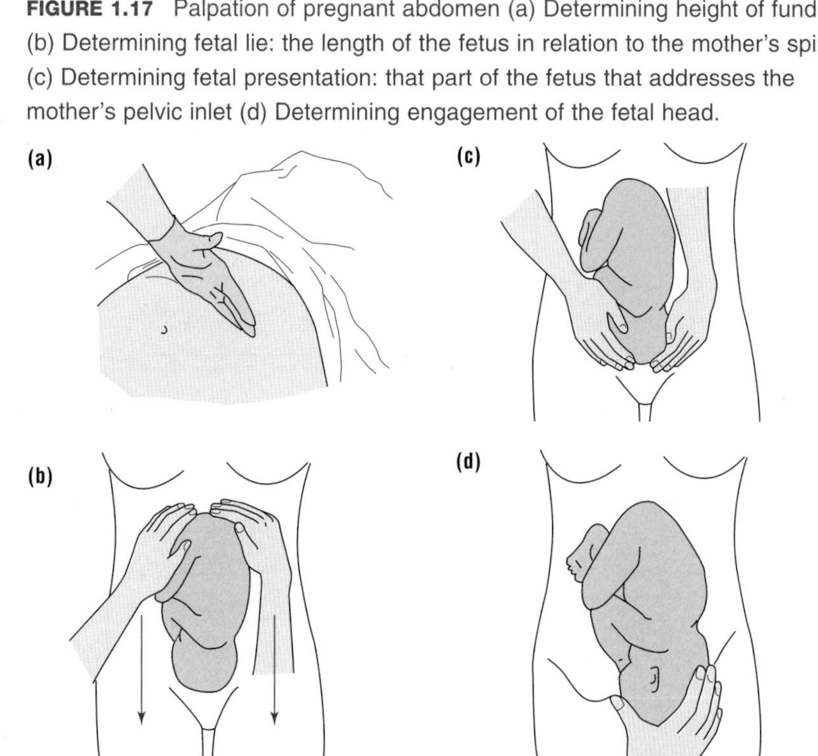

FIGURE 1.18 Determining height of the fundus

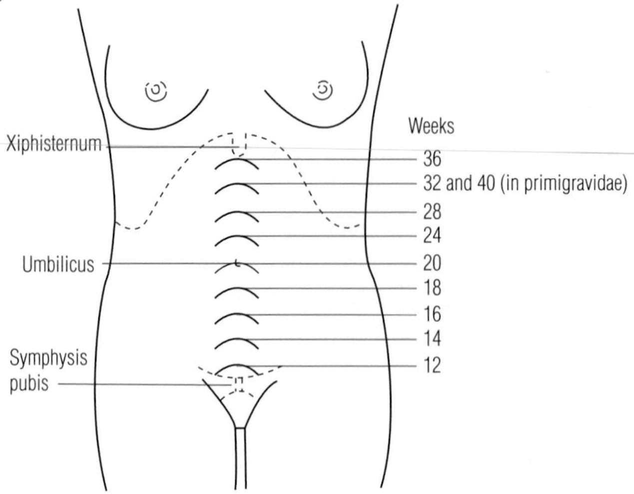

FIGURE 1.19 Lie and presentation (a) Cephalic presentation, longitudinal lie 95% (b) Breech presentation, longitudinal lie 4% (c) Oblique lie, shoulder presentation (d) Transverse lie, back presenting

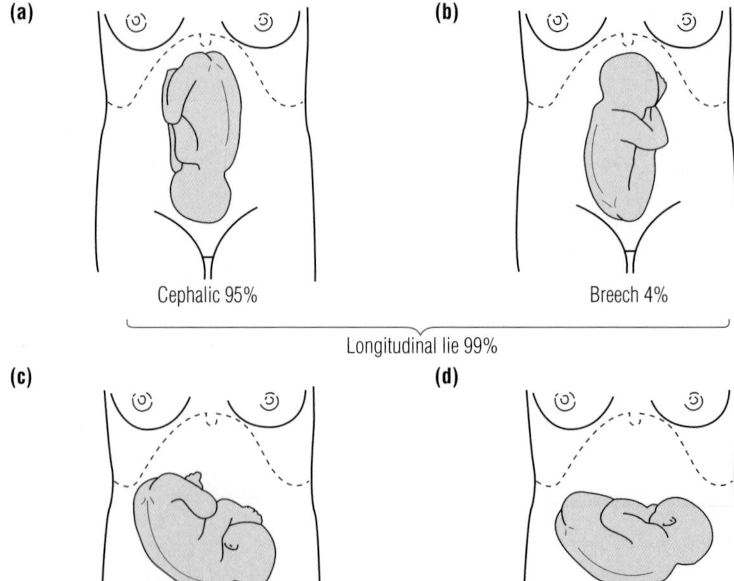

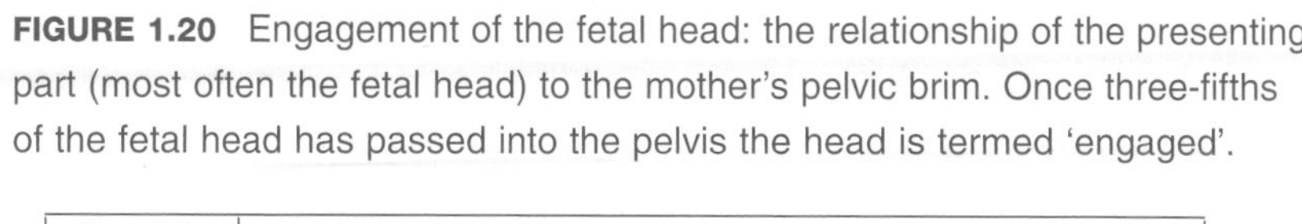

FIGURE 1.20 Engagement of the fetal head: the relationship of the presenting part (most often the fetal head) to the mother's pelvic brim. Once three-fifths of the fetal head has passed into the pelvis the head is termed 'engaged'.

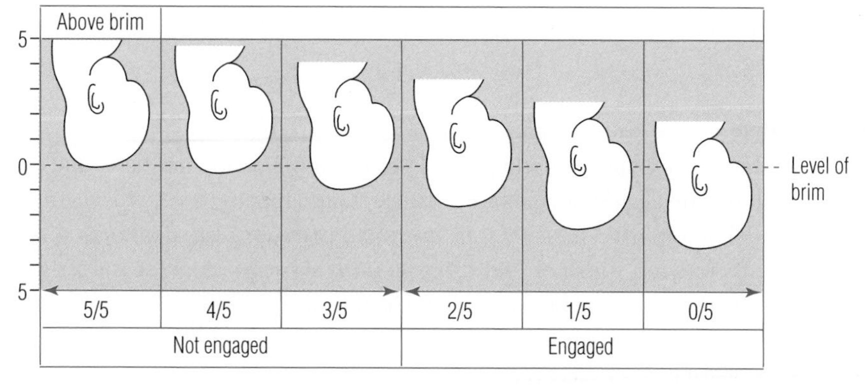

Auscultation

- Check the fetal heart rate. In early pregnancy this is heard midline over the uterus; later, near the position of the anterior shoulder of the fetus. A normal fetal heart rate is 110–160 beats per minute.

Vaginal examination

A speculum examination may be undertaken if the Pap test is due, the woman complains of an abnormal vaginal discharge, or the cervix needs to be inspected for size and length. The increased vascularity to the cervix in pregnancy is said to cause the cervix to look blue in colour. Also the high oestrogen levels of pregnancy cause the squamo-columnar junction to move laterally and away from the external cervical os, giving the appearance of an 'erosion' or reddened area surrounding the os.

Bimanual examination

A bimanual examination can assess:

- Size of the uterus (described in the number of weeks of pregnancy)
- Shape of the uterus (note any possible congenital abnormalities or masses such as fibroids)
- Consistency (firm in the non-pregnant state; soft in pregnancy)
- Position (anteverted, retroverted, axial)
- Fornices: to detect any enlargement of the ovaries.

Investigations

All pregnant women have a number of routine screening tests and additional tests specific for individual risks (Section 6).

Model of antenatal care

This is decided once the woman has been assessed for any specific risks that may be present for herself and the baby. A woman with a low-risk pregnancy may choose her care. The options could involve the hospital obstetrician or midwife, community doctor or midwife, or sharing between these professionals. A woman with a particular problem that needs medical monitoring may be advised to have mainly hospital care.

Documentation

All the history, examination findings, results of investigation to date and those requested should be clearly documented. These should be discussed with the mother and the model of antenatal care agreed. In many institutions the mother is given all the documents to keep with her and bring to each subsequent antenatal visit. This enhances the communication between all the health care professionals involved in the woman's care and the woman herself, and will be useful should the woman need to seek medical assistance elsewhere.

Prescribing for women

Differences between men and women

Women visit their doctor more often than men. They receive more prescribed drugs and are more likely to self-medicate and be influenced by the media, word of mouth and advice from health professionals. Factors contributing to the pharmaco-epidemiology of drug use include the following.

1 Medicines information-seeking behaviour

Market research identifies three categories of health consumers:[18]

- Passive consumers who rarely seek health information or use complementary therapies
- Concerned consumers who sometimes seek out a second opinion but mostly follow their health practitioner's advice
- Health-active consumers who are highly motivated and determined to play a role in their own health. They challenge their health advisers and frequently choose alternative health strategies.

Data from the Queensland Medication Helpline confirms that females are more proactive medicines information-seekers.[19] The service cites a female:male caller ratio of approximately 3:1, yet the ratio approximates 1:1 for patient gender involved in the enquiry.

2 Self-medication

The widespread use of complementary medicines is demonstrated by a survey of 3004 households in South Australia, where 48.5 per cent of individuals had used one form of complementary medicine in the previous year.[20] Usage was highest in females and increased with age. In the United States between 1992 and 1996, alternative medicine use increased from 34 to 42 per cent, with out-of-pocket expenses equalling the amount spent on conventional therapy. Women were the highest users, at 49 per cent.[21] In the United Kingdom it has been estimated that lifetime use of complementary medicine is 46 per cent, with women the most common users.[22]

Why do women use complementary medicines (CAMs)? A survey concluded that the increasing popularity of CAMs is a result of:

- Dissatisfaction with mainstream medicine
- The desire for autonomy over health decisions
- Their ready access
- A general belief that 'natural remedies are more compatible with health (than drugs)'.[23]

However, a drug is defined in medical dictionaries as 'anything which is taken to change the way the body works normally'. Thus, if a CAM is purported to have activity, irrespective of origin, it is a drug, with a chemical structure, pharmacological and side effect profile. A natural origin does not correlate with drug safety. Some of the most potent drugs used today are of plant origin, eg digoxin from the foxglove (*Digitalis purpura*) and morphine, an alkaloid from the opium poppy (*Papaver somniferum*). Also these preparations may not be pure or have standardised bioavailability between preparations and may have unknown short- and long-term side effects. Complementary medicines must therefore be judged by the same evidence-based standards as any other drug.

3 Pharmacokinetics/pharmacodynamics

Gender can play a role in the individualisation of drug therapy, especially in determining the dose of drugs with a low therapeutic index. Parameters influenced by gender include:

- *Body composition.* Women have a higher percentage of body fat and this can affect the volume of distribution of lipophilic drugs such as alfentanyl.[24]
- *Intestinal transit time.* Gastric emptying and intestinal transit time are slower in women than in men, possibly due to differences in steroid hormone levels.[25]
- *Drug metabolism.* Most significant gender differences are due to differences in activity of cytochrome P450 (CYP) isoenzymes.[25]
- *Renal excretion.* When normalised for body surface area, women have approximately 10 per cent lower glomerular filtration rate.[26] This would explain the lower clearance of drugs eliminated primarily via the kidneys, such as digoxin and gentamicin, in women than in men.[27]
- *P-glycoprotein.* The human multidrug-resistance gene 1 (MDR 1) gene product P-glycoprotein has recently been identified as a significant determinant in drug pharmacokinetics. Women express only one-third to one-half of the hepatic glycoprotein level of men.[28] The clinical significance of this in relation to individual drugs requires further investigation.

- *Female-specific issues* such as menstruation, contraceptive use, pregnancy and menopause also affect drug metabolism. Contraceptive use can interfere with the metabolism of many drugs, impairing the activity of one or both agents.[29]

Therapeutic classes that highlight these gender differences include the selective serotonin reuptake inhibitors (SSRIs) such as fluvoxamine and antihypertensive drugs, eg beta blockers and verapamil.[30] These differences may explain the higher incidence of drug-induced side effects seen in women.[24]

Drugs and pregnancy

All drugs have the potential to affect the fetus (heparin, which has a large molecule and does not cross the placental barrier, is an exception). However, contrary to popular belief there are few proven human teratogens. The risk of exposure to drugs, chemicals and other environmental agents during pregnancy is in addition to the general underlying risk of malformation (3 per cent of live births) and the risk of miscarriage (approximately 15 per cent). Women with a concern about drug ingestion should be given appropriate counselling and advice after a thorough history has been taken. This must include the date of the last menstrual period, the timing and dosage of the drug involved, and other potentially confounding factors: regular and other medications, social drugs, over-the-counter drugs and herbal medications. An understanding of changes in maternal physiology, developmental phases of the embryo, fetal drug toxicity, and the variable effect of the same drug at different stages of pregnancy assists in medication risk-benefit assessment (Figure 1.21).

FIGURE 1.21 Embryonic and fetal development: drug impact

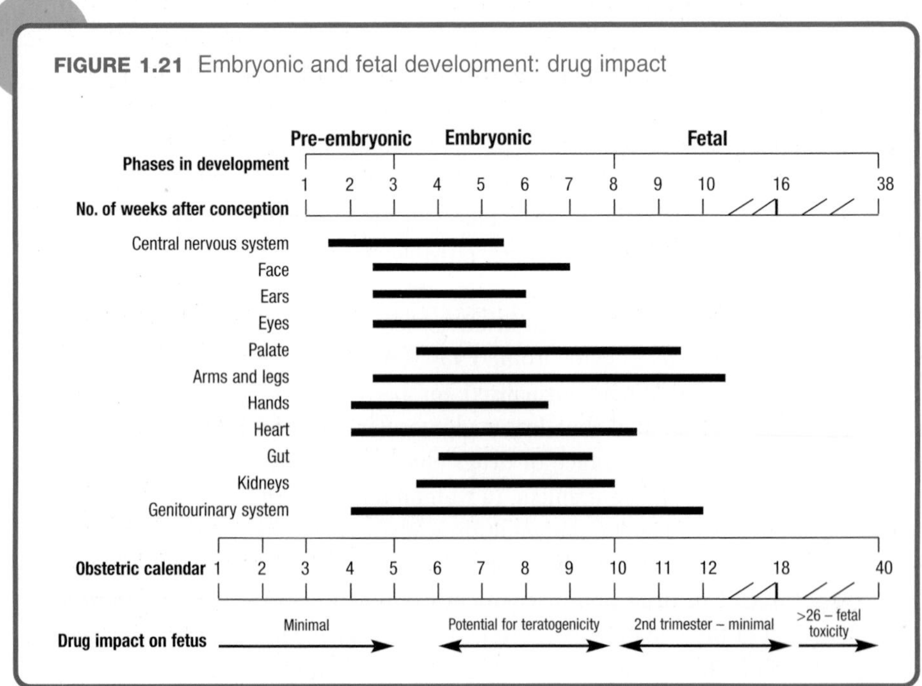

Physiological changes in pregnancy affecting drugs

Pregnant women have an increased cardiac output and renal function. Drugs with a high renal clearance may need a dosage increase, while drugs with a high hepatic clearance require no dose change (as maternal liver size and hepatic blood flow remain unchanged). An increase in plasma volume effectively decreases drug concentration: anticoagulants and antidepressants should therefore be monitored with blood levels. In contrast, there is a decrease in plasma albumin; and plasma protein bound drugs such as phenytoin may need to be reduced in dose. Gastro-intestinal transit time is prolonged and this may be clinically relevant towards the end of pregnancy and in labour when drugs may require parenteral administration.

Classification of drug risk in pregnancy

Drugs have been categorised for use in pregnancy (Box 1.17).[31] These classifications are only a guide. They do not cover infectious or environmental agents, herbal preparations or street drugs.

The drug effects on a pregnancy can be divided into:

- *Teratogen:* this interferes with the development of the fetus, causing a major anatomical defect. For a drug to be implicated as a teratogen, it must

BOX 1.17 ADEC categorisation of drugs in pregnancy[31]

A Drugs which have been taken by a large number of pregnant women and women of childbearing age without any proven increase in the frequency of malformations or other direct or indirect harmful effects on the fetus having been observed.

C Drugs which, owing to their pharmacological effects, have caused or may be suspected of causing harmful effects on the human fetus or neonate without causing malformations. These effects may be reversible. Accompanying texts should be consulted for further details.

B Drugs which have been taken by only a limited number of pregnant women and women of childbearing age, without an increase in the frequency of malformation or other direct or indirect harmful effects on the human fetus having been observed. As experience of effects of drugs in this category in humans is limited, results of toxicological studies to date (including reproduction studies in animals) are indicated by allocation to one of three subgroups:

B1 Studies in animals have not shown evidence of an increased occurrence of fetal damage.

B2 Studies in animals are inadequate or may be lacking, but available data show no evidence of an increased occurrence of fetal damage.

B3 Studies in animals have shown evidence of an increased occurrence of fetal damage, the significance of which is considered uncertain in humans.

D Drugs which have caused, are suspected to have caused, or may be expected to cause an increased incidence of human fetal malformations or irreversible damage. These drugs may also have adverse pharmacological effects. Accompanying texts should be consulted for further details.

X Drugs that have such a high risk of causing permanent damage to the fetus that they should not be used in pregnancy or when there is a possibility of pregnancy.

cause a dose-related, consistent pattern of anomaly in response to maternal exposure during organogenesis. Drugs in this category include: warfarin, danazol, phenytoin, carbamazepine, lithium and sodium valproate. Sometimes a course of treatment may be completed before conception but the drug may still be in the body during organogenesis (eg retinoids).

- *Hadegen:* this interferes with the maturation and development of the fetus to cause a functional impairment (eg deafness) without an obvious structural abnormality.
- *Fetotoxic:* this causes growth restriction and death (eg ACE inhibitors in the second and third trimesters).

Some drugs may have more than one effect or different effects at different stages of fetal development.

Information requested by pregnant women about drug use

This falls into three main categories:

1. *Medicines used to treat for chronic conditions.* Women with chronic conditions such as epilepsy, depression or asthma are likely to be on drug therapy when they fall pregnant.
2. *Medicines to treat pregnancy-associated conditions.* Pregnant women are likely to suffer from nausea. In randomised controlled trials, ginger, pyridoxine (vitamin B6), cyanocobalamin (vitamin B12), antihistamines and phenothiazines were found to reduce nausea.[32]
3. *Self-medication.* Women do self-medicate during their pregnancy, although reports vary on the extent of use and outcome. Lifestyle drugs such as caffeine, cigarettes and alcohol should also be included in this category. Over-the-counter drugs commonly taken include vitamins, iron, mild analgesics, antiemetics and laxatives. There are potential risks—a little may be safe but more may cause risks—such as excessive use of vitamin A or D. Many herbal products and other alternative medicines are used during pregnancy with the assumption that 'natural' is synonymous with 'safe'. There is limited quality research into efficacy or safety with these products.

Lactation

Although most drugs cross over into the breast milk, generally the effect on the baby is minimal as the drug is diluted in the mother's body and little is swallowed by the baby.

A guide should include:[33, 34]

- Use the lowest effective dose.
- Use older rather than newer drugs.
- Avoid polypharmacy.
- Avoid over-the-counter and CAM preparations.
- Balance the above with appropriate control and treatment of the condition.

Drugs and the elderly

In the older patient, absorption may be slightly slower due to changes in gastro-intestinal blood flow and motility. Distribution is influenced by decrease in lean body mass and total body water and an increase in body fat; lipid-soluble drugs have a larger volume of distribution and water-soluble drugs have a smaller volume of distribution. Hence standard doses of drugs should be reduced, especially the loading doses of water-soluble preparations. Plasma albumin levels tend to be well maintained in the healthy elderly, but may be reduced in chronic disease or acute illness, leading to significant changes in the proportion of unbound (free) drug in the case of highly protein-bound drugs, such as warfarin.

Metabolism is also reduced due to reduction in liver mass and blood flow. Therefore, metabolic inactivation of drugs is slower and drugs that normally undergo extensive first-pass metabolism (eg propranalol, verapamil, warfarin) appear in higher concentration in the systemic circulation and persist longer. Elimination of drugs is also altered. Renal blood flow, glomerular filtration and tubular secretion decrease with age after 35 years. This decline is not marked by raised serum creatinine concentrations due to diminished production of this metabolite, since muscle mass is decreased. Thus a normal serum creatinine level may be seen when a significant reduction of creatinine clearance or glomerular filtration is present. Particular risks of adverse effects arise with the drugs excreted mainly by the kidney and also having a small therapeutic ratio (eg aminoglycocides, chlorpropamide, digoxin, lithium).

Pharmacodynamic response may alter with ageing, leading to either greater or lesser effects than would be anticipated in healthy younger adults. Drugs acting on the central nervous system produce exaggerated responses in relation to those expected. Sedatives and hypnotics may cause pronounced hangover effects and are also more likely to depress respiration in the elderly with reduced vital capacity and maximum breathing capacity. Response to beta-adrenoceptor agonists and antagonists appears to be blunted in old age, probably due to altered sensitivity and reduction in number of receptors. Baroreceptor sensitivity is reduced, leading to the potential for orthostatic hypotension with antihypertensive therapy.

In general, when prescribing for older people:

- Use as few drugs as possible.
- Start with low doses; if required, increase the dose slowly and carefully.
- Select easily swallowed formulations.
- Keep drug regimens as simple as possible.
- Assume that any new symptoms may be due to drug-related effects.
- Take a careful drug history, check compliance and also enquire about substances the patient may be taking without your knowledge, such as over-the-counter medications or herbal preparations.
- Remember that stopping a drug is as important as starting it!

In some cases, such as osteoarthritis, measures such as gentle exercises and weight reduction may be effective alternatives, without the risk of drug side effects and the potential to start 'the prescribing cascade', wherein an adverse drug reaction is misinterpreted as a new medical condition and a new drug is prescribed for the 'new' condition.

Conclusion

Every time a drug is prescribed it is prudent to ask: 'Do I need to modify or change this prescription in view of the patient's age, gender, current medications or general condition?' In addition, at the time of a patient review, ask: 'Does this woman still need this medication?'

Screening

Preventing illness before it presents clinically is an attractive idea: finding disease before it is too advanced, allowing simpler and more effective treatment. While much screening is worthwhile, it is intrinsically more difficult than first appears. Unless carefully targeted, screening can be useless or even harmful, and divert effort that could be more usefully spent elsewhere in health care. This section gives a brief background of the science of screening, to give an overview and assist readers to interpret the detail in other sections.

Screening is defined as using a test to divide a population into groups with a high and a low probability of the disease.[35] The 'test' may be a question (Do you smoke?), an examination (blood pressure or spinal curvature), a laboratory test or imaging procedure. Screening tests are not diagnostic in themselves. If positive, they lead to further actions to make the diagnosis that leads to management. Screening may be done for whole populations, or as part of individual health care, tailored to patient characteristics and needs. This is called 'case-finding' but uses the same information and probabilities as screening the population from which that patient comes.

Many screening tests have been suggested over the years. Often enthusiastic protagonists market a test to the profession and public, then it fades away after belated evaluation. Only a few screening programs have proved valuable in the long term. Some screening tests simply do not produce the promised benefits, while others do, but insufficient to counterbalance the harm also caused and the costs entailed. Others that should be effective do not achieve their purpose because they are poorly applied. For example, for many years most of the effort in cervical screening was focused on annual screening of young, low-risk groups while neglecting older women at much higher risk. The national program was established to rectify this problem.[36] Therefore we must be sceptical and demand high standards of evaluation and monitoring for screening tests before diverting effort and resources to them.

Benefits of screening

The value of a screening program should be measured not by the number of cases found, but the number who benefit. Treatment may cure some, and defer death for others, but often people whose disease is detected will still develop advanced disease and die, depending on the type of disease and treatment available. Thus long-term outcomes must be measured carefully. The 'number needed to screen' (NNS) is a useful way to express how many must be tested to obtain benefit for one. Because screening deals with normal people, most of whom would never develop the disease, and usually must be conducted repeatedly over a long time, NNS is usually of the order of several thousands of people per year to prevent one death.[37]

Harms from screening

Screening programs inevitably also cause harm: physical, psychological and costs. While harms are usually minor, at times they are severe or even fatal. Many tests or their follow-up procedures cause physical harm; for example, finding a small shadow on a chest X-ray may lead to bronchoscopy, needle biopsy or partial lung resection to treat a mass that may turn out to be benign or already have metastasised so that treatment is ineffective. People treated for hypertension may develop severe side effects from the drugs they are given: this would be worthwhile if they were saved from stroke but not if they would never have developed any complications of the hypertension. Psychological harm may occur, by being informed of possible cancer or heart disease that needs investigation and treatment. For example, positive cervical smears can cause some women to change their self-perception and relationships in negative ways. The upset may persist in some people long after follow-up provides reassurance that no disease was found. Investigations of positive tests cost time, effort and money from the patient, the health care system or both. Given the shortage of resources in health care, this time, effort or money could have been used in some other way, possibly to greater effect.

Deciding on screening programs

Never think of screening tests, only of screening programs.[38]

Developing and using effective screening programs in practice is difficult, balancing the benefits against the three types of harms described above. The whole screening process must be considered; failure or inaccuracy at any step reduces the value of the process. The ideal assessment of screening tests is a randomised controlled trial (RCT) using mortality as an outcome.[38] This ideal is somewhat impractical since even 'common' diseases are relatively rare in an asymptomatic population. For example, diabetes may develop in up to 20 per cent of people between the ages of 30 and 70 years of age—an incidence of 0.5 per cent per year. Most other diseases are much less common. Consequently very large trials are needed to obtain sufficient people with the disease, and their outcome must be observed over many years to determine whether early treatment of screen-detected patients gives better outcomes compared to patients who present clinically and are treated at a later stage of disease.

To assess new tests in the absence of an RCT, or to decide whether performing an RCT is appropriate, a list of criteria is often used (Box 1.18). These address each step in the screening pathway, providing a logical chain that cannot be stronger than its weakest link. If any one is doubtful, the whole case for screening is questionable.

BOX 1.18 Criteria for appraising a screening program

- The condition
  - The condition should be an important health problem.
  - The epidemiology and natural history of the condition, including development from latent to declared disease, should be adequately understood and there should be a detectable risk factor, disease marker, latent period or early symptomatic stage.
  - All the cost-effective primary prevention interventions should have been implemented as far as practicable.
- The test
  - There should be a simple, safe, precise and validated screening test.
  - The distribution of test values in the target population should be known and a suitable cut-off level defined and agreed.
  - The test should be acceptable to the population.
  - There should be an agreed policy on the further diagnostic investigation of individuals with a positive test result and on the choices available to those individuals.
- The treatment
  - There should be an effective treatment or intervention for patients identified through early detection, with evidence of early treatment leading to better outcomes than late treatment.
  - There should be agreed evidence-based policies covering which individuals should be offered treatment and the appropriate treatment to be offered.
  - Clinical management of the condition and patient outcomes should be optimised by all health care providers prior to participation in a screening program.
- The screening program
  - There should be evidence that the complete screening program (test, diagnostic procedures, treatment/intervention) is clinically, socially and ethically acceptable to health professionals and the public.
  - The benefit from the screening program should outweigh the physical and psychological harm (caused by the test, diagnostic procedures and treatment).

Adapted from the UK National Screening Guidelines, National Screening Committee, UK, www.nsc.nhs.uk.

Developers of new screening programs understandably tend to be enthusiasts, impatient to provide benefits to those at risk. Thus many screening tests are publicised and disseminated before adequate evaluation. Then trials are even more difficult to establish, since they require some participants to be controls who do not receive 'benefits' of the program. When many doctors or patients already believe that the program is effective, they will not accept randomisation into the trial. Consequently, many screening tests are still controversial because appropriate trials were not instituted early.

The test

The transfer from laboratory to effective screening test is difficult for several reasons. While advanced disease may be obvious, early disease produces smaller changes in whatever measurement is being used, so it is often difficult to differentiate from normal variation. Diagnosing early changes has a high chance of error, especially for tests requiring human assessment, as in cytology or radiology. Thus extra training and quality assurance procedures are needed for screening, compared to ordinary diagnostic assessment. Even for tests such as laboratory measurements that do not require judgements, the cut-off point for the test poses difficulty. A screening test must be sensitive to detect early disease, but setting the characteristics and cut-off level to be sensitive usually loses specificity—the ability to exclude normal people. The chosen threshold value represents a balance between high sensitivity and high specificity. Thus screening procedures misclassify a small proportion of normal people with a positive test. Because community prevalence is low, the effort to produce one benefit is much higher than in the diagnostic situation, where patients attending with symptoms have a high probability of disease. A hypothetical diagnostic test in a screening setting demonstrates how performance in terms of predictive value apparently deteriorates because of the low prevalence (Box 1.19). Thus further tests are necessary to exclude people who do not have the disease.

BOX 1.19 Behaviour of a test in diagnostic and screening settings

We examine a hypothetical test, omphalo-DNA, for the feared disease omphalosarcoma.

Diagnostic setting

- Ten per cent of patients with certain clinical signs have omphalosarcoma.
- Omphalo-DNA test is 95% *sensitive*—i.e. it detects 19 of 20 patients with omphalosarcoma.
- Omphalo-DNA is 98% *specific*—2 in 100 patients without the disease will have a positive result.

If we test 1000 patients *with those clinical signs*, we obtain the result:

		Omphalosarcoma		
		+	–	Total
Omphalo-DNA test	+	95	18	113
	–	5	882	887
	Total	100	900	1000

One hundred and thirteen of the patients have a positive result on the test and 95 have the disease, but 18 have a 'false positive' result. Of the 113 patients with a positive result, 95 have the disease (*positive predictive value* 84%). Of the 887 with a negative test, only five have the disease and 882 do not (*negative predictive value* 99.4%).

The test has improved the probability of people who you suspect might have the disease from 1 in 10 to 95 in 113. The likelihood ratio = 95/100 X 900/18 = 47.5

(continued overleaf)

BOX 1.19 **continued**

Screening setting

In the general population, aged between 30 and 60, omphalosarcoma is a feared disease, but only occurs with an incidence of one in 1000 in each year. Thus in our population of 100 000 people, the results would be:

		Omphalosarcoma		
		+	−	Total
Omphalo-DNA	+	95	1 998	2 093
test	−	5	97 902	97 907
	Total	100	99 900	100 000

That is, 2093 people will have a positive test, but only 95 of these have the disease (positive predictive value 4.5%), and 1998 have a 'false positive' result. Of the 97 907 people with a negative test, only five have the disease. The likelihood ratio is 95/100 X 1998/99 900 = 47.5; the same as before. However, among the 2093 with positive tests, only 95 have the disease; about one in 20. Thus further testing is needed to determine those with disease.

Definitions

Sensitivity: The proportion of people with the disease who have a positive test result

Specificity: The proportion of people without the disease who have a negative test result

Positive predictive value: The proportion of people with a positive test result who truly have the disease

Negative predictive value: The proportion of people with a negative test result who truly do not have the disease

False positive: The test is positive but the disease is not present

False negative: The test is negative but the disease is present

Likelihood ratio: $= \dfrac{\text{probability of a positive test among those with disease}}{\text{probability of a positive test among those without disease}} = \dfrac{\text{post-test odds}}{\text{pre-test odds}}$

Effects on management

Some minor pathological changes that do not advance or even return to normal are difficult to distinguish from early disease. Indeed, screening programs often discover new pathological entities whose biological behaviour is uncertain, but which doctors feel obliged to treat. Examples are some cervical dysplasias or 'impaired glucose tolerance'. For some diseases such as cervical cancer, 'cure' of early disease reduces mortality by 90 per cent, but for others the effectiveness of treatment is much lower. It has been demonstrated that for 10 000 women having mammography, 400 are recalled for further testing and 80 have a biopsy, to detect about 30 cancers and eight ductal carcinoma in situ (DCIS). At best estimate one-third of breast cancer deaths are avoided—thus 10 women benefit from all this work (NNS 1000).[39] Chronic disease often can only be controlled by long-term treatment, not cured. After diagnosis such people become 'patients' under lifelong treatment, which is likely to improve outcomes if they comply, but commonly at the cost of side effects.

A screening program

Simply assessing that it is worth screening for a disease is only the start (Box 1.18). It is necessary to decide who should be screened, when to start and when to stop, how often, who should do it and how all aspects of the program are to be organised. These are not easy decisions, and the scientific evidence is often obscured by emotional and political overlay, as shown by controversy over the interval and age groups for cervical screening.[40] A screening program must be managed with obsessive attention to detail because of the small benefit and ease of causing harm; because of the difficulty of getting all aspects right, we must expect regular 'scandals' such as laboratory errors as part of the price to pay.

Applying screening to women

The decision to screen or not for any specific disease must be made on the best evidence for the particular population, not just wishing to 'do something'. Younger people generally have very low prevalence of disease, rising with age. Testing should start after crossing the threshold when benefit is greater than harm. These are probability judgements, and inevitably some cases occur outside the chosen range. Many women get breast cancer in their forties, so some argue for screening starting then, but it appears that mammography has less effect for those aged under 50 years, so screening young women may be misplaced energy, although further data should clarify the issue. Mammography screening of Asian women is likely to be less valuable because their breast cancer incidence is lower than that of Western women. If a doctor advised them not to attend, because their risk of harm overshadows their chance of benefit, it would be sound advice, not racial discrimination.[41]

Because women often have a lower or later rise in incidence for many diseases than men, decisions about screening often should be correspondingly different. For example, in Hong Kong the incidence of primary liver cancer among people with chronic hepatitis B was examined.[42] While the benefits of screening for men can be argued, the potential gain for women is small, so the balance of benefit and harm is clearly against screening women. The argument that we should screen men for prostate cancer because women are being screened for breast and cervical cancer fails, not on grounds of fairness, but simply because prostate screening is unlikely to be effective, given the uncertain value of treatment.[43]

Reliable sources of information

Assessment of screening tests requires collation of all available evidence, a time-consuming and difficult task. The methods for doing so were worked out by the Canadian Task Force on Preventive Health Care. Their work is updated regularly, and can be found on their website, at www.ctfphc.org. The United States Preventive Services Task Force (www.ahcpr.gov/clinic/uspstfix.htm) collaborates with them but is more interventionist in approach. Many other countries now produce evidence-based guidelines, either performing primary data reviews or adapting those of others to their own epidemiology and health care system. Guidelines vary, even after viewing the same evidence, because of different interpretations and beliefs about medical care.[44]

Evidence for making clinical decisions

A new skill has emerged in the twenty-first century. It is finding the best information for making clinical decisions. As information is becoming so much easier to find, so the problem has changed emphasis, from finding *any* information to deciding which information is the best to use. When trying to assist a woman with her health problem, clinicians must draw on their clinical knowledge. What causes the illness? Why does it manifest this way? Untreated, what will it do? Will it get better? Is it the prelude to something more sinister? Is there effective treatment? Which is best of several options? And so on. Each of these questions falls into a number of different *question types*. The means by which we find the best answer is called *evidence-based practice*.[45] Evidence-based practice provides a means to assist the practitioner to answer these clinical questions based on a systematic review of the scientific evidence.[46]

Evidence-based medicine

Evidence-based medicine arose out of the realisation that research was being published and stored (in libraries) with no influence on clinical practice: we were still practising as if the information was not available. Sometimes patients were harmed by not being offered effective treatment. Sometimes patients were harmed by the treatment provided for them! Evidence-based medicine is simply the finding of the best available evidence for answering clinical questions. In some respects it is nothing new. In others it represents another way (thinking less pathophysiologically and more empirically). It involves a number of steps.

1 Asking the question

This is the process of appraising the problem and one's knowledge about it. As such it can be very difficult to adjust to. Challenging one's knowledge base is a skill that is hard to develop. So much of what we do is set in tradition. It is hard to re-think the cognitive processes to decide whether or not any one of the many clinical decisions we make is the right one.

Dr Sheila Brown hesitated before hitting the print button for the prescription on screen. The prescription was for the combined oral contraceptive pill (OCP).

'Yes,' repeated Angela, 'I have had quite nasty migraines in the past.'

It was a routine visit for contraception. She had been prescribed the OCP by another doctor before moving to this town recently.

Was there not a contraindication to using the OCP in women with migraine?

'Ah,' said Sheila, 'I think we may need to think of an alternative.'

'Oh no,' was Angela's response. 'The pill suits me so well...'

Should the oral contraceptive pill be prescribed for Angela?

2 Turning the question into an answerable question

This step is to turn the question into something easily answered by searching the literature. This usually involves disciplining oneself to address several elements of the question. This can be best undertaken by using the 'PICO' mnemonic (Box 1.20).

BOX 1.20 PICO: a mnemonic for breaking up a question into its components

P Patients or Population
I Intervention or Indicator
C Comparator or Controls
O Outcome

This helps one address each of the different categories: which patient/population does your question relate to? And what is the intervention or indicator of interest? Then think about what it is you are comparing it to. Is it nothing, or an alternative treatment, for example? And what is the outcome you are interested in? First we need to think what sort of risk we are talking about. What is the untoward outcome we are worried about?

Answer: stroke.

As an example, try the initial question along these lines.

Modified question:
'Should the oral contraceptive pill be prescribed for Angela?'

P In women with a previous history of migraine …
I … does using the OCP …
C … compared to not using the OCP …
O … result in more strokes?

It is also worth thinking about the type of question being asked. This will determine the type of research study that will provide the best answers (Figure 1.22).

Questions:

- Diagnostic ('What is the value of the test? How much added information does it give?')
- Aetiological ('Does this factor cause that disease?')
- Prognostic ('What happens to this condition with time?')
- Interventional ('Which is the best treatment?)
- Epidemiological—the frequency ('How many cases of X disease accompany Y clinical presentations?')
- Clinical phenomena ('Why do people feel this way with that disease?')

Most doctors ask 'intervention' questions, and the best evidence for these comes from randomised controlled trials (RCTs) or, even better, systematic reviews of RCTs.

FIGURE 1.22 Different question types are best answered by different types of research.

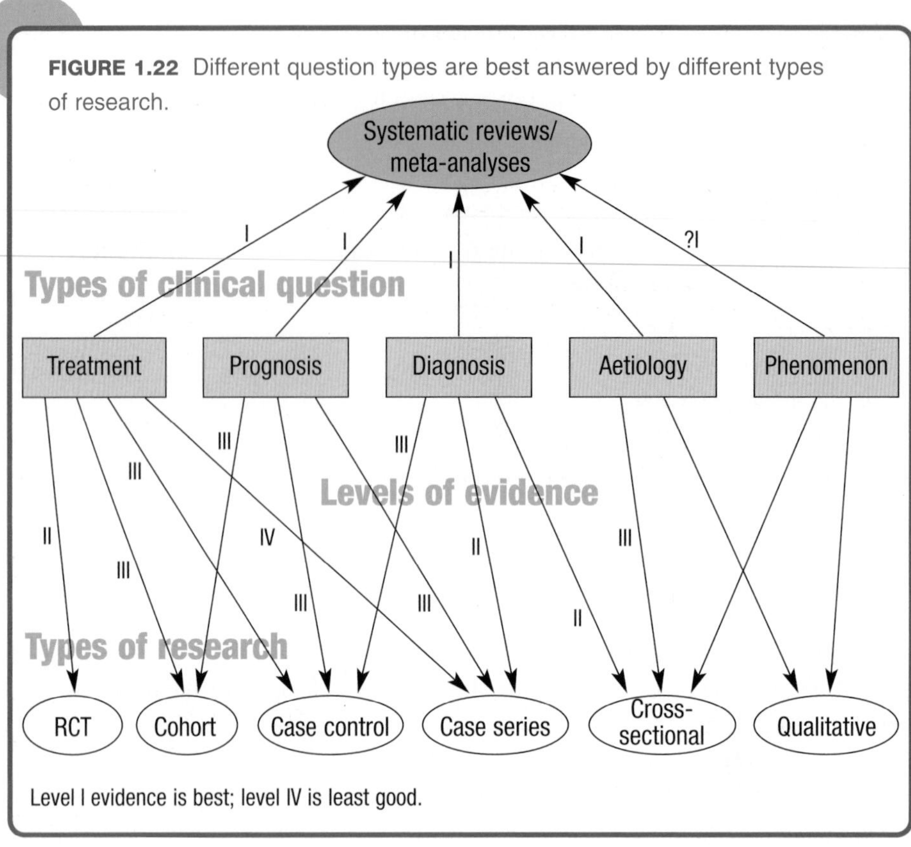

The question about Angela is a type of aetiology question. The best answer then would come from a cohort study. This would mean following up a large number of women put on the OCP and comparing them with others using different contraception, and then seeing which women developed strokes. A moment's reflection would have one realise that stroke is such a rare event that it would be almost impossible to set up such a study. Failing that, the next-best evidence would come from a cohort or case-control study.

(Notice that it is often useful to imagine the sort of research you would design to answer the question: people good at designing research are good at answering clinical questions, and vice versa.)

3 Searching for the evidence

Now you need to find what research has been done. There are many sources of evidence. Initially the pre-appraised evidence may be the simplest to digest (Table 1.1).

Many clinicians find that the easiest place to search is the electronic version of MEDLINE®, called PubMed® (a free service maintained by the National Library of Medicine® in Washington, USA). This has many clinical studies available on it. There is a special interface for clinicians within PubMed which makes much of the searching much easier (Figure 1.23). Searching for 'migraine AND stroke' gets about 24 'hits'. Most of these are irrelevant, but some would seem to be just what we had previously decided to find.

TABLE 1.1 Some sources of evidence

Type or source	Format	Advantages	Disadvantages
Critically appraised topic (CAT)	Website, http://cebm.jr2.ox.ac.uk – or your own!	Pre-appraised summaries for a clinical question	One study per CAT. Time-limited. Quality control
Clinical evidence	Book, BMJ Publishing Group	A compendium of the evidence designed for clinicians	Very brief. Therapeutic interventions only.
Best evidence	CD ROM, online	Pre-appraised summaries filtered for clinical relevance	Limited coverage
Cochrane library	CD ROM, online	High quality systematic reviews covering a complete topic	Limited coverage, time lag, learning curve to use. Therapeutic interventions only.
Bibliographic databases (Medline, CINAHL, PSYCHLIT, EMBASE etc)	CD ROM, online	Original research, up to date. Free for some databases (eg PubMed interface of Medline)	Need to learn to search effectively. No quality filtering.

4 Evaluating the quality of the evidence

Here are the relevant studies we found (dispensing with a lot of irrelevant material):

- *In a recent study, 291 women in eight European cities aged 20–44 years with ischaemic, haemorrhagic or unclassified arterial stroke were compared with 736 age- and hospital-matched controls. Adjusted odds ratios associated with a personal history of migraine were 1.78 (95% CI 1.14 to 2.77), 3.54 (1.30 to 9.61) and 1.10 (0.63 to 1.94) for all stroke, ischaemic stroke and haemorrhagic stroke respectively. Odds ratios for ischaemic stroke were similar for classical migraine (with aura) (3.81, 95% CI 1.26 to 11.5) and simple migraine (without aura) (2.9, 95% CI 0.66 to 13.5). A family history of migraine, irrespective of personal history, was also associated with increased odds ratios for ischaemic stroke and haemorrhagic stroke. After adjustment for a personal history of migraine this association was reduced but odds ratios remained significantly*

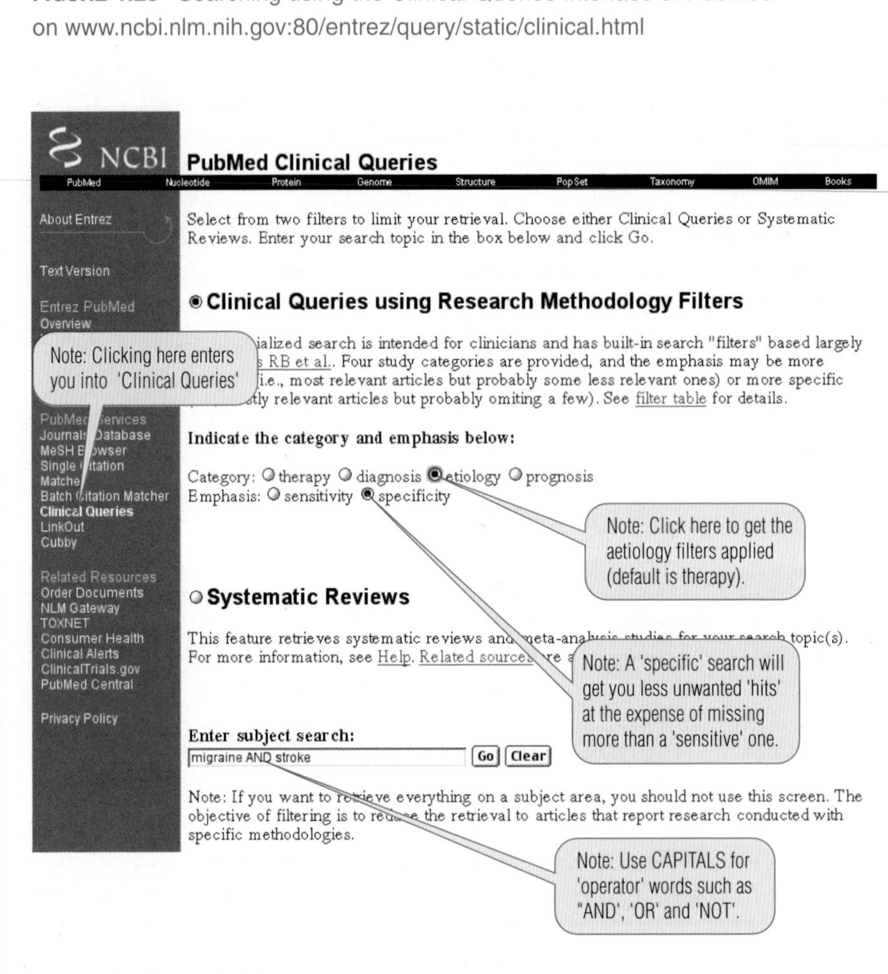

FIGURE 1.23 Searching using the Clinical Queries interface of PubMed on www.ncbi.nlm.nih.gov:80/entrez/query/static/clinical.html

increased: 2.07 (95% CI 1.31 to 3.26), 3.62 (95% CI 1.37 to 9.58) and 2.22 (1.26 to 3.90) for all stroke, ischaemic stroke and haemorrhagic stroke respectively. In migrainous women, coexistent use of oral contraceptives or smoking had greater than multiplicative effects on the odds ratios for ischaemic stroke associated with migraine alone. Odds ratios associated with migraine and oral contraceptive use and migraine and smoking were 6.95 (95% CI 0.79 to 54.8) and 7.39 (95% CI 2.14 to 25.5) respectively. In women without migraine, the odds ratios for ischaemic stroke associated with oral contraceptive use were 2.76 (95% CI 1.01 to 7.55) and 0.82 (95% CI 0.36 to 1.89) for smoking. Compared with women who did not smoke, did not use oral contraceptives, and did not report a history of migraine, the odds ratio for ischaemic stroke associated with use of oral contraceptives in current smokers with a history of migraine based on nine cases and two controls was 34.4 (95% CI 3.27 to 361) (Level III-2).[47]

- *In another case-control study, 72 women under age 45 with ischaemic stroke confirmed by cerebral computerised tomography or magnetic resonance imaging were compared with 173 hospitalised controls. Ischaemic stroke was strongly associated with migraine, both migraine without aura (odds ratio 3.0, 95% DI 1.5 to 5.8) and migraine with aura (6.2, 95% CI 2.1 to 18.0). The risk of ischaemic stroke was substantially increased for migrainous women who were using oral contraceptives (odds ratio 13.9) or who were heavy smokers (≥ 20 cigarettes/day) (odds ratio 10.2) (Level III-2).*[48]
- A *case control study of 178 control subjects and 89 cases aged between 15 and 65 with ischaemic stroke found a significant association between migraine and ischaemic stroke only in patients with classic migraine (odds ratio 2.6, 95% CI 1.1 to 6.6). Classic migraine did not increase ischaemic stroke risk when smoking was present (Level III-2).*[49]
- *Schwartz and colleagues (1998) conducted a pooled analysis of data from two US-based case-control studies examining the association between low-dose oral contraceptive pill use and ischaemic stroke. Data from 175 ischaemic stroke cases, 198 haemorrhagic stroke cases and 1191 control subjects from 18 to 44 years of age was analysed. For ischaemic stroke, the pooled odds ratio adjusted for stroke risk factors for current use of low dose oral contraceptives compared with women who had never used oral contraceptives was 0.66 (95% CI 0.29 to 1.47) and compared with women not currently using oral contraceptives; the pooled odds ratio was 1.09 (95% CI 0.54 to 2.21). For haemorrhagic stroke, the pooled odds ratio for current use of low dose oral contraceptive pills compared with never users was 0.95 (95% CI 0.46 to 1.93) and compared with non-users the pooled odds ratio was 1.11 (95% CI 0.61 to 2.01). The pooled odds ratios for current low-dose oral contraceptive use and either stroke type were not elevated among women who were ≥ 35 years or cigarette smokers (Level III-2).*
- *In an international comparative hospital-based case control study, the risk of ischaemic stroke in association with current use of combined oral contraceptives in 697 cases aged 20 to 44 years and 1962 age-matched hospital controls was reported. The diagnosis of ischaemic stroke was based on computerised tomography, magnetic resonance imaging or cerebral angiography. The overall odds ratio of ischaemic stroke was 2.99 (95% CI 1.65 to 5.40) in European countries. Odds ratios were lower in women who did not smoke (Level III-3).*[50]
- *In a second international hospital-based case control study, the risk of haemorrhagic stroke in association with current use of combined oral contraceptives was examined. This study comprised 1068 cases aged 20 to 44 years and 2910 age-matched controls. Current use of combined oral contraceptives was associated with slightly increased risk of haemorrhagic*

> *stroke; the increase was not significant in Europe (1.38, 95% CI 0.84 to 2.25). Odds ratios among current oral contraceptive users who were also current cigarette smokers were greater than 3 (Level III-3).*[51]

We can summarise this information as follows:

There is good evidence of an association between migraine and stroke (the odds are about double), especially for ischaemic stroke (the odds rise to triple, or more if the migraine is described as classic). There is also good evidence that the oral contraceptive pill increases the risk of stroke (the odds rise to about triple) for ischaemic but not haemorrhagic stroke (where the odds were not significantly different).

5 Putting the evidence into practice

Knowing the *absolute* risk of stroke among women of this age would also assist us in evaluating this information. For example, the annual rate of stroke among women aged 30 to 45 is about 25–50 per 100 000 women in many Western countries (from www.aihw.gov.au in Australia. Other similar sites are, for example, www.cdc.gov/nchs/ in the USA and www.statistics.gov.uk in the UK; other rates can be found for many countries from government health statistics websites). This means that the absolute rate would increase from (say) a baseline of 30/100 000 to 90/100 000 women by using the OCP (a risk we have hitherto regarded as acceptable). The risk is roughly triple that again (210/100 000) if they have classic migraine. The difference (that is, the extra strokes caused by women who have migraine and use the OCP) is 120/100 000, which is about double that we tolerate for using the OCP in healthy women at no extra risk.

What do these numbers mean, and how do we use them? That depends on one's own values. What risks, such as inconvenience, the risk of pregnancy and so on, is the patient (and her doctor!) prepared to increase in order to reduce the risk of stroke? There can be no 'right' answer. We can only look at the figures and try and relate them to the multitude of risks we take every day as part of normal living, and decide if this is acceptable or not.

Many new questions might arise, such as: Does the risk increase much if the woman smokes? (Angela does not.) Should we check for Leiden factor? And so on.

6 Incorporating this into quality assurance

One final step would be to evaluate how to use this sort of information in daily practice. How you go about this depends on how much effort you are prepared to put into audits and getting feedback.

One important consideration is the need to keep track of the process. What questions have been asked? What did you do with the results? Sackett liked to store this information as 'critically appraised topics' (CATs), a sort of little black book with one page per question addressed.[46] And his group would often go back to look the information up again. Some have tried to turn this into an industry with electronic CATs and retrieval systems—and even a website where they can be uploaded (including such refinements as software for helping extract the necessary data, and for calculating useful data such as the NNT automatically).

If you find all this a rather daunting and lonely prospect, it might be worth thinking about ways of doing it as a team. Groups of health professionals often meet to work through a question or two each week, sometimes even doing the searching together. Most clinicians find this fun, and find they replace some other Continuing Medical Education (CME) with this.[52]

If you do not have time to learn the searching skills, and have access to an evidence-based literature search service, another option is available to you. These exist in different parts of the world, and save time. They invite you to address your clinical question to a team skilled at finding evidence-based answers. However, you still have the responsibility to initiate and refine the evidence-based question, and work out how to apply the results in your clinical practice.[53,54] The final step of seeing if your practice is meeting the standards of quality you would like for your patients is of course quite another subject.

Implications and conclusions

We have seen how it is possible to find information to help make the best clinical decision. Learning how to do this effectively and confidently is a skill that has to be practised, like any other. It is becoming increasingly important as information becomes more freely available.

Indeed there are signs that as professionals, doctors and other health workers are undergoing a revolution in the very essence of 'professionalism': the professions can no longer ration information to their clients and patients. After all, information is freely available in unimaginably vast quantities to anyone who has access to, and has only primitive searching ability on, a computer online. Rather, we have a new role with information, as brokers of it, guiding people to the best sources, steering them from the worst, interpreting and explaining it. Perhaps we have become 'information managers'.[55]

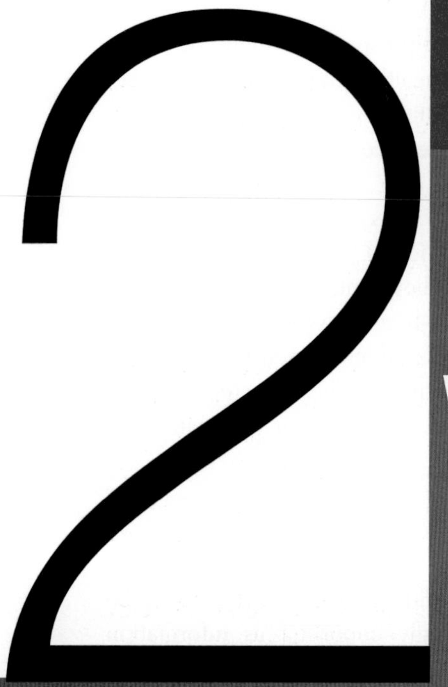

SECTION 2

Women and health

Gender and health

Developing gender-sensitive health care for women

Around the world, the different needs of women and men are beginning to receive greater attention in the planning of health services. The growing recognition of these gender differences derives mainly from the campaigning activities of women who have drawn attention to their sexual and reproductive health needs and also to the insensitivity that still characterises many of their medical encounters.[1–5] More recently, some men have begun to express similar concerns on their own behalf, highlighting the difficulties they face in obtaining effective and appropriate health care.[6–9]

This is an introductory account of the impact of gender on the health and health care of women. It begins with a conceptual clarification of the differences between biological sex and social gender and then explores the implications of each of these in the shaping of female experiences of morbidity and mortality. This is followed by an analysis of evidence relating to gender inequalities in access to services and quality of care. The section concludes by examining the implications of this analysis for the development of gender-sensitive health care. The focus is on issues in developed countries such as Australia, the UK and the US. These countries have different health care systems but, as we shall see, the challenges faced in developing gender-sensitive services are very similar.

Defining terms: sex, gender and health

The term 'gender' is increasingly used in debates about health care but its meaning is often imprecise. Indeed, it is often used interchangeably with the term 'sex' when the two actually refer to very different things.[10,11] Though they are closely interconnected, it is essential to distinguish between the biological (or sex) differences between women and men on the one hand and the social (or gender) differences on the other. Both are important in understanding human health and illness but their policy implications may be very different. And both need to be taken seriously if services are to meet the needs of women as well as those of men.

Sex differences in health and illness

The most immediately obvious differences between the sexes are biological, with their distinctive reproductive systems capable of generating specific health problems.[12] Cancers of the prostate and cervix are obvious examples. However, women's capacity for pregnancy and childbirth can generate additional problems during the reproductive process. Unless they are able to control their fertility and give birth safely women can determine little else about their lives. They therefore have 'special needs' for health care and this is reflected in their greater use of services. In both Australia and the UK contraceptive use is by far the commonest reason for women visiting their general practitioners, while childbirth is the major reason for hospital stays.

The importance of meeting women's reproductive health needs has been widely recognised, and pregnant women receive a great deal of attention in the health care systems of developed countries. As a result, the specialty of obstetrics and gynaecology has become a powerful force in the medical arena, and has played its part in ensuring that Britain and Australia now have among the lowest maternal and infant mortality rates in the world. However, this should not be taken as an indication that all the health needs specific to women (or men) have been met. Much remains to be done in guaranteeing all women appropriate methods of fertility control, for example. Other differences between males and females are now being identified beyond the reproductive arena. There is growing evidence that a very wide range of biological differences between men and women are involved in shaping their characteristic patterns of health and illness.[12] We know, for example, that men typically develop heart disease ten years earlier than women, that women are at least twice as likely as men to develop an autoimmune disease and that male-to-female infection with HIV is nearly twice as efficient as female-to-male infection.[12,13] Recent studies suggest that these differences are due in large part to previously unrecognised genetic, hormonal and metabolic differences between the sexes. As yet, these differences have received relatively little attention from researchers. Instead there has been a continuing presumption that women are the same as men except in the sphere of reproduction. However, it is increasingly clear that the confinement of 'female problems' to the specialty of obstetrics and gynaecology leaves other important sex differences in biological functioning unacknowledged and unexplored.

Gender, women and health

However seriously we take the biological differences between the sexes, this can provide only a partial picture of the impact of femaleness and maleness on health and illness. Gender or social differences also have an important role and need equally careful exploration.[14,15] All cultures assign particular characteristics to those they define as female and those they define as male.[1] Men and women are seen as different types of beings with different duties, different responsibilities and different rights and rewards.[16] In most societies these are not merely differences but inequalities, with women having less access than men to a whole variety of economic and social resources.[17]

The reality of these gender divisions is apparent in the different lives led by women and men, and these can influence health in a number of ways.[18] They may be exposed to different health risks, both physical and psychological. They have access to different amounts and types of resources for maintaining or promoting their own health and may also have different levels of responsibility for the care of others. If they become ill they may have very different strategies for coping. They may define their symptoms in very different ways, will probably seek help from different sources and may respond differently to treatment.

Of central importance here is the division between 'public and 'private' worlds. In most cultures women are allocated the responsibility for household duties—for the wide range of 'caring' that ensures family survival and well-being. Too often these duties are not accompanied by entitlement to the relevant resources. Excessive work can be both physically and emotionally debilitating, especially for those with the fewest resources on which to call. Migrant women may be especially vulnerable in these settings where their traditional networks have disappeared or been seriously eroded.[19,20]

The low status of household work, the material dependence of many women on the state or on a male partner, and the broader cultural devaluation of what is 'female' go some way towards explaining why women in most communities continue to report about twice as much anxiety and depression as men.[21–23] In a recent national survey, 12.5 per cent of Australian women reported anxiety disorders compared to only 7 per cent of men, while the figures for depression were 7 per cent and 4 per cent respectively.[24] The effects of these pressures may continue to be significant even after the period of child-bearing. A recent report from the Longitudinal Study on Women's Health Australia indicated that one in five mid-age women (aged 45–50) felt 'rushed, pressured or too busy' every day and 38 per cent felt 'more rushed than five years ago.[25] Those women with major responsibility for family caregiving were found to be at especially high risk of emotional problems.[26] The study found that these women rated their health lower than other respondents, reported more physical symptoms and scored lower on standard physical and mental health measures.[27,28]

The fear or the reality of domestic violence can also be a source of danger in women's domestic lives. Far from being a haven in a cruel world, households are too often the place in which women are most vulnerable to their 'nearest and dearest'. Figures from both the UK and Australia indicate the widespread nature of this problem. The Women's Safety Survey carried out in Australia in 1996 found that among women who had ever been married or in a de facto relationship, 23 per cent had experienced violence from their partner at some time in the relationship.[29] The British Crime Survey of 1996 found exactly the same proportion of UK women reporting violence from a partner at some point in their lives.[30] In both countries these attacks seemed to be especially common during pregnancy.[31]

Thus, both their biological characteristics and the similarities in their social circumstances mean that women have certain health needs in common and that these are sometimes different from those of men. However, this should not lead us to assume that they can be treated as a homogeneous group. Though sex and gender are clearly important determinants of health and illness, their influence can only be understood in the context of the wider economic, social and cultural factors that separate different groups of women from each other. These differences too will have to be taken seriously if the health care needs of all women are to receive equal attention.

Women and health: dimensions of diversity

The health status and health needs of women (and men) will vary markedly across the lifespan. The physiological processes of ageing are undeniable and women in particular experience major bodily changes as they move through different stages of their reproductive cycle. However, the ageing process is also shaped by life experiences and by social attitudes towards people of different ages.[32] The stereotype of older people in general is too often a negative one and older women may be treated especially badly. As a result, the low income and lack of support experienced by many older women can contribute directly to physical and psychological ill health.[33] Women's health status will also vary with their economic and social status. Despite the existence of the National Health Service (NHS), a British woman in social class I or II still has almost four years greater life expectancy than her compatriot in social class IV or V. She will also have significantly less chance of dying during pregnancy or childbirth.[34] Of the 70 major causes of death in women, 64 are more common in those married to men in unskilled or semi-skilled occupations, with breast cancer being the only major exception.[34] These differences are also reflected in patterns of morbidity, with 15 per cent of professional women reporting limiting and long-standing illness compared with 31 per cent of women in unskilled occupations.[35] Figures from Australia show a similar pattern. In 1995, 22 per cent of those adults (15+) living in the most disadvantaged areas rated their health as only fair or poor compared with only 12 per cent in the least disadvantaged areas.[36]

Race and ethnicity also affect health status in a variety of ways.[37] Racist and discriminatory practices are one element in the structural disadvantage that members of many ethnic minority communities still experience. Different cultural beliefs, demographic structures and levels of access to a range of economic and social resources also contribute to the variations in patterns of health and illness found between ethnic groups. As yet there have been few attempts to explore the influence of gender on these complex processes but some interesting findings are now beginning to emerge. In the UK, for instance, there is growing evidence of the mental health problems facing young women of South Asian background who have to develop their identity against what are often very conflicting demands and expectations.[37,38]

Issues relating to ethnicity have been high on the agenda in Australia with research relating to the health of both Indigenous and migrant communities. Again, these links have not always been explored with gender in mind but a number of important studies provide evidence of its significance. We know for example that the life expectancy of Aboriginal and Torres Strait Islander women is 15–20 years less than that of non-Indigenous women.[39] A recent study of the reproductive health of women in a remote Indigenous community in the Northern Territory found it to be extremely poor. Rates of pelvic inflammatory disease and sexually transmitted diseases such as gonorrhoea (at 32 per cent and 27 per cent respectively) were very high, as were rates of infertility.[40]

It is clear that women's health needs are sometimes different from those of men but that women are not a single homogeneous group. They have extremely varied experiences, interests, needs and desires. Any policy designed to meet the needs of all women will therefore need to take the differences between them as seriously as the similarities. However, there is evidence from both Australia and the UK that some aspects of health care systems serve not to reduce but to reinforce existing inequalities both between women and men and between different groups of women.

Inequalities and discrimination in health care

These continuing gender inequalities are sustained by a range of discriminatory practices which act as an arbitrary constraint on the benefits women can obtain from health services. Of course the origins of these practices and the motivations of those who carry them out are often complex and sometimes contradictory. Indeed they will sometimes be designed to meet what are genuinely perceived to be women's 'real' needs. But whatever the subjective intentions of those involved, their objective effects can be damaging. In their attempts to map the impact of this discrimination on service users, women's health advocates have focused on two key issues: access and quality of care.

Gender inequalities in access to care

Around the world, many millions of women continue to be denied access to basic health care as a result of social, economic and cultural inequalities.[14] One of the main achievements of the health care systems in the UK and Australia has been to remove obstacles of this kind so that most women receive at least a basic level of care. Indeed, in the first years after the creation of the NHS, it was working-class women who were among the main beneficiaries as their pent-up need for items such as gynaecological surgery, dental care and spectacles was at last met. However, this does not mean that access is no longer a problem.

Some women in the UK still have difficulty in obtaining appropriate care, with lack of transport and responsibility for dependants posing significant obstacles. Many of these problems have intensified as the pressures on NHS spending have increased. Though waiting lists and other symptoms of financial strain have an impact on both sexes there is evidence that women are disproportionately affected in particular areas. Family planning services, for instance, have been significantly reduced in many parts of the UK.[41] Similarly, a recent Australian study showed that public abortion services in Melbourne were not sufficient to meet the demand and that many low-income women were being forced to use the private sector.[42]

Research in Australia has also highlighted the impact of socio-economic status on the uptake of cervical screening services.[43] Women with a gross annual income of less than $20 000 were significantly less likely to have been tested than those earning $40 000 or more. A similar study carried out in New South Wales found that the lowest uptake of Pap screening in rural populations was in the most remote areas with the highest proportion of Indigenous women. For urban NESB (non-English-speaking) women, the biennial Pap test rate was estimated as 50 per cent and for rural Indigenous women 29 per cent, compared with the New South Wales average of 59 per cent.[44] Australian research has also shown that despite the existence of Medicare, those women living in more remote areas have higher out-of-pocket costs and poorer access to general practitioner services.[45]

Gender differences in quality of care

When they do receive services, there is evidence that women may experience particular problems in their relations with those who are paid to care for them.

Though men may also find it difficult to communicate with health workers, women seem to face additional difficulties, reflecting both their own socialisation and the stereotypical views that others may hold of them.[1,46] Poor women in particular, as well as those from ethnic minorities, are sometimes treated by health workers as though they are less rational, less capable of complex decision making and sometimes as simply less valuable than men.[47–49] A recent survey of Australian women's experiences of general practice did find the overall levels of satisfaction to be good, though many were not satisfied with the help offered in relation to headaches, tiredness and related chronic symptoms. Young women were particularly dissatisfied with the doctor's skills at explaining their problems.[50]

A number of Australian studies have also highlighted the importance of respecting cultural preferences in the design and delivery of services. A recent study of Islamic women in Melbourne found that while they valued the quality of care they were given, they still expressed dissatisfaction with some aspects of it.[51] They reported that cultural differences often made communication difficult and many made clear their preferences for women doctors. In the sphere of prevention, a study in Brisbane identified significant cultural barriers to cervical and breast screening among Thai women which needed to be tackled if the services were to be equitably distributed.[52]

These issues have generated particular concern in the context of reproductive health care where the price paid for access to technology can be loss of autonomy.[53–55] Women seeking to use modern methods of fertility control may need to negotiate with a doctor whose personal judgements about the appropriateness of particular methods may constrain the woman's own choice. This appears to be especially true of some younger women.[56] In surgery too, women are sometimes denied the opportunity to participate fully in treatment decisions. In the case of breast cancer surgery and hysterectomy in particular, many still report lack of support in their attempts to make an informed choice.[57]

Concerns about the quality of caring relationships continue to be high on the agenda of women's health advocates in both the UK and Australia. Their implications were highlighted in a recent study of women's health centres in Australia.[58] This confirmed the high value women still place on these 'alternative' services in an increasingly conservative environment. Their appeal appears to be based in particular on their willingness and ability to provide sympathetic care for clients who find it difficult to obtain good care elsewhere, time for complex or especially distressing health problems and the opportunities for active and sometimes collective strategies for health development.

Gender bias in clinical practice

But alongside these more qualitative concerns there has also been a growing debate about the technical quality of women's health care. This has been especially evident in the context of reproductive health. It is clear that the development of contraceptive devices is often influenced more by effectiveness and cost criteria than by concern for women's health. As a result women may be prescribed devices that prevent them from conceiving but only at significant cost to their well-being. Though these criticisms are most frequently levelled at services in the developing countries, it is clear that in the developed countries too, there are women who have difficulty finding a contraceptive that meets all their needs. And these are likely to be the most deprived women.

However, in recent years these criticisms about quality of clinical care have not been confined to specialist 'women's' areas. Studies of cardiac care in particular have found evidence of gender bias.[59,60] Research in the USA has shown that the normal diagnostic process is not as accurate in women as in men. This is turn may contribute to the tendency among clinicians to order fewer invasive diagnostic tests such as angiography for their female patients.[61,62] Similar problems have been identified in the UK, where men in one region were found to be 60 per cent more likely to be given an angiogram than women with the same condition.[63,64]

Once they receive a diagnosis women may also receive less effective treatment than men with symptoms of the same severity. A recent study in New South Wales showed that women were less likely than men to be treated with preferred drugs such as aspirin, heparin and beta blockers and were also less likely to receive coronary angiography.[65] In Western Australia a study has shown that at all ages women with a ruptured abdominal aortic aneurysm are more likely to die than men with a similar condition.[66] Bias of this kind stems in part from the sex and gender blindness of many clinicians, a pattern which is reflected in medical education and in research.[67]

Towards a more gender-sensitive approach

This brief analysis has highlighted the complex links between biological sex, social gender and health. It has also demonstrated the major differences between the health status and health care needs of different groups of women. If these insights are to be translated into more equitable and effective health care services, greater sensitivity to sex and gender concerns will be needed. This will need to be reflected in research, in the planning and delivery of services and in wider social and economic policies.

If gender bias is to be tackled in medical research, measures will need to be taken to ensure that priorities are determined in ways that more closely reflect the needs of women as well as men. It will also be essential that study designs include both sex and gender as key variables whenever appropriate. This would promote greater equity through filling the gaps that currently exist in our knowledge of women's health. In the longer term it would improve the overall quality of medical science and would therefore benefit men too.

To improve access to services, many women will need better transport and child care arrangements as well as more effective financial support. Across the range of health care settings it is also important that women and men be treated with respect. Women should not be humiliated by sexist behaviour, for example, or be damaged by discriminatory practices. Men, on the other hand, should not be expected to live up to stereotypical concepts of masculinity and heterosexuality. The economic, social and cultural characteristics of different groups of women (and men) also need to be understood and their implications for appropriate care respected.

Health promotion policies in particular need to be gender sensitive if their messages are to be heard. Too many campaigns are addressed to women in their roles as the carers of others while ignoring their own well-being. Conversely, men too often feel that health is women's business and that health promotion is nothing to do with them. If this is to change, campaigns need to be designed in ways that encourage both women and men to look after themselves and each other.

Looking at the more technical aspects of care, health care workers also need to be more aware of the importance of both sex and gender issues in developing appropriate treatment strategies. Greater knowledge of sex differences in the aetiology, symptomatology and prognosis of problems such as heart disease and HIV/AIDS will be required. Similarly there will need to be a clearer understanding and acceptance of the ways in which gender differences in daily life can have a major impact on experiences of health and illness and hence on the effectiveness or otherwise of medical responses.

Finally, links will need to be made between health services and wider economic and social policies. The further development of gender equality policies in both the UK and Australia would be of value in tackling the poverty that continues to have a negative impact on many women's health. Similarly, more effective policies for prevention and for the identification and support of survivors could reduce some of the huge burden of distress and disability currently resulting from gender violence.

At the same time, strategies could be devised to help reshape unequal patterns of gender relations. More flexible working hours, for example, as well as more generous parental leave for both women and men would provide the opportunity for reshaping the gender division of labour. Changes of this kind will not be easy to achieve since they would involve a redefinition of some of the most intimate areas of human life. But unless they are tackled, gender inequalities will continue to constrain both women and men in their attempts to realise their full potential for health.[68]

Ethics and women's health

Women's health and the provision of health care to women are topics which raise many ethical issues. Health care has the goals of promoting good health, treating diseases, and decreasing the burdens of illness and disability. These are moral goals, concerning the welfare of others. The actions of health care professionals (HCPs) have ethical content, because, through their actions, HCPs have the potential to affect other people for better or worse, to improve or harm their health in various ways, and to provide a better or worse experience in accessing health care.

What is ethics?

Health care professionals are frequently faced with the question: 'What is the right thing to do in this situation, for this patient?' Part of the answer to this question will be technical, but an important part of it will be ethical, thinking about the values which will come into play and making judgements about which are most important in this case. Ethics is the study of these values, equipping HCPs with the tools to recognise ethical issues and to respond to ethical questions in a systematic way. Ethical analysis involves identifying the important elements in a situation, looking at the whole range of possible actions and assessing how these affect the people involved.

There are a number of well-recognised values which are important in health care decisions, and which HCPs have a duty to consider when making decisions. These include:

- *Patient autonomy*, which is the value we place upon allowing people to make their own decisions without being manipulated or coerced by other people. Respecting autonomy requires that HCPs be honest with patients and help them to understand all the information they need to make decisions. Another part of respecting autonomy requires that HCPs maintain confidentiality about their patients and do not disclose that a consultation has occurred, any possible diagnoses, or results from investigations unless the patient has given consent for this to occur.
- *The welfare of the patient*, which is usually the focus of health care. Promoting patients' welfare creates two duties for HCPs. The first is to do no harm, also known as non-maleficence. Sometimes well-intended actions can harm patients (for example, if the side effects of a treatment are worse than the original illness), so the duty of non-maleficence reminds HCPs to look for the potential bad effects of their actions. The second duty is a positive one, to act for the good of the patient, also known as beneficence. The duty of beneficence requires that HCPs make choices which benefit the patient rather than anyone else.
- *Justice*, which is to do with the fairness of health care. The duty to act justly requires us to ask questions about the distribution of health care, and whether everyone with the same needs has the same access to treatment.

It is important for the HCP to start by looking at his/her own beliefs: What are they? How have they developed? Who has influenced the development of these beliefs? Is this what I really believe?

Good practice is ethical practice

Being a good practitioner requires the ability to identify and deliberate about ethical issues, as well as having clinical skills and technical knowledge. Health care decisions involve value judgements, starting with the basic assumption that good health is generally a more valuable state than ill health. Ethical skills help practitioners to identify the values behind judgements, and to see where points of agreement and disagreement occur. Much of the time patients and HCPs share values about health care, but at times competing values influence women's decisions about health services. For example, a woman with disseminated breast cancer may choose not to have further chemotherapy because she wishes to spend the last few months of her life with her family rather than in and out of hospital; for her the intrusions and side effects of chemotherapy are not worth the possibility of prolonging her life. It is important for HCPs to be able to recognise the advantages and disadvantages of various courses of action in both clinical and moral terms. Discussing the harms and benefits of treatments requires the capacity to identify empathically with others, and to recognise that other people may not share your views about what to do. Ethical skills also include being able to recognise and discuss difficult issues which may arise in the course of delivering health care. Many ethical dilemmas can and should be pre-empted by thoughtful and well-planned practice.[69]

The ethical aspects of health care are magnified when we realise that good or bad health is not just a matter of luck or accident of our genes. For women, both biological sex and social gender create excess burdens of ill health and contribute to the need for health care. This creates an imperative to look beyond the good or harm which may be achieved in individual consultations to the wider social context and to the patterns of poverty, oppression and discrimination which limit the health potential of many women.

Values in women's health

What are the important values in women's health? Control over decision making (*autonomy*) is a central issue. Historically women have been exploited in or excluded from research, given unnecessary surgery, and treated without consent or with experimental therapies.[70–73] In particular, women have often been treated in ways which have not recognised or respected their capacity for making choices about treatments.[74]

Informed consent is a process for trying to ensure that decisions about health care are voluntary and made by competent people who fully understand the issues involved. These are demanding requirements. Voluntariness may be compromised by subtle means, such as expressing disapproval of a woman's choice or ignoring requests for specific interventions, as well as by more coercive actions such as agreeing to a termination of pregnancy on condition that sterilisation is performed at the same time.[69] A person is competent to make a health care decision if she can understand the relevant information and make an informed choice on the basis of that understanding. Understanding can be helped by providing information in a form that the person can understand (size of print, language level) and, where possible, should be given far enough in advance to allow the person to think about the issues, ask questions, and discuss with family or friends before making their decision. It may be necessary to provide an interpreter for patients from a non-English-speaking background, or a tape if the person is illiterate.

How much information does a patient need to make an informed decision? There is no easy answer to this question, but in general, standards for informed consent require that patients be told everything that a reasonable patient would want to know in the circumstances, and anything that would be relevant to this particular patient. There may be a temptation to withhold information because the HCP judges that it is too complex or may be upsetting for the patient, but this is rarely, if ever, justified.

Competent decisions, whether to consent to or refuse a recommended treatment, must be respected even if they are not shared or understood by HCPs.[75] As long as the person involved understands the risks and implications of her choice, she is competent to make that decision, even if she is not competent in some other areas of her life.

Respecting women's right to make decisions about their health care is one part of respecting autonomy, but we also need to look beyond the consultation to a wider understanding of the relationship between women and health care. Who decides which treatments are to be offered, or even which conditions count as diseases? For example, women with fertility problems have little option but to remain childless or to seek technical medical interventions as other solutions, such as adoption, are not easily available. The range of treatments offered in the consultation has been shaped by previous professional interests and research funding, and may not represent anything like an ideal set of choices.

Acting in the patient's best interests (*beneficence*) is a central value in health care. Practitioners' views of patients' interests are shaped by their training, clinical experience and professional expertise. Evidence plays an increasing role in medical expertise, helping us to answer clinical questions such as the best way to do an operation or the best drug treatment for a disease. However, it is important to remember that evidence is limited by the current boundaries of medical and scientific knowledge. Evidence is one component in clinical decision making but evidence alone cannot tell us the right thing to do.

Beneficence is an important ethical consideration when patients cannot discuss their own preferences, for example if they are unconscious or too ill to talk. In these situations the HCP should talk to family or others who know the woman, check whether she has made an Advance Health Directive or appointed someone to have enduring power of attorney for health, and try to understand what the person would want for herself. Other people may be better equipped than the HCP to advise a woman in these situations. Beneficence can slip over into paternalism when HCPs ignore the preferences of women who are able to make their own decisions, and instead make decisions based solely upon the HCP's view about what is best for this person.

Access to health care raises issues of *justice*: are resources distributed fairly in the community and do they reach those who need them most? Much ill health reflects socio-economic inequalities and yet it is often the poorest communities which have the least access to health care. Sometimes there is a tension between doing the greatest good for the greatest number and making health inequalities worse. Screening programs and lifestyle interventions tend to have the least health impact upon the most deprived sections of society while improving the health of others who are better off. Expensive technological interventions may divert resources away from basic health care in other areas. For any intervention, it is worth asking what the impact is upon deprived or marginalised groups. At the same time, advances in science and medicine have the potential to increase knowledge and patient choice.

In Australia there are waiting lists for treatment in public hospitals, and at times public facilities are used for privately insured patients rather than those with the most urgent needs. We may question the fairness of this where hospitals are funded from the public purse.

Ethical issues in women's health

Many decisions about the health and well-being of women involve ethical deliberations as illustrated by the following brief discussions.

Fertility

Women may seek either to avoid pregnancy or to become pregnant. Unless women have access to safe, reliable contraception, their opportunities for having control over other aspects of their life such as employment and relationships are limited. Not all women have access to contraceptive services or can find a method which suits them; some may disagree with the use of contraception. Should the right to control fertility extend to abortion? One of the arguments in support of open access to abortions is that there are harmful consequences for women if they are forced to continue unwanted pregnancies. Without the freedom to end pregnancies, women may damage their health, be unable to care for existing children and have their opportunities in life reduced. For women who suffer failures of contraception or who are forced to have sex, abortion offers a way to avoid unplanned consequences.[76] However, people who believe that performing an abortion is equivalent to killing a person are strongly opposed to abortion, even if the woman's health and other interests are at risk.[77]

Technology

New technologies raise new ethical dilemmas. Reproductive technologies are no exception, from extracorporeal fertilisation to genetic manipulation of fertilised embryos and the non-reproductive use of spare embryos. Is infertility a natural misfortune? Does our culture put pressure on women to undergo risky and often unsuccessful medical treatment for the 'disease' of infertility, or is the restriction of access to fertility treatments an unfair restriction on women's choices? The risks and benefits to the individual can be considerable: the chance of a healthy baby versus the increased risks of ectopic pregnancy and multiple births, the stress and anxiety generated, and the costs involved. Should access to reproductive technologies be restricted to socially approved women, excluding those who do not fit into traditional family patterns?[78] Many people feel that having children is a fundamental part of human life, and that it is wrong to deny people the chance to try for a family. Using reproductive technologies may avoid harms such as some genetic diseases, or allow parents greater choice about the children they have—should this extend to choice of gender or other attributes such as hair or eye colour? Where does this lead?

Pregnancy

Most pregnant women wish for the best possible outcome for their pregnancy. Screening offers a way to identify pregnancies at risk for fetal disease, and can reassure women about the health of their potential child. A decision about antenatal screening may depend on a number of values including the desire for information, views about having a child with a disability, risks of screening, and the acceptability of abortion.

Conflicts between the interests of the mother and those of the fetus are rare, but can be very challenging to deal with. Maternal drug addiction and alcoholism can damage the fetus; in these situations it is better to offer comprehensive support to the woman involved rather than adopt a punitive attitude.[79] Is it ever right to force a woman to have treatment for the sake of her unborn child? The answer to this question is generally 'no'. It is not right to impose treatments such as fetal surgery or caesarean sections on women, even if the treatment is necessary for the well-being of the fetus. Women have the right to accept or refuse any medical treatments, regardless of fetal outcome.[80] However, this can be very difficult to accept for HCPs who are also concerned about the well-being of the fetus. Refusals of treatment are rare, making it very important to make sure that those involved understand exactly what is going on and what the consequences may be.

Healthy women

Health care institutions and practices are powerful in shaping societies' views about health and illness and about what is normal or abnormal. Many health care practices such as cervical and breast cancer screening, lifestyle advice, contraception, antenatal and intrapartum care, and hormone replacement therapy are offered to healthy women rather than in response to ill health. The aim of these practices is well motivated, to prevent future ill health, but some may consider them an unwelcome medicalisation of women's lives. For example, many women go through the menopause in good health with a minimum of troubling symptoms. However, the widespread promotion of hormone replacement therapy and the labelling of the post-menopause as an oestrogen deficiency disease can change women's perceptions about their health.[81] Any decisions must involve the provision of high-quality information, and a balancing of benefits and burdens for the individual woman.

Screening aims to identify specific diseases in the presymptomatic stages and offer a better chance of cure. The benefits of early diagnosis and cure have to be weighed up against the harms of screening. Screening may carry its own risks including false positives and false negatives, as well as costs in terms of resources and inconvenience to those screened. Some screening programs such as regular Pap smears for the detection of cervical cancer have not been tested in a randomised controlled trial to see how effective they are, and for others such as breast cancer screening the costs and benefits are hard to work out.[82] These factors make it crucial to give women the best possible information to help them make informed choices about screening. Health care practitioners have an obligation to be up to date with the evidence available and to present complex information as clearly and fairly as possible.

Culture

Different cultures may have different beliefs and values. These are thrown into sharp relief when people migrate from their countries of origin to Northern and Western countries, where the prevailing norms may be at odds with the traditions of migrants. Conflicts often arise for the children and grandchildren of migrants who may wish to follow the lifestyle of the new country but who also have to remain mindful of the original traditions and attitudes of their families. At times HCPs become involved in these conflicts, for example in the reconstruction of the hymens of young women who are no longer virgins but who wish to appear so for their wedding night. The family will be shamed if the bride cannot show her bloody sheet after the wedding night, and this may lead to serious consequences for the woman and her family. How should the potential harms of a medically unnecessary operation be balanced against the non-medical harms to the woman if she does not have a reconstruction? Should this be treated as a form of cosmetic surgery, in which the wishes of the patient are paramount?

Female genital mutilation raises more serious questions. Here the physical harms to the patient are immediate, serious and far-reaching and the patient, usually an infant, is not able to give informed consent. Health care practitioners are not justified in supporting these practices, despite any conflicts which may ensue with the parents or communities involved.

Research

Research involving women has the potential to increase our knowledge about health and disease and to identify new treatments, which are important benefits. As with other areas, the ethical issues can be difficult. Current research agendas tend to focus on disorders which are related to women's reproductive systems. However, defining women's health as a single risk category associated with reproductive biology ignores the ways in which the social, rather than the biological, effects of gender affect women's health.[83] The focus on women as reproducers seems to exhaust research interest in women's health, leading to gender blindness with regard to other health problems which have recognised sex differences, such as HIV/AIDS, coronary heart disease, depression, tropical infectious diseases and tuberculosis.[84] Research agendas reflect the interests of funding bodies, including pharmaceutical companies, rather than those of women as patients. Where possible, all research should analyse by gender to determine whether this is significant for presentation, diagnosis, management or outcome. In addition, age is important—results from younger women cannot necessarily be extrapolated to older women. As with all medical research, high standards of informed consent and confidentiality must be maintained in research with women.

Conclusion

Ethics cuts across all aspects of women's health. There may not be definitive answers to all ethical dilemmas but thinking about ethics can support good practice. It is important to consider what we believe, and where our values come from. Examining the reasons we offer for our actions and testing them against recognised values helps to ensure that our actions meet the highest possible ethical standards.

Women in minority groups

A significant number of women of all ages are isolated from mainstream society as a consequence of their geographic location, religion, disabilities, ethnicity, sexuality, social strata, particular family circumstances or occupation. A greater proportion of women in some of these isolated groups have lower socio-economic status. While poverty itself does not cause disease, it is associated with a lifestyle that has many health consequences. Reduced education and income are associated with less opportunity to make lifestyle choices. These include smoking, alcohol, less healthy foods and less physical activity. Many of these women have problems with confidentiality and access to services.[85,86]

Indigenous women

Many of the issues involving the health of Aboriginal women in Australia apply to the health of other indigenous groups in the world. The health of Aboriginal women should be viewed against a background of historical events.[87] Although Aboriginal people shared a similar way of life and similar religious beliefs, they belonged to separate groups that had their own languages, land, legends and ceremonies. The concept of health held by Aboriginal and Torres Strait Islander communities is a holistic one. It includes 'social, emotional, spiritual and cultural well-being', with health represented as the outcome of the interdependence of body, land and spirit.[88] This is a whole-of-life view and it also includes the concept of life–death–life.

As with other women, Aboriginal and Torres Strait Islander women are the major carers of children, spouses and elderly people, but they also play an important part in maintaining the mental and emotional health of their communities. Women may not always come forward to seek primary health services for their own health problems or for preventive health measures, because of their focus on caring for others. Aboriginal women may also face a lack of accessible and culturally appropriate service, which is also sensitive to gender issues.

In Aboriginal society, women's business and men's business are quite separate, and are governed by strict social rules. Aboriginal women may feel particular 'shame' or embarrassment when dealing with a male practitioner, although this will depend on the relationship between patient and doctor.[89] In addition, the causes of illness may be differently defined. The cause of an illness must be viewed in a broader context to involve all aspects of the illness that may have meaning for the Aboriginal woman; strong emotions, for example, can cause distress that may be somatised.[90] Communication must also take a different approach: information exchange is usually two-way, so an Aboriginal woman may appear reluctant to answer a direct question, and non-verbal communication is important, so episodes of silence are to be expected in social interactions. Social responsibilities take priority and appointments for health care might not be kept if other issues arise.

Child-bearing among Aboriginal women starts earlier, with high fertility at young ages. The average age of Indigenous mothers is 24.5 years (compared to 29 years in the total population) and 22 per cent are teenagers.[91] Twice as many Indigenous babies are born with a weight below 2500 grams. Perinatal mortality among the

Indigenous community varies across Australia but is substantially greater than in the non-Indigenous community. Neonatal mortality is twice that of non-Aboriginals. In 1994–96 the fetal death rate among births to Indigenous women was 13.0 per 1000 births compared to 6.7 per 1000 non-Indigenous births.[92]

Sexually transmitted infections (STIs) are common in the Indigenous community. Gonorrhoea, syphilis, donovanosis and chlamydia are now hyperendemic in many Aboriginal communities in the Northern Territory, far north Queensland and some regions of Western Australia. Over 90 per cent of syphilis in Australia occurs in Aboriginal communities, with attack rates over 100 times the rates in non-Indigenous communities. The sequelae of STIs for women (pelvic pain, ectopic pregnancy and infertility) are therefore more common. There is strong evidence that STIs facilitate HIV transmission. The rate of HIV infection in the early 1990s in the Indigenous population approximated that of the non-Aboriginal population, but it is commonly accepted that the potential exists for an Indigenous HIV epidemic. The mortality from cervical cancer among Indigenous women is four times that of non-Indigenous women Australia-wide, and even higher in some states. This is related to many factors, including access to appropriate services and reluctance to attend for cervical screening. Barriers to participation in screening by Indigenous women have been explored and programs recommended to overcome some of these.[93]

The psychological impact of menopause is strongly influenced by the importance attached by a particular culture to procreation, fertility, ageing and female roles. Cross-cultural studies have shown that menopause is indeed experienced differently in different cultures. There is little work on the experience of menopause amongst Indigenous women in Australia. However, some research suggests that the menopause was not traditionally an important phase in women's lives.

Immigrant women

Many women may feel powerless in a medical setting; this may be increased for women from a different cultural or non-English-speaking background.[94] Access to health care for women from some ethnic backgrounds may be limited by difficulty in communicating in English or by male family 'gatekeepers', such as husbands, fathers or brothers. Whilst interpreters can be used in many circumstances, some women may be reluctant to discuss personal medical issues when a stranger is present, or gynaecological issues when a male family member is interpreting. At the same time, many immigrants bring with them the beliefs and practices of their culture. These concern the nature and causes of illness as well as the best means of dealing with conditions. The concepts of health promotion and disease prevention may not be understood; for example, a visit to a health care professional when the woman is well for screening purposes may take additional explanation. People, including health care professionals, tend to develop powerful mental images of other cultural groups. A perceived cultural image may affect the provision of optimum care; it can contribute to misdiagnosis (for example, an intense reaction to a symptom may be attributed to the person's cultural background rather than the severity of the symptom) and provide a barrier to women from other cultural groups from accessing services.

Women coming to a country as immigrants or refugees have already been through many stresses.[95] Refugee women may have experienced additional problems: 77 per cent of refugee women in Australia reported some form of trauma or torture.[96] Particular sensitivity is required when offering health care to these women.

Lesbian women

There is a tendency in most societies to view a heterosexual orientation as the 'norm' and assume all people fit into this category. Yet estimates of the proportion of women who identify as lesbian range from 3 to 10 per cent, depending on whether 'lesbian' is defined by sexual behaviour, orientation or identity. Any person who has a non-exclusively heterosexual orientation must go through an active process of adjustment, seeking role models for this equally normal, yet stigmatised orientation. Few people who identify as gay, lesbian or bisexual completely escape the effects of negative attitudes within society, which are reflected within health policy, the health care, welfare and school systems, the workforce and the media.

Lesbian women are constantly aware of the assumption of heterosexuality that pervades both social interactions and interactions with healthcare providers. The latter can result in avoidance of health care or create a barrier to the development of a trusting relationship with their health care professional.[97] By contrast, facilitation of disclosure of lesbian or bisexual identity will improve the practitioner's understanding of the wider context in which this person lives. It will also improve the health care provided if the practitioner has knowledge of the specific issues relevant to lesbians.[98] These include sexual health, screening, mental health, relationship issues and parenting.[99]

With regard to sexual health, there is the misperception that sexually active lesbian women are not at risk of developing sexually transmitted infections. But this is not the case. It is essential that the health care provider understand this and be able to offer advice about safe sex practices. Similarly, consumers and health care providers alike believe that lesbians do not require cervical screening. Lesbians have reported being given incorrect advice by health care professionals and have even been refused Pap smears by treating practitioners because they were lesbian. Lesbians tend to access health care less frequently and therefore should be targeted as one of the under-screened populations.

Lesbians are known to be at higher risk of mental health problems including depression, anxiety and associated drug and alcohol misuse.[100,101] Causative factors include experiences of discrimination, lack of family support, homelessness and isolation. Young people are particularly vulnerable, with a disproportionately high number of same-sex-attracted youth represented among those who suicide or have suicidal thoughts.[102] Domestic violence can be another consequence of isolation, the prevalence of which approximates that found in heterosexual relationships. The issue has been silenced, however, within the lesbian community due to fear of increased stigmatisation of same-sex relationships if the issue is recognised.[103] Health care providers should be aware of the prevalence of these issues and ensure they are able to detect and manage such conditions for their lesbian patients.

Finally, many lesbians are parents within our society. Blended family formation has been common, where children from a previous heterosexual relationship are brought into a new lesbian relationship. Lesbians are increasingly seeking to become parents within the context of their same-sex relationship. A survey of Victorian same-sex couples showed that 41 per cent were hoping to have children, with 63 per cent of those aged under 30 planning families.[104] There is now excellent evidence that children raised in lesbian families are equal to those in heterosexual families in terms of psychological development, social function, gender and sexuality formation. Despite this, lesbian-led families experience discrimination within the legal, welfare, school and health care systems.[105] The HCP can assist by offering support, advice or referral when needed to assist in overcoming such negative experiences.

Women with disabilities

The World Health Organization defines impairment and disability in the following way:

- *Impairment:* any loss or abnormality of psychological, physiological, or anatomical structure or function.
- *Disability:* any restriction or lack (resulting from impairment) of ability to perform an activity in the manner or within the range considered normal for a human being.

Women with disabilities are often invisible. They are not seen in public places, and are devalued and excluded.[106] They have little voice, role or place in the 'well world'. Related to this is the fact that women with disabilities are often portrayed as asexual. This often presents these women with problems associated with relationships and parenting. Women with disabilities are actively discouraged from bearing and raising children. Often society suggests sterilisation and abortion as preferred options. These women's disabilities may also result in poverty, abuse and exploitation; and access to rehabilitation and technology is more limited for them than for their male counterparts. Women with intellectual disabilities are particularly vulnerable to abuse from an early age. Abusive practices have been identified in professional, institutional and social aspects of these women's lives.

Practitioners may be confronted with particular difficulties when delivering care. Some problems that can arise involve difficulties in diagnosing gynaecological disorders, as history details may not be easily obtained from either the woman or her carer. Menstrual charting will often be useful to aid diagnosis, and with appropriate preparation vaginal examination may be possible. There may, however, be difficulties in performing a vaginal examination. Symptoms indicating pathology will warrant examination under anaesthesia if it cannot be achieved in the surgery. Ultrasound may help clarify the clinical picture but will usually be limited to abdominal ultrasound.

Homeless women

Youth homelessness is a significant problem in many Western countries. In young women in particular, the consequences of homelessness on their health and well-being is of major concern. They are vulnerable to drug abuse, sexual abuse and to using prostitution and unsafe sexual practices to support themselves.[107] They have little support and minimal chance of gaining employment. Although some young homeless people are still at school the majority leave school early and without a complete education.[108] Homeless young people are at high risk of depression and other mental health problems.

Factors contributing to homelessness have been identified as:[109]

- Problems within families, including communication and interaction difficulties within families and family breakdown
- Physical, emotional and sexual abuse
- Personality factors, such as mental illness
- Low self-esteem. This can be an antecedent of homelessness, but is more likely to be a consequence.

Providing health services for these young people may need authorities to take a broader, less conventional approach.[110] Once homelessness becomes 'chronic' there emerges an underclass of 'street kids' and the long-term homeless. This has been described in the UK and the USA.

Women in prison

There are a number of issues that affect the health and well-being of women prisoners. Some of these are present when the women enter prison, and some arise during the time they are imprisoned.[111] For instance:

- An estimated 79–85 per cent of incarcerated women have a history of drug addiction.
- Estimates also suggest that a similar percentage of women in prison are victims of childhood incest or other abuse and/or abuse as adults.
- Between 50 and 70 per cent of women in prison have dependent children. The separation from their children is described by these women as one of the worst aspects of their incarceration.[112]
- Health care whilst in prison is seen as inadequate and difficult to access by women. This includes access to gynaecologists and psychologists.
- Treatment for substance abuse is inadequate and illegal drugs are often freely available in prisons.
- Sexuality issues, including sexual relations with other women, have a significant impact on the ability of women to survive their time in prison.

Sex workers

Female sex workers face the same health issues as the general female population. However, they may be less able or willing to access health services to address these, because of the stigma attached to the work they do. They also face a range of health issues related directly to their work, to which other women are not exposed. These include sexually transmitted infections, diseases spread through injecting drugs, violence, emotional and psychological problems. A woman may become a sex worker for a variety of reasons: she may use it as a short-term way of financing her studies or acquiring property; it may be a choice that offers well-paid work with flexible hours;

she may have been forced into the work by someone else (in the case of women illegally entering the country) or to provide income for a family left at home.[113] Not all women in the sex industry want to stay in this area, but it is difficult for these women to train for and be accepted into other professions. A woman may or may not choose to disclose her occupation. This may depend on the approach of the HCP and how the woman perceives the HCP's reaction.

Abuse in women from minority groups

Particular groups of women from minority groups may be more exposed to abuse by nature of their isolation. Culturally specific forms of violence against women (Section 3) include female genital mutilation (Section 6), dowry deaths, murder of women who have allegedly brought shame to their family, sex-selective abortion and female infanticide, and geographically specific forms of violence such as trafficking, forced prostitution and debt bondage.[114] Trafficking victims (over 800 000 per year) come from Asia, the former Soviet Union, central and eastern Europe, Latin America and Africa, with many women being confined, beaten and raped.

In all cultures, many teenage women become homeless in their attempts to escape sexual abuse in the home. They are then exposed to further physical and sexual violence in the streets. Sex workers are also vulnerable to violence by the nature of their work and experience a high rate of physical and sexual abuse. Similarly, there is a high rate of past abuse in women in prisons, and further abuse, from physical or verbal harassment to sexual and physical torture, can occur in custody and in detention centres. The psychological and physical sequelae of this violence for these already vulnerable women are further compounded by a general unavailability of medical care and support services.

Conclusion

Health inequalities in society will continue until the social inequalities are adequately addressed. It is essential that anyone caring for women be sensitive to the woman's background, beliefs and current circumstances when discussing health options.

Lifestyle issues

Alcohol and drug use

Tobacco, drugs and alcohol can all affect women's health and the health of their children before and after birth. Smoking is medically damaging, while problem (heavy and/or chaotic) drug or alcohol use is both medically and socially harmful and can compromise parenting. These drugs are commonly used but patterns of use vary throughout society. Smoking is more prevalent among lower socio-economic groups and problem drug use closely correlates with socio-economic deprivation.[115,116] While alcohol consumption does not show the same inverse relationship with social class, problem alcohol use is often especially damaging among more disadvantaged women.[117] Socio-economic deprivation is associated with poorer health and less effective use of services, especially those providing screening and preventive health care, and both are exacerbated by problem substance use. Reproductive health care services must therefore address not only problem substance use but also the social factors that predispose to and are a consequence of such use.

Smoking

Tobacco smoking is the largest single preventable cause of death and disease in developed countries today.[118] Nearly one-fifth of deaths in the population are due to drugs and of these, 80 per cent are due to tobacco.[119] Smoking has declined in women in the UK from 41 per cent in 1974 to 26 per cent in 1998; for men this was 51 per cent to 28 per cent respectively.[120] This decline is in all age groups except for young women. Explanations for a smaller decline in smoking rate for women than for men are complex and include:

- Smoking as a demonstration of female emancipation
- Early health messages targeting men (initial high prevalence of male smokers allowed observation of health effects)
- Using smoking as a means of controlling body weight. Nicotine affects body metabolism and food intake; smokers weigh on average 3 kg less than non-smokers.
- Advertising by targeting of women (particularly young women) by cigarette manufacturers. The majority of women who smoke regularly began smoking before 18 years of age.

Women appear to be at risk for the same health problems from smoking as men. Cigarette smoking is responsible for over half the cancer deaths in women, with lung cancer and breast cancer the leading causes of cancer deaths.[121] Breast cancer death rates are steady or slowly declining as the diagnosis is being made at earlier stages that are amenable to treatment. Lung cancer deaths, on the other hand, are likely to rise, because more young women continue to smoke and the disease is not amenable to early diagnosis or treatment. Between 1950 and 1985 there was a 500 per cent increase in lung cancer deaths in women, with smoking the primary risk factor.[122] In the UK deaths due to smoking peaked in 1990 at 2.24 per thousand but have decreased since, with 1.88 deaths from lung cancer in women reported in 1999 (compared to a level of 1.08 deaths per 1000 in men).[120]

Women also have some gender-specific risks to themselves and their children, born and unborn, from smoking. These include:

- Increased Pap smear abnormalities and cancer of the cervix than non-smokers[123]
- Thromboembolic disease (associated with pregnancy and the oral contraceptive pill)
- Earlier menopause
- Increased incidence of osteoporosis
- Earlier appearance of ageing: skin shows discoloration and deep lining
- Reduced fertility (in both women and men).[124]

Once pregnant, the smoking woman encounters more problems (Box 2.1) and the baby has an increased risk of perinatal death.[125] Nicotine, carbon monoxide and cyanide in tobacco smoke cross the placenta readily and are thought to have the greatest adverse effect on the fetus. Nicotine is also found in breast milk.

BOX 2.1 **Smoking effects on pregnancy**[126]

The effects of smoking in pregnancy include an increased risk of:

- Spontaneous abortion
- Ectopic pregnancy
- Vaginal bleeding: abruptio placentae and placenta praevia
- Preterm delivery
- Small for gestational age
- Increased perinatal mortality
- Sudden infant death syndrome (SIDS)
- Childhood respiratory illness and asthma.

According to the 1990 report of the US Surgeon-General, 'smoking is probably the most important modifiable cause of poor pregnancy outcome among women…'. There is a link between the likelihood of a child becoming a smoker and the smoking status of the parents, so the problems are perpetuated.

The effects of smoking are dose-related, so for women unable to stop completely, any reduction could be beneficial. Smoking cessation can improve perinatal outcome,[126] and therefore identifying smoking and alerting the woman to the facts about smoking is an important step for all health professionals in contact with women. It is necessary to assess tobacco use by the woman's past and current use and level of addiction (Table 2.1).

Nicotine is highly addictive and regular smokers are dependent on smoking. Nicotine activates the brain-reward system by increasing dopamine release—the pathway for all pleasurable activities and addictions.[127,128] After rising to a peak, the plasma nicotine levels fall and give rise to withdrawal that is relieved by the next cigarette.[129] Nicotine replacement therapy assists quitting smoking by maintaining the plasma nicotine levels above the withdrawal threshold; the number needed to treat to achieve one person quitting is ten.[130] Quitting smoking is difficult and women find it harder to quit than men do. A number of reasons have been postulated for the gender difference in quitting rates,[131] including firstly, the targeting of women by advertising to allay health fears, and secondly, the disproportionate number of female smokers who have low incomes, low-status jobs or are unemployed, are single parents or divorced, and have low levels of academic achievement. It is suggested that these women smoke because of their belief that cigarettes help them to cope with stress and boredom, and to regulate their weight. Women who manage to quit smoking can expect to increase their weight by an average of 2 kg.[132] Advising women about

TABLE 2.1 Questions on nicotine dependence[133]

Question	Answer	Score
How soon after you wake do you smoke your first cigarette?	Within 5 minutes	3
	5–30 minutes	2
	31–60 minutes	1
	> 60 minutes	0
Do you find it difficult to refrain from smoking in places where it is forbidden?	Yes	1
	No	0
Which cigarette would you hate most to give up?	The first in the morning	1
	Any other	0
How many cigarettes a day do you smoke?	1–10	0
	11–20	1
	21–30	2
	> 30	3
Do you smoke more frequently during the first hours after waking than during the rest of the day?	Yes	1
	No	0
Do you smoke if you are so ill that you are in bed most of the day?	Yes	1
	No	0

SCORE	RATING	SCORE	RATING
0 to 2	Very low dependence	6 to 7	High dependence
3 to 4	Low dependence	8 to 10	Very high dependence
5	Medium dependence		

the health benefits of smoking cessation is essential.[134] The principles to follow are the five 'A's.[135]

- Ask about smoking.
- Advise quitting.
- Assess current willingness to quit.
- Assist in the quit attempt.
- Arrange timely follow-up.

Women who smoked in the past should be congratulated for quitting and reminded that relapse is possible after many years of abstinence.

Alcohol

The prevalence of alcohol consumption among women varies with age, country and socio-economic status. In England and Wales in 1994, 13 per cent of women exceeded 'sensible limits' of alcohol consumption, the highest proportion of heavy drinking occurring in the 35–44 year age group.[136] Most women who experience alcohol-related accidents, health problems or family difficulties do not meet the criteria for alcoholism: they just drink too much, often in high-risk situations. The definition of 'at-risk alcohol use' is based on the relationship of a given quantity of alcohol used to a number of health effects.[137] Many factors correlate with problem drinking in women. These include:

- Physical or sexual abuse in childhood
- Involvement with a partner who drinks heavily
- Social isolation and dependence on other substances
- Depression or anxiety
- Bulimic women
- Women experiencing chronic sexual difficulties.

Young women experience drinking-related problems at high rates. They are especially prone to episodes of heavy drinking (binge drinking), putting them at increased risk of engaging in drunk driving and becoming victims of violence, including sexual assault.

Non-dependent drinkers can be influenced in their consumptive habits by general practitioners.[138] A number of screening questions for identifying those with alcohol problems have been tested and validated in clinical settings and evaluated for use with women.[139] The AUDIT questionnaire has been accepted as an appropriate screening tool in general practice to identify people with alcohol-related problems.

A brief intervention can be incorporated into routine practice. This would involve the following:

- Identify hazardous or harmful alcohol intake.
- Assess the woman's readiness to change.
- If she is contemplating or has decided to change, discuss the health-related and other benefits.
- Discuss possible strategies to reduce her consumption, taking social and lifestyle factors into account. This may require a team approach with a variety of expertise including counselling, support groups or pharmacotherapy.
- Negotiate and set achievable goals.
- Decide on frequency and nature of follow-up.

There are some gender differences in the health consequences of problem alcohol use.[140] Women who are alcoholics die at higher rates than male alcoholics with the same drinking habits. They are more likely to develop alcoholic hepatitis or cirrhosis of the liver, and their liver disease seems to progress especially rapidly. Women are also more susceptible to alcohol-related cardiomyopathy.

Alcohol and pregnancy

Although the effects of in utero alcohol exposure had been suspected for years, fetal alcohol syndrome (FAS) was first described in 1968 in France[141] and 1973 in the USA.[142] The diagnosis of FAS varies as there are racial variations in susceptibility. One generally accepted definition of FAS is a child who, in conjunction with maternal alcohol exposure, has three of the four components of the syndrome: growth restriction, facial abnormalities, CNS impairment, and other physical effects. Fetal alcohol effect (FAE) is considered if two of the four findings are present (Box 2.2).

BOX 2.2 Fetal alcohol syndrome

- Growth restriction:
  - Prenatal onset
  - Postnatal onset
- Facial dysmorphia:
  - Short palpebral fissures
  - Low-set ears
  - Mid-face hypoplasia
  - Smooth philtrum
  - Thin upper lip
- Central nervous system impairments:
  - Microcephaly
  - Mental retardation
  - Attention deficit disorders
- Physical effects:
  - Minor skeletal anomalies of the spine and hands
  - Nail hypoplasia
  - Ophthalmologic effects
  - Increased frequency of cardiac malformations

The embryo or fetus is susceptible to alcohol's toxicity throughout its development, but structural anomalies arise primarily when exposure occurs during 'critical periods' of development. The second to eighth week of gestation is a time when bodily organs and appendages are forming and observable malformations are due to exposure at this time. Exposure of the fetus to high levels of alcohol before and after this period has other effects. Female fetuses are more resistant to exposure to alcohol than males, although the mechanism of resistance is not known.[143] The effects of alcohol are not uniform and the reason that some fetuses are affected and not others from the same alcohol exposure is not understood. The extent of alcohol consumption that increases a woman's risk for FAS has been difficult to establish. Among women identified as having chronic alcoholism, the risk of FAS varies from 6 per cent to 50 per cent. In addition, daily drinking is not essential for the effects of in utero alcohol exposure.

In pregnancy many women decrease their alcohol, tobacco and coffee intake in the first trimester. These behavioural changes are often associated with nausea and loss of taste at this stage of pregnancy.[144] However, women who are the heaviest drinkers before pregnancy are less likely to modify their behaviour.[145]

There is no 'safe' time to drink in pregnancy. Similarly, there may not be a 'safe' level but this has not yet been determined. A threshold exists for all teratogens, below which they do not produce adverse effects. It appears that 'binge drinking' (more than five drinks at one sitting) with episodes of high blood alcohol are particularly damaging.[146] While it might seem reasonable to advise women to abstain from alcohol during pregnancy, increased risk to the fetus from social drinking has not been proved, so abstinence should not be presented as the only acceptable option. Aggressively counselling total abstinence may cause undue anxiety to those women who may have engaged in 'social' drinking prior to learning of the pregnancy. It is worth remembering that more than half of young women drink socially, with many young women involved in binge drinking, and more than half of pregnancies are unplanned. Discussing the issues pre pregnancy could be useful.

Other drugs in pregnancy

It is often difficult to determine whether or not illicit drugs are being used. The socio-economic status is not reliable in predicting this—particularly for expensive drugs. Studies have shown that recreational drug use is common and can often be undertaken while leading a normal lifestyle, including full-time employment. It can be incorporated into daily activities and may not be regarded by the user as anything other than normal. Specific enquiry into drug use therefore needs to be undertaken. Intravenous drug use increases the risk of becoming infected with blood-borne viruses including HIV, HCV and HBV.

Marijuana is a drug prepared from the plant *Cannabis sativa*. It contains more than 400 chemicals including tetrahydrocannabinol (THC), its psychoactive component, which is rapidly absorbed from the lungs into the bloodstream and is metabolised primarily by the liver. Prolonged fetal exposure can occur if the mother is a regular user because THC crosses the placenta, and detectable levels can be found in various tissues up to 30 days after a single use. Marijuana is not established as a human teratogen, although recent studies suggest it might have subtle negative effects on neurobehavioural outcomes but the information is not consistent.[147] There is increasing evidence that cannabis use may be associated with the development of schizophrenia and depression in a dose-response relationship in young people.[148] This could produce further problems for young women who are already at increased risk of depression.

Cannabis may be most frequently used but opiates/opioids cause more maternal and fetal mortality and morbidity as well as social morbidity and loss of child custody. They also cost the health and social services much more than cannabis use does. Heroin can cause amenorrhoea with or without anovulation, and can consequently reduce fertility but not necessarily cause absolute infertility. Methadone does not have this effect so it is important to remember that when women are stabilised on methadone their fertility will increase. Methadone is also socially stabilising and general health is improved by increased contact with services. Stabilisation on methadone prior to pregnancy is therefore beneficial. In addition, while all opiates/opioids affect pregnancy and increase the risk of SIDS, methadone does not increase the risk of preterm delivery but does cause withdrawal symptoms in the neonate. Substitution methadone therapy is therefore especially beneficial for women of childbearing age but should be maintained at the lowest dose compatible with stability.

Evidence suggests that benzodiazepines increase the risk of major malformations including cleft lip-palate and are also extremely socially destabilising.[149] Any reduction in use before and during pregnancy is therefore helpful but there is no evidence of benefit from substitution therapy.

Amphetamines and other chemically related drugs (such as 'ecstasy') have adverse pregnancy outcomes and may be associated with an excess rate of fetal anomaly.[150] In addition, amphetamine use can cause acute health problems, although this is rare.

Cocaine exposure in pregnancy is associated with serious health hazards to the fetus.[151] These seem to be largely restricted to heavy, chaotic and/or injecting use and especially use of crack cocaine. Medical effects of cocaine/crack cocaine on women's reproductive health are probably less than reported and are secondary to the social effects, which are extremely significant.

The study of adverse effects of drugs during pregnancy on the fetus and newborn is fraught with difficulties; many women in the studies conducted were users of a number of drugs, and there were many other confounders such as inadequate nutrition and social factors.[152]

Planning of pregnancies

It is important that women with problem substance use receive help to deal with their use before they become pregnant and that their pregnancies are intended and at a time of their choosing. Appropriate, effective contraception is therefore essential but may be difficult to deliver if lifestyles are chaotic. Imaginative community-based services with easy access are essential. Entry into drug and alcohol treatment services can provide an ideal opportunity to provide family planning. The most appropriate methods include long-acting progestogens either by injection, implant or intrauterine device. However, none of the methods providing reliable contraception also provide reliable protection against sexually transmitted infections, so this issue must be addressed separately. Women with problem drug and/or alcohol use are at particular risk if they finance their habit by prostitution. This carries risk of sexually transmitted infections, unplanned pregnancy and violence, both from those who control their prostitution and/or partners, and from clients.

Social factors and service delivery

Housing, finance and relationship problems are common, and are either due to or exacerbated by substance use. In addition to making service delivery difficult, they can make women isolated and unsupported and increase the risk of loss of child custody.

Women with problem substance use need multidisciplinary care that deals with both medical and social problems. Such services should as far as possible be community based and accessible by any route including self-referral. Perhaps most importantly they should deliver non-judgemental care that, while not condoning their problems, does not condemn such women, recognising that their aspirations and motivation are no different from those of other women.

Weight and nutrition

Human requirements for nutrients vary with age, size and gender. Women's nutritional requirements can differ greatly from those of men, as the different phases of a woman's reproductive life—adolescence, menstruation, pregnancy, lactation and menopause—affect her nutritional needs. The importance of body image in modern society leads many women to follow 'fad' diets, often at the expense of nutritional well-being. An understanding of the specific nutritional needs associated with the various aspects of a woman's life cycle will greatly enhance her ability to maintain optimum health through an adequate and well-balanced diet.

Healthy weight

A 'healthy weight range' can be defined as the body weight, adjusted for height, which is associated with longest high-quality life expectancy. The body mass index (BMI) provides a useful indication of the range of healthy body weight (Table 2.2). The BMI is an indirect measure of body composition based on a height/weight ratio. However, the BMI is not a suitable index for anyone under 18, pregnant or nursing women, frail and sedentary elderly people, competitive athletes or body builders. It should be noted that the BMI associated with the lowest mortality increases with age, being 19–24 kg/m^2 in the 19–24 year age-group and rising gradually to 24–29 kg/m^2 in those above 65 years of age. The Australian Longitudinal Study on Women's Health found an optimal range for BMI of 19–24 kg/m^2 in women aged 45–49 years. Low and high BMI were associated with decreased vitality and poorer mental health.[153] Body mass index does not, however, take into account the proportion of muscle or fat; individuals with the same BMI can differ in body fat content.

TABLE 2.2 Classification of size

Classification	Body mass index (BMI) kg/m^2	Waist measurement (cm)
Underweight	< 85	
Normal range	18.5–24.9	
Overweight	≥ 25.0	72–79
• Pre-obese	25.0–29.9	80–87
• Obese class I	30.0–34.9	≥ 88
• Obese class II	35.0–39.9	
• Obese class III	≥ 40.0	

The total amount of fat and its distribution are an important risk to health. Fat in a central or upper body distribution is a particular indicator of health risk. A measurement that may be of greater clinical use in assessing abdominal fat and therefore health risk is the waist measurement. Waist circumference is simple to assess, correlates well with BMI, and can identify those at risk from either central obesity or increased weight.[154] In women a waist measurement ≥ 80 cm (90 cm in men) is a risk factor for cardiovascular disease, insulin resistance and diabetes mellitus.[155] Hip and waist circumferences measure different aspects of body composition and fat distribution: a narrow waist and large hips are the ideal that suggest a lower likelihood of cardiovascular disease.[156]

Energy

Energy requirements vary greatly from person to person, and are affected by factors such as:

- genetic predisposition
- build—greater muscle mass burns more kilojoules
- gender—women have greater energy requirements during the pre-menstrual phase and also during pregnancy and lactation
- age—reduced activity levels and loss of muscle tissue decrease energy requirements
- metabolism
- lifestyle.

Food provides the body with the necessary 'fuel' for energy, growth and repair. A kilojoule is a measurement used to describe the amount of energy a food contains and the amount burned up by a particular exercise. The amount of energy provided by a particular food depends on its carbohydrate, protein and fat content (Table 2.3). Excess body weight results from regularly consuming more food energy than the body needs. The excess energy is stored in the fat cells.

TABLE 2.3 Kilojoules per gram provided by various food components

Category	Kilojoules per gram
Fat	37
Alcohol	29
Carbohydrates	16
Protein	17
Dietary fibre	13*
Water	0

* If fermented by bacteria in the large intestine.

(Table compiled from information in 'Kilojoules and calories explained', http://www.betterhealth.vic.gov.au.)

The largest component of energy expenditure is the basal metabolic rate (BMR). Basal metabolic rate is the energy expenditure of a subject after a 12–14 hour fast (usually overnight) who is mentally and physically at rest in a thermoneutral environment. It is related to height, weight, age and sex. In general it increases with body size, decreases with age, and is higher in men than women. The energy cost of growth relative to total energy requirement can be as much as 30 per cent of energy intake in infants under 2 months, falling to below 10 per cent after 4 months, below 5 per cent in children 10–15 years, and less than 1 per cent at 17–18 years. The theoretical energy cost of pregnancy in women who do not alter their level of activity and who gain 10–12 kg in weight is about 850–1100 kJ/day (averaged over 40 weeks of pregnancy).

Recommended dietary intake

The recommended dietary intake (RDI) is used to measure the amount of essential nutrients necessary to meet the daily nutritional requirements of healthy people. Not all nutrients are needed every day, however, as many can be stored in the body. The RDI as a measure refers only to the nutrient intake recommended to maintain health under 'normal' circumstances and does not take into account factors such as chronic illness, prolonged periods of increased demand, medications or the effects of smoking and alcohol abuse. In women there are particular requirements at different times.

Folate

Folate is the commonly used group name for folic add (pteroyl glutamic acid, PGA) and all its derivatives with similar activity. Folate is involved in many one-carbon transfers in the body, including purine synthesis. In particular, it is essential for DNA synthesis, so without folate, living cells cannot divide. The need for folate is consequently greater whenever cell turnover is increased. Folate requirements:

- The amount of absorbed folate to treat or fully prevent folate deficiency disease in non-pregnant adults is 100 µg/day.
- In pregnancy or for treatment of folate-deficient megaloblastic anaemia, about 200 µg PGA is required.
- The average absorption of folate from food is 50 per cent.

Folate is found in fortified breakfast cereals and bread, liver, black-eyed beans, brussels spouts, peanuts, spinach, broccoli and chickpeas. It is not possible to obtain an excess of folate from food. There is nothing to be gained from taking supplements above a dosage of 0.5 mg/day except in certain conditions (such as malabsorption) for which medical supervision is required. Folate is particularly important for women. All women who could become pregnant should be advised to take folate; this should be continued in the early months of pregnancy and is associated with a decreased risk of having a baby with a neural tube defect (Section 6).

Vitamin D

Vitamin D is the precursor of a steroid hormone, 1,25-dihydroxycholecalciferol, which mediates the vitamin D function in whole-body calcium homeostasis. The levels of 25-hydroxyvitamin D3 indicate vitamin D status. Some foods contain vitamin D (mainly fish with a high fat content). The average daily intake for women is estimated at 2.0–2.2 µg/day and the recommended daily intake is a minimum of 5.0 µg/day.[157] In some countries foods such as margarine are fortified with vitamin D.

In children, deficiency of vitamin D causes the condition rickets and in adults, osteomalacia. Those who are housebound, such as the elderly in nursing homes, could benefit from an oral intake of 10 mg of vitamin D per day if they are not exposed to direct sunlight for 1–2 hours per week in summer. This is important for women in nursing homes who are at risk for osteoporosis. Other women at risk are those who are dark-skinned and veiled; a study of Muslim women in Australia found a severe vitamin D deficiency in 68 per cent.[158]

Calcium

There is some uncertainty about what constitutes the true nutritional 'requirement' for calcium. Part of the uncertainty resides in the definition of 'dietary calcium deficiency'. First, with the possible exception of osteoporosis, no clinical syndrome or biochemical test caused solely by low calcium intake provides a marker of a deficiency state which can then be used to define the dietary requirement. Second, the body can adapt to a low intake by absorbing a greater fraction of the calcium from the intestine when intake is low. This adaptation declines with advancing age and is dependent on 1,25-dihydroxyvitamin D synthesis. A dietary intake regarded as deficient in a person with impaired adaptive mechanisms may be adequate in another with normal intestinal adaptive mechanisms. Calcium balance exists when the calcium absorbed in the intestine is equal to that lost in the urine, faeces and skin.

The 'dietary calcium requirement' is defined as the amount of calcium in the diet that will maintain calcium balance and so prevent skeletal calcium being called upon to maintain ionised calcium.[159] There is a net obligatory (irretrievable) loss of calcium of about 100–150 mg daily. To compensate for this obligatory loss, the diet must contain at least five times this amount, 500–750 mg daily, because only about one-fifth of the dietary calcium consumed is absorbed. This is the dietary calcium 'requirement'. The 'recommended dietary intake' of calcium is set higher than the 'requirement' to ensure that 95 per cent of the population receives a diet containing sufficient calcium. The National Health and Medical Research Council of Australia (NHMRC) recommended dietary intake of dietary calcium is 800 mg daily for premenopausal women, 1000 mg for postmenopausal women and 1200 mg daily at ages 12–15 years.

The guidelines are important as large doses of calcium may result in temporary hypercalcaemia, hypercalciuria, increase the risk of renal stones and produce gastrointestinal side effects including constipation. There is an increase in calcium absorption and bone calcium deposition associated with early puberty. Bone calcium deposition reaches a maximum in females shortly before menarche when it is five times that of adulthood. However, 40 per cent of teenage girls have less than 70 per cent RDI of calcium. This is probably associated with the attempt to reduce fat intake in relation to maintaining a 'slimming' diet. During pregnancy, increased intestinal absorption of calcium by the mother provides much of the calcium supplied to the fetus.[160] Dairy products provide the best source of calcium; dairy protein and lactose improve calcium absorption, and caffeine interferes with calcium absorption.

Iron

Iron is present in the body in haemoglobin, myoglobin, cytochromes and various enzymes; it is also stored as ferritin haemosiderin in the liver and reticulo-endothelial system. Measured iron loss in adult males and post-menopausal women is 1 mg/day. Additional iron losses associated with menstruation vary, but a loss of 40 mg of iron per cycle (averaged at 1.35 mg/day) will cover 90 per cent of women. Phases of rapid growth such as early childhood and puberty create peaks of iron requirements; this is a consequence of rapid expansion of the blood volume as well as gain in body mass.

Both factors are also operative in pregnancy. During the second and third trimesters large increases in the blood volume of the mother and fetus accompany fetal growth and necessitate an extra 1000–1300 mg of absorbed iron, translating into 5–7 mg of absorbed iron daily. Dietary iron intake, therefore, is capable of meeting all physiological requirements except in pregnancy, where diet alone will not reliably meets the needs of all women, and small supplements of iron may be necessary to maintain iron status.

Many women are deficient in iron from:

- excessive menstrual loss
- breastfeeding
- pregnancy—particularly multiparous women
- inadequate diet
- weight loss/weight control programs
- vegetarian diet that is incorrectly followed
- athletic activity.

The main source of iron is meat. Phytates (fibre) and polyphenols (tea) limit iron absorption and vitamin C enhances the absorption of non-haem iron.

Other vitamins

There is little evidence for other supplements of vitamins for the healthy woman. It is important because of the risk of birth defects and toxicity that high doses of vitamin A are avoided in pregnancy (excess accumulation may cause birth defects) and large doses of fat-soluble vitamins at any time.[161]

Fats

Of all the diet myths the notion that all fat is bad is the most persevering. Fats are the most energy-dense of all the food categories and as such provide much of the 'fuel' for the body. Unsaturated fats contained in foods like nuts, avocados and fish are essential fats and provide important nutrients to the body and help build hormones and cells. Although low animal fat diets are promoted, few trials have been for long enough to assess whether or not this is useful in the long term. Diets high in fat do not appear to account for the obesity epidemic in many countries.[162]

Obesity

Prevalence

The Australian Diabetes Study of 1999–2000 found that of all adult Australians over 25 years of age, 60 per cent were overweight with a BMI of 25 or more. Of these, 20 per cent were obese with a BMI of 30 or more. Although women are more concerned about their weight than men, men are more likely to be overweight, with 67 per cent of men over 25 years and 53 per cent of women being overweight. However, women have a higher proportion of both extremes of the BMI distribution, and proportionally more women are obese. The particularly high prevalence of underweight among younger women (29 per cent at 20–24 years) is important in view of eating disorders in young women.[163]

Significantly, the proportion of overweight and obese Australians has increased over the past 20 years, with women weighing on average 4.8 kg more than their 1980 counterparts. In New Zealand the BMI has increased in the last two decades and there has been an increasing trend towards central obesity.[164] In England most adults are overweight and one in five are obese, with 30 000 deaths a year linked to obesity.[165] Similar patterns are found in the USA.[166]

The prevalence of obesity in children has also trebled in 20 years[167] and a reference standard for childhood obesity has been established internationally.[168] The relationship between obesity and socio-economic status varies across countries—in some countries obese children are in more affluent families, and in other countries the reverse is true.[169]

Aboriginal women

Aboriginal women are particularly vulnerable to obesity-related health problems. Available evidence indicates that prior to European colonisation, Aboriginal people in Australia were lean, physically fit and free of 'lifestyle diseases'. Aboriginal and Torres Strait Islander people (both men and women) develop android obesity when they gain weight and have very high prevalence rates of non-insulin-dependent diabetes, hypertension and coronary heart disease. These problems are seen in many Indigenous communities that undergo lifestyle changes under Western influence. There is strong rationale for the development of specific, culturally appropriate, community-based intervention programs aimed at lifestyle modification (diet, exercise) by the communities themselves, with advice from outside experts as required.

Causes of obesity

Excess fat deposition occurs when energy intake exceeds energy expenditure. This may be related to a number of factors.

Genetic

Studies on twins have highlighted the important role of genetic factors in determining the predisposition to obesity. The pattern of inheritance suggests that the effect is polygenic with at least two distinct subtypes: general obesity and abdominal obesity.[170] However, obesity is strongly influenced by environmental factors.

Environmental

The main contributing environmental factors are:

- *Lack of physical activity.* There is no doubt that this is one of the largest contributing factors to obesity. Using a car, a computer for recreation, watching television and the fact that remote control devices do not even require moving from a chair, contribute to inactivity. In a 15-year study in Finland, leisure time physical activity, vegetable and bread consumption were all inversely associated with obesity in women aged 25–64 years.[171]
- *Inappropriate diet.* There are now specially prepared foods available for babies and children of all ages. Promotion and marketing are geared

towards the young and the busy mother. Much of the food promoted is high in fat, sugar and salt and rarely includes vegetables or fruit. Overweight is a problem that now has its beginnings in childhood. Babies that are breastfed may have a lower prevalence of overweight in childhood.[172,173]

Metabolic/hormonal

Obesity can be:

- drug-induced, by glucocorticoids
- secondary to neuroendocrine disorders (Cushing's syndrome, polycystic ovary syndrome).

Leptin is the humoral protein product identified from studies with the genetically obese (ob/ob) mouse model. It is presumed that leptin is the signal molecule from body stores to the brain, responding with receptors in the hypothalamus that regulate appetite.[174] It was hoped that administration of leptin might become a method of medical management of obesity in humans, but not all subjects appear to respond.[175] In addition there are gender differences in the relationship between leptin and adiposity. It would appear that leptin also has a role in puberty, fertility, pregnancy and genetics.

Health risks

Obesity is a complex, chronic disease with significant health risks.

Physical risks

Obesity is a risk factor for hypertension, type 2 diabetes, coronary heart disease, respiratory problems and sleep apnoea.[176] In women with a BMI > 27 kg/m^2 there is a high risk of co-morbidities (hypertension, dyslipidaemia and type 2 diabetes). A BMI > 25 kg/m^2 in women on the oral contraceptive pill is associated with an increased risk of venous thromboembolism.[177] Some cancers have been linked to obesity. A correlation has been reported between relative body weight and cancer of the colon, rectum and prostate in men, and the breast and endometrium in women.[178] The relationship between breast and genital tract cancer and dietary fats is unconfirmed. Various theories have been advanced to explain the relationship between obesity and cancer, including:

- Excess energy may increase cell growth and multiplication.
- Increased oestrogen levels in obese women (from metabolism of androstenedione in adipose tissue) may stimulate the growth of tumours in the breast or uterus.

It has proved difficult to differentiate between the effects of calories, dietary fat and obesity.

Psychological risks

Added to the possible physiological problems and not to be underestimated are social and psychological problems including stigmatisation and depression.

Risks in pregnancy

The woman entering pregnancy with obesity is at an increasing risk for complications during pregnancy and childbirth with increasing weight. This includes gestational diabetes, proteinuric pre-eclampsia and postpartum haemorrhage.[179] Obese women have larger babies, which may lead to relative pelvic disproportion, difficulty with the delivery of the baby's shoulders and a greater chance of delivery by caesarean section. Post partum the obese woman is at greater risk for thromboembolic disease and wound infections.

Risks in surgery

Obesity is a risk factor for complications of surgery. Intubating and ventilating an obese woman may be a problem for the anaesthetist; access for abdominal operations is difficult for the surgeon, and postoperatively the obese woman has increased risk for chest infection, wound dehiscence and thromboembolic disease.

Insulin resistance

In insulin resistance, greater than normal amounts of insulin are required to perform the usual metabolic tasks. This is associated with a number of conditions:

- adiposity
- some diseases (see Polycystic ovarian disease, Section 14)
- pregnancy
- illness and operations
- infection
- stress.

Assessment

Assessment of patients for obesity should include BMI, waist circumference, associated risk factors and motivation to lose weight.

Management

While the health risks of obesity are well known, managing the condition is often problematic. The overall goal for managing obesity is weight loss, but for women in particular, the issue of weight management is often linked to negative body image and with failed past attempts at weight loss. Many women spend years on a rollercoaster ride of weight loss and gain. This can be related to pregnancy, changes in lifestyle and the onset of middle-age and menopause. Changing insulin resistance involves diet (low glucose, low fat, energy restriction), increased physical activity, anti-obesity drugs (metformin, orlistat, sibutramine, thiazolidinediones)[180] and gastric surgery as a last resort.

The initial aim should be to encourage the loss of 10 per cent of weight over up to six months through promotion of healthy eating and physical activity. Once this has been maintained, a further effort to reduce another 10 per cent should be made, and so on. The health professional needs to negotiate an agreed plan acceptable to the woman.[181]

Dietary therapy

There is a great deal of data based on self-reported food intake indicating that overweight people do not eat more, and frequently eat less, than people of normal weight. However, others suggest that overweight people consistently under-report their usual food intake, or unconsciously reduce their actual food intake over the measurement period. This correlates with the finding that energy expenditure in overweight people is related to their lean body mass and is therefore usually higher than that of lean subjects with a lower lean body mass. Dieting to reduce body weight forms the basis of a major industry in developed societies. The strength of this industry is based on the unfortunate reality that most dieters eventually regain the weight that they lose and that many women undergo frequent cycles of weight loss and gain. There are no long-term randomised controlled trials to support a particular program for weight loss. Low-fat and low-carbohydrate diets are equally effective for losing weight when combined with exercise for 6 to 18 months.[182]

Altering physical activity patterns

The most important factor in losing weight and reducing body fat is physical activity. Physical activity can initially be at a slow pace to prevent injury to joints. Quite apart from disease prevention or amelioration, exercise has many other bonuses. Redistribution of weight (not necessarily weight loss initially) results in decreased fat and increased muscle, improving body shape and tone. Production of endorphins during exercise is mood-elevating. Improved body image and self-esteem will follow. Realistic goals should be set for women and the influence of factors such as work and family on their time and their own body image should be taken into consideration. Many women resist exercise because of worry about their appearance and the need to wear shorts, swimsuits or leotards. Most importantly there is a need to find any activity that the woman can enjoy. Any increase in physical activity (as opposed to exercise) will have benefits on health. Seemingly small changes, such as using stairs instead of the lift or parking the car a little further away from a venue, have been shown to be beneficial. Encouraging women to make their own health a priority can be supportive. The elderly can participate in programs of low-intensity exercise such as brisk walking or swimming, with benefits not only in relation to controlling body weight and related disorders, but also in reducing the severity of conditions such as arthritis.

Behaviour therapy

This should be included as part of a weight loss program. It includes counselling not only on eating behaviour, but also exercise, nutrition, relationships and self-esteem.[183] Support from family and friends or health professionals can provide encouragement to start and maintain a weight loss program.

Pharmacotherapy

A number of products are under research or are in current use to assist the obese to lose weight. These include sibutramine, which promotes a feeling of being full, as does PYY3-36, a hormone that has been shown to reduce the appetite by one-third.[184] Orlistat acts locally on the gastrointestinal tract to inhibit lipase and thereby inhibits fat absorption by 30 per cent.[185] Treatment results in obese people losing on average 3–4 per cent more of their initial body weight than through diet alone in a two-year period.[186]

Surgery

A National Institutes of Health Consensus Panel reviewed the indications and types of operations, concluding that banded gastroplasty and gastric bypass were acceptable operations for treating seriously obese patients.[187] A surgical option is not without significant morbidity and occasional mortality.

Conclusion

Obesity has become epidemic in the Western world and a major public health problem requiring urgent attention.[188–190] A combination of programs may be the most effective treatment.[191] However, more research is needed on the effectiveness of interventions for preventing obesity, particularly in children.[192] In addition, treatments need to be assessed for long-term effectiveness and possible harms.[193,194]

Physical activity

Physical activity is an essential requirement for good health in all human beings and all body systems thrive on regular participation in appropriate physical activities. The active, hunter-gatherer way of life to which we have evolved gave way to the development of agriculture about 10 000 years ago. Subsequently, the development of cities, organised societies, the Industrial Revolution and the communications/computer revolution have each contributed to the increasingly sedentary way of life that now exists in Western industrialised nations. We have, essentially, successfully engineered physical activity out of daily life to an extent that is having profound effects on health, function and well-being. Daily energy flux is now so low that many people cannot remain in energy balance (maintain normal weight) and maintain optimal nutrition. For women, there are compelling reasons to be active, possibly even more so than for men. The social influences, benefits, risks and barriers to leading an active lifestyle are considered below.

Social influences on women's physical activity

Body image

Physical activity and women's health have to be considered within wider social discourses of the body and self-identity. In the developed countries, a woman's sense of satisfaction with her body has a central bearing on her cognitions, feelings and behaviours.

Gender

In the world of sport, individual gendered identities are expected to conform to social norms that are essentially male. In other words, for girls and women to be 'equals in sport' they have to become more like boys and men. Liberal approaches aim to provide female participants with access to the same activities as boys and men, while the system remains for the most part unchanged. For example, liberal approaches do not address the emphasis on hierarchy, competitiveness and aggression that exist in sport.[195]

Social class

Social class has a relationship with physical activity and health that influences the type and nature of sporting activities practised by both men and women. Socio-economic status and education also significantly influence who exercises and what sorts of exercise they engage in.[196] Non-white race, lower educational levels and older age are most often associated with lower levels of activity.[197,198]

Age

Physical activity in children is reduced with increasing age and is influenced by the physical activity of the parents. The falling level of physical activity in recent times is related to the epidemic of obesity in children.[199] Physical activity offers an opportunity to reshape one's body and replace unwanted fat with more desirable muscle. For individuals of both genders who are approaching middle age, physical activity may signify an attempt to secure youth and attractiveness within a culture which views an ageing or overweight body as physically unattractive. When these cultural meanings are examined, the desire for good health becomes a minor component of people's reasons for engaging in physical activity—however, any reason that increases physical activity should be encouraged.

Barriers to women's physical activity

Physical problems

Physical problems include:

- *Injury*—musculoskeletal injuries may have a negative impact on continued participation in sport: a third of participants reported stopping the exercise program permanently after injury.[200] The fear of falling is also associated with reduced physical activity in elderly women (70–85 years).[201]
- *Urinary incontinence*—this is reported in women of all ages and prevalence increases with age. The Australian Longitudinal Study on Women's Health reported urinary incontinence in 13 per cent of young women (18–23 years) and over a third of women aged over 45 years. More than a third of mid-aged and a quarter of older-aged women reported avoiding physical activity because of leaking urine.[202]

Time

Many women are involved in full-time employment in addition to other roles—partner, housekeeper, mother and carer. Physical activity may be seen as a personal indulgence and availability of time may restrict these activities.[203] Improving women's knowledge about the benefits of increased physical activity to their everyday life might assist them in prioritising these activities.

Environment

Access and the aesthetics and convenience of facilities influence physical activity.[204] Australian adults were less likely to walk for exercise and recreation if the facilities did not provide these.[205] In addition, safety issues are important for women and they are less likely to walk without company or a pet to walk.[206]

Biological reasons to be active

In both men and women, regular physical activity reduces the risk of coronary heart disease, stroke, diabetes, obesity, osteoporosis and depression. Low to moderate levels of physical activity also improve mental well-being, tiredness, low back pain and constipation.[207]

Coronary heart disease

Possibly the most important reason for any adult to be active is that risk of coronary heart disease (CHD) is halved.[208] It is now accepted that the risks from lack of physical fitness in relation to CHD are no less than the risks of obesity, hypertension, high cholesterol levels and smoking cigarettes—the other main risk factors for CHD.[209] Physical activity also directly affects some of these other risk factors (eg reduces blood pressure,[210] improves blood lipid profile[211]).

Insulin resistance and diabetes mellitus

Insulin resistance is related to many problems for women. Both resistive and aerobic forms of exercise have been shown to modify insulin resistance.[212] Regular walking is associated with higher insulin sensitivity, even after controlling for fatness. Physical inactivity is a major risk factor for the development of type 2 diabetes, with observed relationships between physical inactivity and both impaired glucose tolerance and the development of type 2 diabetes.

Cancer

Physical activity protects against both lung cancer and bowel cancer.[213,214] There is some evidence that physical activity during puberty protects against later development of breast cancer, but it is more likely that activity in adulthood and particularly throughout the lifetime are most protective, although the evidence is not consistent.[215] The frequency of activity seems to be a more important protective factor than the intensity of activity.[216]

Osteoporosis

Physical activity can prevent problems with osteoporosis, which afflicts one in three women and one in twelve men. Vigorous physical activity can increase bone mineral density (BMD) in adolescents, maintain it in young adults, and slow its decline in old age. However, it is doubtful whether physical activity can reverse advanced bone loss.

The effect is local, being greatest in the bones most heavily loaded. Bone mineral density is not increased at all by low-impact exercises such as swimming. The ideal is muscle resistance exercise, which is known to increase bone mass in both men and women.[217]

Rapid BMD gains can occur in childhood and adolescence and may be the most profitable focus for prevention through physical activity, as higher BMD levels are seen in active children.[218] Most bone is accumulated in the two years surrounding peak height velocity and 95 per cent of peak bone mass is in place by age twenty.

Regular physical activity also helps to maintain balance mechanisms and develop muscle power, which may prevent falling. A reduction of 14 per cent in the annual fall rate was found in people aged 70 years and over with an intervention of exercise, home hazard management and vision improvement; the interventions without the exercise component showed no significant effect.[219]

Mental health

Physical activity can reduce clinical depression, generalised anxiety disorder, phobias, panic attacks and stress disorders, and can improve subjective well-being, mood and emotions.[220] Physical activity can make people simply feel better about themselves, possibly through the production of endogenous diamorphine. This is seen in positive changes in body image or physical self-worth.

Conclusion

The benefits of physical activity cannot be stored and only operate during physically active periods of life. Relapsing to a sedentary lifestyle means that health risks return. Conversely, individuals who take up a more active way of life at any stage of the life course gain protection irrespective of the extent of their previous sedentary habits. Therefore, it is never too late to take up an active lifestyle.

Body image

The way women feel about their bodies has become the focus of psychological, sociological and medical research over the past decade and a number of medical conditions including anorexia nervosa and bulimia have been linked to negative body image. While particular attention has been paid to such illnesses among young women, negative body image is not confined to any particular age group but is prevalent in women from all socio-economic groups and across the lifespan.

Background

Body image is how an individual conceptualises her personal appearance including the size, shape and weight of her body. A woman's body image is not static over time and is dependent on cultural and social norms, individual attitudes, biological and psychological factors. Once established, body image dissatisfaction can continue through adult life. While on average women weigh more than they did 20 years ago, the perceived 'ideal' body is thinner.

The way that women, especially younger women, feel about their bodies is influenced by the images they see around them, in advertising and other media. The body has become a very public site and is projected as a mirror through which other facets of ourselves are displayed. Thus, for instance a taut and tanned body reflects an image of health, well-being and self-control, whilst an overweight body suggests poor health, poor eating habits and lack of self-control. For many women, these images and the messages they project have made it hard for them to comfortably inhabit their own body.

Recent research shows that the media has a stronger influence on the body image of adolescent girls than on adolescent boys.[221] Furthermore, other research has found that, having viewed advertising images of thin young women, some girls are more susceptible to body image disturbance than others who have viewed them.[222] What we don't yet know is why this is so.

Thus, the images of women that we are presented with are out of the reach of most Western women. This leads inevitably to women striving to achieve the impossible through unhealthy weight loss strategies and increasingly, it seems, surgical intervention. There is a body of evidence now available that shows that most women in Western cultures are dissatisfied with their bodies. Evidence from America, Britain and Australia indicates that when shown silhouettes of female figures (Figure 2.1), women rated their figures both as substantially larger than the ideal figure and what they thought would be most attractive to men.[223–228]

Negative body image can also result from changes to the body as a result of childbearing, weight gain, ageing or surgery as well as from other significant events

FIGURE 2.1 Body image silhouettes for women[227]

Mature women						
BMI:	20	24	28	30	33	38
Waist:	65 cm	76 cm	89 cm	80 cm	102 cm	101 cm
Waist/height ratio	0.71	0.79	0.88	0.73	0.90	0.93
Age	30	42	64	47	54	54

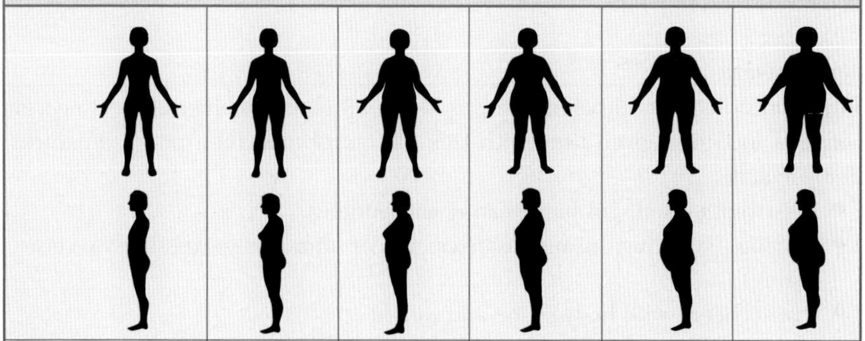

such as physical or psychological abuse or trauma. For health professionals, health issues arising from negative or distorted body image can be significant and complex, and can manifest in physical or psychological ways.

Eating disorders

Eating disorders can affect women and girls from a very young age. Research to date suggests that adolescent girls who have body dissatisfaction begin dieting and move into bulimia, and are unlikely to stop this behaviour unless there is timely intervention. A high proportion of adolescent girls diet at some stage in their teenage years and most do not become anorexic or bulimic. Those who do diet excessively have increased levels of depression and low self-esteem. This pattern may start in girls as young as eight years old and may be correlated with high parental concern about weight and diet, and it is important to consider parental attitudes and behaviour when dealing with dieting and body image issues in young girls and adolescents.

Anorexia nervosa

Features of anorexia nervosa include:

- Large weight loss, 25 per cent of original body weight
- Refusal to eat or strict dieting to maintain an unduly low weight (BMI < 17.5 kg)
- Intense fear of gaining weight
- Distorted body image—feeling fat even when quite emaciated
- Cessation of menstruation
- Thinness as the primary reference point for self-worth.

Those suffering from anorexia fail to see the long-term physical risks they face, including organ damage, destruction of tooth enamel, malnutrition and, possibly, death. It has been estimated that up to 10 per cent of those diagnosed with anorexia may die, and the disease is recognised as one of the few psychiatric disorders that has a significant mortality rate.

Bulimia nervosa

While anorexic women starve themselves, those with bulimia binge eat (eating a large amount of food in a given time with lack of control) and then purge. Features of bulimia include:

- Recurrent episodes of binge eating and purging
- Purging (vomiting, using laxatives and/or diuretics, excessive exercise, fasting)
- Over-concern with body shape and weight
- Frequent dieting.

Bulimic women see their behaviour as an ideal way to maintain a low weight whilst also being able to eat high-calorie foods. It has been estimated that bulimia occurs in 1–5 per cent of young women in their late teens and early twenties. The physical consequences of binge eating can include hypoglycaemia and neurological abnormalities. Purging is known to cause bleeding in the oesophagus, hiatus hernia, intestinal distress and inflammatory bowel disease, mineral deficiencies that result in kidney malfunction, loss of skin elasticity and low blood pressure.

Treating the primary problems associated with bulimia and anorexia often requires specialist medical and psychological intervention. The goals should be:

- Weight gain
- Correcting malnutrition
- Addressing any underlying psychological problems.

Eating disorders are serious psychiatric illnesses needing long-term, coordinated care with a multidisciplinary team involving general practitioners, psychiatrists, dieticians, paediatricians, physicians and psychologists.

Cosmetic surgery

Over the past few years cosmetic surgery has been used increasingly by women. In fact, it has become a growth industry in the developed countries. There has been very little academic research that looks at why women are accessing cosmetic surgery at an increasing rate. However, the work that has been carried out[229] has found that women who undergo a cosmetic procedure do so:

- For themselves and not for a partner
- To correct a feature that has bothered them for a long time (eg a big nose)
- To correct changes in the body due to pregnancy, weight loss or gain
- To address the consequences of ageing—when they looked in the mirror they didn't look as they felt. They wanted to look fresher and some wanted to compete more effectively in the labour market.

The public perception of cosmetic surgery is that it is quick and easy. In fact most cosmetic surgery operations are complex and require a high degree of surgical skill as well as aesthetic appreciation. There are significant risks associated with cosmetic procedures. These include the usual risks of any surgical procedure, the risk that the outcome is not what the woman wanted, the pain and discomfort associated with many procedures and the risk that something may go wrong with the procedure that leaves the patient feeling and looking worse that they did before. Women who undergo cosmetic surgery often receive little sympathy from the general medical community if things do go wrong. It is therefore important that women:

- Understand clearly the possible implications of their decision to undergo a procedure and are aware of *all* the possible risks
- Speak to a number of practitioners before undergoing a procedure
- Ensure that the practitioner they choose is able to spend adequate time with them in consultation
- Feel that they have a good relationship with the practitioner they have chosen.

Pregnancy

For many women pregnancy enhances body image by making them feel that their body is functioning as expected. With other women the physical changes of pregnancy destroy a positive body image that rested on maintaining a trim waistline, clear skin and small nipples. After childbirth some women may have trouble adjusting to their fuller or altered figure (broader hips, thicker waist, fuller breasts) or to stretch marks or to scars left by caesarean section. Others begin to dislike their body as they struggle to lose the excess pounds gained during pregnancy or discover that leaking milk and engorged breasts make them feel that they have no control over their body. Traumatic events associated with reproduction such as miscarriage, stillbirth or genetic defects can be devastating to a woman's body image.

Even when all events proceed as expected, the new maternal role does not 'come naturally'. The beautiful, clean, smiling baby in the magazines that she was led to expect is replaced by reality—crying, frequent nappy changing, wind and night feeds. A new mother may find that she has less control over these events than she imagined and she may feel inadequate in what is considered a woman's most basic biological role. Professional women who had previously been organised and capable may now find themselves with something 'beyond their control'. Associated problems with self-esteem and tiredness may lead to sexual dysfunction and other marital difficulties.

Ageing

Ageing is currently not particularly fashionable in Western societies and the esteem and respect that getting older once brought with it seems to have dissipated. For women ageing brings with it menopause and the end of reproduction. Many women pass through the menopause with ease whilst others suffer various unpleasant symptoms, including tiredness, weight gain, lack of sexual interest, hot flushes and so on. After menopause, collagen is lost, resulting in the thin, translucent skin of old age, brittle nails, hair loss and the development of osteoporosis. The musculoskeletal system changes with age: lean muscle mass decreases due to loss in size and number of myocytes; the subcutaneous fat diminishes, there are degenerative bone and tendon problems, and impaired balance and neuromuscular coordination.

It is therefore of little surprise that for many older women body image issues affect their quality of life. Encouraging activities and interests to maintain and improve both the body and the mind can assist women as they age and maintain physical and psychological fitness.

Conclusion

Body image is a pertinent issue for women across the life cycle. The factors that influence body image are complex and varied, but can have a very real effect on self-esteem and quality of life for many women.

Sexuality

Sexuality can be defined as sexual expression, in terms of both the individual concept of one's own sexual identity, and its expression with other people in social and intimate relationships. Sensuality and desire are part of this expression, and can exist whether or not a person is in a sexual relationship. Sexuality has physical, social and psychological manifestations and is closely related to the health and well-being of the whole person. Development of sexuality begins during early childhood and progresses through adolescence to old age, its expression changing through different life stages. It is influenced by physical effects such as sex hormones, socially via role modelling, ethical, spiritual and moral positions, and emotionally through one's sense of self-esteem and the experience of intimate relationships.

Sexual orientation, identity and behaviour

Sexuality is expressed in various ways. The self-definition of aspects of sexuality depends on three factors: sexual orientation, sexual identity and sexual behaviour.

Sexual orientation

Sexual orientation can be defined as attraction, or sexual feelings, thoughts and fantasies towards people of a particular gender. This does not necessarily correspond with sexual behaviour. Heterosexual orientation is a sexual attraction to people of the opposite gender, homosexual orientation is to people of the same gender (sometimes called same-sex attraction) and bisexual orientation is an attraction to both genders.

Sexual identity

Sexual identity is the self-recognition of the meanings that result from that person's sexual orientation and behaviour. This again may not correspond with orientation or behaviour. Our sexual identity develops over a period of time.

Many people developing a homosexual identity experience homophobia and marginalisation. Few people who identify as gay, lesbian or bisexual completely escape the effects of negative attitudes within society, which are reflected within health policy, the health care, welfare and school systems, and the workforce and media.[230] As a result, homosexual identity formation is a process of overcoming such negative stereotypes held among family and friends, and frequently held by the person themselves (internalised homophobia). Six phases of sexual identity formation in this developmental process have been described.[231] There is initial identity confusion; then comparing oneself to others; next tolerance followed by acceptance; then pride, often including public demonstration of one's identity. The final phase is synthesis, which is a reintegration of sexual identity into a more complete sense of self. This developmental process may begin at various, often transitional life stages, including adolescence, after family formation within a heterosexual relationship or after the death of a spouse. Not all people go through all of these phases, but the model provides a guide to the practitioner and patient when dealing with identity issues.

Sexual behaviour

This is defined by the sexual activities a person has and the gender of the person with whom they occur. This behaviour will vary according to social circumstances, peer pressure and personal attitudes. Some people maintain behaviour that is inconsistent with their sexual attractions throughout their life in order to maintain an intimate relationship or for other reasons of personal choice.

Asking about behaviour

The answer to the opening question 'Are you sexually active?' must be interpreted in light of the person's own definition of what sexual activity is for her. For example, some women define sexual activity as anything that creates sexual pleasure, including masturbation, sensual touch, oral–genital stimulation, and vaginal and anal penetration. For other women, vaginal penetration is the only activity they define as sexual whether or not they engage in other activities. Table 2.4 lists a range of sexual activities for women of any sexual orientation. Sexual behaviour is influenced by a wide range of physical, social and psychological factors (Table 2.5), any of which may

TABLE 2.4 Sexual terms and activities

Sexual term/activity	Meaning
Masturbation	Stimulation of one's own clitoris/vagina
Mutual masturbation	Stimulation of one's own and another person's clitoris/vagina/penis
Monogamy	Sexual relationship with one person at a time
Polygamy	Sexual relationship with more than one person in the same time period or at the same time
Sexual intercourse	Penis-vagina contact. Broad definition: any form of physical contact involving the genital area of at least one partner
Unprotected sex	Sex where transmission of body fluids can occur including vaginal fluid, semen, saliva, faeces, blood
Protected sex	Sexual contact involving the use of a barrier to prevent exchange of body fluids
Condom	Latex barrier placed on the penis
Dam	Rectangular piece of thin latex, applied as a barrier to the vulva and/or anus during oral sex
Vaginal sex	Penetration of the vagina with a penis, sex toy, fingers or hand (fisting)
Anal sex	Penetration of the anus with a penis, sex toy, fingers or hand
Fellatio	Licking or sucking of the penis
Cunnilingus	Licking or sucking of the clitoris/vulva
Anilingus	Licking or sucking around the anus
Sex aids/toys	Items for stimulation through vaginal or anal penetration
Orgasm	Climax of sexual excitement: 'an explosive discharge of neuromuscular tension'[232]
Ejaculation	Release of semen during orgasm
Frottage or tribadism	Rubbing genitals or genital region against any part of the other person's body for sexual pleasure

emerge during a discussion of sexual activity.[233] Health care providers should be prepared to broaden any discussion regarding sexual behaviour beyond physical issues to incorporate these broad influences and gain a more complete understanding of their patient's experience of her sexuality.

TABLE 2.5 Influences on sexual behaviour

Source of	Positive influences: enhancers of sexual behaviour	Negative influences: inhibitors of sexual behaviour
Family of origin	Open communication Sharing of information at appropriate developmental stages	Sexually repressive attitudes Child sexual abuse within the family or unrecognised by family
Self-concept	Completed identity formation Sense of choice Freedom of expression	Sexual identity confusion Low self-esteem Poor body image
Intimate relationship	Receiving affirmation Trust Connectedness with partner Mutual desire, consensuality	Lack of affirmation Unbalanced desire Sexual coercion Domestic violence (past, present or threatened; sexual, physical or emotional violence)
Fertility	Being in control of fertility: • effective contraception • attempting conception	Lack of access to reliable contraception Pressure to conceive
Health	Physical, psychological and emotional well-being	Illness: physical or psychological Recent surgery Sexual problem: primary or secondary to other influences Risk or perceived risk of sexual transmission of infection
Society	Relationship affirmation Public celebration of diversity Cultural encouragers of sexual activity	Homophobia, discrimination, misogyny Sexual violence including rape Moral, religious or cultural restrictions on sexual functioning

The impact of sexuality on health

The expression of sexuality may have a positive or negative impact on health. Self-determination and control are underlying components of healthy sexual expression. For example, an active choice to remain or become celibate can enhance a sense of control and well-being. Equally, comfort with sexual expression within an intimate relationship can enhance and strengthen that relationship.

Conversely, any negative influences can not only inhibit sexual behaviour and trigger or perpetuate sexual health problems but lead to a wider range of negative health consequences including mental health problems (depression, anxiety, social isolation) and risk-taking behaviour (unprotected sex, drug and alcohol misuse). Health-related risk factors are more prevalent among sexual minority groups. Studies comparing patterns of risk factors and subgroups of lesbian and gay people show that experiences of discrimination and marginalisation are key determinants of such risk factors.[234]

The most common sexual problems for women are lack of arousal, difficulty reaching orgasm, vaginismus and low libido (Section 12).[235]

The impact of health and illness on sexuality

Sexual behaviour and expression are often affected by acute or chronic illness (Table 2.6), but patients can be reluctant to discuss such issues with their health care provider. This reluctance in spite of the significant impact of sexual restrictions on health and well-being provides a rationale for including screening questions regarding sexual health for most patients. Of particular concern is the effect of chronic, life-long conditions on sexual expression. This may be due to a direct effect of the illness, such as a spinal cord lesion preventing genital arousal, or indirect effects such as altered body image, pain, restricted range of movement, depression or side effects of medication affecting sexual response.

For women, positive body image is an important determinant of self-esteem and positive expression of sexuality. For example, healthy sexuality for many women is connected with breast and uterine health. A woman's body image can be affected by pathological change (surgery to the breasts) or physiological change (changes in the breasts associated with pregnancy and breastfeeding). The latter may be a positive experience, but for some women it can inhibit sexual expression and/or desire. The cessation of menstruation at menopause again may enhance or inhibit sexual well-being. For some women, menstruation is an outward sign of femininity and many require a period of transition including positive affirmation from a sexual partner to regain a positive outlook on their sexuality after menopause.[236] The area of sexuality and ageing is neglected by health care providers. We tend to ignore the fact that many of our older patients remain sexually active, and so fail, for example, to warn them of the sexual side effects of medication, or even to enquire after their sexual health. This is further exacerbated when people enter supported aged care housing, where there is no provision of privacy for the expression of intimacy. Health care providers have a role in advocacy for the recognition of sexual and sensual expression amongst older people.

TABLE 2.6 Impact of health and illness on sexuality[237]

Underlying issue	Impact on sexual function of sexual behaviour	Management for improved sexual health (include sexual partner)
Arthritis	Pain, difficulty achieving certain sexual positions	Analgesia Advice regarding position
Asthma	Sexual activity may trigger asthma; subsequent fear restricts sexual arousal	Pre-treatment of asthma prior to sexual activity Improve asthma control
Cancer: • pain • surgery • chemotherapy • radiotherapy • loss of fertility	Altered body image Sexual partner afraid to cause harm Vaginal dryness and dyspareunia	Counselling for both parties Pre-treatment advice regarding conservation of fertility (ovarian section freezing, egg harvesting)
Depression: • primary effect • antidepressant medication	Loss of libido, reduced sexual arousal Reduced libido and anorgasmia	Optimise treatment of depression, exclude underlying sexual abuse Change antidepressant
Recurrent genital herpes (or other chronic STI)	Guilt, fear of infecting sexual partner Post-attack neuralgia	Counselling both regarding reduction of STI transmission Analgesia
Ischaemic heart disease	Pain with sexual activity, fear of pain or collapse	Adequate ischaemia prophylaxis prior to sex
Drug and alcohol misuse	Reduced libido, reduced orgasm	Drug and alcohol counselling
Neurological disease including MS, spinal cord defect	Reduced sexual arousal; demyelination can lead to anorgasmia	Adequate lubrication, non-genital arousal techniques
Renal disease	Loss of libido, anorgasmia	Optimise renal function
Chronic vaginitis: candida, bacterial vaginosis	Superficial dyspareunia Fear and vaginismus	Systemic treatment, address vaginal pH Focus on non-penetrative activities
Chronic vulval conditions: lichen sclerosis	Superficial dyspareunia, vaginismus, vaginal stenosis	Optimise treatment of condition, lubrication
Vaginal atrophy: postmenopausal	Superficial dyspareunia, vaginal stenosis	Topical oestrogen, HRT

SECTION

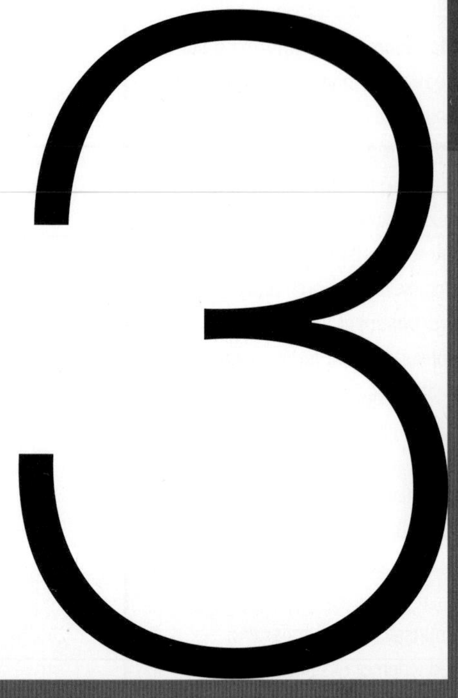

Behavioural and mental health issues

Abuse

Violence against women encompasses many forms of abuse and includes prevalent forms such as child abuse, domestic violence and rape as well as culturally specific forms such as female genital mutilation and sex-selective abortion.[1] This section concentrates on partner abuse (physical, emotional and sexual abuse by a partner or ex-partner) and adult survivors of child sexual abuse, as both forms of violence cause significant psychological and physical morbidity and mortality for many women around the world.[2]

From a health perspective, domestic violence is best understood as a chronic syndrome characterised not by the episodes of physical violence that punctuate the problem but by the emotional and psychological abuse that the perpetrator uses to maintain power.[3] Examples of abusive behaviour that women describe at the hands of their partners are:[4]

- *Physical abuse* ranging from slaps, punches and kicks to assaults with a weapon, violence to property or animals, and murder
- *Sexual abuse* including forced sex or forced participation in degrading sexual acts
- *Verbal abuse* designed to humiliate, degrade, intimidate or subjugate, including threat of violence
- *Economic abuse* including deprivation of basic necessities, seizure of income or assets, unreasonable denial of the means necessary for participation in social life
- *Social abuse* through isolation, control of all social activity, deprivation of liberty, denial of needed medical care or the deliberate creation of unreasonable dependence.

A recent review of more than 50 population-based surveys indicated that 10–50 per cent of women who had ever had partners have been hit or otherwise physically assaulted.[5] The only Australian population-based study found that 2.6 per cent of women in current relationships had experienced an incident of violence in the previous 12 months and 8.0 per cent at some stage in their relationship.[6] Most of this violence occurred only once (49.8%) or rarely (26.2%). However, 42.4 per cent of women reported violence by a previous partner and overall, 22.5 per cent of women who currently or had ever had a partner had experienced physical violence. Twelve-month prevalence in women attending clinical practice (Figure 3.1) is also high, ranging from 5.5 to 17 per cent experiencing violence by partners or ex-partners.

Child sexual abuse includes contact (sexual touching, attempted intercourse and penetration) and non-contact (solicitations, flashing, exposure to pornography) and the most common perpetrator is a father or another male family member.[1] Rates of childhood sexual abuse vary from 7 to 36 per cent across studies from 20 countries.[7]

How do domestic violence and adult survivors of child sexual abuse present in clinical practice?

Women present to a wide range of doctors with a variety of complaints without disclosing that there is a background of abuse (Table 3.1). Hence, women may present with overt physical injuries but more commonly with a large range of chronic symptoms to unsuspecting health care practitioners. Women with a past history of child sexual abuse are particularly prone to chronic pelvic pain, sexual problems and the psychological consequences listed in Table 3.1 and Section 12.

The identification of domestic violence is a challenge to all doctors in clinical practice and practitioners need to be aware of general clinical indicators.[2]

FIGURE 3.1 Prevalence rates of physical violence in women attending selected clinical settings

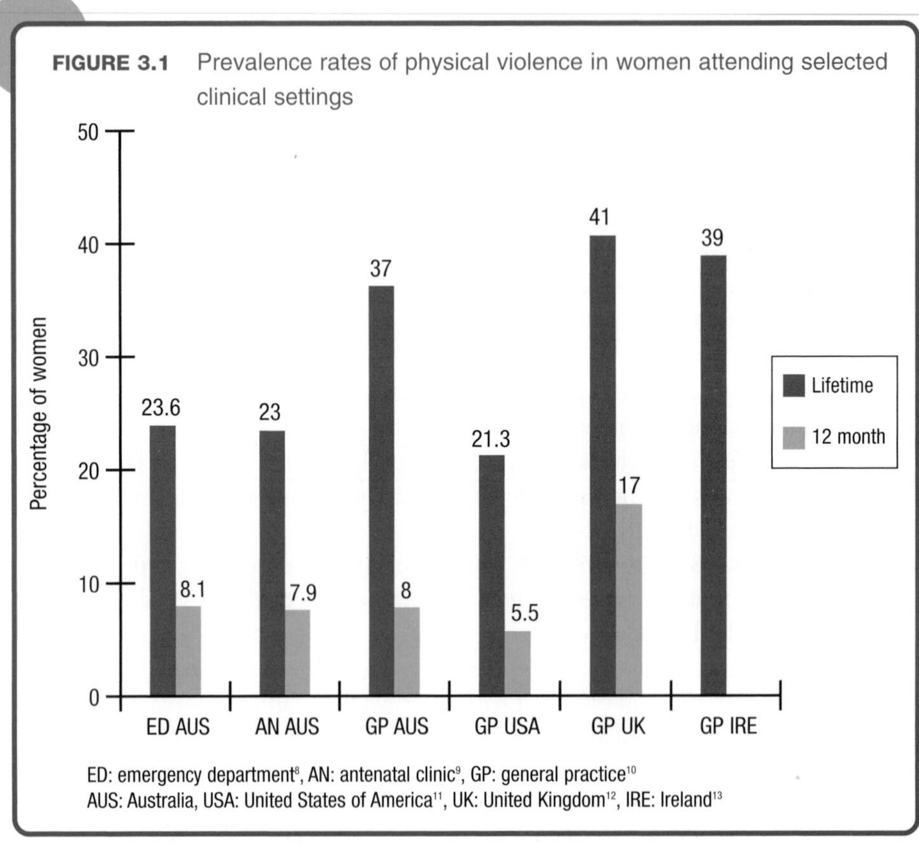

ED: emergency department[8], AN: antenatal clinic[9], GP: general practice[10]
AUS: Australia, USA: United States of America[11], UK: United Kingdom[12], IRE: Ireland[13]

TABLE 3.1 Potential presentations of women experiencing partner abuse[14]

Psychological	Physical
Insomnia	Obvious injuries, especially to the head and neck or multiple areas
Depression	Bruises in various stages of healing
Suicidal ideation	Sexual assault
Anxiety symptoms and panic disorder	Sexually transmitted diseases
Somatiform disorder	Chronic pelvic or abdominal pain
Post-traumatic stress disorder	Chronic headaches or back pain
Eating disorders	Lethargy
Drug and alcohol abuse	

General clinical indicators of partner abuse:

- Delay in seeking treatment or inconsistent explanation of injuries
- Multiple presentations and non-compliance with treatment and attendances
- Accompanying partner who is over-attentive
- Recent separation or divorce
- Past history of child abuse or abuse of a child in the family
- Age less than 40.

Talking to doctors

Women are more likely to disclose about abuse if their doctor has good communication skills, ensures confidentiality and is perceived as being able to help.[15] They are much more likely to tell doctors who ask directly about abuse.

Possible questions to ask if you suspect abuse:[10]

'Has your partner or someone close to you ever physically threatened or hurt you?'

'Is there a lot of tension in your relationship? How do you resolve arguments?'

'Sometimes partners react strongly in arguments and use physical force. Is this happening to you?'

'Are you afraid of your partner?'

'Have you ever experienced sexual abuse?'

'Violence and abuse are very common in the home. I ask a lot of my patients about abuse because no one should have to live in fear of their partner or family.'

Barriers to disclosure

There are, however, major barriers to women disclosing. Reasons given by women include:

- fear, denial, isolation, depression and stress
- emotional bonds to partner/family, commitment to marriage/parents
- hope for change and staying for the sake of the children
- 'normalisation' of violence (coming from a background of abuse)
- feeling that they will not be believed, or that doctors are not interested or able to help.

Despite this, doctors are the major professional group to whom women disclose and thus clinical settings are a potential location for assisting women.

Management

Women understand that there are limits on how the doctor can help them. By using simple skills, doctors can ensure that women feel supported and can act as an advocate for them. No interventions have been evaluated to any great extent but the recommendations below are a compilation of what women say they would like and what the literature says might work. Women want to be listened to and believed, and reassured that abuse is common and that help is available. They want whatever they say to be kept confidential, and they want to be supported and encouraged in whatever they choose to do. Doctors need to assess the woman's current state of change—staying, about to leave, ready to leave (Table 3.2)—and be able to discuss options if the woman is ready.

TABLE 3.2 Stages of change

Stage		Response by HCP
Pre-contemplative	Unaware that she has a problem	Suggest the possibility of a connection between symptoms and problems at home.
Contemplation	Has identified a problem but remains ambivalent about whether or not she wants and is able to make any changes	Encourage the possibilities for change should she decide to do anything and that you are available to help.
Decision	Some catalyst for change eg children have reached teenage years	Explore resources within the women's network and the local community. Respect her decision about what she wants to change.
Action	Plan devised in above stage is put into action	Discuss plan of: • talking to family and friends or counsellor, • leaving the relationship, • taking out a restraining order, or • reporting to the police.
Maintenance		Praise whatever she has managed to do and support her decision.
Relapse	May feel compelled to reverse above action because too stressful; no access to children	Need to support her if she does return to relationship or doesn't see counsellor or doesn't report.

Adapted from RACGP Women and Violence Project, *Women and Violence*, 2nd edn, 1998.

Why do women stay in abusive relationships?

Reasons include: fear of escalation of violence; lack of real alternatives for housing and employment; and low self-esteem, so she believes the violence is her fault. This may be reinforced by cultural or religious views and many women still have an emotional attachment to their partner. Women often stay for the sake of their children, so a strong message for change is about the detrimental effect of their children witnessing and hearing the abuse.

In addition to the above, doctors need to document injuries (history, frequency, severity, clear descriptions of any injuries and how they happened) and be able to assess the safety of women and children by asking the following questions:

- How safe does she feel?
- What does she need in order to feel safe?
- Have the frequency and severity of the violence increased?
- Is he obsessive about her?
- Has she been threatened with a weapon or is there one in the house?

What community resources are available?

At some point the woman may want referral for domestic violence counselling in the community or advice about contacting police, the courts or alternative housing such as women's refuges.

Resources:

- Police and community legal services
- Crisis service (24-hour, 7-day crisis line)—usually crisis counselling, referral, support and advocacy, contact point for women's refuges, referral to other short-term crisis accommodation and local domestic violence services
- Immigrant or migrant women's domestic violence service and telephone interpreter service
- Sexual assault services or rape crisis centre
- Domestic violence resource centre
- Private counsellors and psychologists
- Women's information services and women's community health centres
- General 24-hour counselling telephone lines.

Domestic violence and the law

Assault by a partner is a crime and should be reported to the police, resulting in criminal charges and restraining orders that restrict the partner's ability to have contact. A woman can apply for a restraining order if she has recently been assaulted, threatened or harassed and is fearful of it happening in the future. In some places other persons such as doctors and police can take out orders. It is helpful to provide information and a message that what is happening to her is not her fault, that it is in fact a crime.

An acronym has been developed by the Royal Australian College of General Practitioners Women and Violence project that will help practitioners when taking a history of abuse:

H E L P

H Hear what the woman has to say about her **HISTORY**

- what effect the violence and abuse has had
- onset and pattern of abuse
- worst case of abuse and greatest fear

E Assess the woman's self-**ESTEEM**

- sense of self-worth and control over her life
- has this changed since the abuse

L Assess her **LIFE** situation

- does she have a regular partner, any children
- any supportive people
- financial situation

P **PRAISE** her efforts so far for whatever she has done.

KEY POINT

- **Abuse is common in women attending clinical practice who are divorced, have a previous history of abuse, or present with psychological symptoms or chronic pain.**
- **Good communication skills elicit disclosure.**
- **Management involves believing, validating, supporting and advocating for the abused woman.**

Sexual assault

Sexual assault is a problem of global proportions. No age, gender, race, country or society is free of this problem. Sexual assault has been considered a crime by all societies and the penal codes of most countries criminalise rape and sexual assault.[16] It is mostly women and female children who suffer sexual violence at the hands of men and adolescent males. These simple facts are inescapable; however, they conceal the complexity involved in gaining an understanding of sexual assault. This section describes some of the key responsibilities for health professionals in this area.

Definition

Defining sexual assault is more difficult than it may seem. The term 'sexual violence' is being increasingly used as it draws domestic violence in with the events of sexual assault. Counselling/advocacy bodies include sexual harassment as sexual assault.[17] It is useful to refer to the local legislation for a working definition of sexual assault as these concepts have been tested and subject to repeated scrutiny and law reform, and have practical relevance.

The major sexual offences are rape, indecent assault, incest and sexual penetration of young people and children. In Australia, the *Crimes Act of Victoria 1958* s.38(2) states that:

> *A person commits rape if he or she intentionally sexually penetrates another person without that person's consent while being aware that the person is not consenting or might not be consenting.*

The offence is made up of three elements:

1 sexual penetration (the physical element)
2 lack of consent (the consent element)

3 the intention of the accused person in sexually penetrating without consent (the mental element).

'Sexual penetration' is defined as penile penetration of the vagina, anus or mouth; or penetration of the vagina or anus by any other part of the body or an object.

'Consent' means free agreement. Circumstances in which a person does not freely agree to an act include the following:

The person:

(a) submits because of force/harm or the fear of force/harm to that person or someone else
(b) submits because she or he is unlawfully detained; is asleep, unconscious, or so affected by alcohol or another drug as to be incapable of freely agreeing
(c) is incapable of understanding the sexual nature of the act
(d) is mistaken about the sexual nature of the act or the identity of the person, or mistakenly believes that the act is for medical or hygienic purposes.

Closer reading of the elements of the offence of sexual assault will reveal that gender-neutral language has been adopted, which reflects the reality that both men and women can be offenders and victims. Similarly the list of circumstances in which consent is deemed not to be present is designed to make it clear that rape can occur in a variety of circumstances and not only those where strangers, threat or violence are involved.[18] Rape, sexual assault, sexual abuse and sexual violence are terms that are often used interchangeably. Therefore, it is important for health care professionals to know the legal definition of sexual assault in their particular jurisdiction. The derivative of the term 'rape' is from the Latin word *rapere* which means 'to steal, seize or carry away'. In essence, rape means being sexually penetrated against your will.

Incidence

The pyramid diagram of measures of the incidence of sexual assault (Figure 3.2)[19] illustrates three key areas where data is collected. Official crime statistics are collected by the key criminal justice agencies, namely the police, the courts and the prisons. The most frequently used data is the number of cases becoming known to the police. This gives a rate of sexual assault per 100 000 persons. In 1999 Queensland recorded a rate of sexual assault per 100 000 persons of 100.2. To put this in context, the Department of Justice in the USA reported that the annual incidence of sexual assault was 80 per 100 000 women and accounted for seven per cent of all violent crimes.[20]

Victimisation surveys aim to provide accurate data on the prevalence of crime victimisation in the community for selected offences. The Australian Bureau of Statistics conducted the Women's Safety Survey in 1996. This survey made a significant contribution to our understanding of women's experience of violence and sexual assault, and represents the best source of data available so far on the topic in Australia (Box 3.1).[21]

Sexual assault is a common crime with far-reaching consequences for the victims, but it is vastly under-reported, so the true incidence is difficult to encompass.

FIGURE 3.2 A pyramid of measures of the incidence of sexual assault

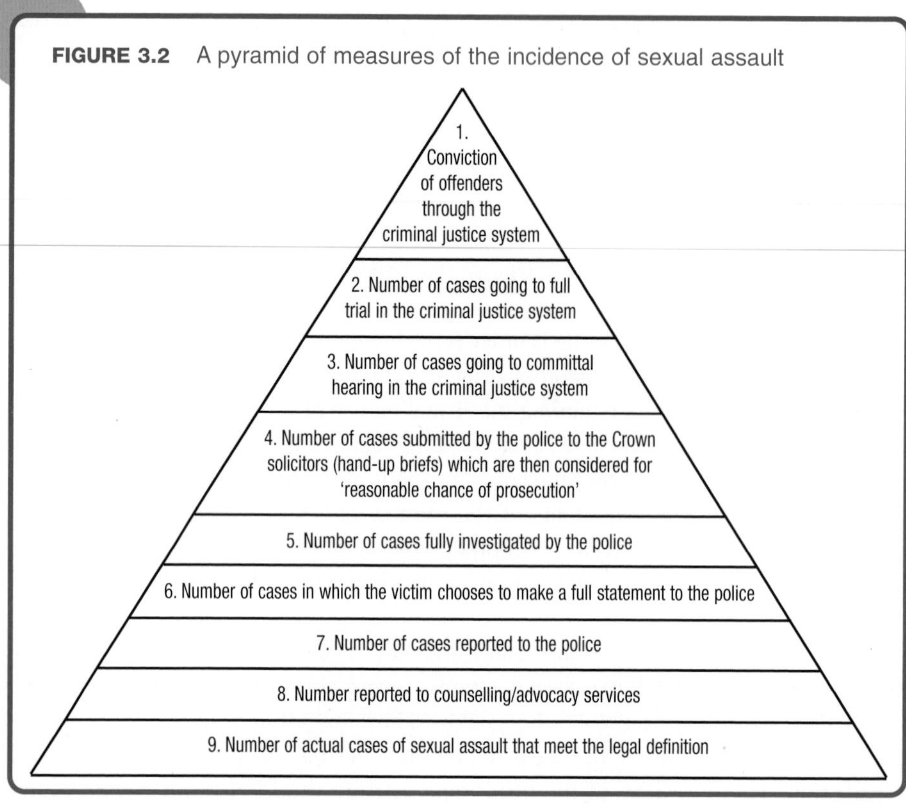

BOX 3.1 The Australian Bureau of Statistics 1996 Women's Safety Survey

- The Australian Bureau of Statistics 1996 Women's Safety Survey found:
  - An estimated 1.5% of women over 18 years of age were victims of sexual assault in the 12 months preceding the survey. This was an estimated 100 000 women in Australia in 1996.
  - An estimated 15.5% of women had experienced sexual assault since the age of 15 years.
  - For those women who were allegedly the victims of a sexual assault in the last 12 months, the overwhelming majority (85.1%) did not report the most recent incident to the police.
  - Of those who had experienced sexual assault by a male perpetrator since the age of 15, one-third indicated that the perpetrator was a known male, 22.8% involved a previous partner and 11% were assaulted by a stranger.

Experience of sexual assault

The far-reaching consequences of sexual assault include the effects on the victim, her children and family and the society and community in which she lives. Society's stereotype of rape is a physically violent assault committed by a stranger in a dark or dangerous place. Sexual assault is violent, but the violence is often psychological rather than physical.[22]

Rape trauma syndrome was described in 1974 by Burgess and Holstrom.[23] This variant of post-traumatic stress disorder describes an acute phase with:

- haunting intrusive recollections
- a numbing of feelings
- generalised hypersensitivity to environmental stimuli;

followed by a long-term reorganisation phase that may take years, and includes:

- periods of denial
- emergence of anger
- possible suicide attempts
- sexual dysfunction
- psychiatric problems
- chronic pelvic pain.

John Briere makes the point that any psychotherapeutic treatment of sexual assault victims must address any underlying issues resulting from child sexual abuse.[24] This highlights the fact that victims of childhood assault are more prone to sexual assault as adults. Vulnerable subgroups include: Indigenous women, adolescents, sex workers, the intellectually impaired and the psychiatrically impaired.

Sex offenders

A sex offender is 'a person who has been legally convicted as the result of an overt act, committed by him for his own immediate sexual gratification, which is contrary to the prevailing sexual mores of the society in which he lives and/or is legally punishable'.[25]

Sex offences have assumed an unprecedented profile in recent years, with high-ranked members of the church in particular facing accusations of historical sexual assault of children. A study of sex offenders in a treatment program offered confidentiality to the participants and asked them about their offending. The paedophiles reported having multiple victims and engaging in other types of sex offending such as voyeurism and exhibitionism. In this study, the 453 offenders admitted to molesting a stunning 67 112 victims.[26] Paedophiles target children who are vulnerable. They groom their victim by winning their affection and trust. Implied force and threats are more characteristic of their abuse patterns than violence and explicit coercion.[27] The sexually deviant can be found in all walks of life. The popular notion of seedy-looking men in trench coats lurking in playgrounds has little basis in reality. Sex offenders may be doctors, lawyers or politicians.

Many deviant sexual behaviours commence during or, in the case of fetishism, prior to adolescence. Adolescents account for a substantial portion of sexual offences, conservatively estimated to be around 20 per cent of all cases and 30–50 per cent of child molestation cases.[28] Sexual offending by juveniles can no longer be dismissed as adolescent sexual curiosity or experimentation. It is increasingly recognised in criminal justice and treatment circles that early intervention is essential in order to halt the young offender's offending career and prevent multiple further victims.

Adolescents are even less likely than adult perpetrators to seek treatment voluntarily, and they may be directed by the Court to participate in specialised adolescent sex offender group programs.[29]

Rapists are distinguished here from paedophiles by defining them as perpetrators of penetrative sexual assaults on adult victims. Attempts have been made to describe the cognitive distortions that distinguish them from non-rapists. Polaschek and Ward describe rape-supportive beliefs that support offending.[30] These include the following:

- Women are unknowable. Believing that women are inherently different facilitates harm towards women because it is easier to harm someone who is perceived as unlike oneself.
- Women exist in a state of continual sexual reception and are sex objects.
- Male sex drive is uncontrollable.
- Men should have their sexual needs met on demand.

Management

As Figure 3.3 indicates, when a patient presents to a health professional stating that they have been raped, the first and overwhelming priority is to determine their medical status and attend to any medical needs.

FIGURE 3.3 Pathway for the health professional in a case of reported sexual assault

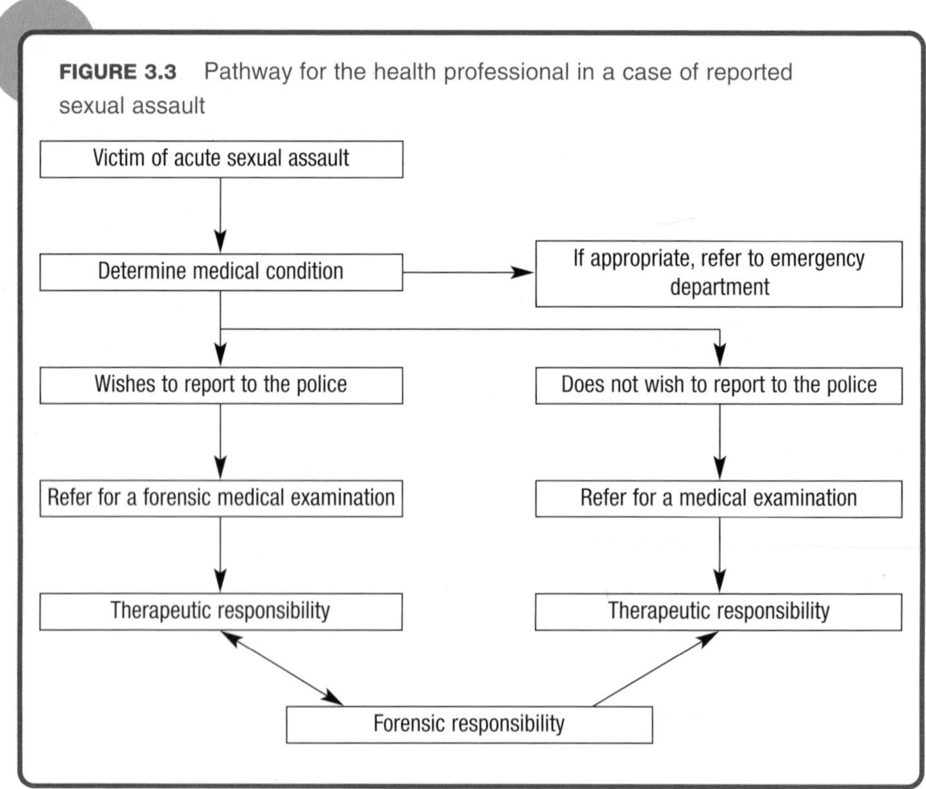

The doctor's responsibility is first and foremost to care for the well-being of the patient. The health professional should be alert to the following possibilities while maintaining clinical acumen for the full range of medical emergencies.[31]

1 Conditions that may preclude an immediate forensic assessment:
   - Head injury
   - Impaired conscious state
   - Untreated pain from injuries or fractures
   - Shock from concealed blood loss
2 Conditions that may affect the person's ability to provide informed consent:
   - Psychiatric conditions
   - Intellectual disability
   - Intoxication
3 Conditions that warrant special medical consideration:
   - Pre-existing pregnancy.

Informed consent

The next responsibility is to ask the patient what her main three concerns are as a result of the sexual assault. This means the patient's needs may be incorporated into any management plan and a locus of control can be returned to her. The process of explaining her options will provide the patient with an environment in which to provide informed consent. Time spent on informed consent is never wasted.

Supporting the patient

Remember, there is no typical victim. A chaperone, preferably a trained health worker, provides comfort and support for the patient. In addition, the chaperone also protects the health worker in the event that the patient alleges that the examining health worker behaved in an unprofessional manner.

The examination is performed in a setting with light, warmth, cleanliness and privacy for undressing (screen). If the clothing removed was that worn in the assault then the patient needs to undress over a sheet of paper so that trace evidence can be collected. Each item of clothing needs to be placed by the examiner's gloved hand into a paper bag.

Give the patient the opportunity to stop the examination if necessary. Use a calm tone of voice. Ask the patient's permission to touch her before you do so, and explain every stage of the examination. Give the patient a chance to ask any questions. Address patient questions and concerns in a non-judgemental, emphatic manner.

Genital injury after non-consensual penetration

> *'The rape victim often needs an unusual degree of professional reassurance, acceptance and understanding in regard to the therapeutic examination.'*[32]

Not all women who allege sexual assault will have genital injury on genito-anal examination performed without magnification. Indeed, in many cases none would be expected. If a mature, sexually active woman does not resist through fear of force or harm and penile penetration of her vagina occurs, then there may be no genital injuries evident on genito-anal examination. This finding does *not* disprove her claim. This issue is of fundamental importance in sexual assault medicine. Forceful penetration of the female genitalia and anus can cause injury (Figures 3.4 and 3.5). The penetration may be by the erect or semi-erect male penis, other parts of the body including the fingers and tongue, or by objects of various dimensions and characteristics.

The act of penetration causes the soft tissues around the orifice to stretch. The likelihood and extent of genital injuries thus depends on the:

- state of the tissues—size/lubrication/durability
- size and characteristics of the penetrating object
- amount of force used.

Common sites of injury include:

- posterior fourchette
- labia minora and majora
- hymen
- perianal folds.

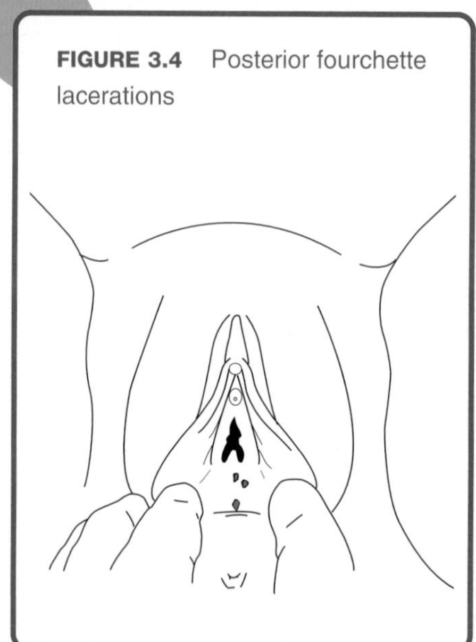

FIGURE 3.4 Posterior fourchette lacerations

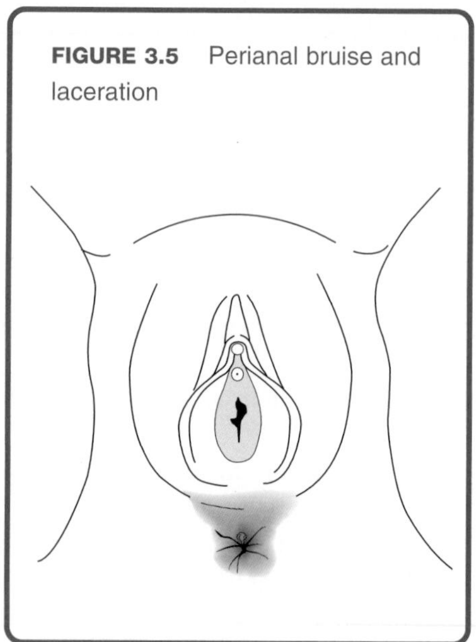

FIGURE 3.5 Perianal bruise and laceration

Forensic issues

Definition of a forensic examination: 'A medical examination conducted in the knowledge of the possibility of judicial proceedings in the future requiring medical opinion' (Box 3.2).

BOX 3.2 The forensic examination

How does the forensic examination differ from a normal medical examination?

1 A consent form may be required. Information gained with the informed consent may be provided to other parties, most typically law enforcement (police) and the criminal justice system.
2 The doctor will usually be meeting the patient for the first time. The patient will be suffering the emotional reactions of the assault.
3 Examination takes time and usually consists of a 'top-to-toe' inspection of the skin and a genito-anal examination.
4 Detailed documentation is required. Information is recorded so that it may be used in criminal proceedings.
5 Unusual body areas are inspected and are of interest, for example, the axilla, behind the ears, in the mouth and the soles of the feet.
6 Unusual specimens are collected during the examination, such as clothing, drop sheets and hair.
7 Chain of custody of specimens must be documented.
8 Therapeutic opportunities should be maximised as follow-up examinations may not occur.
9 The patient usually does not pay money to the doctor for the forensic examination.

How do I learn how to conduct a forensic examination?

1 Obtain training.
2 Have access to written material to refer to during and after training.
3 Understand the components of the examination.
4 Perform an examination under supervision.
5 Perform an examination alone.

What does a forensic examination consist of?

- Provision of informed consent using a consent form
- Taking a history or obtaining an account of the events described as sexual violence
- 'Top-to-toe' physical examination (Figure 3.6)
- Genito-anal examination
- Collection of forensic specimens. In practice, these are collected at the time of the examination
- Labelling and packaging of forensic specimens
- Therapeutic opportunities
- Arrange follow-up care
- Storage of documentation
- Provision of medico-legal report

FIGURE 3.6 'Top-to-toe' physical examination. Start with the patient's hands. This will reassure the patient. Then conduct a sensitive, systematic examination from 1 to 11.

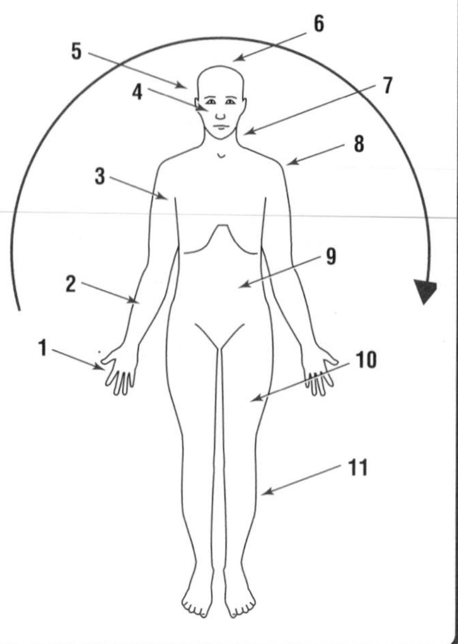

Injury patterns in sexual assault

Table 3.3 describes assaulting physical actions and their injury sequelae on body sites.[33] The information in this table should be of use in the medical examination of not only sexual assault victims, but domestic violence victims as well.

TABLE 3.3 Assaultive injury patterns[33]

Action	Site	Possible injuries
Bite	Neck	Bite marks: bruising, abrasions Suction type petechial bruising
	Breasts	Bite marks, abrasions/lacerations to nipples
Blows	Scalp	Bruising (including haematomas), lacerations
	Face	Fractures (cheek, jaw, nose) Dental trauma Intraoral bruises, abrasions, frenulum damage Facial bruises: slap marks
	Eyes	Periorbital haematomas (black eyes) Subconjunctival haemorrhage (bleeding into the white of the eye)
	Ears	Eardrum perforation (usually slapping) Bruises/lacerations to ear Bruises on scalp behind ear

TABLE 3.3 continued

Action	Site	Possible injuries
	Neck	Laryngeal skeleton trauma Voice changes (hoarseness, dysphonia), or difficulty with swallowing
	Hands	Knuckle abrasions (punching) bruising, lacerations or fractures
	Limbs	Bruises, abrasions, lacerations and fractures
	Trunk	Bruises, abrasions, fractures (especially ribs)
Burns: cigarette		Circular burns 5–15 mm in size, on any part of the body Partial or full thickness. Flame, scald contact
Defensive responses	Limbs	Bruising (especially on medial and lateral aspects of forearms, hand), 'warding off' type injuries Incised wounds (knife, bottle) Lacerations and fractures (blunt implements)
	Hands	Incised wounds to palms and web space (grasping sharp weapon) Incised wounds and bruises to dorsum (deflecting blows) Nail damage (may also occur in counter-assault, eg scratching)
Dragging	Limbs	Abrasions and bruises on exposed skin surfaces.
	Trunk	Embedded foreign material
Falls	Limbs	Abrasions and bruising especially to bony prominences; elbows, knees and heel of hands, lacerations, fractures
Fingernail scratches		Linear scratch abrasions to any part of body
Flight	Limbs	Linear curved scratch abrasions from contact with vegetation Bruises from contact with other objects Abrasions and bruises on knees, elbows, hands and hips from falls
Grasping	Ears	Bruising Trauma secondary to earring contact/loss
	Limbs	Fingertip bruises, especially to medial aspect of upper arms and forearms and medial thighs
Hair pulling		Hair follicle haematomas, bald patches, tenderness
Injections	Upper limbs	Puncture site over the course of a vein
Kissing	Multiple sites	Contact with whiskers may cause superficial abrasions and erythema

(continued overleaf)

TABLE 3.3 continued

Action	Site	Possible injuries
Ligature/manual compression	Neck	Ligature marks or imprint bruising (necklace, clothing) Fingertip bruises, abrasions (due to fingernails) Facial petechiae, intraoral petechiae, conjunctival haemorrhages
Penetration	Mouth	Pharyngeal bruising, palate bruising, frenulum trauma
Restraint	Limbs	Ligature marks (wrists and ankles), fingertip bruising
Squeezing/pinching	Breasts	Bruising
Whipping with rope/cord	Trunk/limbs	Linear, curved or looped bruising, abrasions Trainline bruises

Conclusion

Sexual abuse is common in communities. Health professionals need to be alert and facilitate disclosure of sexual abuse, as there are significant social and health sequelae for victims. The initial response to the victim's disclosure substantially affects recovery.

Mental health and illness

The importance of mental health has been recognised and promoted in recent times. In the past, to suffer from a mental disorder was regarded as shameful. The stigmatisation of psychiatric problems has led to barriers to mental health care, reluctance to seek appropriate care, delay in return to well-being, and discrimination in allocation of resources.[34] Unfortunately, this is still apparent in many societies; but now that there is effective treatment for many conditions, it is important to improve the awareness and understanding of both the general public and health professionals in order to reduce prejudice and assist those with a mental illness to seek help and improve their quality of life.[35,36]

The burden of mental illness

Neuropsychiatric disorders and suicide have been estimated by the World Health Organization to account for 12.7 per cent of the global burden of disease.[37] In 1990 it was estimated that mental and neurological disorders accounted for 10 per cent of the total daily adjusted life years (DALYs) lost due to all diseases and injuries. This was 12 per cent in 2000. It is projected that by 2020 the burden of these disorders will have increased to 15 per cent. Mental and behavioural disorders:

- Affect more than 25 per cent of all people at some time during their lives and 10 per cent of the population at any point in time
- Affect people of all countries and societies, individuals of all ages, women and men, the rich and the poor, from urban and rural environments
- Have an economic impact on societies
- Affect the quality of life of individuals and families.

Gender and mental illness

Women's mental health and well-being across the life cycle are linked not only to hormonal or biological factors, but also to women's roles in the family and in society generally. Thus, biological, psychological and social factors interact to affect vulnerability to mental health problems. The traditional and the changing roles of women in society expose women to great stresses. It is within this context that women's mental health and well-being need to be understood and responded to. Some mental disorders are more prevalent among women, others among men. Mood swings related to hormonal changes as part of the menstrual cycle and following childbirth are well documented. In addition, women suffer a high rate of both domestic violence and sexual abuse, both childhood and adult, affecting long-term mental health.[38–40] Comorbidity is more common among women than men. This often consists of a combination of a mental and a somatiform disorder, the latter being the presence of physical symptoms that are not accounted for by physical diseases.

Women are also higher users of psychotropic medication. This higher use of drugs may be partly explained by the higher prevalence of common mental disorders and a higher rate of help-seeking behaviour (Section 1). It is also influenced by the prescribing behaviour of physicians, who may take prescribing as an easier path when faced with a complex psychosocial situation.

Women are most often the ones to take on care for the mentally ill within the family. This is an important additional stressful role, as more and more individuals with chronic mental disorders are being looked after in the community.

What is mental health?

Everyone experiences peaks and troughs of emotion. For most women these are of short duration and are manageable. When any psychological disturbance interferes with the quality of life for a longer term it could be regarded as a mental or psychological disorder. The range from 'normal' experiences to disorder is wide and there is often no dividing line between the two. For the individual woman this may also vary during the life cycle and will be influenced by genetic predisposition, neurohormonal factors, life experiences, and developmental and psychosocial factors. Maintaining mental health for women thus consists of more than solely dealing with major psychiatric disorders, and must include attention to the daily stresses and concerns influencing their well-being.

Gender and brain function

Research is increasingly revealing that gender differences exist in brain physiology, and that male and female reproductive hormones have psychoactive effects. The psychoactive effects of oestrogen and progesterone have received particular attention. The antidopaminergic and serotonin-enhancing effects of oestrogen, and modulation of gamma-aminobutyric (GABA) receptors by metabolites of progesterone, may play a role in psychiatric disorders in women.

Receptors for oestrogen are found predominantly in the pituitary, hypothalamus, limbic forebrain and cerebral cortex. A number of neurotransmitter systems, including the serotonergic, GABA and opioid systems, have been suggested to respond to oestrogen. Receptors for testosterone are predominantly found in the pre-optic area of the hypothalamus, with smaller concentrations in the limbic system and in the cerebral cortex. The brain contains aromatising enzymes necessary to convert androgens to oestrogens. Thus, it is clear that the sex steroids exert direct actions on portions of the brain thought to subserve emotion and sexuality. In addition it is suggested that oestrogen is associated with verbal fluency and verbal representations in memory.[41,42]

Psychiatric assessment of women

Clinicians should be alert to the elements of the history that are specifically relevant to women patients.[43]

Present history

Menstrual and reproductive history may be relevant to the presentation of the condition or possible treatment. For example, it is important to assess the relationship of the patient's symptoms to her menstrual cycle, to enquire about the possibility that she may be pregnant, and to ask about the use of contraception. It is also important to ask about the patient's plans regarding pregnancy, because this may influence the choice of treatment. In the middle-aged woman reporting sleep impairment, it is important to consider that perimenopausal night sweats might be disrupting her sleep in addition to, or instead of, an underlying mental or physical disorder. Seasonality of mood symptoms should be explored, as seasonal affective disorder predominates in women.

Past history

Women with a history of psychiatric symptoms occurring in relation to one reproductive life event are at risk for the development of psychiatric symptoms during subsequent reproductive events. Women who have experienced a termination of pregnancy or delayed child-bearing may be left with residual anger, guilt or sadness if they are unable to conceive or retain a pregnancy, as may those women whose infertility is related to sexually transmitted disease. Gynaecological conditions (such as genital warts, genital herpes and cervical smear abnormalities) may affect women's sexual functioning and mental well-being. Breast surgery and hysterectomy may influence a woman's body image and affect her relationship with her partner.

Family history

Mood disorders related to reproductive events often run in families, and therefore a family history of premenstrual dysphoric disorder or postnatal depression should be obtained. In addition, the presence of a mood disorder in a family member may influence the woman's attitude and approach to a condition in herself.

Social history

Treating clinicians should also be aware of the social roles and pressures that may influence a woman's coping capacity and vulnerability to psychopathology. Economic conditions frequently dictate access to health care in general and to mental health care in particular. The greater number of female-headed households and the lower salaries for women than men continue to place increasing economic stress on women. Elderly women are particularly affected by economic difficulties. As they live longer, commonly their increased risk of illness further stresses their financial resources.

Alcohol and drug abuse, although less prevalent in women than in men, are a significant problem for some women. A woman may need encouragement to discuss strains in her life, such as family or marital conflict, domestic violence, or exhausting care-taking responsibilities, because she may feel guilty or disloyal about voicing her own needs when they conflict with those of other family members.

Stressful events

It has been suggested that accumulation of daily hassles is an even greater predictor of emotional and physical health than are major life events in women's lives.[44] Common psychological stressors on women's lives include excessive demands, boredom, frustration, conflict and discrimination. Emotional responses to stress may include anxiety, anger, withdrawal and apathy, and depression.

Major life events are those which have a strong impact and long-term consequences—examples are the birth of a baby, the death of someone close, being a victim of serious crime, or inability to pursue a career choice. It is difficult to estimate the impact of such events on the individual as most women cope with such events without becoming ill. However, there does seem to be a relationship between life changes and health. Catastrophic events in life are outside most women's range of life experiences but when they occur they may have a profound impact.

Depression and anxiety

Mental health issues are common and are associated with considerable morbidity for women and their families, but the diagnosis may not always be initially apparent. Health professionals across all disciplines should be proactive in considering the possibility of these conditions, rather than merely making the diagnosis by exclusion, in view of the suffering they engender, and the highly effective treatments available.

Depression

Depression is a major public health issue for women. Previous assessment of the impact of disease has focused on survival statistics, but new approaches have used the concept of disability to examine the impact of disease. Such research reports that for women, depression currently poses the largest single disease burden world-wide.[45] Although patterns of help-seeking may affect diagnostic rates,[46] there is general consensus that depression is twice as common in women as in men, occurring most commonly between the ages of 25 and 40 years.[47]

CLINICAL PRESENTATION

Despite evidence about the prevalence of depression, rates of detection and treatment are suboptimal, due at least in part to the attitudes and training of health professionals.[48] The attitudes of women themselves may compound the problem, particularly if they are reticent about expressing the full nature of their emotional concerns. For example, less than half of a group of clinically depressed women attending an outpatient gynaecology clinic identified themselves as having depression, although the majority were prepared to acknowledge that they were 'distressed'.[49] Shame and guilt about being depressed may make the woman reluctant to seek help, and in some contexts such as in the postpartum period, the sense of being unworthy as a mother may lead to secrecy about the real level of emotional distress.

Depression should be considered in women who present with marked irritability (often expressed in relation to partner or children), feelings of profound low self-esteem, of being overwhelmed, social withdrawal, and lack of capacity for pleasure. The otherwise unexplained exacerbation of previously stable physical symptoms should also flag the possibility of depression.

History

Exploration of psychological symptoms may seem difficult, especially if the woman has presented with predominantly somatic symptoms. Comments such as 'I can imagine that all of these issues must be tough for you emotionally, too. Can you tell me how you have been feeling?' may provide an introduction. Exploration of depressive cognitions (negative thoughts of oneself, critical appraisal of personal or professional performance, helplessness) is a necessary adjunct to questioning about sleep, appetite, energy, and concentration and functional ability, providing a guide to the severity of depression.

To make a diagnosis of major depressive episode according to DSM-IV,[50] five or more of the symptoms listed in Box 3.3 must have been present during the same two-week period.

An important aspect of the history is clarification of antecedents to this episode of depression. The postpartum period is a time of particular vulnerability.[51] Other pathways to depression in women include:

- Poverty[52]—breakdown of relationships leading not only to financial strain, but to a cascading series of losses, with more minor stressors exerting a powerful negative impact on mental health[53]
- Sexual abuse[54]
- Domestic violence[55]
- Being a caregiver[56]

BOX 3.3 Symptoms of a major depressive episode

- Depressed mood for most of the day, nearly every day
- Markedly diminished interest or pleasure in almost all activities most of the day
- Significant weight loss or gain
- Insomnia or hypersomnia
- Psychomotor agitation or retardation
- Fatigue or loss of energy nearly every day
- Feelings of worthlessness or excessive guilt
- Inability to think or concentrate, indecisiveness
- Recurrent thoughts of death, suicidal ideation

- Experiencing a stillbirth, neonatal death[57] or other type of loss
- Medical condition such as breast cancer.[58]

Examination

Key features of mental status examination are retardation or agitation, stooped posture, poor eye contact, and pervasive sadness or irritability, with a reduced range of normal affective responses.

Differential diagnosis

The major differential diagnosis is with adjustment disorder, in which the mood disturbance is less severe and less pervasive. There is also often overlap with anxiety disorders. It may be that depression is a more common pathway to alcohol abuse for women than men.[59] However, social stereotypes and the guilt felt by women themselves may reduce the chance of alcohol abuse being detected and responded to. Reliance solely on screening tools is likely to be associated with reduced rates of detection of alcohol abuse in women.[60]

The presentation of an atypical depression, such as occurring for the first time later in life or without apparent environmental or personal contributory factors, warrants consideration of other diagnoses such as hypothyroidism or other systemic disease.

Tests

Investigations should be considered on a case-by-case basis, as above. Useful investigations include thyroid function tests, full blood count, electrolytes and liver function tests, and CXR and ECG in the older woman or one with known heart disease. Results will influence drug dosage (for example with hepatic impairment) or drug selection (for example, tricyclic antidepressants are associated with cardiac side effects).

Management

Ensuring the safety of the woman is the first priority. Lack of hope for the future is a predictor for suicide, risk being increased in women whose depression is complicated by anxiety.[61] Active suicidal ideation is a psychiatric emergency, and specialist review should be obtained urgently.

Effective treatment of depression is underpinned by the establishment of a therapeutic relationship, in which the woman is provided with information about the condition and supported to explore loss and grief and other issues pertinent to her presentation.

There is broad consensus that for mild to moderate depression, cognitive-behavioural therapy is as effective as antidepressants, with some evidence that it may be efficacious even in more severe depression.[62] For more severe or persistent depression, selective serotonin reuptake inhibitors (SSRIs) are generally regarded as the first treatment choice[63,64] taking into account differences in drug deposition in women, and cyclical alterations in drug levels and action.[65] There is no clear evidence of the superiority of one agent over another,[66] but weight gain is of concern to women, and may limit adherence to treatment.[67] The tricyclic antidepressants (TCAs) are highly effective antidepressants, but their side-effect burden is considerable compared with SSRIs, and they are also more likely to be lethal in overdose.

The stigma of mental illness may limit acceptance of treatment. Drawing a comparison with other conditions may facilitate discussion: 'Most women feel that they should sort out their emotional concerns themselves, and accepting treatment seems hard. Yet we all accept that we need help if we have medical problems like diabetes or heart disease…'.

Emerging issues

Adverse physical health impact

Evidence is emerging that depression may be associated with adverse effects on physical health. Population-based research has found that men who have been depressed within the preceding ten years are three times more likely to develop ischaemic heart disease.[68] There is no comparable data for women, but some research has found that past or current depression is associated with decreased bone mineral density in women.[69]

Impact on children

The impact of maternal depression on children is increasingly being recognised.[70] In part this is mediated biologically; however, negative maternal cognitions potentially affect the confidence of children, and undermine the development of strong self-efficacy and a sense of mastery. This evidence further strengthens the argument in favour of aggressive treatment of depression.

Chronicity and relapse

Depression was previously regarded as an episodic disorder, from which the majority recovered, with up to 50 per cent experiencing a further episode. Newer data suggests that rates of recurrence are in fact considerably higher, with up to 25 per cent of patients developing chronic depression.[71] Observational follow-up over 15 years has found that women are more likely to relapse than men.[72] This research raises concerns about the standard approach of treating each episode of depression 'on its merits'. Those who fail to achieve complete remission continue to experience the corrosive effects of low self-esteem, reduced sense of self-efficacy, and relationship and occupational difficulties, but over time such problems may come to be seen as 'normal' by the woman, and even health professionals, and so less worthy of treatment. Recognition of these issues has prompted discussion of the need to review acute treatment models, and to establish a more proactive, long-term approach in order to improve outcomes.[73]

Anxiety

Women have higher rates of generalised anxiety disorder than men. The condition is less common in adolescents, and prevalence increases with age, affecting up to 10 per cent of women over 40 years of age.[74] Anxiety tends to be a long-term condition, with exacerbations often in relation to external events, and in some cases to menstrual cycle.[75] In addition to generalised anxiety, women are affected by panic disorder twice as commonly as men.

CLINICAL PRESENTATION

Typically, anxiety symptoms have been present for many months or even years before the woman expresses emotional distress. There may be repeated presentations with somatic symptoms or sleep disturbance before the diagnosis becomes clear. In panic disorder, the woman presents with extreme distress, sweating, tachycardia and hyperventilation, often initially arousing concerns that this is a medical emergency.

History

There will often be a positive family history of generalised anxiety disorder, phobias and panic disorder, with biological factors exerting a major influence in these conditions.[76] However, early developmental and traumatic experiences, drugs, illness and psychosocial factors may also contribute to and exacerbate anxiety disorders.[77]

Generalised anxiety disorder is defined as excessive worry and tension on most days, for at least six months, along with at least three of:[50]

- restlessness
- being easily fatigued
- difficulty concentrating
- irritability
- muscle tension
- sleep disturbance.

A panic attack is an intense exacerbation of anxiety associated with palpitations, shortness of breath, feeling light-headed, chest tightness, tingling around mouth and fingertips, and sweating. Psychological symptoms include a sense of impending doom, fear of losing control or collapsing, or a sense of detachment from the environment. The intensity of the experience is such that the woman feels overwhelmed, or fearful that she is 'going mad', leading to avoidance of situations in which such an episode might occur, or from which she could not escape if one did occur.

Self-medication with alcohol is a common complication of anxiety disorders. Women face particular risk because of lower rates of detection of abuse, and their increased susceptibility to the adverse physical consequences of alcohol abuse.

Examination

Key features of anxiety are restlessness, being easily startled, preoccupation with physical symptoms, and apprehension.

Differential diagnosis

Particularly when somatic symptoms are prominent, conditions such as hyperthyroidism, cardiac conditions, drug intoxication or withdrawal should be considered. Rarely, anxiety symptoms may be the presentation of conditions such as phaeochromocytoma or carcinoid syndrome.

Tests

It is important initially to exclude medical causes of symptoms; however, repeated physical examination and investigations may compound anxiety, reinforcing the idea in the woman's mind that there is a serious but as yet undiagnosed medical problem.

Management

For many patients, the distress and dysfunction related to anxiety and panic are compounded by unrealistic expectations of coping. The cornerstone of management is education about the nature of anxiety, including discussion about the potential benefits of some stress in promoting enhanced performance and productivity.

Cognitive behaviour therapy is an effective treatment modality for those with anxiety disorders[78] and panic disorder.[79] Graded exposure is a specific behavioural technique, the premise of which is that anxiety will diminish through incremental exposure to a hierarchy of stressful situations over which the woman gradually gains mastery. Structured problem-solving is especially useful when the woman's level of distress is high and she feels overwhelmed, posing the risk of poor decision making. Specific training in these techniques is often valuable for general practitioners.

For the woman with long-standing anxiety, apprehension about perceived threats may lead to a constricted lifestyle in which the normal validation and 'reality checks' afforded by social supports is lost. A structured approach in which the woman documents her thoughts and feelings in a diary provides the opportunity for a health practitioner to gently challenge her thoughts and fears, introducing strategies such as distraction and thought-stopping. This technique also allows identification of unrealistic and negative 'automatic thoughts'. 'Homework' between sessions includes critical appraisal of these thoughts, so that more appropriate interpretations and responses can be made.

There is a role for medication in the treatment of anxiety disorders. Traditionally the TCAs have been effective, but their side-effect profile and lethality in overdose has meant that SSRIs are increasingly seen as the treatment of choice for more severe disorder. Benzodiazepines are useful as an acute treatment for extreme distress, but this benefit comes at the cost of dependence, sedation, impaired motor coordination and confusion in the elderly, in whom half-life is prolonged.

Emerging issues

Research into responses to the diagnosis of breast cancer demonstrates high levels of anxiety, traumatic imagery and intrusive thoughts about the diagnosis, with younger women appearing more vulnerable.[80] The suggestion that this distress relates to the diagnosis itself[81] raises implications about the way the diagnosis is communicated, and interventions to support women in adjusting.

Hormonal-related mood changes in the life cycle

Premenstrual syndrome (PMS) in some form and in some cycles is experienced by 75 per cent of women. Only 3–8 per cent of women suffer the severe form called premenstrual dysphoric disorder.[82] The peak age for PMS is the late twenties to thirties. Premenstrual syndrome has an association with postnatal depression and other mood disorders.[83]

Premenstrual syndrome

CLINICAL PRESENTATION

Premenstrual syndrome is a condition in which symptoms commonly occur about seven days before the period starts. There are both physical and mood changes described (Box 3.4).

BOX 3.4 PMS symptoms

- Mood changes:
  - irritability
  - tension
  - aggression
  - depression
  - loss of self-esteem/no confidence
  - weepiness
  - sleep disturbance
- Physical symptoms:
  - headaches
  - pains in the legs, arms, back etc
  - nausea
  - food cravings
  - binge eating
- Fluid retention:
  - bloating of the stomach
  - swelling and soreness of the breasts
  - swelling of the ankles, hands and face

History

It is important to establish the relationship of the symptoms to the cycle. Asking the woman to chart her symptoms for one or more cycles is invaluable in making the diagnosis and then useful to observe the response to treatment[84] (Figure 3.7). The syndrome is associated with cyclical ovarian activity and does not occur before puberty, during pregnancy or after menopause. It does not occur in women who are not ovulating. It will still occur in a woman after hysterectomy in whom the ovaries are preserved—an important discussion point for a woman contemplating hysterectomy.

FIGURE 3.7 Premenstrual syndrome daily symptom rating chart

Month beginning ....

My last period started on

......../......../20......

Each night before retiring, please record your experience during the day of the feelings and sensations listed here. Write a number in the box opposite the item to indicate how intensely this symptom or feeling was experienced.

Not at all 0
Very little 1
Moderate amount 2
More than moderate 3
Great deal 4
Couldn't be worse 5

DATE	WEEK 1						
1 Restlessness							
2 Headache							
3 Breast soreness							
4 Depression							
5 Verbal aggression							
6 Physical aggression							
7 Feelings of well-being							
8 Irritability feelings							
9 Tiredness							
10 Swelling of abdomen, hands, legs							
11 Other:							
12 Tampon/pads: number used							

Investigations

Some premenstrual symptoms can be attributed to a response to the physiological production of progesterone in the luteal phase of the cycle. Thus cyclical mastalgia is related to the effect on the breasts of oestradiol followed by that of progesterone. Progesterone also has an inhibitory effect on the smooth muscle of the gut and may therefore cause symptoms of bloatedness and constipation. However, there are no known abnormalities of gonadal-steroid levels or menstrual cycle physiology that characterise women with PMS. A diagnosis is made on the history and the review of the symptom diary.

Management

A range of options have been suggested according to the severity of the symptoms and the wishes of the woman, although few long-term well-conducted trials exist.

1 *Lifestyle modification:* there have been modest improvements with aerobic exercise. Dietary modification and supplementation (calcium, evening primrose oil and vitamin B6) have not been shown to be better than placebo.
2 *Medical therapy:* often by the time a woman seeks medical assistance, she has tried all the suggested remedies from friends, family and women's magazines. After discussion, she may wish to discuss medical options. For a woman who does not respond or who prefers non-hormonal treatment, the serotonin-acting agents have been shown to be effective.

The use of a continuous oral monophasic contraceptive to suppress ovulation may be useful, particularly where contraception is also required. This can be taken continuously long term, although the woman may experience occasional light unpredictable bleeding with this approach. To avoid this she may choose to break for a few days once or twice a year.

Premenstrual dysphoric disorder

CLINICAL PRESENTATION

Premenstrual dysphoric disorder (PMDD) is characterised by distressing emotional and behavioural symptoms included in the DSM-IV (Box 3.5). The boundary between severe PMS and PMDD may not be clear but can be related to the severity and number of the symptoms.

BOX 3.5 Diagnostic criteria for premenstrual dysphoric disorder[50]

- Symptoms:
  - Have occurred cyclically in most cycles in the past year
  - Present for the last week of the luteal phase, remitting within a few days of the follicular phase, and absent in the week post menses
  - Are confirmed by prospective daily ratings through two cycles
  - Are serious enough to interfere with activities and relationships
  - Are not an exacerbation of an underlying disorder
- At least five of the following are present (including at least one of the first four):
  1 Anxiety and tension
  2 Depressed mood, feelings of hopelessness, or self-deprecating thoughts
  3 Anger or irritability or increased interpersonal conflicts
  4 Affective lability
  5 Decreased interest in usual activities
  6 Lethargy, lack of energy, easily tired
  7 Appetite change: overeating or food cravings
  8 Insomnia or hypersomnia
  9 Subjective sense of difficulty in concentrating
  10 Physical symptoms: breast pain, bloating, headaches

Aetiology of PMS and PMDD

The exact aetiology is unknown. A likely hypothesis is that women with PMS have an altered sensitivity of central neurotransmitters, particularly serotonergic, to the normal circulating levels of oestrogen and progesterone.[85,86] This is supported by the use of serotonin agents in treating PMDD.

Management

Serotonin-acting agents are the mainstay of treatment.[87] Treatment can be daily or intermittent with selective SSRIs. The intermittent therapy is commenced premenstrually with the onset of symptoms and is continued until the onset of menses; this regimen is effective and acceptable to women.[88]

Psychological aspects of pregnancy and post partum

Pregnancy

Pregnancy, even when planned and wanted and a healthy baby results, is both exciting and anxiety-provoking. All women are aware at some level of the hazards inherent in child-bearing for themselves and their offspring. Miscarriages, premature births, developmental disability, cot deaths are matters of common knowledge and all parents check the appearance of their baby when they first see the infant.

Underlying these concerns are the specific meanings of the pregnancy for the individual woman in the context of her psychological development. Historically, conception and achieving motherhood have been considered a socially sanctioned, positive maturational step, allaying feelings of insecurity about femininity, personal identity and life goals. Countering this, there is increasing evidence that women who have experienced childhood adversity, including abuse, may find parenting a difficult task.

Parenthood

A commitment to parenthood is a lifetime decision and it closes off many options. This, and the other losses inherent in or cued by the event, must be adequately worked through. As in other transitional stages:

- The opportunity arises to review and possibly resolve previous conflicts, especially in close relationships, including with oneself.
- Anxiety and mood instability are expected. In those who are vulnerable for genetic, psychological or social reasons, mental health problems or actual illness may result. Psychological growth and maturation, decompensation and various combinations are possible outcomes. The doubts and fears connected with inexperience of the task, unrealistic expectations, and fatigue, will particularly test the coping strategies and threaten the self-esteem of the first-time mother and father. The changes in identity, interpersonal activity, social and occupational roles, body image and internal sensations, emotionality, physical health, life options, have their most profound impact during the course of the first transition to parenthood. The arrival of any subsequent child, particularly if unwanted, also alters family dynamics.

Support

Many societies devise rituals to support women during this upheaval; however, in many developed countries, the rituals offered by healthcare systems are system-defined interventions which fail to take account of the complex personal, social and family needs of the woman. Increased social mobility, limited family size, migration and financial pressures may further compound the isolation and lack of support available for women at this time. Comprehensive care requires attention to psychological and social well-being.

History

Perinatal risk and protective factors should be reviewed.[89] Enquiry should be made concerning:

- Pregnancy: whether it is wanted, and by whom
- Current mental state: thought processes, mood, appetite, sleep pattern, energy level, productive activity, interest and enjoyment. Assess distress level and depressive symptoms by use of a simple screening scale such as the Edinburgh Postnatal Depression Scale (Figure 3.8, on page 130).[90]
- Mental health problems or actual illness (and treatments): personal or family history of any mental health problem. In particular, any history of a previous pregnancy-related mental health problem.
- Drug use: cigarettes, alcohol, other substances
- Support: whether there is a partner who is likely to be emotionally and instrumentally supportive. His mental health. Are there other supports?
- Relationship with her mother and the availability of maternal emotional and practical support
- Social situation: adequacy of language skills, housing, income, transport
- Abuse: current or past domestic violence
- Adverse childhood circumstances: physical, sexual or emotional abuse, neglect, early loss of a parent through separation, divorce, illness or death
- Loss: other bereavements, losses or traumas.

Exploration of these aspects of history requires sensitivity, and staff training and education are necessary. Ongoing clinical supervision and support for staff should be provided, since doctors, nurses and their families also experience the problems listed. Resources should be available to manage any problems identified.

Identification of problems

Ambivalence is normal though often denied. Also common are acute or chronic anxiety and depressive difficulties ranging from mild to severe. Some 13.5 per cent of women will screen positive for significant depression at 32 weeks of pregnancy[91] and a similar or greater percentage for anxiety.[92] These problems may be associated with cognitive, behavioural and emotional problems in the offspring.[92,93] Women with a prior history of anxiety or depression are at risk of exacerbation or recurrence, while for some women pregnancy may include their first experience of disorder. Actual anxiety (panic, obsessive-compulsive, generalised anxiety, post-traumatic stress, phobic) or depressive (major, minor, dysthymic) disorder may be diagnosable in some 10–15 per cent of women. Anxiety and depression often occur together.

Management during pregnancy

Antenatal classes should include discussion of the practical points and relevant mental health issues listed in Box 3.6.[94]

If symptomatology results in dysfunction in the woman's daily activities, treatment is necessary. This may consist of:

- Extra visits to the health professional to provide support.
- Linkage to community resources.
- Medication. Prescription of medication[89] requires careful discussion. The effects of medication should be balanced with the possible consequences of untreated anxiety and depression—for example, a failure to attend antenatal care, smoking and other substance use—that may result.
- Referral to other professionals for specific management such as (individual or group) non-directive counselling, cognitive-behaviour therapy, interpersonal psychotherapy, relationship counselling or some combination of these.

Additional support should automatically be provided where there is a history of obstetric problems such as infertility, miscarriage, prematurity, stillbirth, that raise anxiety levels.

Women already receiving specialist psychiatric care for bipolar disorder, recurrent depressive episodes, schizophrenia, personality disorder, should be managed in collaboration with a psychiatrist.

BOX 3.6 Practical discussion points for antenatal classes

1 The responsibilities of being a mother (and not a martyr) are learned, hence get help and advice.
2 Make friends of other couples who are experienced with young children.
3 Don't overload yourself with unimportant tasks.
4 Don't move house soon after the baby arrives.
5 Don't be too concerned with keeping up appearances.
6 Get plenty of rest.
7 Don't be a nurse to elderly relatives at this time.
8 Confer and consult with husband and family and experienced friends and discuss your plans and worries.
9 Don't give up your outside interests but cut down the responsibilities and rearrange your schedules.
10 Arrange for babysitters in advance.
11 Get a driving licence.
12 Get a family doctor now.

Post partum

The postpartum period is stressful as so many adjustments are required and the new responsibilities can seem overwhelming. Sleep deprivation plays a significant role, especially in those with genetic vulnerability to psychological or psychiatric disorder. Practical strategies for managing sleep deprivation are an obvious requirement for all parents with a new baby.

CLINICAL PRESENTATION

Self-reported depressive symptoms are noted in some 25 per cent,[95] and although with diagnostic interviewing not all such women will be accorded a formal psychiatric diagnosis, the dysphoria may be sufficient to affect the woman and her relationships with infant and partner.

History

Detailed enquiry should be made regarding the birth experience, feelings about the infant and partner, mental state, rest and respite arrangements, and availability of emotional and practical support.

Investigations

The Edinburgh Postnatal Depression Scale (Figure 3.8) is widely used as a screening test for depression.[90] Postpartum mood difficulties are customarily divided into 'the blues', postnatal depression (PND; non-psychotic depression) and postpartum psychosis.[94] The validation study showed that mothers who scored above threshold 92.3 per cent were likely to be suffering from a depressive illness of varying severity. Nevertheless the score should not override clinical judgement. A careful clinical assessment should be carried out to confirm the diagnosis.[90]

Postpartum mood disorders

'The blues'

'The blues' are noted by some 30–80 per cent of women, who report tearfulness, lability, sadness, irritability, low mood, sleep problems and somatic symptoms occurring from around the third day post partum. In some women, the mood is euphoric rather than low and this may be termed 'the highs' or 'pinks'. Symptoms should resolve spontaneously within a week. Severe or longer-lasting symptoms may presage the development of clinical depression.

Postpartum psychosis

Postpartum psychosis (PPP) is at the other end of the spectrum. It is rare (0.3%) and constitutes a psychiatric emergency. Prodromal symptoms may have been present antenatally and misconstrued (eg elevated mood, severe, symptomatic anxiety), but onset is usually reported within three weeks of delivery.

By convention, PPP includes mania, depression, mixed states and schizo-affective disorder. Thinking and behaviour are markedly disorganised and bizarre ideas concerning the infant may be expressed. Suicide and infanticide may occur.

FIGURE 3.8 Edinburgh Postnatal Depression Scale[90]

This scale indicates how the mother has felt during the previous week and in doubtful cases it may be usefully repeated after two weeks.

Instructions for users

1 The mother is asked to underline the response which comes closest to how she has been feeling in the previous seven days.
2 All ten items must be completed.
3 Care should be taken to avoid the possibility of the mother discussing her answers with others.
4 The mother should complete the scale herself, unless she has limited English or has difficulty with reading.
5 The EPDS may be used to screen postnatal women. The child health clinic, postnatal check-up or a home visit may provide suitable opportunities for its completion.

As you have recently had a baby, we would like to know how you are feeling. Please UNDERLINE the answer which comes closest to how you have felt IN THE PAST 7 DAYS, not just how you feel today.

1 I have been able to laugh and see the funny side of things.
- ☐ As much as I always could
- ☐ Not quite so much now
- ☐ Definitely not so much now
- ☐ Not at all

2 I have looked forward with enjoyment to things.
- ☐ As much as I ever did
- ☐ Rather less than I used to
- ☐ Definitely less than I used to
- ☐ Hardly at all

3 I have blamed myself unnecessarily when things went wrong.*
- ☐ Yes, most of the time
- ☐ Yes, some of the time
- ☐ Not very often
- ☐ No, never

4 I have been anxious or worried for no good reason.
- ☐ No, not at all
- ☐ Hardly ever
- ☐ Yes, sometimes
- ☐ Yes, very often

5 I have felt scared or panicky for no very good reason.*
- ☐ Yes, quite a lot
- ☐ Yes, sometimes
- ☐ No, not much
- ☐ No, not at all

6 Things have been getting on top of me.*
- ☐ Yes, most of the time I haven't been able to cope at all
- ☐ Yes, sometimes I haven't been coping as well as usual
- ☐ No, most of the time I have coped quite well
- ☐ No, I have been coping as well as ever

7 I have been so unhappy that I have had difficulty sleeping.*
- ☐ Yes, most of the time
- ☐ Yes, sometimes
- ☐ Not very often
- ☐ No, not at all

8 I have felt sad or miserable.*
- ☐ Yes, most of the time
- ☐ Yes, quite often
- ☐ Not very often
- ☐ No, not at all

9 I have been so unhappy that I have been crying.*
- ☐ Yes, most of the time
- ☐ Yes, quite often
- ☐ Only occasionally
- ☐ No, never

10 The thought of harming myself has occurred to me.*
- ☐ Yes, quite often
- ☐ Sometimes
- ☐ Hardly ever
- ☐ Never

Response categories are scored 0, 1, 2 and 3 according to increased severity of the symptoms. Items marked with an asterisk are reverse scored (ie 3, 2, 1 and 0). The total score is calculated by adding together the scores for each of the ten items. Major depression is likely if score is > 12.

Postpartum psychosis is more frequently reported in primiparae (so obtaining a family history may be critical) following caesarean section, if the infant is sick or dies, and if there is no partner at the time of delivery. Subsequent pregnancies should be managed in collaboration with a psychiatrist, as the recurrence rate is high. Recurrence at other times (eg with jet lag, following viral illness or severe stress) is also possible.

Postnatal depression

Postnatal depression (PND) occurs in 10–15 per cent of new mothers,[96] with a higher rate reported in some studies and in particular groups (eg women with a history of childhood abuse, refugees and recent migrants who do not speak English). The recurrence rate in subsequent pregnancies may be as high as 40 per cent.

Diagnosis

Postnatal depression is defined as a non-psychotic depressive episode, beginning in or extending into the postnatal period and meeting standardised DSM-IV-R criteria for major or minor depressive disorder. Less than 50 per cent of cases are identified unless routine, universal assessment is in place. In practice, a variety of diagnoses and problems will be found under this label. Several subtypes may be distinguished:

- Postnatal depression only
- Ongoing depression from the antenatal period
- Dysthymia (chronic depression)
- Major depression, with or without melancholic features, superimposed upon dysthymia or personality disorder.

Comorbid anxiety disorders and personality difficulties are common.

Consequences of PND

Postnatal depression may have profound effects on the woman, the child and the family as a whole. Social, emotional and cognitive development of the child may be adversely affected, with the longer-term possibility of vulnerability to and inter-generational transmission of mental health problems.

Postnatal depression is not limited to the Western world; careful assessment reveals its presence in other cultures. Similar genetic, personality and contextual aspects are reported, including: isolation; lack of support; financial strain; marital conflict, including domestic violence; experience of loss or abuse; and previous history of mental health problems. It is important to consider additional factors affecting women from culturally and linguistically diverse backgrounds:

- Language difficulties
- Previous experience of torture and trauma
- Thoughtless or disrespectful professional care
- Cultural expectations regarding the gender of the child or the gender of professionals
- Cultural stigma regarding mental illness
- Punitive or guilt-inducing cultural interpretations of the woman's misery.

Management

Management varies according to the diagnosis and must include attention to the mother's significant relationships (infant, partner and other children) and other circumstances. Sub-syndromal symptoms ('not a case') should not be dismissed; the context must be explored and appropriate supports arranged. Practical strategies for rest and respite are essential. Management of 'the blues' includes anticipation, understanding and acknowledgement of the woman's concerns, following adequate antenatal discussion of the syndrome. Schizophrenia and postpartum psychosis require specialist mental health consultation.

Treatment

Non-directive psychotherapy, interpersonal psychotherapy, cognitive-behavioural counselling, group therapies and mother–infant therapies have all been used singly or in combination, with some success.[97,98] As noted earlier, treatment that reduces maternal depression but does not address relationship difficulties (infant, partner) or chronic problems such as anxiety, is not sufficient.

Hoffbrand and colleagues[96] reviewed all trials where women with depression in the first six months post partum were randomised to receive antidepressants with or without any other treatment, and concluded that only one trial met the criteria. In this study, fluoxetine was significantly more effective than placebo and, after an initial session of counselling, as effective as a full course of cognitive-behavioural counselling in the treatment of PND.[99] This was a small, short-term study where women had to agree not to breastfeed before being included in the trial.

Ethical consideration may preclude randomised controlled trials in pregnant and lactating women. Nevertheless, many antidepressant medications have been used and the usual advice is: discuss their use carefully with the mother; be cautious; avoid the first trimester where possible; avoid combinations of medication; reduce dosage prior to delivery; avoid medication if the infant is premature or otherwise unwell, and monitor the infant.[89,100] The tricyclic, dothiepin, which has useful sedating properties, and various SSRIs have been widely used though some, mostly minor, adverse effects have been reported. Benzodiazepines should be avoided. Most antidepressants are also anxiolytic. Access to an up-to-date, professional resource is recommended.[101]

Perimenopause and menopause

Women's mental and emotional well-being in mid-life is affected by a number of factors. These include relationships, growing children, work, ageing parents and the menopause (Figure 3.9). Women who have ageing parents or in-laws are far more likely than men to be responsible for their care and to spend more time caring for parents than children. This role is usually undertaken during the middle years of a woman's life when other responsibilities converge. Stress and conflict in marriage are more likely to lead to depressive episodes in women than in men. Indeed, there is now substantial research to show that marriage offers men more emotional protection than it does women. It is during this complex time that women reach menopause.

CLINICAL PRESENTATION

Menopausal symptoms can include sleeplessness, irritability, fatigue and other mood changes. The psychological symptoms experienced by women around this time of life, particularly in the three to five years preceding the last menstrual period, can be most disturbing. Irrational moods, anxiety and sudden memory loss are a few examples of psychological symptoms that can lead some women to think that they may have a serious mental disorder. Although depressed mood may occur around menopause, clinical depression is not considered to be more prevalent than at other times in a woman's life. However, women with a previous history of depression may be at risk for relapse at this time.

FIGURE 3.9 In mid-life a woman is affected by many factors. These cause varying stresses that may influence any symptom.

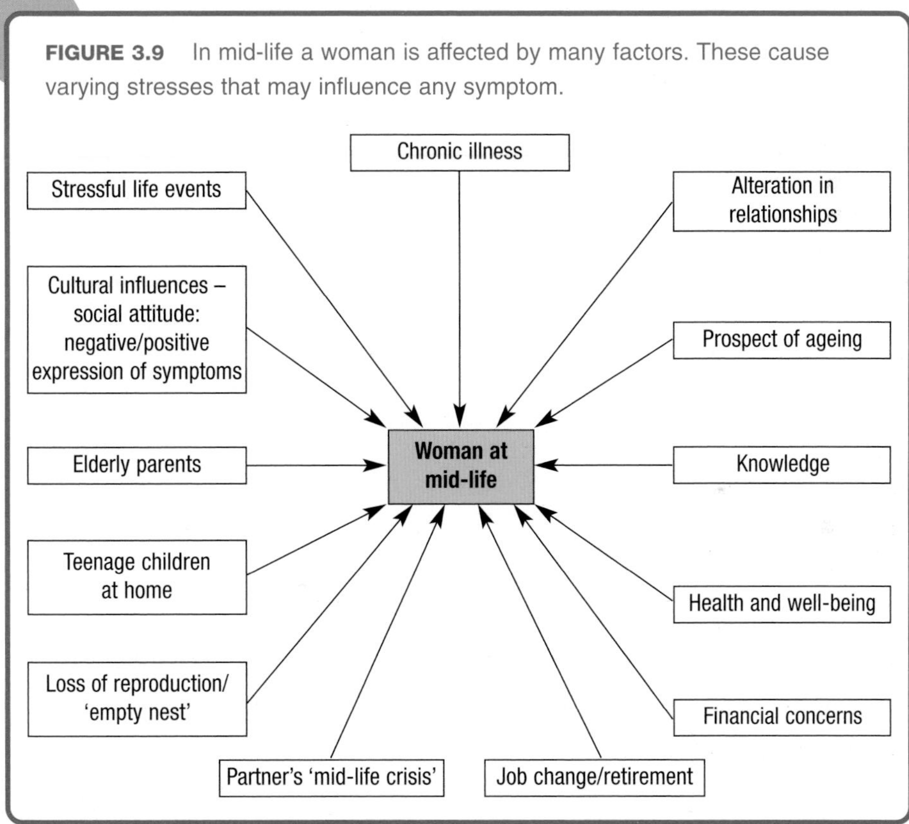

Hormone treatment

The value of hormone replacement therapy around the menopause to treat these mood changes is not clear. There are plausible mechanisms that would support the use of oestrogen for mood disorders. However, mood disorders based on oestrogen fluctuation or deficiency have not been demonstrated. Many of the trials have methodological problems and a significant difference between treatment and placebo effect over time has not been clearly demonstrated.

Many women are relieved once they understand that this may be related to the stresses of their multiple roles at this time, and is likely to be temporary and unrelated to the development of dementia long term. The relief of other menopausal symptoms, in particular the vasomotor ones that may interfere with sleep, may improve well-being and the ability to cope with stress.

Ageing and mental health

The physical health of older adults appears to be linked to their mental health.[102] Positive mental health in older age is often related to individual characteristics and patterns of coping that have been present throughout life.[103] Mental health problems experienced by older women can be the result of:

- lifelong mental health problems
- dementia
- stress arising from caring for a spouse or other dependent family member.

Lifelong problems

Women who have a history of mental health problems may have their symptoms exacerbated by widowhood, loneliness, isolation, increasing frailty, lack of adequate nutrition and altered pharmacokinetics. Psychotropic drug use, in particular the benzodiazepines, is more common in older women than older men. Confusion can lead to mistakenly taking extra doses and can cause physical and psychological problems, altering the mental state, which may lead to further depression and anxiety.

Dementia

As the population ages and life expectancy increases, dementia, particularly Alzheimer's disease and multi-infarct dementia, is becoming more common (Section 17). Women's increased life expectancy means that there is more opportunity for these conditions to occur. Figures suggest that at least 5 per cent of women aged over 65 years have severe or moderate dementia, with this figure rising to 20–30 per cent for women over 80 years. The rising numbers of mentally frail older people has been described as a 'silent epidemic' that has implications for carers, health professionals and government alike.

Carer's health

The prevalence of dementia in people with Down syndrome is not thought to be higher than in the general population, but the age of onset is approximately two decades earlier. This may also have implications for carers.

Conclusion

Health professionals involved in the clinical care of women are in a powerful position to positively influence the mental health and well-being of women. It is thus crucial to look beyond the obvious biological determinants, and recognise the dynamic interplay of personal and social relationships and roles of women in shaping not only the development of, but also responses to, mental illness. This section provides clear information about the detection and treatment of disorder. However, comprehensive care implies more than just detection and treatment—it must also include identification of those who are at increased risk, and the development of supportive interventions which aim to reduce distress, improve well-being and promote optimal functioning.

Loss and grief

Simply because they are human beings, women will experience loss. Loss through death and other sorrows will enter their lives as it does the lives of men and children. It is important to recognise the individual and personal journey through grief and not assume that all women grieve in exactly the same way.

Where are we in our knowledge?

Many people considering women and loss or grief confine their understanding to bereavement and perhaps divorce. However, a much broader definition of loss should be used in clinical practice, incorporating awareness of the meaning of change in women's lives. An apparently similar change in the lives of different women may be interpreted quite differently—for one it may be positive, for another highly negative. An event is not considered a 'loss' until it is interpreted as such by the person experiencing it. Any event that causes distress for the person experiencing it, such as a relationship breakdown, can be defined as a loss. While scientific knowledge has contributed greatly to our understanding of the grieving process, it is important to remember that loss is a normal life event.

Some definitions

While the words 'loss', 'grief' and 'mourning' are commonly used by professionals and the broader community, there is often a lack of consensus on what is meant by these terms. To ensure a commonality of language, the term 'grief' is considered here to represent manifestations of reactions to loss. While the term 'grieving' is similar to 'mourning', it is used here to refer to the process of dealing with losses other than bereavement.

Losses in the lives of women

There are many events in the lives of women in which issues of loss are implicated. Some losses in the lives of women will occur more or less by chance or are losses over which women may have little control. In contrast, developmental losses are associated with the normal physical and social changes associated with human and social development. Some losses in the lives of women are private, less tangible, less easily observable losses. Finally some losses are associated with deprivation in the life of a woman (Table 3.4).

Loss plays a significant role in the lives of many women, and for many women presenting to health practitioners, the losses will be complex and multiple, sometimes concurrent. Hence an understanding of loss as a universal concept in adverse life events is a powerful tool for practitioners in understanding the distress being expressed by many women.

TABLE 3.4 Losses in the lives of women

Chance	Life events
Death of loved one	Leaving home/work
Pregnancy loss/infertility	Menopause
Separation/divorce	Retirement/ageing
Victim of crime	Loss of body part (hysterectomy)
Unemployment	Diagnosis of disease (incontinence)
	Physical decline
Private, less tangible	**Deprivation**
Loss of trust from betrayal/abuse	Poverty
Social non-acceptance	Lack of stability
Failure to meet expectations (overweight)	Lack of 'personal' time
Failure of partner to understand one's needs	Partner a 'workaholic'
Disappointment in children	No contact with children/grandchildren

What do we know about loss and grief?

In considering the many adverse life events that affect the lives of women, a number of themes appear to be consistent across such situations of loss.[104]

1 Grieving is a normal process

Grieving is a healing process that allows a person to progress from a state of significant disorganisation to a position of being able to reinvest in life. Many theories have been proposed to explain the mechanism of the grieving process. These theories may guide the understanding of where on the journey of grieving a person may be situated and can assist in reassuring a person of the normality of this often frightening experience. It is essential not to lose sight of the central role of the grieving person in understanding their personal journey through grief, and to be aware of the risk of imposing one's own values. A practitioner must bring to the care of those who grieve a respect for the individual and a willingness to listen.

The experience of loss is integrated into the basis psychological functioning of a person. It is important to remember that there are two sides of loss: growth and deterioration. The likelihood that a person will gain maturity in thought and behaviour (growth) through successful integration of loss will be influenced by the environment in which the person grieves, as well as personal factors. An understanding of loss as being integrated rather than resolved allows acceptance of aspects of loss such as the ongoing relationships that people have with the deceased, known in the literature as 'continuing bonds'.[105] It also acknowledges the concept of chronic sorrow.[106]

2 Dealing with loss is a very individual, mostly private, and even at times lonely experience

Many factors will affect the severity of a person's individual reaction to loss: factors related to the person him- or herself, factors related to the particular situation of loss, and factors external to the person. These may include:

- Where the woman and the 'significant others' in her life are located in the grieving process
- The importance and meaning of the loss in the life of the woman
- The circumstances surrounding the loss. Was the loss sudden or anticipated? Does it remain chronic? Is there guilt, shame or blame associated with the loss?
- The support available. Does the woman perceive that she has sufficient support? Remember that proximity of others does not always mean the provision of emotional support appropriate for the woman's needs.
- The woman herself. Aspects of the person of the woman herself have been found to affect her grieving: her age, personal beliefs, values and attitudes, personality or temperament, and how resilient she has been to past events.
- Individual culture. Each culture will have its own accepted knowledge, values and norms. Whether the 'culture' is that of the family, ethnic background or occupation, each will be moulded into the woman's 'individual culture'. There is a whole feminine culture that influences the way women deal with adversity. Whether it is generic, evolutionary, socialised or imposed on women, such a feminine culture can affect both a woman's interpretation of and reaction to loss.

3 Loss threatens a person's sense of safety, mastery and control

Loss can make the world a less predictable, more fearful place. Care of many of those faced with loss therefore will fundamentally involve trying to rebuild a sense of safety and control within a changed world.

4 Losses rarely exist alone

When loss enters the world of a person, it is not usually an isolated entity divorced from other elements of the person's life. Associated or secondary losses may influence the ability of the person to adapt to the primary loss. Indeed, consequences of divorce such as selling a home, perhaps moving away from friends and supports, financial hardship and estrangement from extended family may profoundly undermine the capacity of the woman to adapt to breakdown of the marriage.

5 A person experiencing loss remains a person

Natural concern by others for the woman experiencing a loss may result in a preoccupation with the loss, and the woman becoming defined by that loss. A woman who suffers from HIV or mental illness will often be defined in the health systems more in terms of her illness than her own person. A number of consequences can occur as a result of a person being defined thus. All actions and behaviours, even normal developmental changes or moods, may be considered a consequence of the loss. As a result, normal behavioural controls may be withdrawn or altered. In addition, with attention focused on the loss, other characteristics of the person, or other activities that could afford her some sense of mastery or control, can be overlooked.

Selected situations of loss

Death

Reactions of individuals to conjugal bereavement vary widely; widows have generally been found to fare better than widowers. Over time, many widows, particularly older widows, while deeply distressed by the death, report increasing levels of self-esteem and well-being as grief abates as the result of growing confidence in their ability to live independently. Ambivalence that existed between spouses prior to the death can affect reactions to bereavement. In this age of growing numbers of separated, divorced, de facto and lesbian relationships, reactions to the death of a spouse or partner can be affected by societal sanctions and confusion about the accepted role and reactions of the 'widow'.

Compared to spousal death, mothers consistently report short- and long-term effects following the death of a child. A mother's whole view of the world is changed by the death of a child. The intensity of the relationship between a mother and child has at times seen mothers describing the loss of a child as a loss of part of the self. Guilt can be a significant part of the grief of parents, particularly in the case of accidental death.

Obstetric losses

It is important to remember that spontaneous abortion (miscarriage), stillbirth and neonatal death for most mothers constitute the death of a child. It has been suggested that childbirth may constitute a traumatic event in cases when there is (a) fear for the life of mother and child, overtaking any feelings of anticipation, (b) inadequate pain control or its intensity is completely unanticipated by the mother, or (c) non-elective, instrument-assisted or surgical delivery.

Parenting losses

Many women dream of becoming mothers. The assumptive world of many women concerning motherhood is related to either their own experiences of being parented, or social or media images of motherhood. Many are not prepared for the realities of motherhood. Many situations of parenting will involve a loss of the assumptions held by many women of idealised parenting. Loss for a mother may occur with the birth of an intellectually or physically impaired child, living with an attention deficit and hyperactivity disorder (ADHD) child or spending a great deal of time dealing with behavioural problems. How this loss is grieved and how meaning is made of these events can have ongoing and serious repercussions for the relationship between mother and child.

Women requiring care and women as carers

In Western cultures, the average life expectancy of women is usually a number of years longer than it is for men. This is likely to lead to differences in care needs and ageing. For example, care facilities for the aged may have a more female focus. Also, a new population mix can emerge in older ages not seen in younger age groups. In addition, offspring are more likely to be called upon to care for mothers, rather than fathers, which can lead to particular social matrix disruptions within the home. With ageing and illness come many losses for women (Section 17).

It is also more common for women to be caregivers of the young, the ill or the older person. As such, women are often socialised to accept the role of carer, as evidenced by the lower tendency for female spousal caregivers to use institutional and respite care for their partners than male spousal caregivers. Female caregivers appear to have higher levels of anxiety, sadness and anger than male caregivers.

Becoming a caregiver can also involve loss: loss of personal time, loss of social interactions if isolated by caregiving demands, loss of financial security, loss of perceived future, and loss of loved one if caring for one suffering a degenerative condition.

Loss and depression/anxiety

It has been suggested that some losses are more likely to lead to depression, in particular those that made a person feel deeply humiliated or diminished in their interactions with others.[107]

Traumatic loss

Some situations of loss in the lives of women that involve trauma are associated with an intense sense of loss of safety. For example, becoming a victim of crime, suffering from domestic violence or being involved in a serious accident or disaster can have both short- and long-term serious effects on women. While many women recover from such situations without serious long-term problems, others may be affected in the long-term through the development of conditions such as post-traumatic stress disorder (PTSD), clinical depression or anxiety disorders.

Conclusion

If a much broader view of loss than only bereavement is taken, it can be seen that loss is an integral part of the lives of all women at some stage. Consequently, loss is an important part of the daily interactions of practitioners with their female patients/clients. Loss is one of the few concepts that can be applied to most of the situations of adversity experienced by women, and understanding this can enhance the care offered to women.

Death and dying

All of us die. As members of Western societies, it is unusual for people to experience death first-hand, and many do not know how to react to death. It is vital that health practitioners respond to death appropriately. The quality of the physical and emotional care offered to a dying person, and of those critical interactions between health professionals and surviving friends and relatives, can affect the long-term psychological well-being of bereaved people.

The four most common causes of death are cancer, cardiovascular disease, cerebrovascular disease and respiratory disease. Death occurring quickly and unexpectedly is thus as common as death with a predictable palliative phase. However, many people suffer a non-fatal cardiovascular event or stroke, then subsequently die of a second event. These people live in the shadow of death, and may also be considered to be 'palliative', but with an unpredictable time course. Quality of life and maximising function are the key issues for health professionals associated with these people. The elements of a 'good' death have been described by Clark (Box 3.7).

BOX 3.7 Elements of a 'good death' in modern Western culture[108]

- Pain-free death
- Open acknowledgement of the imminence of death
- Death at home, surrounded by family and friends
- An 'aware' death in which personal conflicts and unfinished business are resolved
- Death as personal growth
- Death according to personal preference and in a manner that resonates with the person's individuality

Most of the care that palliative care patients receive occurs in the home. Most patients want to die at home, but only 30 per cent actually achieve this. Another third remain at home until the final 1–3 days. Preference for home care falls steadily over the course of the illness as the care increases in intensity. In one study of home care, about three-quarters of patients and half the relatives remained composed and often enjoyed life. About 1 in 20 patients suffered serious depression or anxiety; relatives manifested depression in 1 in 5 cases, and anxiety in 1 in 6 cases. In acute care settings, patients can receive aggressive treatment out of proportion to the likelihood of success or enhanced quality of life. Views of patients about the aims and methods of treatment should be sought in all cases, but in hospitals in particular.

Breaking bad news

Bad news will be delivered to people whose prognosis is poor, and to their relatives and close friends. It will also be delivered to the circle of people around persons who have died, in both expected and unexpected circumstances. People do not remember much of a consultation where bad news is delivered. Practitioners need to ensure that the important messages of the consultation are retained. These are:

- For the person being told of a terminal prognosis:
  - There is nearly always something positive that can be done to minimise symptoms.
  - Help will be available whenever it is needed.
  - The patient and their family are not going to be abandoned.

- Where a patient has died suddenly, the message to be conveyed includes:
  - What happened.
  - That everything reasonable was done to prevent death.
  - What happens now.

The delivery of bad news takes time and foresight. The essential steps are shown in Box 3.8. Try to set aside sufficient time if you know that the consultation is coming up.

BOX 3.8 **Delivering bad news**[109]

- Allow sufficient time.
- Encourage the presence of a friend of close relative.
- Write down the key messages and patient choices.
- Encourage questions—write them down for the next visit.
- Arrange follow-up.

It goes without saying that promised availability and support *must* be backed up with a solid plan to provide the promised support. Whoever has the responsibility to provide that support must ensure that they are reliably available, and that patients have clear instructions on how to contact the support. Locum and after-hours services need enough clinical detail on hand to provide meaningful support.[109] Arrange routine follow-up to bereaved relatives. Use bereavement services and counsellors if they are available.

The experience of dying

Patients who are dying may be aware of what is happening, and health professionals should assume awareness as they manage them and their carers. A study of near-death experiences in cardiac arrest survivors reports that a fifth of patients reported this phenomenon.[110] A core set of experiences including an awareness of being dead, positive emotions and a constellation of experiences described variously as moving through a tunnel, communication with light or colours, and observation of a celestial landscape were described. It is described as a pleasant experience, and survivors lost the fear of death. Some reported an out-of-body experience where they were aware of, and could describe in detail, the process of resuscitation.

Physical symptoms

Death can occur in minutes, or can be the culmination of months of worsening symptoms. Patients who die quickly may have severe distress, or be unconscious and not suffer physically at all. In the acute setting, when patients are clearly at risk of death, it is essential to consider symptomatic treatment at the same time as trying to treat the illness. Adequate analgesia delivered by effective routes can minimise the physical distress. Five milligrams of morphine can be delivered to most adults safely as an intravenous bolus. More should be delivered slowly over 2–5 minutes depending on response. The dose will depend on whether the patient is opioid-naive or not. People on regular opioids may need much larger doses. As a guide, one-sixth of the daily dose is a reasonable bolus dose, with one-third delivered intravenously and the remainder as an intramuscular preparation.[111] It is important to be aware that different opioids and routes of administration have different bioavailabilities, and a conversion chart should be consulted when assessing the correct dose. Appropriate sedation can also be useful when severe symptoms such as choking or massive exsanguination are occurring. In this situation consider intravenous or rectal clonazepam 0.5 mg or diazepam 2.5–5 mg.[111]

Patients at the terminal phase of a long illness still suffer pre-existing symptoms, particularly pain. They should remain on the medication that controlled the symptoms, if this can be delivered appropriately. Systemic routes should be chosen if swallowing is a problem or absorption is questionable. All non-essential medications should be ceased. Two major symptoms are frequently present in the dying person.

1 Altered breathing, particularly rattly breathing, is common. Use subcutaneous or intramuscular anticholinergic agents to minimise this—eg hyoscine hydrobromide 0.4 mg subcutaneously four-hourly, or 0.8–1.6 mg/day as a continuous subcutaneous infusion.[111]
2 Muscle twitching and restlessness. Effective medications for this condition are clonazepam or diazepam in the same dosages as above.[111]

Both of these symptoms can cause considerable distress to onlookers, but are probably not distressing to the patient. Patients are often hypoxic, uraemic and partly conscious at best at this stage.

Psychosocial–spiritual aspects

The threat of death or impending death forces patients to address a series of losses, re-evaluate life goals and achievements, and confront issues of meaning and purpose (Section 17).

What to do when someone dies

Several tasks arise for the health professional at a person's death. The legal requirements differ from jurisdiction to jurisdiction, but the main aspects are:

- Confirming that life is extinct
- Determining a cause of death, confirming that no suspicious circumstances exist, and issuing a death certificate
- Notifying the coroner or police if a death certificate cannot be issued.

The relatives or friends of the deceased person may require considerable support at this time, particularly if the death is unexpected or traumatic. This may involve listening, arranging active support in making funeral arrangements, contacting close friends, and/or religious support if desired.

Death marks closure of relationships. It is important to give relatives and close friends the opportunity to spend time with the body, in order to pay their last respects. Removal of a body need not take place immediately after death. Strong emotions may be exhibited, and the practitioner needs to be prepared for this. Be aware of cultural and personal differences in responses to death.

Caring for bereaved relatives and friends

Bereavement is the task of adjusting psychologically, emotionally and practically to a loss. The process can be abnormal, and this can lead to significant long-term psychosocial morbidity. Also be aware of the increased risk of physical illness, depression and suicide in newly bereaved persons.

It is strongly recommended that relatives or close friends be followed up after death, to monitor this process. Many communities have excellent bereavement support programs and trained bereavement counsellors. Bereaved people can benefit greatly from what they have to offer.

1 Normal anatomy and common conditions

A Vaginal examination in the dorsal position. Using a Sim's speculum: descent of the uterus is seen.

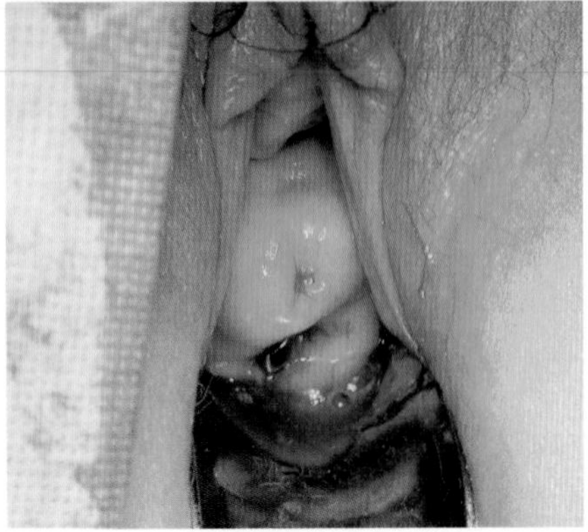

B Vaginal examination in the left lateral position. Using the Sim's speculum: slight anterior wall prolapse is seen.

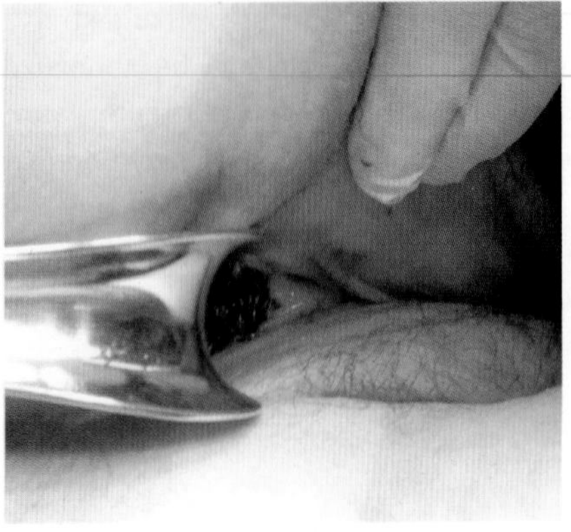

C Nulliparous cervix. The cervical os is rounded. Note 'egg white' ovulating mucus coming from os.

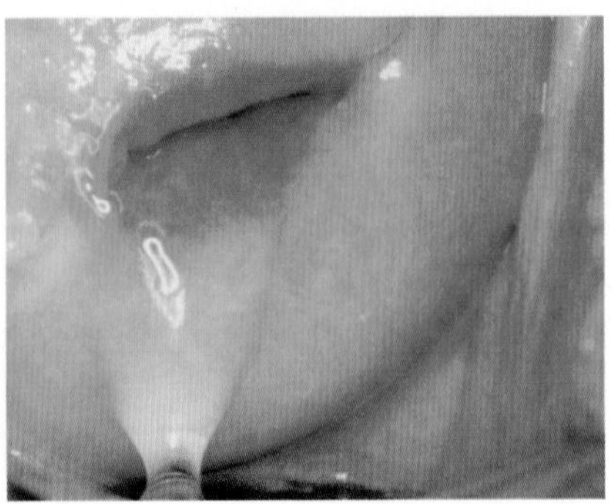

D Multiparous cervix. The cervical os is oval-shaped.

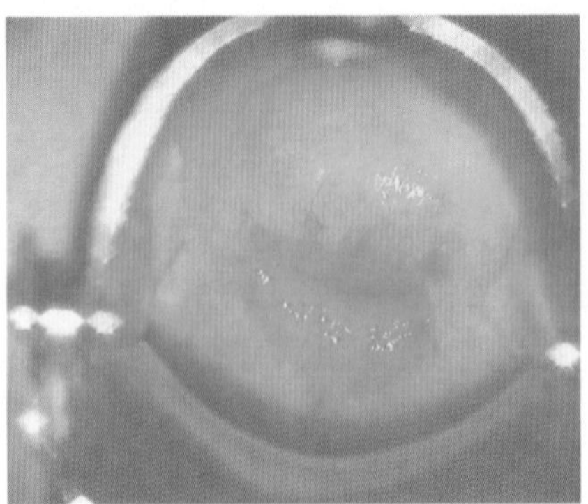

E Postmenopausal cervix. The atrophic tissue shows fine capillaries through the thin surface. The squamo-columnar junction is within the endocervical canal.

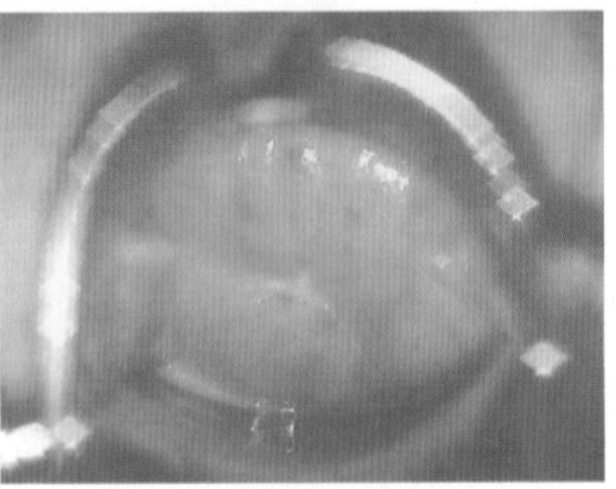

F An irregular squamo-columnar junction (SCJ). This demonstrates the importance of visualising the cervix when taking a Pap test to include the SCJ.

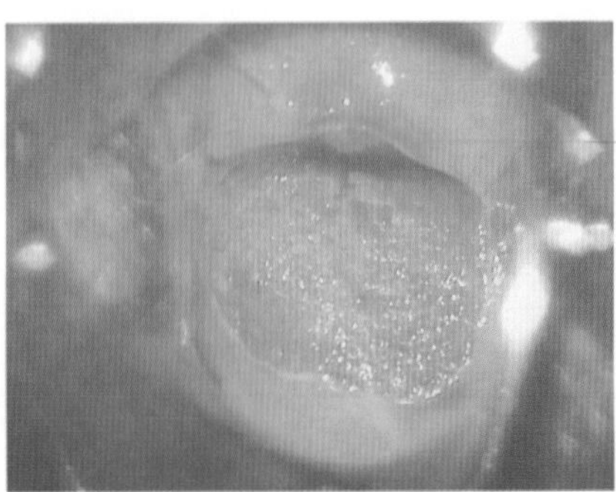

A In the reproductive years, the vulva varies in amount of hair, length of the perineal body, size and shape of the clitoris and labia (frequently varying between sides in the same woman).

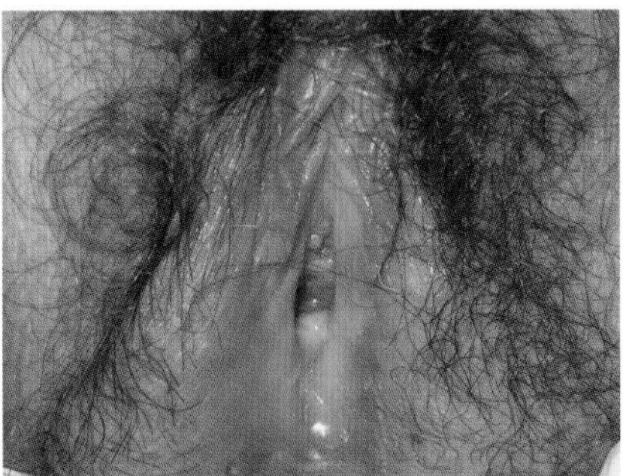

B The vulva in a postmenopausal woman. There is atrophy of the right labia majora, with signs of excoriation from lichen simplex chronicus. Normal thin left labia.

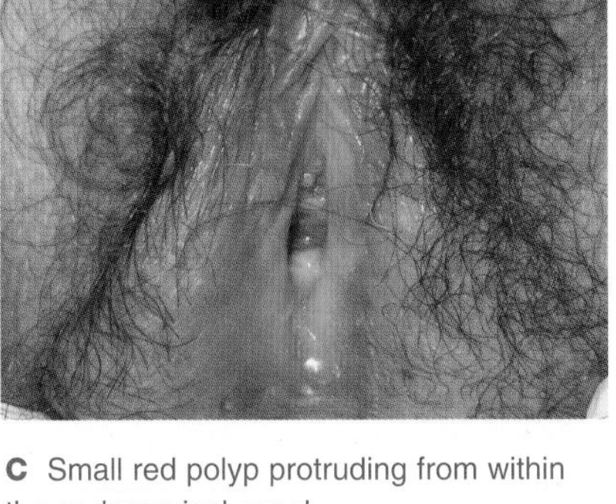

C Small red polyp protruding from within the endocervical canal

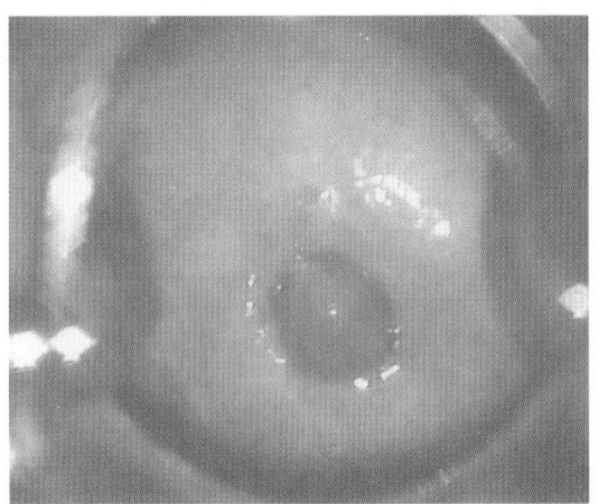

D Procidentia or complete uterine prolapse. The cervix is seen at the tip of the protrusion, with the vaginal wall behind, beneath which lies the uterus.

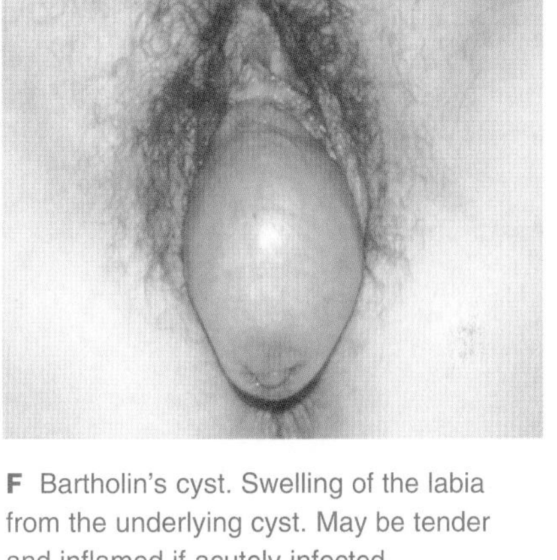

E Pelvic organs seen through the laparoscope. The uterus is midline, with normal ovaries (white) at either side.

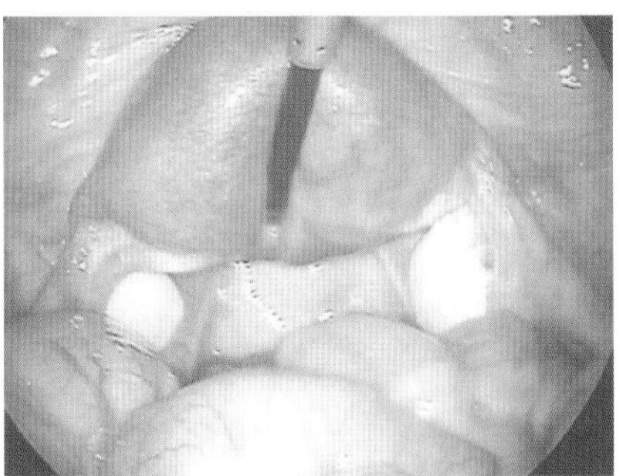

F Bartholin's cyst. Swelling of the labia from the underlying cyst. May be tender and inflamed if acutely infected.

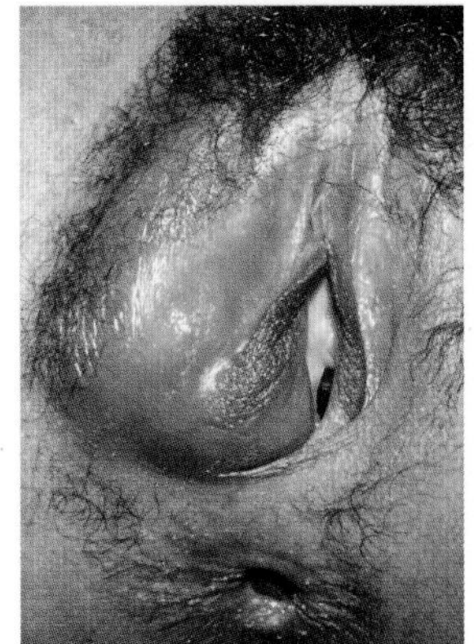

SECTION 4

Part 2
Early life

Hormones and early development

Hormones through the life cycle

Many aspects of female growth, development and adult life, both reproductive and post reproductive, are unequivocally linked to hormonal changes, particularly those of pituitary and ovarian origin. These include pubertal development, ovulation and menstruation, pregnancy and the events surrounding the menopause (Table 4.1).

In the fetus the structural and physiological components of normal function are established and the newborn axis is able to function when separated from the placenta. In infancy and childhood when physical development is the priority, a gradual increase in gonadal function and responsiveness to central stimulation occurs. At a critical stage in this process, puberty is triggered with the development of secondary sexual characteristics and reproductive ability. During the reproductive years a critical decline in primordial follicles ultimately leads to the menopause, from which a hormonal state of oestrogen deficiency ensues.

TABLE 4.1 Women's hormone levels through the menstrual cycle and post menopause

	Early follicular	Mid-cycle	Mid-luteal	Post menopausal
FSH (IU/l)	3–8	10–25	1–6	20–100
LH (IU/l)	3–8	20–80	4–10	10–40
Oestradiol (pmol/l)	100–400	800–1800	300–700	< 20–80
Progesterone (nmol/l)	0.3–3	3–5	15–80	< 1
Testosterone (nmol/l)	0.6–2.2	0.8–2.5	0.8–2.5	0.8–2.5
DHEAS (µmol/l)	3–12	3–12	3–12	2–8
Inhibin A (pg/ml)	< 10	20–45	45–75	< 10
Inhibin B (pg/ml)	72–100	100–150	< 20	< 20
DHEA (nmol/l)	3–35	3–35	3–35	*

* Decreases with age; however, measurement is difficult.

Fetal life

Development and structure of the ovary

In human embryos, primordial germ cells reach the genital ridges from the yolk sac endoderm at 5–6 weeks post fertilisation.[1] The primordial follicles are the basic reproductive units of the ovary. All dominant pre-ovulatory follicles are selected from the pool of germ cells at 24 weeks gestation. Each primordial follicle is composed of an immature oocyte surrounded by a single epithelial cell layer called granulosa (or follicle) cells. These are surrounded by a basal lamina creating a microenvironment that does not directly interact with surrounding cells. All primordial follicles are formed before birth and few remain at menopause[2,3] (Table 4.2).

TABLE 4.2 Development of the ovary and oocytes

Stage	Development
5–6 weeks	Primordial germ cells reach the genital ridges from the yolk sac endoderm
10 weeks	Cells differentiate into oogonia; gradual migration of stromal cells from the medulla. The ovary is morphologically distinguishable
12 weeks	Germ cells in meiosis (oocytes) and interstitial cells begin to appear
20–24 weeks	Primordial follicles are formed
24 weeks	Number of germ cells reaches a peak of approximately 6–7 million
Birth	Two million primordial follicles present
Birth to menarche	Number of primordial follicles decreases from several million to several hundred thousand
Reproductive years	Four hundred will develop to full maturity, reach ovulation and corpus luteum formation; 99.9% become atretic after recruitment
Menopause	Few if any remaining

The fetal hypothalamus and pituitary

Gonadotrophin-releasing hormone (GnRH) is a decapeptide neurohormone produced by neuronal cell bodies within the medial basal hypothalamus. GnRH neurons originate outside the central nervous system in the olfactory placode.[4] They migrate along the olfactory nerve up the nasal septum, through the cribriform plate to the forebrain, eventually reaching the arcuate nucleus. Kallmann's syndrome, which is characterised by anosmia and hypogonadotropic hypogonadism, is an X-linked disorder in which this migratory path is disrupted.

Pulsatile secretion of GnRH is essential to the initiation and maintenance of reproductive functioning in humans and results in secretion of follicle-stimulating hormone (FSH) and luteinising hormone (LH) from the anterior pituitary. By mid-gestation, the GnRH pulse generator and the anterior pituitary have become a functioning unit, the inhibitory feedback mechanisms are developed, the hypothalamus secretes less GnRH and the pituitary gonadotrophin levels decline.[5]

Gonadal steroids

The young ovary is unable to synthesise oestradiol due to a lack of the aromatase enzyme. Therefore, most oestrogen is manufactured by the placenta from androgens produced in the fetal liver and adrenal. Oestriol is the major oestrogen produced by the fetus while in the mother oestrone and 17 β-oestradiol are the major contributors. During late gestation oestrogen levels rise in the fetus and especially in the mother. This elevation is not reflected in a comparable change in bioavailable oestradiol because of the accompanying 5–10 fold increase in maternal sex hormone binding globulin (SHBG) that persists until one week after delivery.[6] Fetal SHBG is only one-twentieth of the maternal level.

The role of hormones in the sexual differentiation of the fetus

In the human, sexual differentiation occurs initially with the development of the gonads, accessory ducts and then external genitalia. The gonads are derived from the coelomic epithelium, the mesenchyme and the primordial germ cells. In the presence of the testis-determining factor, SRY (sex-determining region of the Y chromosome), the bipotential gonad develops into a testis.[7] Normal ovarian development occurs if there is no Y chromosome. The fetal testis produces hormones that stimulate and inhibit the reproductive organs (Figure 4.1). Fetal testosterone secretion is mediated primarily by placental gonadotrophins as normal male sexual differentiation occurs in male apituitary and anencephalic fetuses.[8]

Administration of androgens to the female fetus before 12 weeks gestation results in fusion of the labio-scrotal folds and clitoral enlargement. If exposure occurs after this time, there is only clitoral enlargement.

By late fetal life the reproductive axis is fully developed. The ovaries contain millions of primordial follicles, each encapsulated by theca interna. The growth and maintenance of these follicles requires pituitary gonadotrophin secretion; however, levels remain suppressed by circulating sex steroids of fetal and placental origin. At term the cord blood contains very high placental oestrogen and progesterone levels. The most significant endocrine sex difference is the higher testosterone in the male newborn thought to be mediated by human chorionic gonadotrophin (HCG).[9]

FIGURE 4.1 Hormones and sexual differentiation of the fetus

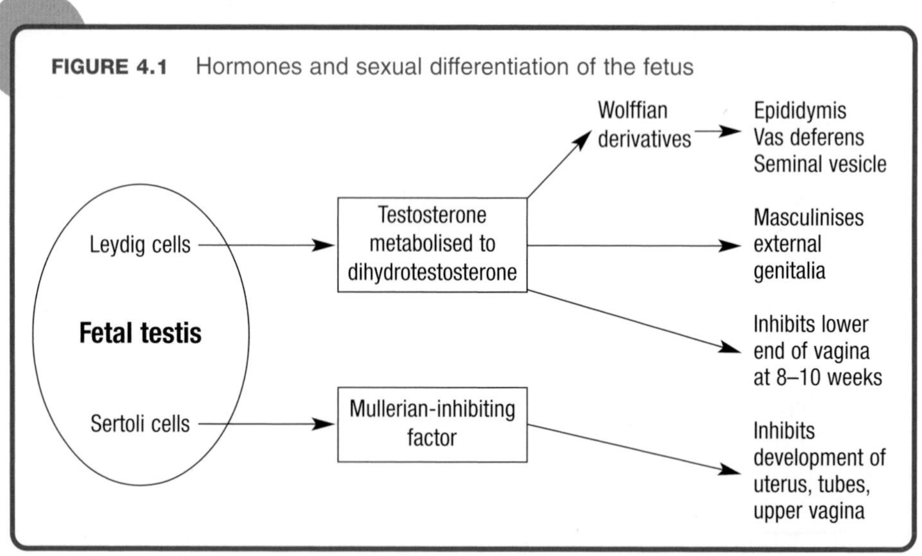

After birth

In the first week following separation of the placenta, HCG, oestrogen and progesterone levels abruptly decline. Testosterone levels in the male fall to levels similar to those in females as HCG is no longer detectable. This precipitous decline results in a gonadotrophin surge as there is no longer suppression from circulating sex steroids. The ovarian response to the gonadotrophin surge is modest. Mean levels of oestradiol are higher in the first four months than in later childhood. A clinical indicator of elevated oestradiol is the frequently seen breast enlargement of infancy, which usually resolves by three years.

In children aged 4 to 8 years, gonadotrophin and sex steroid production is maintained at low levels. However, this stage is far from quiescent in terms of reproductive development. Pulsatile GnRH secretion with low amplitude and long periodicity favours greater FSH than LH responsiveness at the pituitary. There is gradual enlargement of the ovaries, follicular turnover and increase in follicular size with age. Inhibin B and oestradiol are both generally low but measurable in about 50–60 per cent of girls in pre-puberty, indicating that some gonadotrophin-responsive follicular activity is occurring at this stage. Uterine growth occurs from the age of seven with a greater enlargement of the corpus than the cervix.[10–12]

Adrenarche

The adrenal cortex is responsible for the secretion of three different classes of steroid hormones. These are glucocorticoids, mineralocorticoids and adrenal androgens. The adrenal androgens include dehydroepiandrosterone (DHEA), dehydroepiandrosterone sulphate (DHEAS) and androstenedione (which are more correctly termed androgen precursors or pro-androgens) and testosterone. The androgen precursors are rendered biologically active in peripheral tissues (skin and liver) when converted to testosterone and dihydrotestosterone. Adrenarche occurs when the secretion of these hormones is increased, from about the age of six years. The stimulus to this increase is not yet known. Serum levels and urinary secretion rates of DHEA and DHEAS increase progressively from adrenarche, to reach a peak by about the mid-twenties. Adrenarche is independent of adrenocorticotropin (ACTH), gonadotrophin and GnRH secretion.[9]

Female puberty

Puberty is the period that occurs between childhood and adulthood during which secondary sexual characteristics develop and reproductive function is attained. These changes result from an increase in secretion of gonadotrophins and gonadal steroids.

An increase in pulsatile GnRH release occurs, resulting in enhanced LH pulsatility, initially during the night, and later throughout the day. This leads to a gradual increase in gonadal steroid levels. Recent studies of prepubertal Rhesus monkeys have suggested that the central inhibition of GnRH release is due to inhibitory G-aminobutyric acid (GABA) neurotransmission. Why GABA inhibition subsides at the onset of puberty is not yet known.[13]

Age of pubertal onset

Marshall and Tanner's classic studies on height, height velocity and pubertal staging remain the basis for clinical evaluation of puberty in females (Figures 4.2 and 4.3). They described five stages, stage 1 being prepubertal, stage 5 representing adult pattern of pubic hair and breast development and the other three stages being

FIGURE 4.2 Tanner stages of pubertal breast development (1–5)[14]

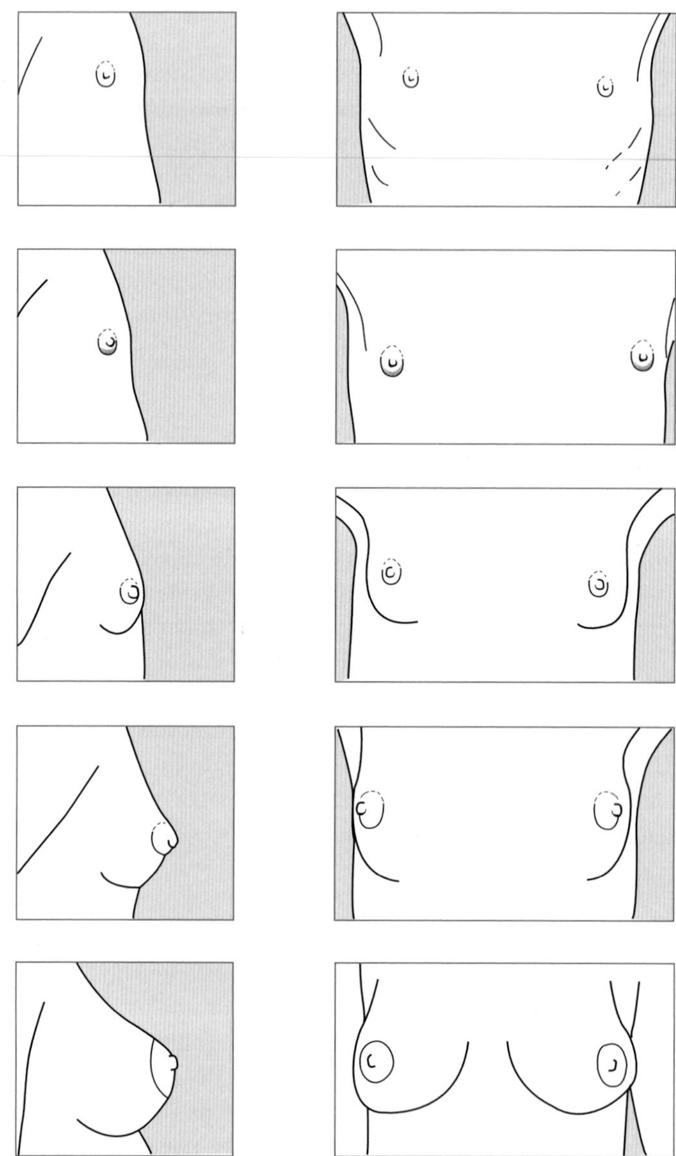

FIGURE 4.3 Tanner stages of pubic hair development in girls (1–5)[14]

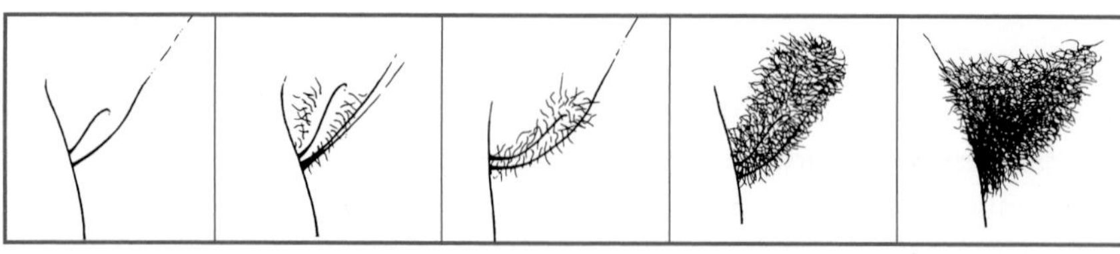

intermediate.[14] During puberty (Tanner stages 2–5) levels of circulating gonadotrophins and sex steroids increase and subsequently show the cyclic pattern characteristic of ovulation and menses.

Cyclic changes in gonadotrophins have been shown to occur even in early puberty and before menarche.[15] This may occur when periodic follicle recruitment successfully results in an increase in oestrogen production. The endometrium may become primed and bleed when the follicles become atretic, resulting in menstrual bleeding without ovulation. Within a year of the first menstrual bleed (menarche), the adult pattern occurs.

Mean oestradiol and testosterone levels increase through puberty. The gonadal steroids, of themselves and through increase in growth hormone secretion, cause the physical manifestations of puberty which include breast development, female fat distribution, vaginal and uterine development, growth velocity and skeletal maturation. Adrenal androgens converted in the periphery to testosterone are mediators of acne, change in pubic hair and accelerated growth velocity of adolescence.

Early studies of girls in puberty showed a progressive increase in immunoreactive inhibin from stage 1 to stage 4 of pubertal development. Later studies, with assays specific for inhibin A and B, have shown that inhibin B increases with progression through puberty (Tanner stages 2–3). This supports the observation that inhibin B is produced by small antral follicles in response to gonadotrophin stimulation. It also suggests that as puberty progresses more antral follicles are recruited.

In Tanner stage 3 all girls had measurable inhibin B and the median level was higher than adult women sampled randomly throughout the menstrual cycle. This would indicate that that there is a period of consistently high ovarian stimulation before onset of menses. In late puberty and adulthood, mean levels decline primarily because of the low concentrations characteristic of the luteal phase of the menstrual cycle. Serum inhibin A levels progressively increase through the Tanner stages, reaching a peak in adulthood. This is consistent with the observation that inhibin A is produced by the dominant follicle and the corpus luteum. In terms of detecting the onset of puberty, measurement of the inhibins does not give additional information beyond that provided by LH and oestradiol.

The reproductive years

From the age of 20 to 40 years, the menstrual cycle is regular, with a median cycle interval of 28 days. For 12–18 months after menarche and 5–8 years before the menopause, these cycle intervals are more variable, frequently with anovulation and irregular menses.[16]

The menstrual cycle is divided into two phases, based primarily on changes in endometrial and ovarian histology coupled with hormonal measurements (Figure 4.4). The follicular phase begins on day 1 and lasts 12–16 days until ovulation occurs. This is followed by the luteal phase, which lasts 10–16 days and is characterised by the development and involution of the corpus luteum. The endometrium undergoes proliferative change in response to rising oestradiol concentration, and secretory change in response to the added action of progesterone provided by the corpus

FIGURE 4.4 The menstrual cycle: endometrial changes, vascular changes of the aterioles in the endometrium, and hormone changes

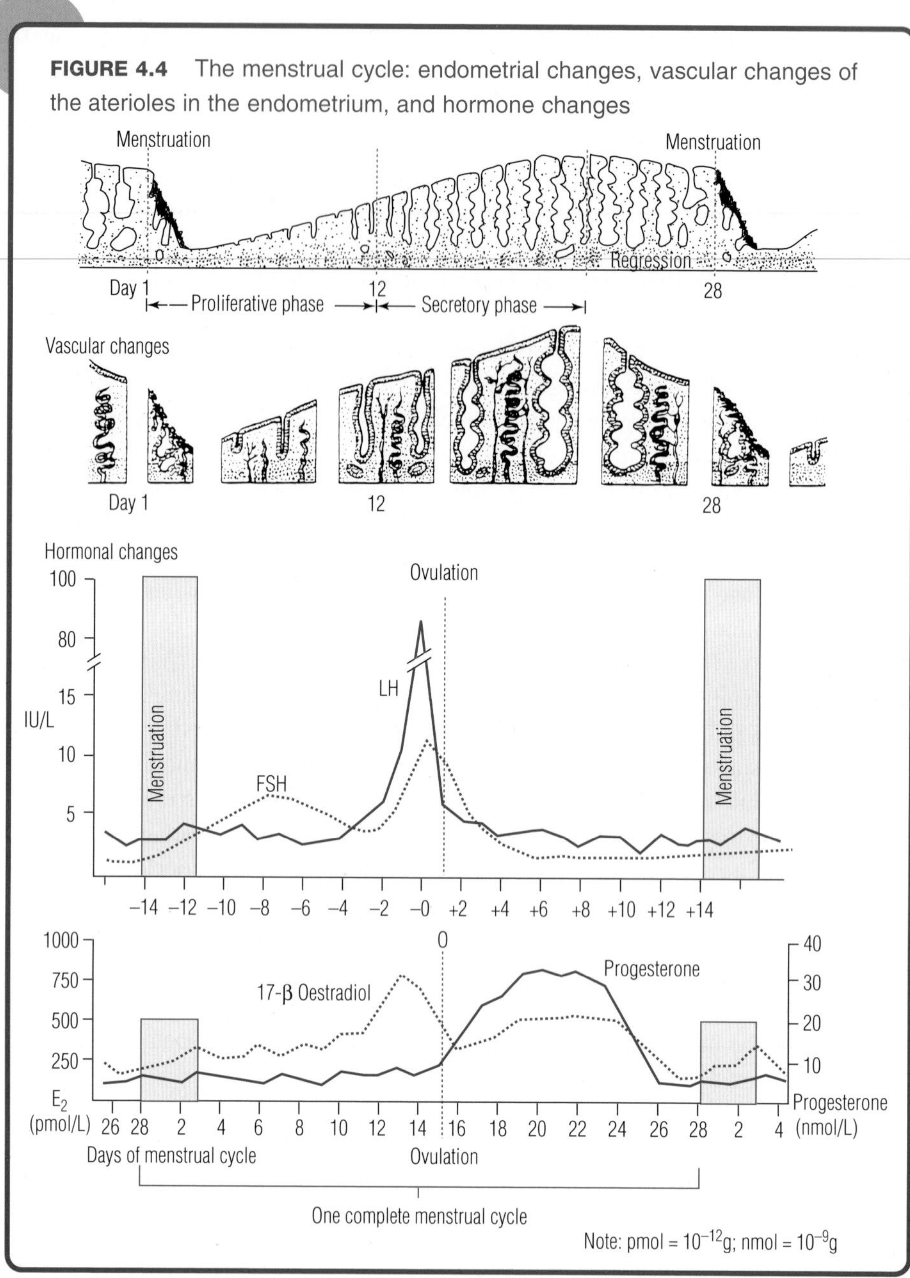

luteum. In the absence of a fertilised ovum, the corpus luteum involutes and shedding of the endometrium occurs.

Hormones during the menstrual cycle

GnRH

GnRH is essential for normal ovarian cyclicity. In humans GnRH pulsatility is inferred from LH measurements. In the early follicular phase, LH pulse amplitude is constant and pulses occur every 1–2 hours. In the luteal phase, LH pulse amplitude is more variable and the frequency slower, with large amplitude peaks occuring every 2–6 hours. However, the mid-cycle gonadotrophin surge is not dependent on variation in frequency or amplitude of the GnRH pulse generator. For example, in hypogonadotropic women who receive GnRH at a fixed hourly interval, the gonadotrophin surge occurs when the oestradiol level reaches a critical threshhold for approximately 36 hours. Ovulation then occurs 24 hours later. This indicates that oestradiol acts directly on the pituitary to permit an LH surge which in turn triggers ovulation.[17]

FSH

FSH level starts to rise during the last two or three days of the preceding menstrual cycle. It peaks early in the follicular phase and then declines due to feedback inhibition from inhibin B, inhibin A and oestradiol.[18,19] There is a pre-ovulatory surge in FSH followed by baseline levels throughout the luteal phase. High FSH levels in the early follicular phase result in recruitment and maturation of a number of follicles. FSH concentration is higher than LH, which is released in pulses every 90–100 minutes. With maturation of the developing follicle the concentration of oestrogen rises slowly then more abruptly to reach peak levels 24–48 hours prior to the LH surge. The increase in serum oestradiol together with a late follicular rise in progesterone acts to increase gonadotrophin responsiveness to GnRH, culminating in the LH surge. This lasts approximately two days and is followed 16–24 hours later by the release of the dominant follicle.

With the LH surge, the oestradiol concentration drops rapidly until corpus luteum functioning is established. Levels then rise for 7–8 days after ovulation and decline in the late luteal phase to low levels as the corpus luteum involutes.[9] Following ovulation, progesterone levels rise to reach a peak in 6–8 days. As the corpus luteum involutes, the progesterone concentration declines to follicular phase levels just prior to menses.[20,21]

The precise factors that determine which of these follicles will become the dominant or ovulatory follicle are not yet known. FSH induces the appearance of LH receptors on granulosa cells. It also increases the presence of aromatase required for the conversion of theca cell produced androstenedione to oestradiol.

Inhibins

Inhibins are glycopeptide hormones produced predominantly in the gonads (though also placental and adrenal tissue), in response to FSH stimulation. Production of the inhibins feeds back onto the pituitary-regulating FSH secretion in a classic endocrine negative feedback loop. In adult females, inhibin A is produced by the dominant follicle and corpus luteum, whilst inhibin B is produced by the pre-ovulatory follicles.[18,22] Inhibins are a peripheral indicator of granulosa cell function.

Prolactin

Prolactin (PRL) is found in the human pituitary from the twelfth week of gestation and levels rise rapidly during the last weeks of intrauterine life.[23] At birth, umbilical vein PRL is higher than maternal serum levels; however, they rapidly decline to reach prepubertal levels at one week after birth. The role of PRL in the fetus is currently thought to relate to lung maturation and fetal osmoregulation. Prolactin levels remain constant throughout childhood, then rise at the onset of puberty in girls only to reach the adult female range. Levels decline after the menopause.

Prolactin is a single polypeptide composed of 198 amino acids. It is secreted by the pituitary lactotrophs which occupy approximately 50 per cent of the pituitary cell population. Prolactin release is predominantly under tonic inhibitory control by prolactin-inhibiting factors (PIF), particularly dopamine. Prolactin release is also possible under situations of maximal inhibitory stimuli, indicating a role for prolactin-releasing factors (PRF). This observation accounts for the elevation in PRL often seen in the clinical setting of hypothyroidism. Prolactin release is not regulated by feedback signals from target tissues; rather, retrograde PRL flow acts on regulatory hypothalamic factors (autoregulation).

Prolactin release is also modified by a number of neurotransmitters, mainly serotonin, though also opioids, histamine, neurotensin and substance P. A number of peripheral hormones are modulators of PRL release. Oestrogen promotes synthesis and release of PRL and elevated PRL is often seen in therapy with the oral contraceptive pill. Progesterone administration after oestrogen priming also effects an increase in PRL levels, whilst exogenous glucocorticoids inhibit PRL gene transcription.

Sex hormone binding globulin (SHBG)

When steroids enter the bloodstream from an endogenous or exogenous source, they interact with plasma steroid-binding proteins. A dynamic equilibrium is established where some of the steroid is bound and the remainder is free in the bloodstream. The free steroid is considered the only portion available for uptake by the target tissues. The main steroid-binding proteins are sex hormone binding globulin (SHBG) and corticosteroid-binding globulin (CBG), both of which are low in concentration but have a high affinity and specificity for the sex steroids; and albumin and orosomucoid, which are in high abundance but have a low affinity for the sex steroids.

Sex hormone binding globulin binds oestradiol and testosterone and has a linear relationship with the free hormones in the bloodstream. It transports these hormones in the blood and plays a key role in the regulation of the free component. Plasma SHBG is produced by hepatocytes but little is known about the mechanisms controlling the expression of the SHBG gene in the liver. Women have about twice the level of serum SHBG of men and have a lower occupancy level of the SHBG steroid-binding site. Some factors are known to influence plasma SHBG levels (Table 4.3). The inverse relationship to body mass index may be related to insulin levels, as insulin reduces SHBG produced by HepG2 cells.[24] As obese women lose weight, the SHBG levels increase. Clinically the administration of the oral contraceptive pill, where the oestrogenic component increases the SHBG with minimal exposure to androgenic progestins, can reduce the free testosterone in the blood and decrease the androgen-dependent hair growth and acne.[25]

TABLE 4.3 Factors influencing SHBG levels in women

Increase	Decrease	No change
Obesity	Anorexia	Age
Hyperthyroidism	Hypothyroidism	Menstrual cycle
Thyroid hormones	Obesity	
Oestrogens	Levonorgestrel	
	Androgens	

Pregnancy and childbirth

While many of the hormone changes that occur during pregnancy are known (Table 4.4), the series of events that initiates the onset of labour is still not fully understood. Measurement of progesterone or oestradiol levels has not been shown to predict the onset of labour. Salivary oestriol is under investigation. Relaxin is produced by the placenta, endometrium, decidua and ovary. Its effects are on collagen and the myometrium, where it inhibits the activity.

Changes in the pituitary-ovarian axis with age

Reproductive ageing is associated with a decline in the follicular pool and a subsequent decline in fertility starting in the third decade and accelerating after the age of 35.[20] The age-related decline in follicular number is associated with a monotropic rise in FSH followed a few years later by an increase in LH. Oestradiol secretion is preserved with increasing age in women who have regular menses and has even been shown to rise during the early follicular phase with age.[21]

The menopausal transition and the menopause

Menopause is the permanent cessation of menstruation resulting from the loss of ovarian follicular activity. The perimenopause (often referred to as the menopausal transition) commences when the first features of the approaching menopause begin until at least one year after the final menstrual period (FMP). The median age of onset of the perimenopause is between 45.5 and 47.5 years, and the average time to final menses is four years.[26] The perimenopause is clinically associated with menstrual irregularity, an increased incidence of dysfunctional uterine bleeding, and the onset of oestrogen deficiency symptoms (Figure 4.5).[27,28]

The increase in FSH with age in regularly cycling women has been shown to be specifically related to a fall in inhibin B, with inhibin A preserved until the later menopausal transition.[29,30] This is in keeping with the understanding that inhibin A together with oestradiol are derived from the dominant follicle and the ensuing corpus luteum. Inhibin B is a secretory product of the small antral follicles and its circulating concentration may reflect the number of follicles recruited from the diminishing follicular pool. It may be the elevated FSH that drives the dominant follicle to secrete adequate oestradiol and inhibin A. The preservation of oestradiol

TABLE 4.4 Hormones in pregnancy

Hormone	HCG	Oestrogen	Progesterone	Prolactin
Origin	Trophoblast cells of embryo then placenta once developed	Corpus luteum then placenta	Corpus luteum until day 35 then placenta	Pituitary
Changes/effects	Maintain corpus luteum. Possible role in regulating placental production of oestrogen.	Reduces adherence of collagen fibres in connective tissue (softens cervix). Increases blood flow to uterus. Breast: increases nipple size, causes duct and alveolar development.	Muscle relaxation: keeps uterus quiescent. Also acts on bowel, stomach, intestines, ureters and veins. Rise in body temperature (0.5–1°C). Relaxant effect on brain.	Acts on alveolar cells to initiate and maintain lactation. Mobilises free fatty acids, stimulates insulin secretion but inhibits its effects at peripheral sites.
Pregnancy	Steady level	Continual rise to term		
Postpartum	Rapid fall at term. No longer detectable by day 10 post partum.	Falls 48 hours after childbirth. Non-pregnant level by day 7. Remains steady if breastfeeding; otherwise rises with follicular growth.	Rapid fall to non-pregnant level by day 7.	Initial fall in levels. Rise following suckling.
Notes	Secreted within 10 days of conception. Basis of pregnancy test.	Concentration of oestrogen (E3:E2:E1): non-pregnant 3:2:1 to pregnant 30:2:1 (E1 = oestrone, E2 = oestradiol, E3 = oestriol).		The effect of the high levels of prolactin during pregnancy on the breast is blocked by oestrogen which occupies the binding sites on the alveoli.

FIGURE 4.5 Hormones around the menopause

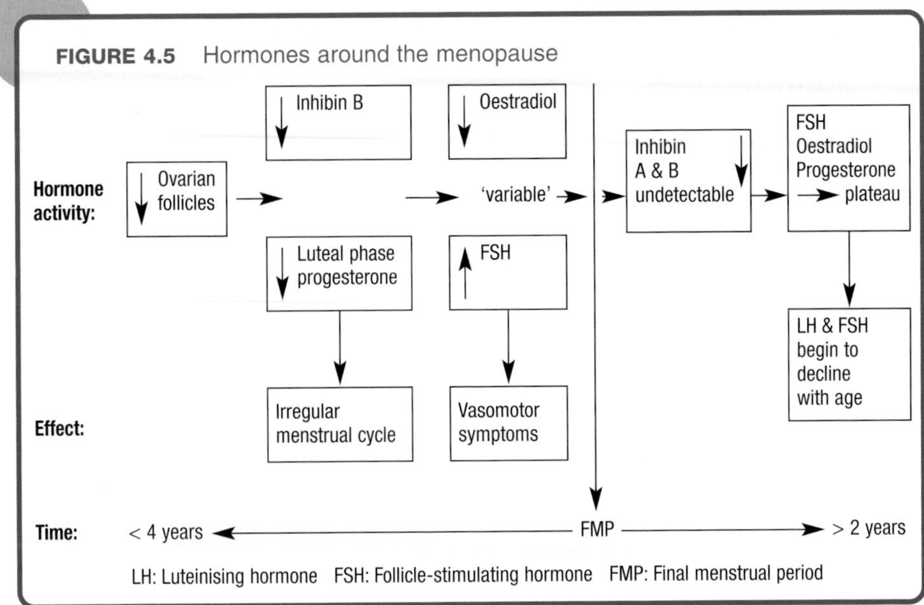

LH: Luteinising hormone FSH: Follicle-stimulating hormone FMP: Final menstrual period

into late reproductive life may be desirable for overall health including vascular and bone function.

A lack of luteal-phase rise in progesterone is a striking feature of the post menopause compared with the reproductive years. Anovulatory cycles become more frequent with increasing age and therefore the frequency of non-detectable luteal phase progesterone increases as the FMP approaches, eventually dropping to post-menopausal levels after the FMP.[31]

KEY POINT

The variability in hormonal levels during the perimenopause makes measurement of these hormones an ineffective tool in the evaluation of ovarian status at the menopausal transition.

Androgen production in women

Androgen production occurs in both the adrenals and the ovaries and is dependent upon stimulation by ACTH (adrenal) and LH (ovary). The major androgens and androgen precursors in adult women listed in descending order of serum concentration are dehydroepiandrosterone sulphate (DHEAS), DHEA, androstenedione, testosterone and dihydrotestosterone (DHT).

- *DHEAS* is produced by the zona reticularis of the adult adrenal. Serum concentrations increase from age 7 to 8 years, peak in the twenties and thirties and decline steadily with age, the rate of decline slowing by the age of 50 to 60.[32] Circulating concentrations show diurnal variation with little change during the menstrual cycle.[33] Concentrations do not change significantly during the menopausal transition and menopause. Clinical deficiency of DHEAS may occur in Addison's disease, hypopituitarism with adrenal involvement, corticosteroid therapy and oestrogen therapy. DHEAS is an important source of peripheral androgen production.

- *DHEA* and *androstenedione* are derived from the ovary and adrenal glands and the levels decline at a steady rate with age. Androstenedione shows circadian variation and a mid-cycle peak in parallel with oestradiol during the menstrual cycle.[34] Oophorectomy in postmenopausal women results in an approximately 30 per cent fall in circulating levels of androstenedione.[35] Levels are reduced in hypopituitarism and with administration of glucocorticoids.
- *Testosterone* is the most potent androgen and is secreted by the zona fasciculata (25%) and ovarian stroma (25%). The rest is derived from circulating androstenedione. Testosterone levels show circadian variation, with the highest level occurring between 4 am and midday.[36] In addition, concentrations are lowest in the early follicular phase, reach a mid-cycle peak and decline to a higher steady state in the luteal phase. Testosterone levels rise at adrenarche, reach a peak in the twenties and decline slowly with age. They do not fall at the menopausal transition or the menopause. Levels are substantially reduced in women with hypopituitarism both pre- and postmenopausally.[37] Testosterone is carried in the peripheral blood substantially bound to SHBG. During the menopausal transition SHBG levels fall substantially, increasing the free testosterone concentration.
- *Dihydrotestosterone (DHT)* is primarily a product of peripheral conversion of testosterone and circulates in low concentrations. A small quantity is secreted by the adrenal zona fasciculata.

Recent studies suggest that the postmenopausal ovary may not be a gonadotrophin-responsive androgen-producing gland as once thought, with most androgens and their precursors produced by the postmenopausal adrenal gland.[38]

Conception and implantation

Reproduction involves steps that pass from the production of ova and sperm, to fertilisation, implantation, fetal development and birth. Each of these steps is influenced by the health or ill-health of the woman. An understanding of the pathway is essential to counsel and assist women in controlling their reproduction.

Folliculogenesis

The female is born with her full stock of potential eggs (oocytes). Following replication by mitosis, the primary oocytes become surrounded by a single layer of cells forming primordial follicles. At this stage, in the month before birth, they enter the prophase of the first meiotic division. They are arrested at this stage until puberty. Most of the two million primordial follicles present at birth degenerate so that at puberty only about 250 000 remain. Of these, about 400 oocytes will ovulate in a lifetime, the rest undergoing degeneration (atresia).

From birth onwards, a large number of follicles exit the primordial pool each day and begin further development (folliculogenesis). The epithelial cell layer (granulosa cells) proliferates, an outer layer or shell is formed from the stroma (theca layer) and oocyte growth occurs. Follicles do not progress beyond this stage until sexual maturity occurs, when monthly cyclical changes take place in the ovary and uterus.

Each month a cohort of about 30 follicles become enlarged in response to rising levels of FSH. A zona pellucida develops around the oocyte and a small fluid-filled cavity (antrum) appears within the granulosa layer. Each follicle has a differing sensitivity to FSH, but the most sensitive follicle becomes the 'dominant' follicle that is destined to ovulate. This follicle secretes increasing concentrations of oestradiol, which leads to a fall in FSH. The remaining follicles, which require increased levels of FSH, thus undergo atresia. The dominant follicle can continue to grow in the face of falling levels of FSH because it has greater sensitivity to FSH and also acquires LH receptors and so has the ability to grow in response to LH. The increasing concentration of oestradiol from the dominant follicle leads to a surge in LH secretion from the pituitary that results in ovulation approximately 24–36 hours later. This pre-ovulatory follicle is now approximately 20 mm in size. The follicle wall ruptures, in part due to release of prostaglandins triggered by the LH surge. The oocyte and its surrounding corona radiata of granulosa cells is expelled. Resumption of meiotic division occurs in the oocyte, giving rise to the ovum and first polar body. Meiosis is arrested for a second time and is not completed until fertilisation takes place.

Formation of the corpus luteum

The ruptured follicle fills with blood from torn theca vessels. The remaining granulosa and theca cells enlarge and are invaded by blood vessels (neovascularisation). These granulosa lutein and theca lutein cells of the corpus luteum produce progesterone. LH sustains the development of the corpus luteum. Carotene is deposited in the cytoplasm of the cells, giving them their characteristic yellow appearance. Maximal progesterone production occurs one week after ovulation. This forms the basis for testing a day 21 serum progesterone level in women, to determine if ovulation has occurred. The corpus luteum has a lifespan of 14–16 days unless fertilisation occurs. Degeneration (luteolysis) gives rise to a pale scar on the ovarian cortex known as the corpus albicans. If fertilisation occurs, then the corpus luteum enlarges and persists under the influence of HCG from the implanting embryo.

The menstrual cycle

The ovary

The granulosa cells produce oestradiol under the influence of FSH, which is converted from an androgen precursor by the action of the enzyme aromatase. The androgen substrate is produced by the theca cells, from blood-borne cholesterol under the influence of LH. It reaches the avascular granulosa layer by diffusion. Thus follicle growth requires two hormones (FSH and LH) and two cell types (granulosa and theca).

The endometrium

Menstruation is the periodic shedding of the lining of the uterus (endometrium). The endometrium grows and matures each month in preparation for implantation of an embryo. In the absence of pregnancy, the endometrium breaks down and is shed. Regeneration and regrowth of the endometrium then begins in preparation for a potentially fertile cycle. Menstruation usually occurs at intervals of 25–35 days (average 28 days), with bleeding for 1–7 days (mean 4 days). Day 1 is defined as the day when menstruation starts. The median blood loss is 35 ml. Only the middle and superficial layers are shed with regrowth from the basal layer. Endometrium consists of glands in a cellular stroma.

- *Proliferative phase:* growth occurs by proliferation of both glands and stroma in response to increasing concentrations of oestradiol secreted by the growing follicles. The endometrium increases in thickness and mitotic figures are apparent in both glands and stroma.
- *Secretory phase:* following ovulation, progesterone secretion from the corpus luteum brings about secretory changes in the endometrium. Glands become tortuous and filled with glycogen-rich secretions, subnuclear vacuoles can be seen in the epithelium of the glands and oedema is evident in the stroma. These secretory changes are necessary if implantation is to be successful.

In the absence of pregnancy, regression of the corpus luteum brings about declining concentrations of progesterone. The withdrawal of progesterone brings about an influx of white cells and a release of prostaglandins and production of cytokines within the endometrium. The net effect is vasospasm of blood vessels in the endometrium, which results in tissue hypoxia and ischaemic necrosis. White cells migrate through capillary walls into the stroma and red cells escape into the interstitial spaces. With this ongoing interstitial leakage, blood is extruded into the uterine cavity. A plane of separation becomes evident between the basal and superficial layers and menstruation ensues (see Figure 4.4).

Conception

Fertilisation is the sequence of events that begins with the contact of the sperm and oocyte and ends with the fusion of their pronuclei (haploid nuclei of sperm and ovum) to produce a fertilised conceptus, known as a zygote (diploid). It takes place in the distal portion of the fallopian tube (ampulla) within 24 hours of ovulation. In order for sperm to penetrate the ovum, enzymes such as hyaluronidase are released from the acrosome cap of the sperm. This leads to sloughing of cells of the corona radiata around the oocyte and facilitates the passage of the sperm through the zona pellucida, the membrane surrounding the oocyte. As soon as a sperm contacts the plasma membrane of the ooctye, changes occur in the zona pellucida, known as the zona reaction, which impedes the entry of other sperm, so preventing polyploidy, which would occur if further sperm fused with the oocyte. Fusion of the sperm and oocyte results in the resumption of meiosis with the expulsion of the second polar body. The two sets of chromosomes align on the metaphase spindle and cell division then proceeds, forming the two-cell embryo.

Implantation

The zygote (fertilised conceptus) reaches the uterine cavity four days later (Figure 4.6). Over this time it has undergone a series of mitotic cell divisions, forming cells known as blastomeres. Once it reaches the uterus it consists of 12–16 blastomeres and is known as a morula. Uterine fluid enters the morula and forms a cavity, in what is now known as a blastocyst. The external cells of the blastocyst form a layer known as the trophoblast. These cells produce the hormone HCG, which is structurally similar to LH. HCG prevents regression of the corpus luteum so the corpus luteum can

FIGURE 4.6 Conception: oocyte and its surrounding layers and the sperm. Fertilisation occurs as the sperm penetrates the zona pellucida. Embryonic cell division is initiated, leading to the formation of the blastocyst, with implantation occurring around day 6 post fertilisation.

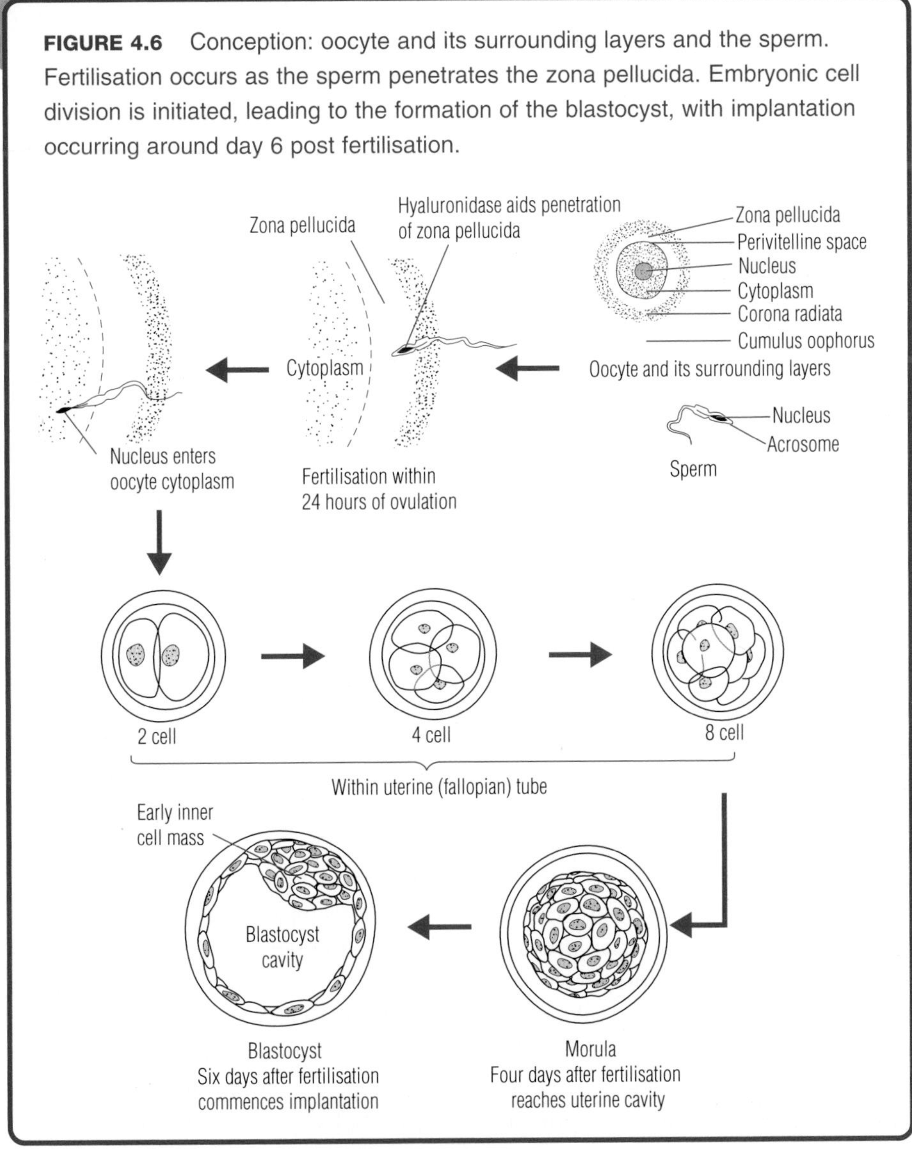

continue to secrete progesterone, which is necessary for the maintenance of pregnancy. The production of progesterone is later taken over by the placenta once it is established at 10–12 weeks gestation.

The blastocyst commences implantation on the sixth day after fertilisation. At this stage the zona pellucida has disappeared. The endometrial glands are at the height of secretory activity and laden with glycogen-rich secretions. Microvilli from the uterine luminal surface, known as pinopodes, are present. It is believed that they differentiate under the influence of progesterone and absorb luminal molecules and fluid to facilitate implantation by drawing the uterus closely around the embryo. A rich vascular capillary plexus is present just beneath the surface epithelium of the endometrium. The endometrial stromal cells in this region have enlarged and give the impression of a distinct superficial compact layer beneath the surface epithelium. The endometrium is thus of sufficient depth, vascularity and nutritional richness to support the conceptus through the early stages of implantation. Further development of the embryo, however, demands an increased supply of food and oxygen, which necessitates access to the maternal blood supply. The attached region of the trophoblast differentiates into an inner cellular layer of cytotrophoblast and an outer layer of syncytiotrophoblast. The syncytiotrophoblast is composed of a syncytium or multinucleate mass, formed from cytotrophoblast cells which have fused and lost the dividing cell membranes. The syncytiotrophoblast invades the endometrium and incorporates cells by fusion and phagocytosis into the trophoblast. The endometrial stromal cells become large and pale and this is known as the decidual reaction. The endometrium of pregnancy is subsequently known as the decidua. The process of implantation is complete by the tenth day after fertilisation. At this time HCG can be detected in the serum and urine of the pregnant woman. This means that a pregnancy test (detects HCG) can be positive even before the expected menstrual period has been missed. Implantation usually occurs in the body of the uterus on the anterior or posterior wall. Occasionally implantation can occur outside the uterus, such as in the fallopian tube, giving rise to an ectopic pregnancy.

Placentation

The inner cells of the blastocyst differentiate to become the inner cell mass that will give rise to the fetus. The inner cell mass develops into a flat, circular plate composed of two layers, an outer ectoderm and inner endoderm. A further layer, the mesoderm, then forms between these and grows outwards to line the blastocyst. The combination of mesoderm and trophoblast is termed the chorion. The amnion, derived from the trophoblast, attaches to the margins of the ectoderm to produce the amniotic sac. As the syncytiotrophoblast expands, small spaces (lacunae) develop that become filled with maternal blood and provide nutrition for the developing embryo. At this stage the lacunae are completely separated off from each other by columns of syncytiotrophoblast (primary villous stems). Maternal blood flows in and out of lacunar networks, establishing a primitive uteroplacental circulation. Continued growth of cytotrophoblast occurs and a mesodermal core appears which later becomes vascularised. These are known as primary stem villi. Subsequent growth and divisions give rise to secondary and tertiary stem villi (Figure 4.7). Each villus is supplied by one artery and drained by one fetal vein. These blood vessels later connect with those in the chorion, connecting stalk (future umbilical cord) and embryo.

The region of the decidua between the blastocyst and myometrium is known as decidua basalis. Chorionic villi in this region increase and become known as villous chorion or chorion frondosum. As the syncytiotrophoblast invades the decidua basalis, large intervillous spaces are formed. Intervening parts of decidua form the placental septae which divide the placenta into compartments known as cotyledons. The placenta is a fetomaternal organ because it is formed from both fetal (villous chorion) and maternal (decidua basalis) tissues. A thin membrane separates fetal blood in the capillaries from maternal blood in the intervillous spaces. This consists of fetal capillary epithelium, connective tissue, cytotrophoblast and syncytiotrophoblast. Deoxygenated fetal blood leaves the fetus in two umbilical arteries in the umbilical cord. On reaching the placenta these divide into branches that enter the chorionic villi. Oxygenated blood returns via veins in the chorionic villi, which join to form the umbilical vein in the umbilical cord.

FIGURE 4.7 Development of the placenta

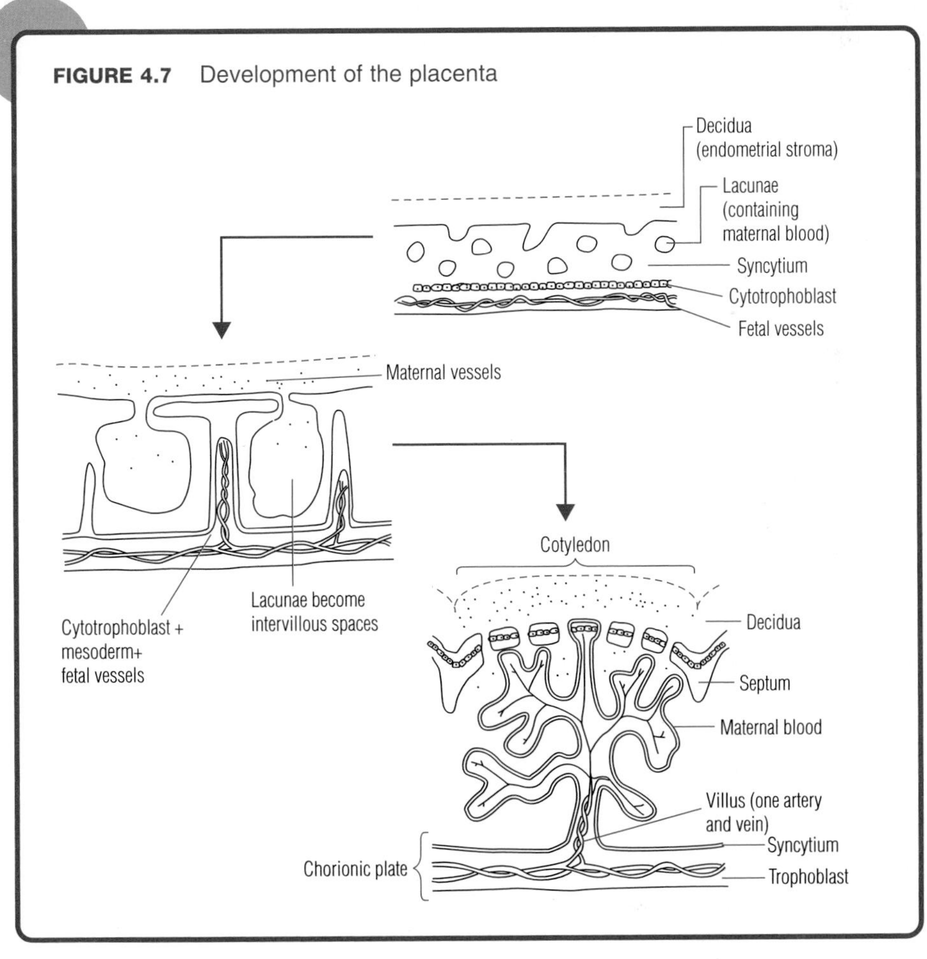

Placental functions

The functions of the placenta are named in Table 4.5.

TABLE 4.5 The functions of the placenta

Respiratory	This relates to the transfer of oxygen from maternal to fetal blood and carbon dioxide from fetal to maternal blood which occurs by simple diffusion. In addition fetal haemoglobin has a greater affinity for oxygen than adult haemoglobin (Figure 4.8, oxygen dissociation curve)
Excretory	The main excretory function of the placenta is the elimination of urea from the fetal circulation.
Nutritional	Carbohydrates, lipids and amino acids are also transferred across the placenta to the fetus, either as a diffusion process or by specific transport mechanisms.
Endocrine	This is the production of the hormones oestrogen, progesterone, HCG, human placental lactogen and corticosteroids.

FIGURE 4.8 Fetal haemoglobin has a greater affinity for oxygen than does adult haemoglobin. The fetal oxygen dissociation curve lies to the left of the maternal curve. This means that, for any given P_{O_2}, fetal blood contains a larger quantity of oxygen than does maternal blood. The transfer of hydrogen ions from fetus to mother across the villus further separates the two curves, thus increasing the oxygen tension gradient between fetal and maternal circulations—this 'double Bohr effect' is unique to the placenta. The greater the separation, the more rapid the transfer of oxygen.

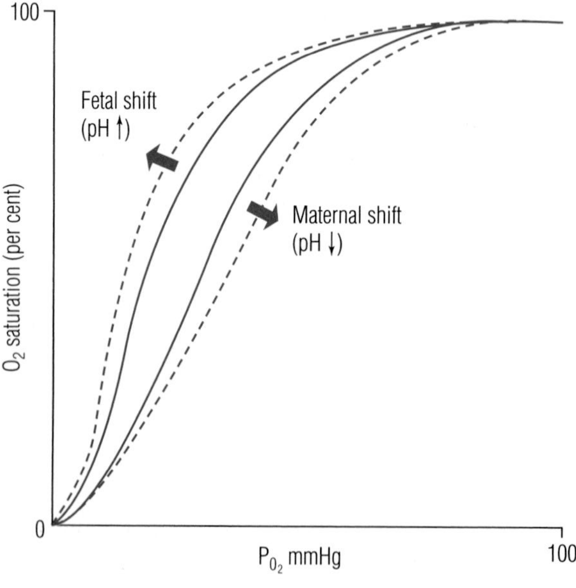

Embryo and fetus

The three primary germ layers of the embryo—ectoderm, mesoderm and endoderm—give rise to the tissues and organs of the fetus (Table 4.6).

Each of the systems develops in parallel but the development is completed for each system at different times (Table 4.7). An understanding of this development is important to:

- Understand how birth defects may occur
- Understand the possible effects of teratogens at different stages of pregnancy
- Appreciate the timing of investigations (eg ultrasonography)
- Answer questions from parents about development.

TABLE 4.6 Tissues derived from the germ layers

Embryonic layer	Derivative
Ectoderm	Skin
	Nervous system
	Sensory epithelium of eyes, ear and nose
	Anterior pituitary and salivary glands
Endoderm	Lining of gastrointestinal tract
	Lining of respiratory tract
Mesoderm	Muscle
	Connective tissue
	Bone
	Blood vessels

TABLE 4.7 Organ development in fetal life

Organ	Complete formation (weeks gestation)
Heart	6
Renal	7
Limbs	8
Genital system	8
Olfactory apparatus	8
Liver	12
Renal system	12
Eyes	20–24
Spinal cord	20
Gastrointestinal system	24
Respiratory system	24–28
Auditory apparatus	24–28
Brain	28

System development

The cardiovascular, central nervous and genital systems are considered here, as they are the systems that produce major congenital anomalies.

Cardiovascular system

Embryonic blood vessels form in plexuses. The heart develops from mesoderm and begins to beat about 21 days following fertilisation. Initially it is only a primitive heart from which blood passes into an aortic sac through branchial arches and into the dorsal aorta. Some blood goes to the brain via the internal carotid arteries but most passes through three major plexuses: the vitelline vessels to the yolk sac and gut, intersegmental arteries and cardinal veins to supply the nervous system and body wall, and the umbilical vessels to the placenta. Blood islands containing red and white stem cells develop on the surface of the yolk sac. Erythropoiesis begins in the liver during the sixth week of conception. It is apparent in the bone marrow at 16 weeks gestation.

Changes at birth

Figure 4.9 shows the changes in the cardiovascular system at birth. Oxygenated blood from the placenta returns to the fetus via the umbilical vein to the liver. Most of this oxygenated blood is directed by the ductus venosus into the inferior vena cava, which is returning non-oxygenated blood from the lower limbs, kidney, liver etc. There is only partial mixing of the two streams and most oxygenated blood is directed from the inferior vena cava through the foramen ovale (a valvular opening in the heart functioning from right to left) into the left atrium. Blood then passes into the left ventricle and aorta. This relatively well-oxygenated blood supplies the head and upper extremities. The remainder of blood from the inferior vena cava mixes with that of the superior vena cava and passes to the right ventricle and so into the pulmonary artery. A very small amount of blood goes to the lungs but most passes via the ductus arteriosus into the aorta. Thereafter it passes down the aorta to supply the viscera and lower extremities. Most of this blood then passes into the umbilical arteries that arise as branches of the left and right internal iliac arteries. At birth the umbilical vessels contract. Breathing helps to create a negative thoracic pressure, so drawing blood from the pulmonary artery into the lungs and diverting it from the ductus arteriosus, which gradually closes. The left atrial pressure rises and closes the foramen ovale.

Central nervous system

During the third week after fertilisation, a central thickening of ectoderm develops, known as the neural plate. This thickening folds to form a tube that will form the future brain and spinal cord. Ectodermal cells, known as neural crest cells, migrate laterally from the neural tube and give rise to structures such as spinal ganglia, ganglia of the autonomic nervous system, meninges and adrenal medulla. The cephalic end of the neural tube forms three distinct dilatations: the forebrain, midbrain and

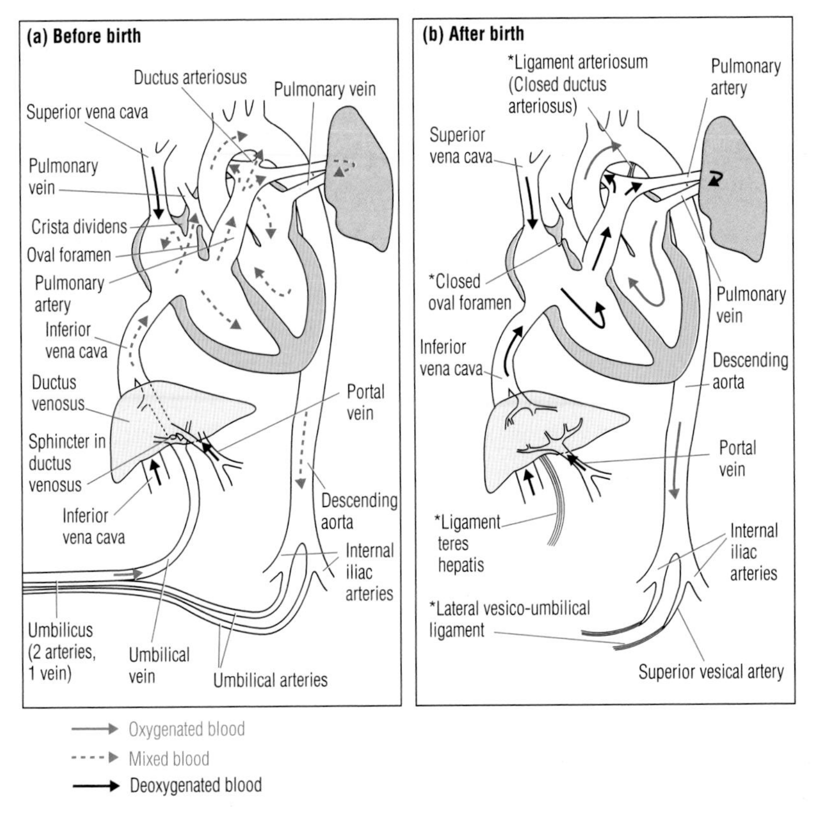

FIGURE 4.9 Plan of human circulation (a) Before birth (b) After birth.* Note the changes occurring as the result of respiration and the interruption of placental blood flow.

hindbrain. The lumen of the vesicles is continuous with the lumen of the spinal cord, allowing the cerebrospinal fluid to circulate freely.

Occasionally the neural tube fails to close. Such a defect may extend the length of the tube or be restricted to a small area. If localised in the region of the spinal cord, the abnormality is termed spina bifida; if in the cephalic region, anencephalus or encephalocoele. Spina bifida covers a wide range of defects (Figure 4.10):

- *Spina bifida occulta:* an abnormality localised in the sacral region, covered by skin and not noticeable on the surface apart from a small tuft of hair.
- *Meningocele:* occurs if one or two vertebrae are involved in the defect, the meninges of the spinal cord bulge through the opening and a sac covered with skin is visible on the surface.
- *Meningomyelocele:* occurs if the sac (in *meningocele* above) is so large that it also contains spinal cord and its nerves. The covering skin is thin and easily torn.

FIGURE 4.10 Schematic drawing showing the various types of spina bifida (a) Spina bifida occulta (b) Meningocele (c) Meningomyelocele

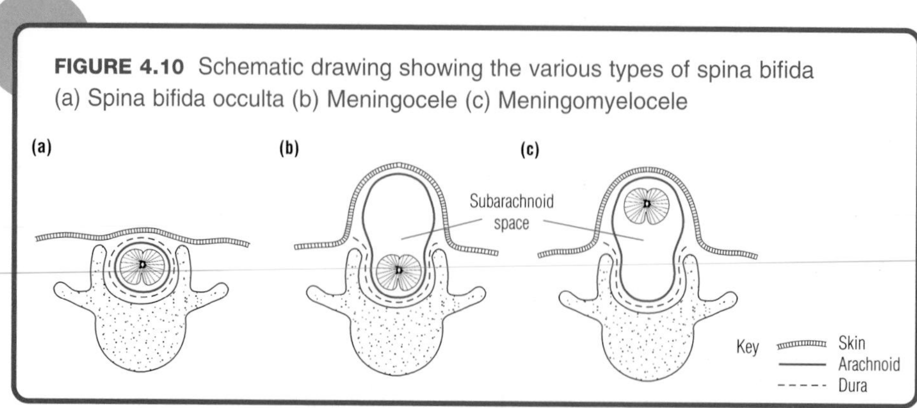

These abnormalities may be diagnosed in the antenatal period on ultrasound if marked. A major defect (anencephaly) is incompatible with life; other defects may be amenable to surgery; spina bifida occulta may be diagnosed on examination of the neonate (Section 8). Ingestion of folic acid by the mother before conception and in the early antenatal period is associated with a decreased risk of these defects (Section 6).

Reproductive tract

Gonads

The renal and genital tract develops from intermediate mesoderm which gives rise to the pronephros, metanephros and mesonephros. A thickened area on the medial mesonephros becomes the gonadal ridge which will form the undifferentiated gonad. Primordial germ cells migrate from the yolk sac to the gonadal ridge. There, in the absence of a Y chromosome, they become surrounded by granulosa-thecal cells arising from ridge somatic tissue. These form the primordial follicles.[39] The primordial germ cells begin to degenerate in large numbers at three months gestation. If all of them degenerate or fail to develop, as in an XO situation, then the gonad becomes a 'streak' of non-functioning tissue. The ovary needs germ cells to develop, in contrast to the testes which do not. At 12 weeks gestation, the primary follicle in the female begins the secretion of hormones which are at relatively high levels at birth, declining only near the second year after birth. These hormones are the androgens (androstenedione, DHEA, DHEAS) progesterone, 17-OH progesterone and oestrogen.[40]

The undifferentiated ovary on the mesodermal ridge will develop into a female gonad without inducement. To become a male gonad at seven weeks gestation, the tissue must be acted upon by testicular-determining factors (TDF), which are products of the SRY (sex-determining region of Y chromosome) gene located on the short arm of the Y chromosome. These factors induce the gonad to produce testosterone from testicular Leydig cells and Müllerian-inhibiting substance or factor (MIS or MIF) from testicular Sertoli cells. Previously, the H-Y gene, which produces a cell antigen, was believed to be the major male sex-determining influence. Now the importance of the testicular-determining factor gene appears to be the major influence and the H-Y antigen is important for its prognostication value of neoplasia in individuals with XO gonadal dysgenesis.[41] Determining the interaction of important factors with TDF acting on the indifferent gonad and on the genital ridge occupies genetic research.

Internal genitalia

There are three duplicated tubular systems:

1 The metanephric system which gives rise to the kidneys and ureters. (The pronephros, which acts as a rudimentary kidney, regresses.)
2 The mesonephric system which, in the presence of testosterone, develops into the seminal vesicles, vas deferens and epididymis. This system regresses in the female. Vestigial remnants may be seen in the female presenting as paratubular cysts (hydatid cyst, Cyst of Morgagni), paravaginal cysts (Gartner's duct cyst) or paraurethral cyst.
3 The paramesonephric duct system which, in the absence of mullerian-inhibiting substance, MIS), will develop into the fallopian tubes and uterus, and contribute to the vagina in the female, but will regress in the male (Figure 4.11).

On either side of the mesonephric duct are the paramesonephric ducts, which arise as an invagination of the coelomic epithelium. The distal ends of the fallopian tubes remain free and communicate with the peritoneal cavity. The lower end of the ducts fuse vertically and laterally, forming a uterovaginal primordium which forms the uterus and cervix and contributes to vaginal formation. It contacts the endoderm of the urogenital sinus leading to the development of the sinovaginal bulbs and the formation of a vaginal plate.[42] This plate extends and canalises to form a single patent vaginal canal. The hymen represents the distal aspect of this union.

Failures on lateral fusion or agenesis of the upper paramesonephric ducts will result in uterine defects such as uteri which are described as being unicornuate (one side only), bicornuate bicollic (didelphic or complete duplication including cervix), bicornuate unicollic (two horns, one cervix) and septate (normal external appearance with internal wall). Occasionally one horn may not develop fully and may or may not communicate with the vagina (Figure 4.12). Particularly in this circumstance, the vagina and renal development are frequently abnormal.

Failure of the vaginal plate to develop or cannulate appropriately leads to vaginal agenesis,[43] and transverse and vertical vaginal septae. These are not detected at birth and present as dyspareunia, failure to obtain an adequate Pap smear or amenorrhea. Usually there is some fenestration of a transverse septum permitting menstruation. They are not resected during pregnancy because of the danger of bleeding. In the Mayer-Rokitansky-Kuster-Hauser syndrome which affects 1/4000 neonates, there is Müllerian agenesis such that the uterus (if present) is bud-like and the entire vagina is absent. Concomitant renal anomalies such as agenesis are seen in up to 43 per cent of these patients.[42]

Failure of canalisation of the hymen leads to an imperforate hymen. If the hymen does not cannulate, cervical and uterine secretion in an otherwise patent system would be obstructed (cryptomenorrhoea). The most common shape for hymenal canalisation is crescentic with the narrow tip pointing posteriorly.

FIGURE 4.11 Development of the genital systems (a) Male genital ducts. Mesonephric system (regresses in female). (b) Female genital ducts. Paramesonephric system (regresses in male). Note the epoophoron, paroophoron and Gartner's cyst, as remnants of the mesonephric system.

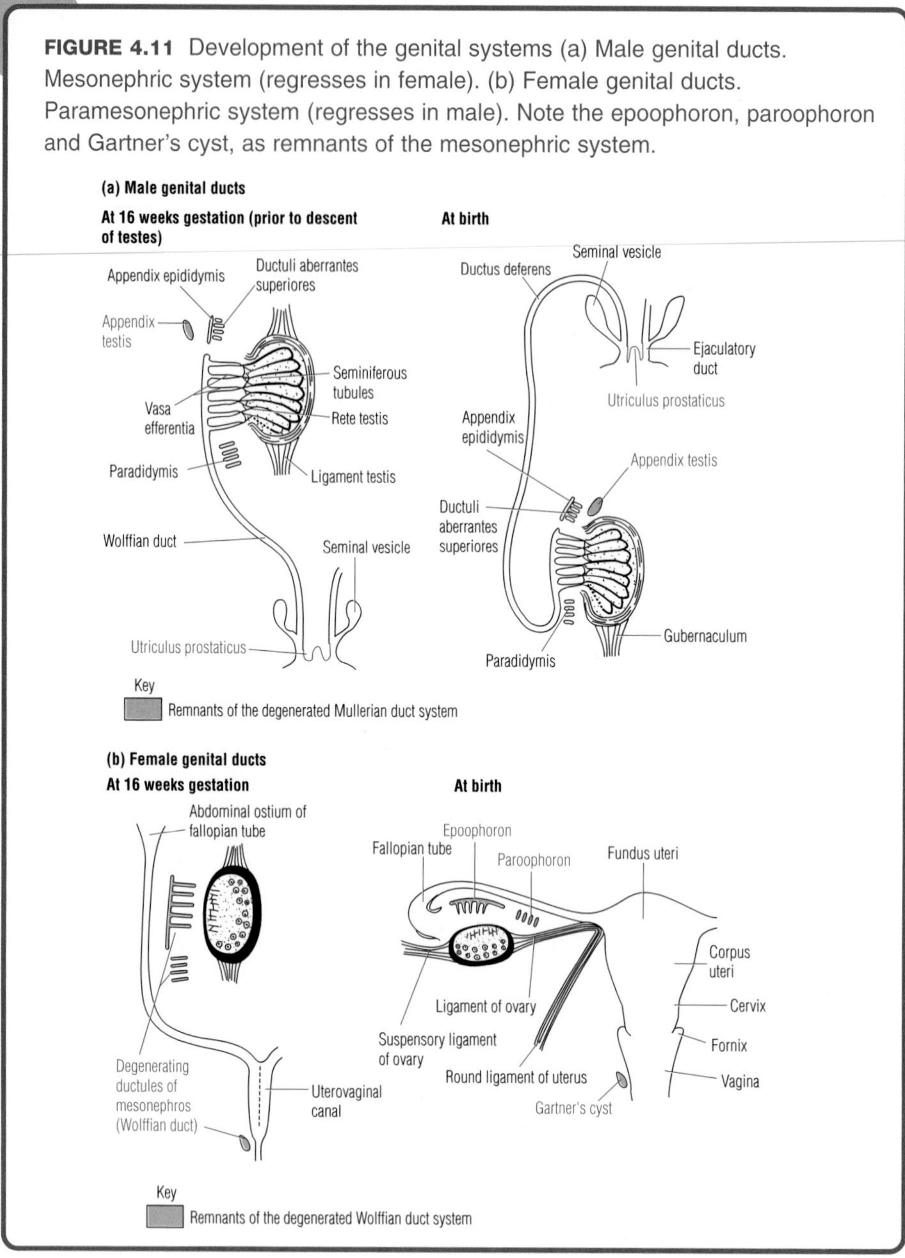

Gently lifting the labia anteriorly may break the suction of the hymen and a very superior opening of the hymen may be revealed in the newborn. After detecting a bulging fluctuating hymenal membrane, hymenotomy can be performed as soon as an accurate diagnosis is made. Hymenotomy consists of making a cruciate incision in the hymen leaving a 0.5 cm margin around the junction of the hymenal membrane and the vaginal wall. The tips of the incision are then sutured back, leaving an orifice large enough for fluid egress. Suprapubic pressure can be used to assist in expulsion of

FIGURE 4.12 Formation of the uterus and vagina (a) Normal. (b) Main abnormalities caused by persistence of the uterovaginal septum or obliteration of the lumen of the uterovaginal canal

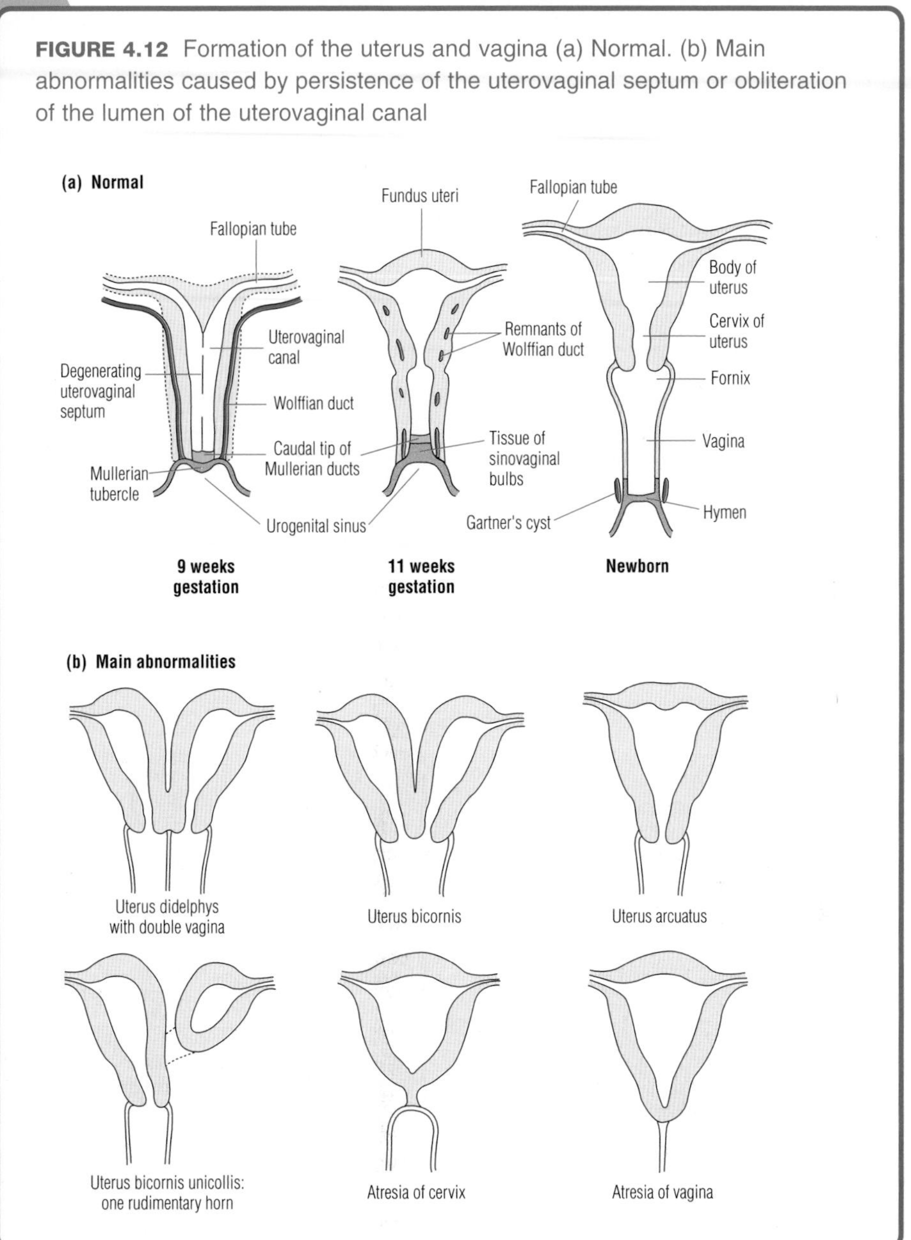

trapped menses but suctioning of the vagina and uterus is not advised. Careful follow-up for orifice stenosis and infection is undertaken.

External genitalia

The external genitalia develop at about 10–12 weeks gestation from a common anlage. If a Y chromosome is present with TDF it will induce the (undifferentiated) gonad to become a testis and secrete testosterone. In the presence of dihydrotestosterone and functioning receptors, the anlage will differentiate along male lines. If absent, the anlage will develop in a feminine manner (Figure 4.13). Development of the internal male structures requires testosterone, whereas the external genitalia require dihydrotestosterone for appropriate male development. This is formed by the action of the 5α-reductase enzyme on testosterone. The genital tubercle which forms the phallus under the influence of androgens, and clitoris in the female, arises from the cranial end of the cloaca. Labial-scrotal folds become the urethra and the genital swellings fuse and become the scrotum. The corresponding female

FIGURE 4.13 The development of the external genitalia. Indifferent stage: at around six weeks the genital swellings develop. These will later become the scrotum in the male or the labia majora in the female. In the male the genital tubercle rapidly elongates to form the phallus. The urethral groove eventually becomes the urethral canal. The glandular portion of the urethra develops later during the fourth month as the ectodermal cells penetrate inwards, canalising and joining up with the urethra. In the female the genital tubercle elongates slightly to form the clitoris. The urethral groove is open to the surface to form the vestibule.

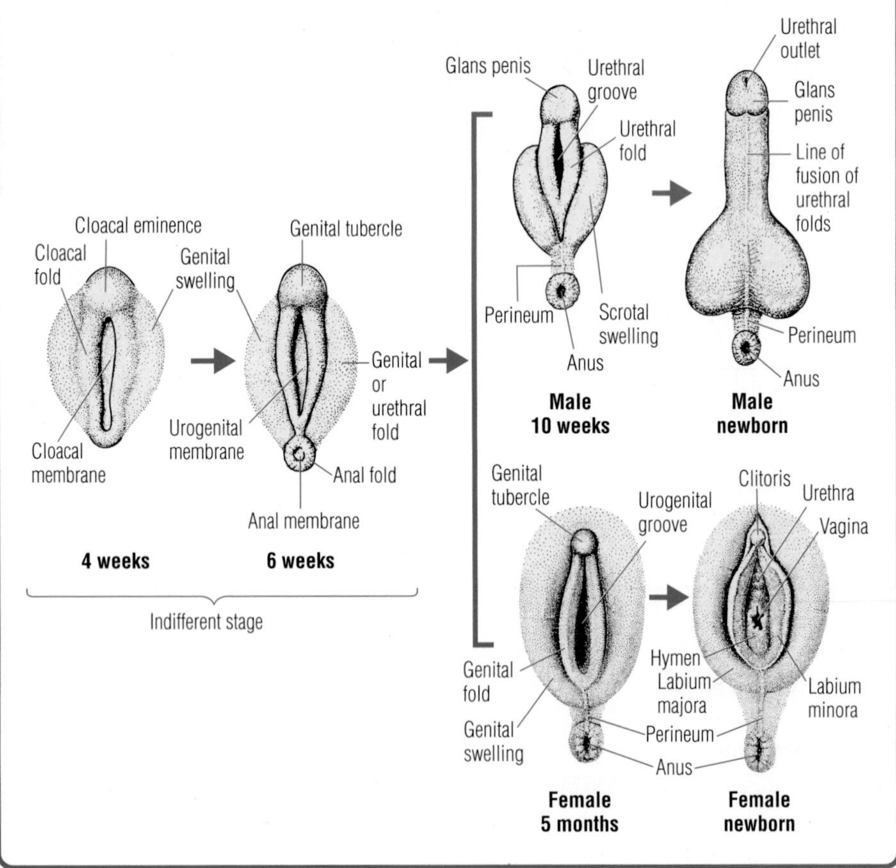

structures are the labia minora and majora respectively. Fusion of the labia is not seen in the female unless androgen has been active in embryonic life. Labial adhesions which represent an agglutination of the labia secondary to irritation should not be confused with fusion. Fusion is present at birth, labial adhesions are not. Unlike labial fusion, labial adhesions consist of a fine filmy membrane responsive to small doses of oestrogen.

Ambiguous genitalia

Ambiguous genitalia at birth present a dilemma for parents and health professionals. The correct assignment of sex at this time must be as accurate and predictive as possible in order to promote bonding and short- and long-term management.

CLINICAL PRESENTATION

Ambiguity noted on routine examination of the newborn.

Examination

Close inspection of the genitalia is mandatory on all newborn examinations. For example, the absent vagina is often not detected until puberty simply because no one has looked to see if it was visible at birth. Gentle traction anteriorly on the labia will usually break the suction of the hymen and permit visualisation of patency beyond.

Management

When a baby is born and the sex is indeterminate, there is a need to:

1 Make certain that the baby does not have a life-threatening condition.
2 Deal with the immediate parental reaction.
3 Diagnose the condition as expediently as possible to promote parental bonding and establish a treatment plan.

Some syndromes are present at birth but are not recognised until later in childhood, at puberty or in adulthood. After gender assignment, usually the parents are more relaxed and can cope with the ensuing care. When the assignment of sex has been inappropriate, changed or when ambiguity is diagnosed retrospectively years later, the problems are focused more on the reaction of the patient. The young child raised as a female will be helped along the way to adjustment, whereas the teen presenting with primary amenorrhea, for example, may face a disastrous shock to her self-esteem, sexual identity and confidence if the situation is mishandled. The assignment of gender is one of the most powerful influences on one's life. Getting it right and offering informed, sensitive counsel is important at any age.

1 Ensuring the baby does not have a life-threatening condition

Congenital adrenal hyperplasia (CAH) 21-hydroxylase deficiency is the most common life-threatening condition leading to ambiguous genitalia.[44] Therefore it is vital to determine immediate sodium, potassium, 17-OH progesterone and glucose levels, to obtain baseline blood pressure, and to prevent dehydration. Electrolytes, glucose and weight are monitored daily for at least seven days.

Ambiguous genitalia can also be associated with cloacal anomalies that require urgent diagnosis such as imperforate anus, prune belly and neurofibromatosis.[45] Immediate bowel-anal re-anastomosis, colostomy and/or renal assessment may be necessary. If there is no life-threatening situation, immediate surgery is rarely necessary at birth. Corrective surgery is often left until the tissues mature and the patient herself perceives the need for surgery. This can be performed at puberty or later.

2 Parental reaction and bonding

Immediately, one can use such terms as 'your baby' or 'little person' to refer to the newborn appropriately. The tone of sincerity, affection, appreciation for life and joy at the birth are often more important than the words. Reassure the parents that the baby appears otherwise healthy if that is so. Using gentle phrases like 'Your baby has not yet finished developing the sexual organs' may soften the news. In the anxiety to assign a name and sex, giving the baby an ambiguous name like Robyn straight away may not be the best long-term decision. Once sex is assigned the baby is referred to as 'him' or 'her'. The name the parents have usually previously considered can now be used and this will assist bonding. It is important that the entire team has a consistent approach to the gender of the baby. The mother is encouraged to breastfeed and perform the usual activities of any new mother in order to focus on the positive aspect of the birth. Reassurance that there is specialist assistance to help the parents, keeping the baby hospitalised in the same room with the parents until the sex is assigned, and informing them of the nature and progress of investigations, also promote bonding. Within a week most of the information is usually obtained. Gender assignment does not rely solely on phallic length, and modern research is increasingly investigating the role of the nervous system and psyche in sexual identity.[46] Cultural expectations can also influence gender assignment.[47] Altering the initially assigned gender can result in severe stress to the patient and the family. Issues of fertility, sexual identity, puberty, sexual function, hormone administration, neoplasia and corrective surgery can occur over time and it is often easier for the parents to focus on one issue at a time. Parental issues such as guilt, anxiety, depression and fatigue can arise. Having a consistent person who has a good rapport with the family will provide continuity of care. It is important that this person is one who can give an accurate interpretation of various specialists' opinions, the treatment plan and ways of dealing with family and members of the community.

3 Diagnosing the condition

Diagnosing the condition begins on the day of birth. A differential diagnosis provides the framework for the history, physical examination and investigations. There are a multitude of classification methods for 'ambiguous genitalia'. A simplified, easily recalled and practical initial approach includes the more common syndromes (Table 4.8). Inclusion of late intersex problems is included to emphasise the fact that sexual ambiguity can present beyond birth.

TABLE 4.8 Common aetiologies of ambiguous genitalia

Classification	Conditions leading to ambiguous genitalia
Masculinised 46 XX female	Maternal drug ingestion: androgens, teratogens
	Maternal androgen-secreting tumour
	Congenital adrenal hyperplasia
	• 21-hydroxylase
	• 1β-hydroxylase
	• 3β-hydroxysteroid dehydrogenase
	Structural defects during embryogenesis
	• absent vagina (Mayer-Rokitansky-Kuster-Hauser Syndrome)
Undermasculinised 46XY male	Total testicular agenesis (agonia)
	Gonadal dysgenesis (Swyer syndrome)
	Deficient testosterone synthesising enzymes
	• 17-ketoreductase
	• 17α-hydroxylase
	Deficient 5α-reductase
	Abnormal testosterone receptor and post-receptor events
	• androgen insensitivity syndrome (partial or complete)
Sex chromosome abnormality	Deletions:
	• X chromosome: Turner XO, 45X0/46XY
	• triploidies
	• mosaicism

The masculinised 46XX female baby

The 46XX female may have masculinised external genitalia due to:

- *maternal ingestion of androgens* such as danazol, progestins, body-building steroids and teratogens
- *maternal androgen-secreting tumour*, for example, an ovarian or Krukenberg tumour. Clinical presentation: increased phallic length and/or fused labia majora. A careful history, the examination, the presence of normal chromosomes and of normal mullerian structures and ovaries would suggest this diagnosis.
- *adrenal enzyme deficits* (Figure 4.14). The clinical presentation can be dehydration, shock and ambiguous genitalia. This may present with varying degrees of phallic enlargement and fusion of the labia majora. In severe cases, abnormal vaginal and urethral emptying into a persistent urogenital sinus can result in extremely complex anatomy. The uterus, tubes and ovaries are normal no matter how ambiguous the external genitalia may appear.

Adrenal enzyme deficits shift the metabolic pathway to favour an increased androgen production. Depending on the enzyme concerned, this shift may result in the lack of production of essential mineralocorticoid and glucocorticoid hormones. The enzyme deficit states of the adrenal are autosomal recessive congenital conditions.[48–50]

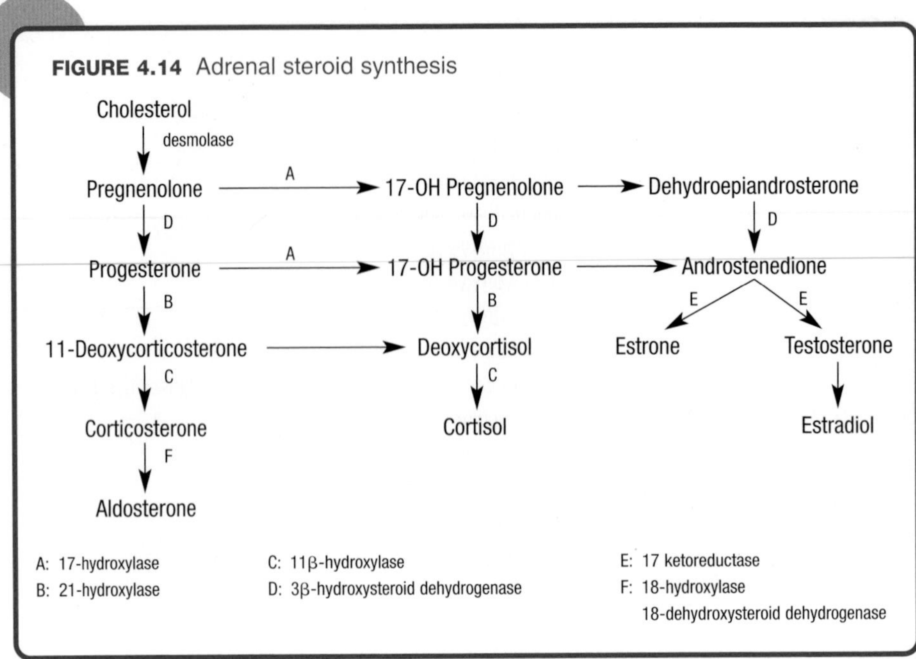

FIGURE 4.14 Adrenal steroid synthesis

The under-masculinised 46XY male baby

This baby has normal 46XY chromosomes, but is deficient in androgen for masculinisation. To induce masculinising changes, testosterone needs to be produced, transported, converted to its usable form and then coupled with a functioning androgen receptor. If any error occurs in this pathway, under-masculinisation can occur. Reasons for deficient testosterone include:

- *Absent or undeveloped testes (gonadal agenesis or dysgenesis).* Clinical presentation of gonadal agenesis: this syndrome is not generally diagnosed at birth. This genetic male phenotypic female presents at puberty with primary amenorrhea, some breast development, poor sexual hair development, streak gonads and an intact mullerian system. This baby appears to be female and is raised as female. Here there is no production of testosterone or mullerian-inhibiting factor (MIF) or oestrogen if the situation is one of total agonia. In the case of Swyer syndrome, largely an X-linked disorder, the testes are streaks (dysgenetic) and the gonads develop as ovarian tissue streaks. Whenever a dysgenetic gonad contains a Y chromosome, there is a 15–30 per cent chance of neoplasia in the form of dysgerminoma or gonadoblastoma and the gonad requires removal. Oestrogen replacement is required after removal of these streaks after puberty. Because of an intact Müllerian system in this case, progesterone must also be added.
- A *defect in enzyme production of testosterone.* 17α-hydroxylase, 17-ketosteroid reductase, 3β-hydroxysteroid dehydrogenase enzymes are examples.

- *A 5α-reductase deficiency.* To become biologically active, testosterone must first be converted to dihydrotestosterone by the 5α-reductase enzyme. Without this enzyme, masculinisation of the external genitalia of the male is not maximised, although internal testosterone structures such as Wolffian ducts (vas and epididymis) are present.
- *'Post-reception' events.* The final step is the reaction of dihydrotestosterone with a functional receptor capable of instigating the appropriate 'post-reception' events. Modern research is identifying the anatomy of the receptor and its gene-coding for DNA and hormone binding. When the androgen receptor fails to permit expression of testosterone, the androgen insensitivity syndrome (AIS) occurs in a complete or partial form. Previously called the testicular feminisation syndrome, this X-linked autosomal recessive condition causes 46XY males to have a female phenotype. Testes are intra-abdominal or inguinal and produce MIF, testosterone and oestrogen.

CLINICAL PRESENTATION OF POST-RECEPTION EVENTS

Patients present with absence of pubic or axillary hair and a short, clitoral-sized phallus because the testosterone cannot induce its changes. Mullerian-inhibiting factor prevents uterine development. Breast development occurs because of the predominance of oestrogen from the testes and adrenals. Usually a short pouch arising from the urogenital sinus is present. The testes are removed, as there is a 15–30 per cent chance of neoplasia arising within them. This is not usually performed until after puberty is complete in order to maximise oestrogenisation and a steady progress through a feminine puberty.

The incomplete form has variable presentations from total masculinisation to total non-masculinisation. Lubs, Reifenstein and Gilbert-Dreyfus syndromes are variations included in partial AIS. Patients may present with complaints of primary amenorrhea, lack of sexual hair and inability to have intercourse. The short urogenital sinus vaginal pouch may be elongated with persistent intercourse and the patient may actually present as an infertility patient. Counselling, often-long term, oestrogen replacement and vaginoplasty or vaginal dilatation are elements of continuing care.

The hermaphrodite baby

The rare true hermaphrodite individual has both ovarian and testicular tissue. Occasionally these two tissues are combined in one gonad. Of eight cases studied,[51] most were 46XX. A few patients are 46XY and others have a mosaic karyotype with at least one XX cell line. Variable phenotypic attributes can be noted. The combination of a unilateral female internal system and a contralateral male ductal system is possible and the degree of external sexual attributes can also be hormonally dependent.

The baby with abnormal sex chromosomes

There are two considerations with regard to the influence of chromosomes on ambiguous genitalia.

- The integrity of the autosomal chromosomes as sources of aberrant loci which can influence genital development must be recognised. As human gene mapping has become refined, loci on autologous chromosomes have demonstrated that aberrations in these non-sex chromosomes can influence final genital structure and function. For example, 21-hydroxylase deficient CAH has been linked to the HLA complex on the short arm of the sixth chromosome.[51] The homozygosity or heterozygosity of alleles can explain the various degrees of disease. The absent vagina syndrome (Mayer-Rokitansky-Kuster-Hauser syndrome) is described as autosomal dominant although the exact genetic nature of this syndrome found in 46XX girls is yet to be elucidated. Deficiency of testosterone-producing enzymes is another area of genetic interest. Enzyme deficiency states are often autosomal recessive.
- Gonadal and hence hormonal development of the individual is governed by the sex chromosomes. Reasons for the gonad not to develop appropriately include inappropriate sex chromosomal division, deletion, loci accidents and the reasons underlying these accidents, such as teratogen exposure and inheritance. If the TDF gene loci and other sex-determining loci are aberrant or missing on the short arm of the Y chromosome, then the gonadal direction along male lines will not occur. In the female, two X chromosomes and oocytes are necessary for the ovary to develop. Loci for ovarian maintenance (not formation) are believed to be contained on both the long and short arms of the X chromosome. In the absence of either loci, gonadal dysgenesis and failure can result.

The classic Turner syndrome presents with webbing of the neck and dorsal pedal oedema in the newborn. Horseshoe kidney occurs in some. There may be congenital heart defects such as co-arctation of the aorta and bicuspid aortic valve. An echocardiogram and X-ray are mandatory in children with this syndrome. Later the child may show a broad ‘shield-like’ chest, widely spaced and hypoplastic nipples, wide carrying angle of the arm (cubitus valgus) and may be of short stature if the 5p portion of the short arm of the X chromosome is damaged or missing. Because of eustachian tube anomalies, otitis media is common.

Turner syndrome has a deletion of X (45X) or a mosaic form (45XO/XY). This syndrome is composed of a variety of chromosomal patterns but all share the lack of ovarian-determining genes.[52] The 45XO/XY ‘mixed’ gonadal dysgenesis consists of one streak on one side and a dysgenetic ovary on the other. Most patients have bilateral streak gonads, a complete Müllerian system and female-appearing genitalia and are thus recognised as and assigned female gender at birth.

Maximal growth is achieved by the use of growth hormone and oxandrolone (an anabolic agent).[52] Surgical extirpation of any gonadal tissue associated with a Y chromosome is undertaken after puberty, as the incidence of gonadal neoplasia also exists at a rate of 15–30 per cent in these patients. Initiation of growth hormone starts when the growth falls below the expected height by 5 percentiles. This can occur as early as age two.[53] Oestrogen is begun once epiphyseal closure is imminent or complete. Progesterone is added, because the uterus is intact.

Investigation and management

In order to work through the diagnosis of the sexual ambiguity, the following investigations are recommended. This part of the management is the least difficult to achieve. The difficult part is counselling the parents through the process and instituting long-term plans for care. Even once satisfactorily through the initial neonatal period, the child and parents will encounter events, body awareness, identity concerns and questions about ultimate successes for sexual function, fertility and genetic inheritance. The problem faced at birth can therefore translate into a lifetime need for sensitive and informed counselling.

Day 1

1 Family history
   - Anomalous genitalia
   - Medication or teratogen exposure
   - Parents' state of health
2 Physical examination
   - General: vital signs, muscle tone, hydration
   - Genitalia: describe, image and measure
   - Abdominal or inguinal masses
3 Observations
   - Urine and meconium output
   - Daily weight, feeding, assessment of hydration
4 Investigation
   - Sodium, potassium, glucose, 17-OH progesterone: repeat daily for 10+ days (CAH mostly presents day 2–6 but some > day 10)
   - Chromosome studies: use blood, amniotic fluid, buccal smear SRY gene on short arm Y; fluorescent long arm Y
5 Establish management team: parents, doctor, geneticist, paediatrician, urologist, gynaecologist, psychologist etc.

Day 2

1 Check: plasma androgens, AE, DHEA, testosterone, dihydrotestosterone (DHT), deoxycortisol 17-OH progesterone, 17-OH pregnenolone and 17-OH progesterone
2 Molecular investigation of the androgen receptor
3 Ultrasound, renal scans or IVP, MRI, vaginoscopy and cystoscopy
4 Establish steroid and mineralocorticoid therapy as indicated.

Conclusion

In summary, the dilemma of ambiguous genitalia at birth requires a specific plan of action (Box 4.1). Late diagnosis requires particular sensitivity and appreciation of the stage of growth and development of the child.

BOX 4.1 Pathway summarised

When encountering ambiguous genitalia at birth:

1 Explain to the parents that the sex of the baby is uncertain at this time but will shortly be known.
2 Examine the newborn.
3 Take a detailed history.
4 Form the easily recalled differential diagnosis:
   - Masculinised female
   - Under-masculinised male
   - Hermaphrodite
   - Sex chromosome anomaly.
5 Rule out life-threatening conditions such as congenital adrenal hyperplasia.
6 Order appropriate investigations, particularly electrolytes, glucose, 17-OH progesterone, ultrasound/MRI and chromosomes.
7 Establish management team, call a team conference.
8 Present a clear plan and keep the parents informed. Support the parents in their own education and their management of family and friends.
9 Provide for long-term follow-up.

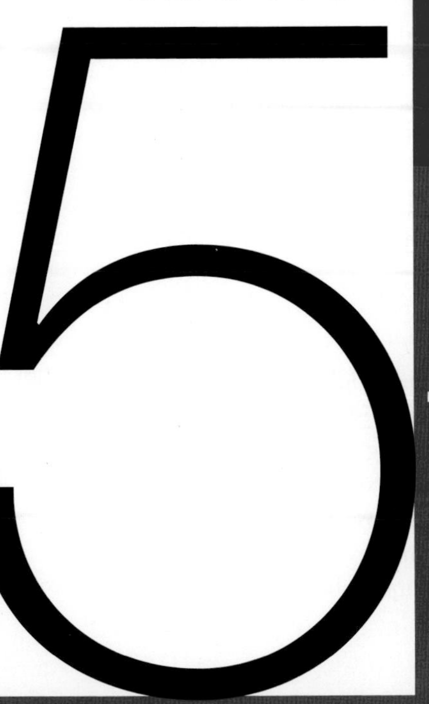

SECTION 5

The female child and adolescent

Development of the female child

After birth, the growth and development of the reproductive tract is due to genetic and hormonal influences. The level of oestrogen is high at birth and remains so for a couple of months. It then declines but remains at relatively high levels for the first two years due to heightened GnRH activity during this time.[1] Following this, the oestrogen levels fall as follicular development declines and do not return to elevated levels again until follicles begin to develop in preparation for puberty. This leads to oestrogenisation of the breasts and vulva early after birth, decline in prominence and then growth again before puberty.

Breasts

The breast buds are palpable at birth. Some infants and toddlers may have transient enlargement of one or both breasts in response to innate oestrogen. This rarely needs investigation unless it is bilateral and accompanied by vaginal bleeding. More common examples of aetiology of the latter include central nervous system dysfunction or ovarian oestrogen-secreting tumours such as the granulosa tumour. Biopsy of the breast bud can result in injury to the bud and later maldevelopment of the breast. Beginning after age six,[2] breast development is more noticeable as it passes through the Tanner stages[1] (Section 4).

Abdomen

With the presence of pelvic organs in the abdomen until they begin to descend into the pelvis at about age 7–8, and with the pelvic bones undeveloped and small, the abdomen remains protuberant until the period of adrenarche—usually after age eight. With longitudinal growth, muscle development, flaring of the ilium and descent of the bowel and genitourinary structures, the abdomen becomes flatter by puberty.

Uterus and tubes

The uterus begins as a flat structure with a cervical/corpus ratio of 2–3:1. As oestrogen promotes growth, the ratio becomes 1:2 by puberty. The fornices are undeveloped, with a flat, button-like cervix seen on vaginoscopy in the prepubertal years. At birth, vaginal bleeding and cervical secretion may lead to 'menses' in the first 10 days of life because of transfer of maternal oestrogen and progesterone.

Beyond that period, investigation is warranted as the causes of vaginal bleeding in children are extensive. Of these, the most commonly encountered vaginal bleeding in prepubertal children will be relative to trauma and precocious puberty. Prior to puberty, the endometrium develops, as does the anterior wall of the corpus. Should the hymen be imperforate, the newborn may present with a 'hydrocolpos' presenting as a bulging vaginal mass which fluctuates with changes in intra-abdominal pressure (when crying, for example). At puberty the bulging of the hymen may have a bluish colour secondary to entrapment of chocolate syrup-like menses (haematometria and/or haematocolpos). If the collection is large enough, an abdominal mass may be palpable or visible at either age. Pain in the teen may be cyclic or constant. A simple, adequate hymenotomy treats the problem.

Ovaries

At birth the ovaries contain follicles usually less than 1 cm in size. Enlarged follicles, which are generally only detected by prenatal ultrasound, may reach several centimetres in size. The majority of enlarged follicles regress after birth; however, expert consultation is required if they persist beyond 6–8 weeks or do not appear to be simple cysts.[3] The postnatal elevation of gonadotrophins may contribute to persistence of these cysts.[1] Ovarian torsion is possible in newborns and also can be seen again in puberty. Ovaries begin their growth after age five.[3] Ovulation usually does not occur until after 12–15 cycles, when menses is well established. As this is not the case in every adolescent, sexual health education would include advising the teen that she may ovulate earlier and that pregnancy precautions should be undertaken.

Vagina

The prepubertal vagina, measuring approximately 4 cm, appears red because of a thin unoestrogenised epithelium permitting the redness of the vasculature to be appreciated. This is often mistaken for infection or abuse. With infection, generally vaginal discharge accompanies this redness and the redness extends beyond the vagina to the vulva. As the tissue becomes oestrogenised and colonised by Döderlein's bacilli, it becomes pinker and thicker and changes from an alkaline to an acidified passage.

The prepubertal clear/milky-looking discharge which precedes menarche may irritate the child and is frequently mistaken for and treated as a yeast infection. It responds to simple hygiene measures as well as an explanation to the child and to the mother about normal puberty. Vulvovaginal irritation is discussed in the section on vulvovaginitis

Hymen

The hymen of the newborn is prominent and oestrogenised and thus appears large. There are a variety of shapes to its canalisation, the most common being crescentic. Gently lifting the labia anteriorly then laterally is often enough to break the hymenal suction and allow the examiner to visualise the lower vagina beyond the hymen. Hymenal tags and cysts are sometimes seen. Tags tend to regress with a decline in hormone. Cysts become relatively smaller and may resolve spontaneously. Only if the tissue is non-homogeneous or interferes significantly with cleansing does it need to be removed with a simple ligation and excision. If a hymenal or lower vaginal cyst fluctuates with intra-abdominal pressure changes, then an ectopic ureter is considered. The hymenal diameter is sometimes used to document the possibility of sexual abuse. It should be noted that the infant's position, fullness of bowel, measuring device, traction on the labia and observer experience can all influence this measurement. Therefore, using this measurement to make claims should be undertaken with caution and with qualification. At puberty, the hymenal opening, which is ordinarily slightly above 1 cm in diameter, soft and distensible, will accept a gently inserted tampon and yet maintain its integrity. Teen-sized tampons are available.

Forgotten tampons lead to very foul-smelling vaginitis and adolescents should be advised to change tampons frequently and to leave the strings outside the vagina so as not to forget that they have one in place.

Vulva

The vulva is hairless until adrenarche when androgens stimulate hair growth through the Tanner stages (Section 4, Figure 4.4). Hair growth and distribution is generally in accord with Tanner stages III–IV[1] by puberty, but racial variations can be seen. At birth and in premature babies, the labia and clitoris appear quite prominent. With pelvic growth and declining oestrogen, the labia become relatively thinner until puberty. Labial asymmetry, hernias, fibromas and lipomas can occur in children. Abnormal androgen secretion can cause aberration in the development of the vulva because receptors for androgens invoke structural change during embryogenesis.

Vulvovaginitis

The most common paediatric gynaecology problem the non-specialist will see is inflammation of the lower vagina and vulva, usually presenting in the toddler age group.

CLINICAL PRESENTATION

1 Rubbing/scratching the genital area
2 Vaginal discharge on underwear, noticed by mother

History

Predisposing factors for the development of this problem are thin genital epithelium, poor hygiene, restrictive moisture-retaining clothing, respiratory infections, antibiotic administration and the presence of allergies and eczema. Sexual abuse is not the most common cause for vulvovaginitis, nor is it seen in all cases of sexual abuse.

Examination

1 Vulvovaginitis presents with varying degrees of erythema of the labia majora and perineum. Vaginitis without vulvar involvement is uncommon in the preschooler. The normal red epithelium of the lower vagina should not be mistaken for infection. Helpful details on how to examine a child are described by Jordan.[4]
2 Discharge may be absent, clear, purulent and with or without odour. A foul-smelling, sometimes bloody, purulent discharge can be associated with a foreign body. To detect a foreign body, milking the vagina through the rectum or lavage of the vagina with a lubricated small feeding tube may prevent the need for vaginoscopy performed in the operating theatre.
3 Ulcerated lesions. Chickenpox and Cocksackie B viral lesions may be confused with herpes.
4 Molluscum contagiosum is not uncommonly seen on children and may or may not be sexually transmitted (Section 12).

Investigation

1 Cultures are best taken with a small 0.25 cm sterile non-bacteriostatic saline swab. It is also possible to collect a sample for *Chlamydia* and other organisms by vaginal washings taken with a small paediatric feeding tube with a syringe attached. It is important to prevent the catheter tip creating suction against the vaginal wall, as this hurts the child. The labia may be held slightly closed and less than 10 cc of saline irrigation used. Dry cotton buds are not used as they are too big and they irritate the dry epithelium. PCR DNA urine testing for *Chlamydia* and *Neisseria gonorrhoeae* is now possible.
2 Ultrasound of the vagina is not always definitive.
3 If a vaginal examination is deemed necessary in the preschooler and non-sexually-active adolescent, this is usually performed in the operating theatre using a hysteroscope or cystoscope. Otoscopes or speculum of any size are traumatic and unnecessary in the young child.
4 Pinworms may be present in the vagina and if not seen, an anal tape test can be undertaken (Figure 5.1).

FIGURE 5.1 Pinworms can be a cause of vulvar irritation.

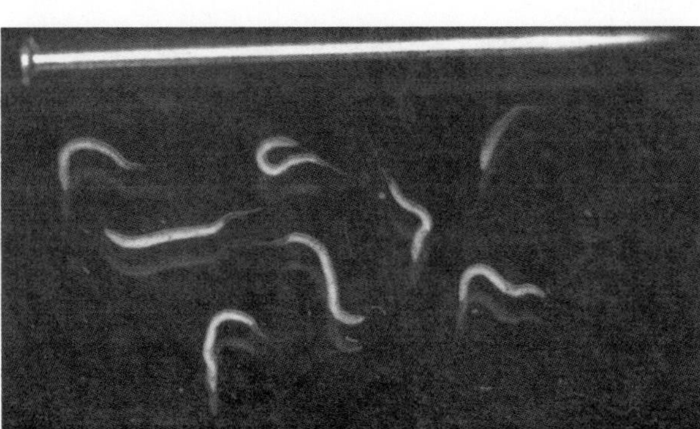

Pathophysiology

Common normal flora of the genitalia in the prepubertal child include diphtheroid, a-haemolytic streptococcus and lactobacillus. In addition, *E. coli*, bacteroides and yeast have also been seen in asymptomatic girls.[5,6]

When cultured, most vulvovaginitis is non-specific for particular organisms and generally only normal flora will be present. Pathogenic organisms associated with infection generally include those associated with respiratory or gastrointestinal disorders. Organisms capable of being sexually transmitted, such as *N. gonorrhoeae*, *Trichomonas vaginalis*, *Gardnerella vaginalis* and viruses such as herpes simplex type 1 and 2, and human papilloma virus (HPV) are associated but not always proof of sexual abuse. Of these *Neisseria* detection mandates an investigation of sexual abuse[7] and the others are suggestive enough to make inquiries. *Chlamydia* is best detected by cell culture rather than direct immunoassay or fluorescent antibody testing. A positive culture may occur up to one year of age if the pathogen was maternally transmitted. Likewise, HPV causing genital warts in the mother is believed to be transmissible for 1–2 years after birth[7,8] but this belief should not prevent appropriate inquiry.

Management

1 Simple cleansing. Most cases of vulvovaginitis, being non-specific, respond to cleansing with a non-irritating/allergenic friction-proof cleanser. Such cleansers are available over the counter. This cleansing should be demonstrated to the mother by parting the labia and explaining the need to cleanse after every toileting. This may be a challenge, especially in the self-toileting toddler in whom the vulvovaginitis occurs most frequently. The normal leucorrhoea that occurs before and after menarche should not be mistaken for an infection such as yeast and usually responds well to appropriate cleansing.
Unresponsive or chronic vulvovaginitis can be seen most commonly with non-compliant cleansing but also in some sexual abuse cases.

2 If a particular organism is identified then paediatric dosing of an appropriate oral and topical antibiotic is appropriate. More details on specific infections are noted in Section 12.

Adolescence

Adolescence is a period of transition between childhood and adulthood. Puberty describes the physiological changes that result in adult size and appearance and the ability to reproduce. Adolescence is a time of very active physiological and psychological growth; however, physical and psychological development may not progress in parallel. This is particularly important to remember when dealing with young women—an adolescent with adult physical characteristics may still be at an early stage of emotional development and vice versa.

Psychological changes

Psychological development consists of cognitive and socio-emotional components. This development is often divided into three stages—early, middle and late—each with its own specific features (Table 5.1). Not only may the physical and psychological development progress at different rates, but the ability of the adolescent to grasp concepts may be highly variable. It cannot, for example, be assumed that the capacity to grasp one concept will mean universal understanding of other concepts. In situations of illness, conflict and stress there will be a tendency to regress to less mature processing, so health professionals must adjust their explanations and interactions accordingly. Identity is the sense of self, separate from others—'who I am'. It involves multiple components including physical, social, sexual, emotional, occupational, intellectual and moral dimensions.

TABLE 5.1 **Psychological development of the adolescent**

Feature	Early adolescence (age 10–14 years)	Mid-adolescence (age 15–18 years)	Late adolescence (age 19–20s)
Cognitive development			
Thought	Concrete thinking	Concrete thinking: fascinated by capacity for new thinking	Ability to think abstractly Recognition of ambiguity Concept of time
Values	Testing of moral system of parents	Self-centred	Able to appreciate things from another's perspective Ability to reason and make decisions
Emotional and social development			
Relationships and peers	Adjustment to new body image Need to be accepted by peers Single-sex groups	Emotional separation from parents 'Adolescent sub-culture' Identification within the group leads to a 'ready-made' identity Mixed-sex groups Increased health risk-taking behaviour	Individuation Independence Social autonomy Sense of personal identity Development of internal controls Need to conform less dominant Formation of intimate relationships (couples)

Social development

This includes negotiation of relationships, moral values and adaptation to expectations and roles within society. Membership of a group may provide a sense of stability and identity, particularly in early and mid-adolescence. Exclusion from peer groups because of disability or other factors such as membership of a cultural minority may profoundly undermine self-esteem and social development.

Self-esteem

This refers to a sense of contentment and self-acceptance. For girls in particular, body image emerges as an issue undermining self-esteem. High self-esteem in parents plays a major influence in the self-esteem of adolescents.

Engaging the adolescent

Communicating with the adolescent should involve a normal approach of confidentiality, dignity and respect. Discussion should be clear and straightforward, without any facade (Box 5.1)—adolescents are quick to reject a non-genuine approach!

BOX 5.1 Engaging the adolescent

Don't assume concrete thinking has disappeared:

'What are your best and worst subjects?' vs 'How is school?'

'What are the best and worst things at home?' vs 'How are things at home?'

Offer choices:

'Did that make you feel happy or sad?' vs 'How did it make you feel?'

Give options:

'When that happened, did you feel stressed or fairly okay?' vs 'How did you feel?'

Talking in general terms can reduce the personal focus:

'Tell me what it's like being a teenager in the 21st century.'

'Can you tell me about how things are for young people who live in big cities?'

Ask before delving into personal issues:

'A lot of young people say that they have ... Have you ever had ...'

'I've heard quite a few people your age say ... I was wondering ...'

Never miss a chance to give a compliment:

'Sounds as though you've given a lot of thought to the problem.'

'You've already come up with some great ideas ... Is there anything else we could add?'

Don't confirm their belief that they are always being told what to do!

'What ideas do you have about what might help?'

Adapted from Sanci & Young 1995.[9]

Recognition of disorder

The popular view that crises are a normal part of adolescence is ill-founded. Severe identity crisis and turmoil are generally symptomatic of a significant underlying disorder which requires careful assessment. Between 4 and 8 per cent of adolescents have a major depressive disorder,[10] although depression in this age group often presents as anger or boredom rather than depressed mood. Treatment of the disorder is essential to reduce the suffering of the individual, the chance of occupational and social dysfunction, and the risk of suicide, which is a major public health problem.

Risk-taking

Healthy risk-taking is a positive tool in an adolescent's life for discovering, developing and consolidating his/her identity. Adolescent risk-taking only becomes negative when the risks are dangerous. Healthy risks—often understood as 'challenges'—can turn unhealthy risks in a more positive direction or prevent them from taking place to begin with.

Unhealthy adolescent risk-taking may appear to be 'rebellion'—an angry gesture specifically directed at parents or adult authority figures. However, risk-taking, whether healthy or unhealthy, is part of a teen's struggle to test out an identity by providing self-definition and separation from others, including parents (Box 5.2).

BOX 5.2 Risk-taking behaviours

- Healthy
  - Participation in sport
  - Development of artistic/creative abilities
  - Community volunteer activities
  - Travel
  - Running for school office
  - Making new friends
- Unhealthy
  - Alcohol use
  - Smoking
  - Drug use
  - Reckless driving
  - Unsafe sexual activity
  - Disordered eating
  - Self-mutilation
  - Running away/truancy
  - Stealing
  - Gang activity

Since adolescents need to take risks, adult carers need to help them find healthy opportunities to do so. Adolescents often offer subtle clues about their negative risk-taking behaviours through what they say about the behaviours of friends and family, including parents. Parents often stay silent about their own histories of risk-taking and experimenting, but it can be important to find ways to share this information with adolescents in order to serve as role models, to let teens view mistakes as a learning experience, and to encourage healthier choices than those the parent may have made during his/her own adolescence.

Parents need to help their teens learn how to evaluate risks and anticipate the consequences of their choices, and develop strategies for diverting their energy into healthier activities when necessary. Parents also need to pay attention to their own current patterns of risk-taking as well, because teenagers watch and imitate.

There is ample evidence that many young people get through their developmental journey without engaging in major life-threatening risk-taking behaviour. Red flags which help identify dangerous adolescent risk-taking can include psychological problems such as persistent depression or anxiety which goes beyond the more typical adolescent 'moodiness', problems at school, engaging in illegal activities, and clusters of unhealthy risk-taking behaviours.

Risky activities

Sexual behaviour

The transmission of sexually transmitted infections (STIs) can occur during any sexual activity. The young women at high risk are those with a number of casual partners who do not practise safe sex. Many young women may not be aware of safe sex practices and may not be consistent in their practice. Even those who have appropriate information often find that they are often not in a position to negotiate safe sex. This is related in part to loss of control where alcohol and drugs are used and the power in the relationship—many young women are in relationships with an older male.

Drugs[11]

In 1998, 25 per cent of young persons aged 14–19 years and 40 per cent of those aged 20–24 years were regular or occasional tobacco smokers. Thirty-eight per cent of young people aged 14–24 years reported using marijuana in the past 12 months. Alcohol dependence was more prevalent than drug dependence, with 12 per cent of males having alcohol dependence compared with 9 per cent for cannabis and opioid dependence. Nearly half of 14–24 year old males and one-third of females of the same age had an alcoholic drink at least once a week. Drug dependence accounted for 7 per cent of youth deaths. Deaths where drugs and medicinal substances were either the underlying or the contributing cause represented 24 per cent of youth deaths. One in five males and one in ten females in the 18–24 years age group were found to have substance use disorders ('harmful use' or 'dependence' on drugs and/or alcohol).

Injury

Injury is the leading cause of death for 12–24 year olds, with two-thirds of all deaths attributed to some form of injury, including accidents and suicide. Injury death rates for 15–24 year olds are higher than for all other age groups under 75 years.

Health promotion activities[11]

Many young women do not take care of themselves. The proportions of young people who reported exercising at a 'vigorous' or 'moderate' level for sport or recreation declines with age, from about 61 per cent of males aged 15–17 to about 44 per cent of males aged 20–24, and from 41 per cent of females aged 15–17 to 31 per cent of those aged 20–24.

Young people aged 15–24 years were less likely (35 per cent) to always use sun protection measures, compared with children under 15 (56 per cent) and adults over 24 years (46 per cent). This may be related to body image concerns.

Young women are often reluctant to obtain Pap smears and checks for STIs. This may be due to lack of knowledge, embarrassment or fear of the procedure or result.

At-risk groups

There are some groups of young people for whom risk-taking behaviour leaves them comparatively worse off. Twenty per cent of unemployed youth in 1995 assessed their health status as being fair or poor, compared with 9 per cent of employed youth and 8 per cent of students. Youth living in rural and remote areas appear to have poorer health compared with those in capital cities and other metropolitan areas—both death rates and hospitalisation rates increase with increasing remoteness. Using recent data, death rates for young Aboriginal and Torres Strait Islander people were found to be 2.8 times higher for males and 2.0 times higher for females than for their non-Indigenous counterparts.[12]

Gender differences

There are also clear differences in risk-taking behaviour between males and females. Among young Australians, there are about three male deaths to every one female death. Higher death rates for young males from accidents and suicide account for most of this difference. The male suicide rate was four times the female rate, but the female hospitalisation rate for parasuicide (attempted suicide) was greater at all ages and more than three times the rate for males at ages 15 and 16. The rate of substance use disorders for males is twice the rate for females. The higher rate of substance use disorders in males is reflected in higher rates of alcohol and drug dependence: 12 per cent of males were alcohol dependent, compared with 4 per cent of females, and 9 per cent of males were cannabis and opioid dependent, compared with 3 per cent of females.[13]

Identifying risk factors

While all young people take risks, specific risk factors that increase the likelihood of some young people engaging in hazardous risk-taking behaviour have been identified.[14]

These risk factors lie within five key realms (Box 5.3):

- the community
- the young person's family
- their school
- the individuals themselves
- their peer interactions.

Many of the risk-taking behaviours engaged in by young people—delinquency, substance abuse, violence, dropping out of school, and teen pregnancy—share many common factors. Reducing those common precipitating factors will have the benefit of reducing the probability of them engaging in problematic risk-taking behaviours.

Protective factors

Some young people who are exposed to multiple risk factors do not become substance abusers, juvenile delinquents, teen parents or school dropouts. Balancing the risk factors are protective factors, those aspects of people's lives that counter risk factors or provide buffers against them. They protect either by reducing the impact of the risks or by changing the way a person responds to the risks. A key strategy to counter risk factors is to enhance protective factors that promote positive behaviour, health, well-being and personal success. Research indicates that protective factors fall into three basic categories (Box 5.4):

- individual characteristics
- bonding
- healthy beliefs and clear standards.

Conclusion

The negative effects of risk factors can be reduced when schools, families and/or peer groups teach children healthy beliefs and set clear standards for their behaviour. Examples of healthy beliefs include believing it is best for children to be drug- and crime-free and to do well in school. Examples of clear standards include establishing clear no-drug and no-alcohol family rules, establishing the expectation that a youngster will do well in school, and having consistent family rules against problem behaviours.

BOX 5.3 Risk factors

- ***Community risk factors***
  - Availability of drugs
  - Availability of firearms
  - Community laws and norms
  - Media portrayals of violence: allows learning of violent problem-solving strategies and decreases sensitivity to violence.
  - Transitions and mobility: communities with high rates of mobility appear to be linked to an increased risk of drug use and crime problems.
  - Neighbourhood attachment and community disorganisation: the most significant issue affecting community attachment is whether residents feel they can make a difference in their own lives.
  - Extreme economic deprivation: children who live in deteriorating and crime-ridden neighbourhoods characterised by extreme poverty are more likely to develop problems.
- ***Family risk factors***
  - Family history of the problem behaviour
  - Family management problems: lack of clear expectations for behaviour, failure of parents to monitor their children, and excessively severe or inconsistent punishment.
  - Family conflict
  - Favourable parental attitudes and behaviour toward drugs, crime and violence influence the attitudes and behaviour of their children.
- ***School risk factors***
  - Early and persistent antisocial behaviour: boys' aggressive behaviour in the early school years, combined with isolation or withdrawal, hyperactivity or attention deficit disorder, increases the risk of problems in adolescence.
  - Academic failure in primary school
  - Lack of commitment to school
- ***Individual risk factors***
  - Alienation, rebelliousness, and lack of bonding to society
  - Favourable attitudes toward the problem behaviour
  - Early initiation of the problem behaviour: young people who initiate drug use before age 15 are at twice the risk of having drug problems of those who wait until after age 19.
  - Constitutional factors: sensation-seeking behaviour, low harm-avoidance behaviour and lack of impulse control.
- ***Peer risk factors***
  - Friends with problem behaviours: this is one of the most consistent predictors for problem behaviours.

Puberty

Normal female maturation involves an elaborate orchestration of the hypothalamic pituitary gonadal axis, although the exact biological events that trigger the onset of puberty are not well understood. The average age of puberty and menarche has

BOX 5.4 Protective factors

- ***Individual characteristics***

  These attributes are considered inherent in the youngster and may be difficult or impossible to change.
  - *Gender:* given equal exposure to risks, girls are less likely to develop health and behaviour problems in adolescence than are boys.
  - *Resilient temperament:* the ability to adjust or recover from misfortune or change.
  - *Positive social orientation:* young people who are 'good-natured', enjoy social interactions and elicit positive attention from others.
  - *Intelligence:* bright children are less likely to become delinquent or drop out of school. However, intelligence does not protect against substance abuse.
- ***Bonding***

  Children who are bonded to others with healthy beliefs are less likely to engage in behaviours that threaten that bond. Positive bonding can balance many other disadvantages caused by other risk factors and environmental circumstances.
  - Strong bonding with positive, pro-social family members, teachers, or other significant adults.
  - Bonding with pro-social friends who are committed to achieving goals.
- ***Healthy beliefs and clear standards***
  - Clear, positive standards for behaviour held by those with whom children are bonded is protective for substance abuse, criminal activity, unprotected sexual activity and school drop-out.

declined steadily over the last century throughout the industrialised world. This has been attributed to improved nutritional and general lifestyle conditions.[15] A recent cross-sectional study in the USA suggested that Caucasian girls on average are now beginning puberty by the age of 10 years. This average is lower for African-American girls, at 8–9 years.[16] A large US study of 10 000 children followed for 10 years reported that parental divorce/separation and the introduction of a non-father male into a household with young females could also be an important factor predisposing towards early puberty.[17] The earlier onset of puberty carries implications for both parental anticipatory counselling and for teaching of sex education in schools. The implications of early puberty for future fertility require further research.

Physical events during adolescence include:

- Changes in hormones
- Growth: initial increase then decrease in the rate of growth
- Changes in major organ systems to meet increased demands from growth
- Development of secondary sex characteristics
- Changes in the distribution of body fat and muscle.

Endocrine changes

The external signs of puberty are acceleration in growth (growth spurt) and the appearance of secondary sexual characteristics. Prior to these appearing a series of hormone changes occur (see Section 4). As puberty progresses there is a gradual increase in the rate and amount of gonadotrophins secreted (FSH and LH) with a resulting surge in ovarian production of androgens and oestrogens. The rise in androgens results in growth of pubic and axillary hair. The rise in oestrogens results in growth in the female reproductive organs: the ovaries, fallopian tubes, uterus and vagina, and priming of the endometrium which leads to menstrual bleeding. Research on leptin (a peptide released from adipose tissue) suggests that once a threshold level of leptin has been reached, puberty proceeds if other control mechanisms are operational.[18] Children with chronic diseases may experience a delayed onset of puberty.[19]

The external signs of puberty

The work of Marshall and Tanner in the 1960s and 1970s documented the sequence of events at puberty (see Section 4). In summary:

- Start of puberty: 10–11 years (range 8–13 years).
- Breast development is one of the earliest signs of the advent of ovarian function and precedes both pubic hair and the growth spurt. It occurs at about 10 or 11 years of age, and is completed some four years later with the appearance of the adult breast. In the early stages, breast development is often asymmetrical and this may initially cause some concern, particularly if it occurs at an earlier age. In these circumstances the young woman (and her mother) can usually be reassured that this is just an early onset of puberty. Mature breast development takes several years to complete, typically at about age 15, but the full adult development of the nipple/areolar complex may not occur until the late teenage years.[20,21] The adolescent breast is very dense in texture with prominent proliferation of fibrous tissue and minimal glandular and ductal development.
- Pubic hair begins 12 months later and starts with lightly pigmented sparse hair along the medial border of the labia majora and ends some three years later with the adult triangular shape of the pubic hair with spread to the medial surface of the thighs.
- Growth spurt: 12 years (range 10–14 years). There is a fairly close relationship between growth velocity and the occurrence of the menarche, with all girls starting to menstruate on the downward part of their growth velocity curve.
- Menarche: 12–13 years. The onset of the first period (menarche) is associated in most girls with Stage 3 pubic hair and Stage 3–4 breast development.

It can be seen that there is a wide range in respect of the age of the girl during which these developments take place (Figure 5.2). Other expected events include the development of acne, dandruff and body odour.

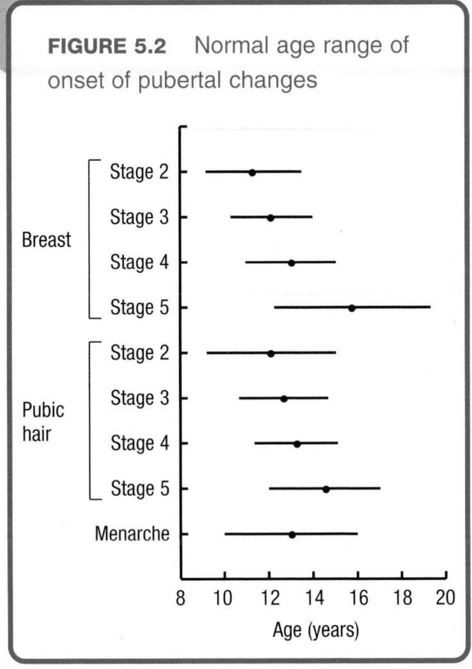

FIGURE 5.2 Normal age range of onset of pubertal changes

Menarche

Menarche is the first menstrual period, an important event in a girl's life, with special significance in many cultures. In developed countries the average age of menarche is around 12.5 years (range 10–16 years).[16] The literature frequently reports a gradual reduction in the age of the menarche during the twentieth century, with a decrease of approximately 3–4 months every decade. Interestingly, there has been a recent upturn in the age of the menarche in the UK and other European countries for reasons that are not clear, although it has been suggested that an increase in exercise and the desire to be slim may be factors. There are a number of factors determining the age of the menarche, including genetic and nutritional factors, socio-economic status, geographic location, general health and exercise. Body weight at menarche has remained constant at 45–47 kg and whether or not age at menarche is related to body weight or percentage of body fat has been the subject of much debate.[22]

The menstrual cycle

The initial cycles are often characterised by anovulatory bleeding which may be heavy and irregular. In the first two years following menarche, 55–82 per cent of cycles in young girls were found to be anovulatory.[23] The average cycle is 28 days (range 21–36) with 5 days of bleeding (range 3–10 days). The normal luteal phase is of constant length (14 ± 2 days) but the follicular phase is of variable duration (Section 4, Figure 4.4).

Clinical issues in the teenage years

CLINICAL PRESENTATION:

Precocious puberty (signs of puberty at less than eight years of age)

The features of puberty sometimes make their appearance in a very young girl and different authors have used different ages at which they would use the term 'precocious puberty'. Given the statistical ranges it would be wise to regard the appearance of any of the physical signs of secondary sexual development before the age of eight or of menstruation before the age of ten as being precocious.

Investigation

In close to 80 per cent of these instances no abnormality is detected on special investigation of these young girls. In other cases:

- The activity of the hypothalamus and pituitary can result from a variety of intracranial lesions, eg meningitis, encephalitis, ventricular hamartoma or other intracerebral tumours.
- Both ovarian tumours and adrenal neoplasms may produce abnormal levels or hormones, which may result in precocious signs.

Any girl with precocious puberty requires specialist investigation.

CLINICAL PRESENTATION: Delayed puberty

Some authorities prefer the term 'delayed puberty' to the more commonly used 'primary amenorrhoea'. The latter focuses attention merely on one of the features of puberty whereas 'delayed puberty' implies an abnormality of the general process of sexual maturation.

A girl aged 16 presents because she has not yet menstruated.

Differential diagnosis

This is not necessarily abnormal given that the normal age range of the first period is 10–16 years. However, an examination should be undertaken to decide:

1 If secondary sexual development is absent or very poor then quite clearly this is abnormal and warrants further investigation. There is likely to be an endocrine cause for the failure—either primary gonadal failure or hypothalamic/pituitary failure. Women without ovaries (or with streak ovaries—see Section 4) require hormone replacement therapy to start and maintain secondary sexual development and protect against osteoporosis. This can result in premature closure of the epiphyses if started too early. Intra-abdominal testes or streak ovaries where there is a Y chromosome on the karyotype should be removed to avoid early-onset gonadal malignancy.

2 If secondary sexual development is good apart from the absence of menstruation.
   - The diagnosis is very probably an anatomical fault in the uterus or vagina, eg imperforate or absent vagina or an absent uterus (see Section 4). Congenital abnormalities of the genital tract are associated with up to a 40 per cent incidence of minor urinary tract abnormalities.
   - Craniopharyngiomas are tumours arising from the remnants of Rathke's pouch and are the most common hypothalamic tumours causing primary amenorrhoea. They commonly present by the age of 14 years but can cause secondary amenorrhoea in young women.

CLINICAL PRESENTATION: Heavy menses (menorrhagia)

Heavy menses is one of the most common reasons for a teenager to present to a gynaecological clinic.

History

1 *Menses.* A careful history is especially important when assessing a young girl with a menstrual complaint. Failure to obtain an objective assessment of the magnitude of the problem and to elect to treat what may well be a normal cycle will confirm to the girl that indeed her menstruation is abnormal, probably with resultant problems in later years.

2 *Sexual activity.* It is important to establish whether the girl is sexually active and requires contraceptive and safe sex advice. This will influence the choice of treatment. This may be best achieved by asking any accompanying person to leave the room while you discuss this.

3 *Mother's fears and expectations.* A well-recognised scenario that requires sensitive handling is the 'I had problems with my periods when I was my daughter's age and I ended up needing a hysterectomy before I was 30 and it seems my daughter is going the same way'.

If the oral contraceptive pill is required to manage a problem of bleeding or pain, it may be necessary to reassure the mother of a girl who is not sexually active that this will not encourage her to be so. Legal issues must be considered where a girl is under the age of consent and at risk from sexual activity (see Teenage pregnancy).

Investigations

1 *Menstrual loss.* Unfortunately there is no simple way of assessing menstrual blood loss. A menstrual diary or pictorial chart can be extremely helpful in long-term management (Figure 5.3).

FIGURE 5.3 Pictorial representation of menstrual blood loss. These symbols, together with icons representing clots equivalent to 1, 3, 5 ml blood, and loss from a sudden 'flood', can be entered onto a daily chart during menstruation to give an estimate of blood loss.

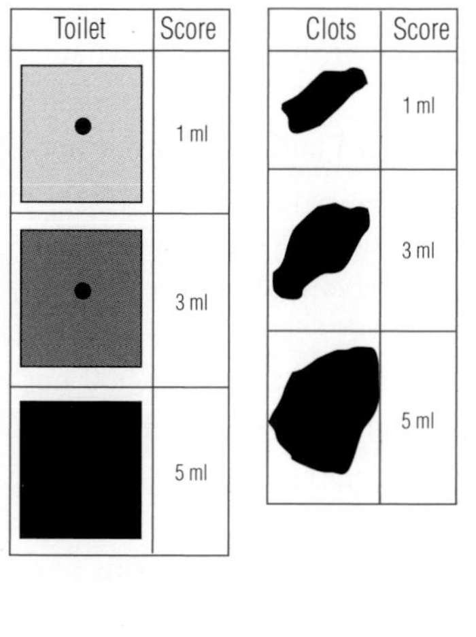

Towel	Type	Score
	Day time	1 ml
	Night time	1 ml
	Day time	2 ml
	Night time	3 ml
	Day time	3 ml
	Night time	6 ml
	Day time	4 ml
	Night time	10 ml
	Day time	5 ml
	Night time	15 ml

Tampon	Type	Score (ml)
	Regular	0.5
	Super	1.0
	Super Plus	1.0
	Regular	1.0
	Super	1.5
	Super Plus	2.0
	Regular	1.5
	Super	3.0
	Super Plus	4.0
	Regular	4.0
	Super	8.0
	Super Plus	12.0

Adapted from Wyatt et al. 2001.[24]

2 *Quality of life.* In taking the history, information such as having to miss school or games because of her period or the necessity to get up at night to change her nightwear or bed sheets may well provide very useful information.
3 *Anaemia.* A check of haemoglobin and ferritin levels is useful (Section 13).

Pathophysiology of heavy and/or irregular periods

It needs to be remembered that in the first year after the menarche only 15 per cent of girls are ovulating regularly. During this time the endometrium is often under the influence of unopposed oestrogen action, resulting in a thick, proliferated and unstable structure. This endometrium will often break down in an irregular and unpredictable fashion, frequently resulting in very heavy and sometimes prolonged menstrual loss. Girls with regular periods are likely to be ovulating, particularly if these patients complain of dysmenorrhoea. Girls who have heavy vaginal losses at the time of menstruation from the menarche onwards, whether their cycles are irregular or regular, should be investigated for a clotting disorder.

Examination

There is no place for either a pelvic or a rectal examination in these girls and an insensitive examination may cause reluctance to attend for checks, including cervical smears, in the future.

Investigation

An abdominal ultrasound examination looking at the uterus and other pelvic structures through a full bladder will provide all the information that is required. Other special investigations would need to be based on features in the history and clinical examination but it is seldom that anything more than a full blood count and serum iron studies is required.

Treatment options

Treatment will be influenced by the presence of anaemia or dysmenorrhoea and the need for contraception.

- In the absence of these, reassurance for both the girl and her mother may well suffice.
- An antifibrinolytic, tranexamic acid for the first three days of bleeding. The dose of the former is 1 g six-hourly and this has been shown to reduce menstrual flow by some 54 per cent.
- A prostaglandin synthetase inhibitor. Mefenamic acid in a dose of 500 mg eight-hourly has been shown to reduce menstrual blood loss by some 20 per cent. If there is any dysmenorrhoea then it is likely to improve or even eliminate it.

  Both these drugs need to be started as soon as menstruation begins and should be continued for three days.
- Should the heavy menstrual blood loss be irregular then the diagnosis of anovulation would be appropriate and treatment with a combined oral

contraceptive pill will impose a regular 28-day withdrawal bleed of a much smaller volume of blood lost. The patient and her mother need to understand, however, that although a combined oral contraceptive pill will give regular withdrawal bleeds that are both predictable and pain-free this will not correct the underlying condition, and it would not be surprising if after stopping therapy there were a recurrence of the irregular menstrual period. The duration of therapy should probably be 6–12 months (assuming no significant side effects) and then it might be wise to stop to see whether the cycles have settled into a regular pattern.

CLINICAL PRESENTATION: Painful menstruation (dysmenorrhoea)

History

This is quite a common symptom in adolescents and teenagers, affecting 60 per cent of young women. Dysmenorrhoea is commonly associated with ovulatory cycles and therefore often commences a few months to a year after menarche.

Pathophysiology of dysmenorrhoea

The cascade of events that results in the shedding of the endometrium produces increased levels of prostaglandins in the endometrium. Prostaglandins have two essential effects within the uterus: first, they cause increased uterine tone and high amplitude contractions, and second, they cause vasodilatation with increased menstrual blood loss. In addition to this normal physiological sequence of events, certain risk factors have been identified which may influence either the occurrence or the severity of dysmenorrhoea. These include:

- weight over the 90th percentile
- alcohol
- smoking
- early age of menarche
- lack of exercise.

Management

1. *Lifestyle factors:* early in the management of a young girl with dysmenorrhoea, recommendations concerning a healthier lifestyle, particularly increasing exercise, may be beneficial.
2. *Prostaglandin synthetase inhibitors* such as Mefenamic acid or Ibuprofen.
3. *Combined oral contraceptive pill* should be the next line of treatment or considered first line if contraception is required.

There are a group of girls who do not respond to treatment and for whom further investigation for underlying causes should be considered. Initially, an ultrasound examination should be requested to exclude a duplex genital tract with one side obstructed, or a uterine anomaly, particularly a rudimentary uterine horn. Then proceed to a diagnostic laparoscopy to look for endometriosis.[25]

CLINICAL PRESENTATION: Sexually transmitted infections

Sexually transmitted infections (see Section 12) may present as a concern, either as a result of sexual behaviour or as a perceived/experienced symptom.

The most common sexually transmitted diseases are the human papilloma virus (HPV), *Chlamydia trachomatis* and herpes simplex virus (HSV); all are acquired predominantly by women less than 25 years of age and have their highest incidence in pregnant teenagers.

Screening for disease in teenagers

STI screening

Chlamydia trachomatis screening is warranted on cost-effectiveness grounds, when the incidence of the disease is greater than 2 per cent in the community. It is most common in young, unmarried, pregnant women who use non-barrier methods of contraception and have more than one simultaneous sexual partner. The incidence of *C. trachomatis* in the general antenatal population ranges from 2 to 10 per cent. However, the incidence in younger teenage mothers has been reported at 26 per cent, more than justifying a routine screening policy.[26] Where the incidence of *C. trachomatis* is in excess of 10 per cent in a community, endocervical screening using gene amplification techniques such as polymerase chain reaction (PCR) is the diagnostic test of choice despite the additional cost. New screening modalities to enhance consumer acceptability of screening for *C. trachomatis* include the use of condoms and patient-collected swabs.

Pap smear screening

The current Australian guidelines for cervical screening state that Pap smears should be performed every two to three years, between the ages of 18 and 70 years or within two years of a woman becoming sexually active, whichever is later. In contrast, in the USA, screening commences at the earlier of these two options and is an annual process, whilst in the Netherlands routine screening does not commence until 35 years of age. In the UK, women between the ages of 20 and 64 are eligible for cervical smear testing every three to five years.

The principal objective of Pap smear screening is to identify high-grade precancerous changes (cervical intraepithelial neoplasia (CIN) 2 and 3) in order to treat these and reduce the incidence of cervical cancer. However, the epidemiology of high-grade Pap smear and cervical biopsy changes has altered. In Australia between 1970 and 1998, the peak incidence of high-grade biopsy-proven CIN rose from 0.5 per cent to 1.3–1.4 per cent of women screened. During the same period, the age of peak incidence of high-grade biopsy-proven CIN fell from 40–49 years in 1970 to 20–24 years in 1998.[27,28] Much of this change has been attributed to the increase in teenage smoking and the spread of HPV infection.

Thus, sexually active teenagers are at particular risk for the subsequent development of cervical cancer and warrant special consideration within formal Pap smear guidelines. Risk factors for cervical cancer include early age of coitarche, smoking and the presence of high-risk HPV infections, features that frequently congregate in pregnant teenagers. In Australia, 38 per cent of pregnant teenagers had an abnormality on Pap smear screening, of which 1 per cent exhibited high-grade abnormalities. Routine screening is therefore recommended.

CLINICAL PRESENTATION: A need for contraception

Condoms are the best method for adolescents at their sexual debut as these offer protection against both pregnancy and the acquisition of an STI. It is necessary to demonstrate correct condom use using a model and to stress that condoms have to be used every time intercourse occurs for effective protection. An emergency contraceptive (ECP) should be given to all condom users as a backup in case of condom rupture or slippage or in cases where unprotected intercourse has occurred. Providing backup ECP does not result in less consistent use of condoms.

Alternatively, the combined oral contraceptive pill can be used for prevention of pregnancy and condoms used simultaneously for protection against STIs in new relationships. When oral contraceptives are prescribed for adolescents it is important to provide information regarding the likelihood of breakthrough bleeding in the first 1–2 cycles and following missed pills. This bleeding, if unexpected, may result in pill cessation and subsequent pregnancy. Low-dose pills may also sometimes result in pill amenorrhoea. Women should be warned not to stop the pill if a withdrawal bleed does not occur until a positive pregnancy test is available.

For adolescents it is particularly important to prescribe a pill that provides reasonably effective cycle control. Adolescents seem to be less tolerant of breakthrough bleeding than older women and tend to stop the pill if this occurs. Ideally, adolescents should be prescribed a monophasic formulation, as the triphasic formulations can be confusing. Concerns that the pill may stunt growth or affect subsequent fertility when prescribed to young adolescents are unfounded.

For adolescents who are inconsistent pill takers a subdermal progestogen implant provides a viable alternative. It is essential to provide detailed counselling about changes in bleeding patterns prior to use and for the practitioner to be readily available to provide support if problems occur. Again, additional condom use should be advised with a new partner or if there are multiple partners.

Depo-Provera is an option for older adolescents who have difficulties in remembering to take oral contraceptives. Change in bleeding patterns and the likelihood of amenorrhoea need to be explained prior to use. In young adolescents (< 16 years), concerns regarding effects on peak bone mass need to be balanced with the obvious benefits of use of a long-acting method.

CLINICAL PRESENTATION: Teenage pregnancy

Teenage pregnancy deserves special consideration in women's health. There are unique issues of consent that can affect patient care and decision making. Pregnancy is often complicated by social and economic disadvantage. Furthermore, young mothers and their offspring are at increased risk of child abuse, non-voluntary foster care and lifelong dependency on government benefits. This makes teenage pregnancy an important medical, social and political issue.

Once ovulation occurs, young women are physically mature and capable of pregnancy. However, pregnancy at a very young age (11–13 years) may have detrimental physical consequences. The size of the birth canal is smaller in the first three years past menarche than at age 18.[29] This will have an impact on the young pregnant teenager. It has also been postulated that competition for nutrients between the fetus and the mother could affect maternal growth.[30,31] Pregnancy after 14 years is not thought to have a direct detrimental physical impact, but is frequently associated with emotional and economic effects.

Younger age (< 17 years) confers an increased risk of specific pregnancy complications. These include preterm birth and intrauterine growth retardation and appear separate from associated deleterious socio-demographic environment of many pregnant teenagers,[32] although studies are conflicting.[33] The risk of caesarean section overall is reduced. Older teenage mothers (aged 18–19 years) often have better than average obstetric outcomes and tend to overshadow poorer outcomes in some younger mothers in population-based demographics, as numbers are proportionally higher.

Antenatal care options for the teenager

Most teenagers access the routine antenatal care clinics. In Australia about 10 per cent of teenagers deliver through a specialised multidisciplinary service—with the involvement of peer educators, education advisers, social workers, dietitians, and midwifery and medical staff, such services allow comprehensive medical and social support. However, these are not always feasible on financial grounds.

Epidemiology of teenage births

Globally, teenage births remain common and account for 10 per cent of all births.[34] Despite the average age of women giving birth in Australia increasing gradually from 27.9 in 1991 to 29.3 in 1999, the proportion of teenage mothers has remained steady. On a national basis, teenage confinements make up 5.1 per cent of all births, with great variation between states.[35] The Australian figures probably underestimate teenage pregnancy as, due to the lack of data, they fail to include induced abortions of unwanted pregnancies.[36]

The USA and the UK have the highest teenage pregnancy rates in the developed world.[37] Roughly three-fifths of teenage pregnancies resulted in a live birth. The abortion rate was highest in the under-16 year age group.[38]

Factors contributing to teenage pregnancy

There is wide variation from country to country in teenage pregnancy and birth rates. The lowest birth rates are sometimes achieved with a higher abortion rate (Denmark and Sweden). Teenagers from more economically deprived areas are more likely to proceed to a live birth.[39] Despite this, these teenagers do not appear to become pregnant in order to receive financial assistance.[40] Some groups within societies may need special provision: Aboriginal teenagers in Australia have a pregnancy rate twice that of non-Aboriginal teenagers; they become pregnant earlier, access less frequent antenatal care and have a neonatal death rate twice that of non-Aboriginals.[41]

The teenage pregnancy rate has been seen to fluctuate with societal attitude, legislation on abortion, availability of contraception, and media reporting. An open societal attitude to teenage sexuality is beneficial to reducing teenage conception rates, while religious sanctions do not seem to be influential.[38] Some countries have seen dramatic falls in pregnancy rates with the improvement in sex education and the liberalisation of contraception.[38] Improving sexual health education with specific programs needs careful evaluation with randomised studies.[42,43] Education should include not only sexual health and contraception, but also preparation to cope with the demands of sexual life and parenting today. Contraception needs to address cost (condoms are available free of charge at family planning clinics in the UK but not at GP surgeries), availability (emergency contraception is available 'over-the-counter' in the UK but only on prescription in Australia), attitude of health professionals and confidentiality.

Educational, cultural and social implications

Specific educational, socio-economic and cultural circumstances are often associated with early pregnancy and parenting.

Education

Young girls who leave school early have been shown to be at high risk of becoming pregnant and there is a higher incidence of teenage pregnancy in low socio-economic areas where levels of education are low.[44,45] Teenage mothers are less likely to complete high school, marry, find stable employment or be self-supporting than older childbearing women. Young girls who drop out of school while pregnant are unlikely to return to any form of training or education within five years. There is a need to develop strategies within the school and community to encourage young women to continue their education during and after pregnancy.

Income and employment

Young mothers are less likely to be employed and, if they are working, are unlikely to remain in a job for longer than a year.[46] In the USA as many as 80 per cent of all teenagers who give birth are living below the poverty line.[34] In Australia, most teenage mothers also live in poverty, are at high risk of homelessness and have an increased chance of being reliant on government benefits.[47]

The children of teenage mothers are also at a disadvantage because they are more likely to grow up in a single-parent household and in adverse economic circumstances. Providing social support to assist young mothers to address the issues of education, income and employment, and housing is therefore a key to improving the outcomes for young women and their children.[48]

Psychosocial problems

The incidence of psychosocial problems such as psychiatric disease, homelessness, domestic violence and social isolation are common companions of teenage pregnancy.[47] The one-year prevalence of psychiatric disorders in the general adolescent population is 10–15 per cent, increasing up to 21 per cent in some inner city areas.[47] However, data suggests that as many as 60 per cent of all young teenage mothers may have a major psychosocial problem.[47] Common psychiatric diagnoses include emotional, conduct and mixed emotional–conduct disorders. Family and social influences are often important; the role of individual illness is less clear.

Domestic violence may complicate up to 30 per cent of teenage pregnancies, and often involves both physical and sexual abuse.[49] These pregnancies are complicated by higher rates of both maternal and newborn morbidity. Intensive postnatal support is important and can help reduce rates of major adverse outcomes for the infant.

Smoking, alcohol, drug use

Baseline levels of smoking, alcohol and illegal drugs use are significantly higher in the subgroup of teenagers who become pregnant than in the general teenage population and the general antenatal population. In Australia, 31 per cent of women aged 16–19 years are smokers. Data on Australian pregnant teenagers suggests that 44 per cent smoke, compared to rates of 27 per cent in the general antenatal population. Twenty-one per cent of pregnant teenagers drink throughout pregnancy, compared to 5 per cent of the general antenatal population. Illicit drug use is also common in pregnant teenagers. Cannabis is the drug most commonly used, with solvent abuse and heroin the next most commonly used agents.

Diet

Pregnant teenagers often have poor diets, and anaemias are common. Usually 50 per cent of pregnant teenagers will be anaemic (haemoglobin < 11.5 g/dl). In addition to screening for iron deficiency, B12 and folate studies may be warranted. Dietary deficiency can persist into the next generation if not corrected with adequate antenatal education. Infants of teenage mothers are at risk of failure to thrive as a result of poor breastfeeding rates, maternal difficulties in preparing formula feeds according to manufacturer's instructions and inappropriate early introduction of solids.

Strategies to prevent teenage pregnancy

These have focused on three main areas, to educate teenagers of both sexes about contraception and sexual education:

- School-based educational programs
- Community programs to promote contraception and sexual education.
- Preventing a second teenage pregnancy. Up to 80 per cent of teenagers will have a second unplanned teenage pregnancy within two years of their first. Teenagers receiving care following termination of pregnancy or birth of a first child should receive detailed contraceptive advice.

Any program introduced needs to be evaluated for both benefits and adverse effects. There is increasing evidence that the leading risk factors for the onset of teenage mothering arise during the early life of the teenage mother and father. These factors include early-life exposure to domestic violence, parental separation/absence, poverty, low educational attainment and coexisting use of illicit drugs.

Ultimately, strategies to prevent the cycle of teenage pregnancy may be best served through expert early intervention services in childhood.

Legal issues surrounding the teenager

Legal issues are complex because they are influenced by social, psychological and ethical questions that can arise when dealing with young people in the context of sexual relationships, marriage and medical procedures. Before treatment decisions are made, it is necessary to know the law of the place in which you practise.

In the area of adolescent medicine, the key issues for teenagers all involve the age at which the law recognises their ability to give effective consent: consent to their own medical treatment, to sexual relationships and to contraceptive advice and abortion.

Medical treatment, contraception, abortion

Young people do not necessarily have full legal capacity either to give or to withhold consent to treatment. The age at which a young person acquires the legal capacity to give consent to medical treatment was considered by the High Court of Australia.[50] The case incorporated a UK decision[51] into Australian common law. The result was that a minor was considered capable of giving informed consent when he or she 'achieves a sufficient understanding and intelligence to enable him or her to understand fully what is proposed'. A practitioner's decision in any given case will therefore depend on the intelligence and maturity of the young person and the nature and seriousness of the treatment.

The law is not entirely clear in the area of prescribing contraception for girls under eighteen. The legality of prescription will depend on the 'informed consent' issues raised above. General advice to medical practitioners is that they may give contraceptive advice to minors, provided:

- the minor is capable of understanding the advice given
- they are unable to be persuaded to talk to their parents/guardians
- they are otherwise likely to engage in sexual activity without contraception, or
- the treatment is required for their physical or mental health and is in their best interests.

Sexual relations

The age at which a young person can enter into a sexual relationship depends on a number of factors, the most important of which is the age at which the law specifies that a young person is able to consent to sexual relations. The law restricts the sexual behaviour of young people by criminalising the behaviour of the person having sexual relations with the young person. In all Australian states, a person who has sexual intercourse with another person who is under a prescribed age can be found to be guilty of an offence.[52] Consent as a defence is often not available under a certain age, usually 14 years, although this varies between the different jurisdictions.

Conclusion

The turbulent teenage years are a normal transition from child to adult. Many of the health problems of this stage are associated with unhealthy risk-taking. Addressing psychosocial problems in childhood, providing early education about these risks, and devising strategies to improve self-esteem may go some way in preventing problems. Health care professionals are key players in the process.

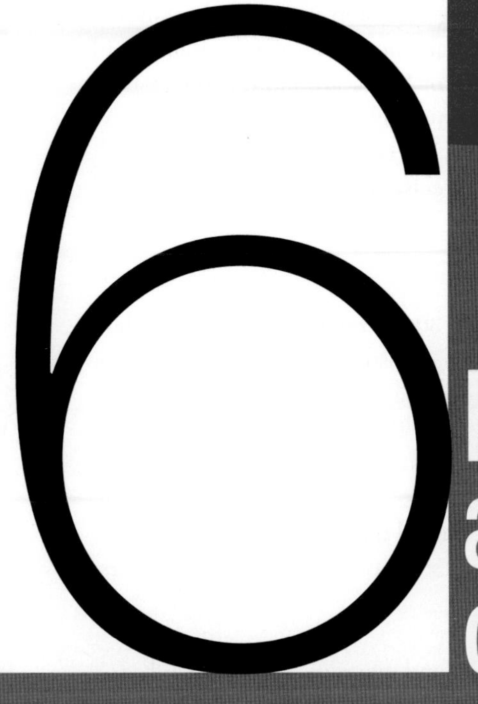

Part 3
The reproductive years

SECTION 6 Pre-pregnancy and antenatal care

Genetics

The mapping of the human genome is an exciting first step in the understanding of our genetic inheritance. However, it is clear that the mode of inheritance and expression of the genes inherited from the mother or father are more complex than originally thought. Inherited susceptibilities and environmental factors affect many common disorders. The notion of a large digital map of chromosomes in which each pair of chromosomes is programmed to work in a precise way and exhibit a particular characteristic is being shown to be too simplistic.

The human genome

The mapping of the human genome located some 30 000 coding genes, fewer than the 100 000 pairs previously proposed. The sequences also provide variants that can be used to track genes through families using genetic studies. It will lead to the development of diagnostic and therapeutic tools and the ability to compare DNA sequences of different racial and ethnic groups. This will lead to understanding of the roles of genes in common diseases. The uses will include diagnosis (eg haemochromatosis), prediction (breast cancer), prenatal diagnosis (eg cystic fibrosis) and therapy (eg immunodeficiency). DNA chips will soon assist in identifying carriers.

Genetic counselling

Genetic factors contribute significantly to morbidity and mortality. Approximately 2–3 per cent of neonates have at least one major congenital abnormality and 2 per cent have either a chromosomal abnormality or a single gene defect. Genetic disorders account for around 50 per cent of severe mental retardation, childhood deafness and blindness. Genetic disorders and congenital malformations are responsible for 40–50 per cent of all childhood deaths. By the age of twenty-five, 5 per cent of the population are affected by a genetic disorder.

In the post-genome era people have an increasing range of screening and diagnostic tests available to them, providing an array of choices for knowing about their health and regarding the child they wish to conceive. A couple may seek screening tests to help maximise their chances of having a healthy child. The practitioner needs to be aware of the available tests and how they can be accessed by the prospective mother, provide information about the benefits of periconceptional folate and potential teratogens such as alcohol. For every couple contemplating a pregnancy, the practitioner needs to review the relevant medical and family information (and construct a three-generation pedigree) to check whether the couple is at average or known increased risk for having a child with birth defects (Figure 6.1 and Box 6.1). This may identify a risk of a genetic disease to the woman herself, to other children or to family members for whom genetic referral may be appropriate. This information should be included in a letter of referral to the geneticist.

In counselling, geneticists aim to establish early in the interview the questions and issues relevant to that individual. It is important to confirm the diagnosis by examining the patient or the patient's records. If the index case (the first known affected individual in the family) is available they are examined together with other

FIGURE 6.1 Constructing a family tree

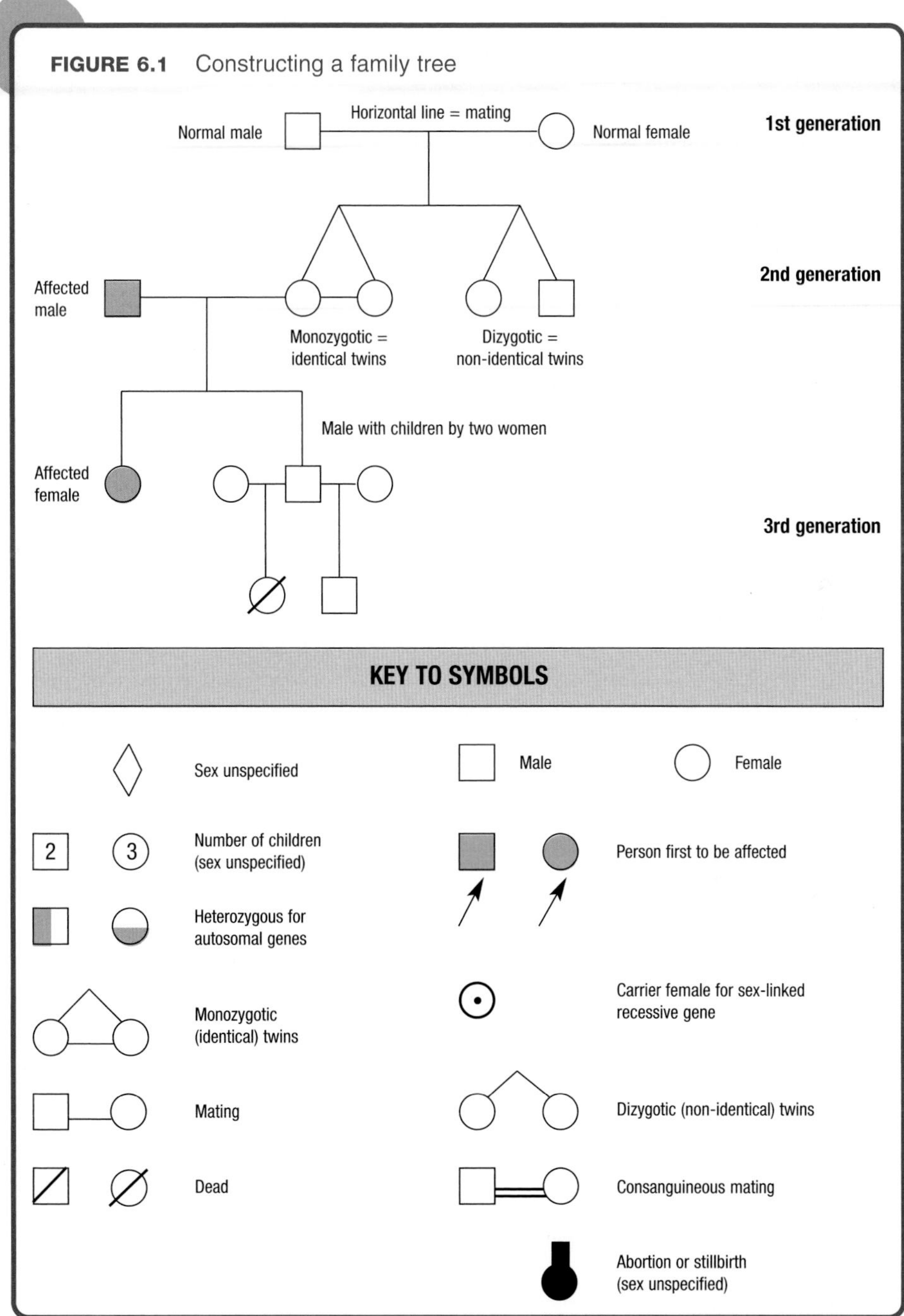

individuals accompanying them who may also be affected, such as parents or siblings. Sometimes further investigations may be needed before the diagnosis can be confirmed. Once the diagnosis is established the family can usually be provided with information about the cause and the likelihood of the condition happening again, and information about the condition itself, which may be helpful in the care of that

BOX 6.1 Reasons for genetic counselling

- A known condition in the family
- The birth of a child with birth defects
- A history of spontaneous fetal losses or perinatal loss—a possible chromosome abnormality
- Advanced maternal age and the risk of trisomy (eg trisomy 21)
- Specific ethnic background needing carrier testing (eg thalassaelmia, Tay-Sachs' disease)
- Inadvertent exposure to potentially harmful substances in pregnancy
- A screening test which identifies increased risk

person. The diagnosis may have implications for other family members. Possible carriers will need investigation and counselling. For some conditions antenatal diagnosis is available for future pregnancies; for others preimplantation genetic diagnosis may be an alternative.

Causes of birth defects (genetic and non-genetic)

There are many causes of birth defects (Box 6.2). Many congenital abnormalities are not inherited and genetic disorders may not be evident at birth. Some anomalies, such as asymmetry or joint contractures, may be the result of deformation (rupture of membranes before the onset of labour; see Section 9) rather than malformation. Infection, drugs or chemicals may disrupt normal embryogenesis, or there may be abnormalities in the programming of development due to genetic causes. There are no simple tests to determine the genetics of a disorder. Genetic factors are deduced from the knowledge of the condition (for example, cystic fibrosis is always recessively inherited), and that in turn is deduced from family studies. Some disorders may be inherited in more than one way. A search for associated distinguishing features and careful family studies may be needed to clarify the mode of inheritance in a particular family.

BOX 6.2 Causes of birth defects

- Chromosomal:
  - Numerical—aneuploidy eg trisomy 21, Turner syndrome
  - Structural—translocations, deletion, duplication, Imprinting
- Single gene disorders :
  - Autosomal dominant, recessive or X-linked
- Multifactorial disorders:
  - Neural tube defects
  - Heart defects
- Teratogens:
  - Infections, drugs, maternal illness
- Disruption/deformation
  - Rupture of membranes before the onset of labour (see Section 9)

Chromosomal problems

Numerical

Trisomy 21

This is the most frequent of the trisomies, occurring in 1:650 births. Most cases of trisomy 21 result from non-dysjunction in the ovum, mainly in the first and sometimes in the second meiotic division. There is a strong association between increased frequency of trisomy 21 and advanced maternal age. Ultrasound examination in the first trimester may alert the obstetrician to potential problems by finding thick nuchal folds. High-risk pregnancies at any maternal age may be identified by triple screening of maternal serum and are tested further by karyotyping CVS or amniotic cells. Later ultrasound findings include a flat occiput and incurved fifth fingers. The risk of recurrence is 1:100 (plus the maternal age-related risk of trisomy 21).

The same phenotype in about 5 per cent of cases is due to translocation. In that case, parental chromosomes should be checked to establish whether one of the parents is a translocation carrier. If this is the case, the risk of recurrence is 12 per cent for maternal and less than 2 per cent for paternal carriers.

Children with trisomy 21 have a distinctive facial appearance, intellectual disability and variable birth defects. Those who do not have cyanotic heart disease and survive the first two years have a normal expectation of survival to adult life.

Turner syndrome, 45X

It has been estimated that 90 per cent of 45X conceptions abort spontaneously and perhaps all survivors are at some level mosaics. The risk of recurrence is low. Turner syndrome may be diagnosed:

- *Incidentally:* the karyotype may be found incidentally when screening the pregnancy for advanced maternal age
- *During pregnancy:* by finding cystic hygroma on ultrasound examination and checking the karyotype
- *In the newborn:* oedema of the hands and feet and congenital heart disease (coarctation of the aorta) may lead to the diagnosis
- *In girls:* girls are diagnosed because of short stature, delayed puberty and variable dysmorphic features, and they are almost all sterile. Intelligence is in the normal range although there may be learning problems. Oestrogen treatment is recommended to achieve secondary sex characteristics. Immaturity often results in social problems.

Only half the girls with Turner syndrome have a 45X karyotype. Others have various/mosaic rearrangements in one of the pair of X chromosomes and may be fertile but at risk of early menopause.

Structural

Imprinting

The following examples are rare but interesting disorders and are another mechanism for variation. It is known that it is essential to inherit one chromosome of a pair from each parent. It appears that a number of chromosomes are imprinted, that is, altered in some way by passage through that parent. The gene appears to carry with it a 'history' of its origin. It has an 'imprint' from conception as to whether it is of maternal or paternal origin. In the cells where the gene is active the 'imprinted' version of the gene is switched on and the other switched off. An example of the complexities of inheritance can be seen by considering chromosome 15.

Prader-Willi and Angelman syndromes

Two conditions exist which are the result of a change in chromosome 15 (chromosome locus 15q.11 affected in both syndromes). In the Prader-Willi syndrome the person has small hands and feet, and underdeveloped sex organs. They also have temper tantrums and are mildly mentally retarded. At birth these children are floppy and pale-skinned, and refuse to suck at the breast, but later the eating pattern is uncontrolled, resulting in obesity. A child with Angelman syndrome, on the other hand, is taut and thin with a small head and long jaw. They are hyperactive and suffer insomnia. They move jerkily, have a happy disposition but never learn to speak and are severely mentally retarded. In both these syndromes part of chromosome 15 is missing. In Prader-Willi syndrome, the missing material is from the father's chromosome, whereas in Angelman syndrome it is from the mother's chromosome.

Imprinted genes seem to evolve quite slowly. There appears to be an 'imprinting centre' which is a small stretch of DNA close to both the relevant genes that somehow places a 'mark' on the chromosome. To add a further complexity to 'imprinting' is the observation that this switches from mother to father. In a man, the maternal copy of chromosome 15 carries a mark that identifies it as coming from his mother, but when that man passes it to his son or daughter it acquires his 'mark'—that is, it identifies it as coming from the father.

Single gene disorders

Fragile Xq27.3

This is the most common form of inherited intellectual disability, affecting about 1:1500 males. It is inherited as an X-linked condition. The alteration in the gene is a triplet repeat expansion of three nucleotides, CGG, and the size of the expansion often increases from parent to child, particularly when transmitted by the mother. The carrier frequency in women may be as high as 1:200. Repeats of 50–200 are considered to be a pre-mutation and over that number a full mutation. The level of fragile X mental retardation protein (FMRP) correlates with the level of disability. DNA diagnosis has replaced chromosome analysis and depends on the estimation of the number of triplet repeats.

Males with this condition are shy and avoid eye contact. They have intellectual disability of variable extent, ADHD, a distinctive facial appearance with a long face, large jaw and large ears as well as large testicles. In females the appearance is more subtle and the developmental effects less than in males. It is important to identify the carrier females in the family to clarify their chances of having an affected child. Prenatal diagnosis is available.

Cystic fibrosis

Cystic fibrosis is inherited in an autosomal recessive fashion. This means that a couple who have had one child with cystic fibrosis have a 1 in 4 chance of recurrence in any pregnancy. Gene frequency in the population is 1:20 (UK) and 1:25 (Australia).

Usual screening is available for:

- delta 508 deletion (70% population)
- exon 11 mutation G551D, G542X, R553X (7% population).

The introduction of gene sequencing technology will facilitate identification of other mutations. If these common mutations are identified the carrier risk is reduced to 1:110. The normal sister of an affected person has a 2 out of 3 chance of being a carrier and her carrier status can be clarified by gene testing if the mutations are known in the family. Her unrelated husband has the population risk of 1 in 25 of being a carrier. There is a 1 in 4 chance that two carriers will have a homozygous and affected baby. The sister of a person with cystic fibrosis has a 1 in 150 risk of having an affected child (2/3 × 1/25 × 1/4) if no carrier gene testing is performed. If both mutations are identified, DNA studies in the sister will clarify whether she is a carrier of one of the mutations and if not, then her residual risk of being a carrier is low. If she is a carrier, then her partner can be screened for the common cystic fibrosis mutations. If no mutation is identified, their risk of an affected child is low. If both are found to be carriers, then antenatal diagnosis may be offered to them. A chorionic villus sampling at 11 weeks of pregnancy provides sufficient DNA for testing and the result is usually available in two weeks. If the result is positive for homozygous mutations, the couple have the option of interrupting the pregnancy.

Multifactorial

Neural tube defects

Neural tube defects (NTDs) include anencephaly, spina bifida, some encephaloceles and hydrocephalus. They are the second most frequent serious malformation, surpassed only by congenital heart defects. Neural tube defects are a heterogenous group of disorders that result from failure of the neural tube to close normally between the third and fourth week of embryological development. During development, the cranial end of the neural tube becomes the forebrain, mid-brain and hind-brain; a failure here results in anencephaly. A failure of closure distal to this region usually results in spina bifida. A third type of NTD, an encephalocele, is an extrusion of brain tissue through a skull defect, usually covered by overlying skin. The aetiology is multifactorial, including both genetic and environmental factors. Population studies point to environmental and nutritional factors. There is now good evidence that when at-risk pregnancies are treated with folate before conception and through the first trimester of pregnancy, up to an 80 per cent reduction in the development of neural tube defects can be achieved.

When there is an open neural tube defect, elevated levels of alpha fetoprotein (AFP) may be detected in maternal serum and amniotic fluid. Amniotic AFP levels can be normal when the neural tube defect is covered by skin. A careful ultrasound examination in expert hands can detect most cases of anencephaly and spina bifida by

18–20 weeks of pregnancy. Anencephaly may be detected as early as 10 weeks of pregnancy by vaginal ultrasound examination. When an encephalocele is found, one must look for other birth defects to establish the cause. Associated multiple birth defects may point to a chromosomal cause, as in the recessively inherited Meckel syndrome where there is also polydactyly and large polycystic kidneys.

Teratogenesis

Teratogens are agents which disrupt normal embryogenesis. These include intrauterine infections, drugs, chemicals and radiation (Table 6.1). Not all fetuses are equally vulnerable to damage and the vulnerability is related to the time of exposure in relation to gestation and possible maternal factors, such as whether or not the mother has immune antibodies to a virus. The teratogenic pathogenesis is agent-specific and tissue-specific. For example, retinoic acid interferes with cranial neural crest development and therefore affects structures derived from these tissues.

TABLE 6.1 Examples of teratogenic agents

Teratogen	Timing	Result	Notes
Infections			
Syphilis	First 20 weeks	Rhinitis, depressed nasal bridge, cartilage and bone defects, skin rash and mucosal defects, lymphadenopathy and hepatosplenomegaly. Subsequent dentition shows notched incisors.	Prevented with routine maternal antenatal serological screening Treatment is chemotherapy with penicillin before the fourth month.
Toxoplasmosis	First trimester greatest risk of clinically severe disease	Fetal death or severely affected with convulsions, hepatosplenomegaly, microcephaly and mental retardation	Good hygiene and avoid exposure to faeces and undercooked meat during pregnancy. Chemotherapy with sulphonamide and pyrimethamine
Varicella	First 20 weeks	Congenital varicella syndrome in 2–3% of fetuses involving CNS, eye and limb malformations	Requires primary maternal exposure and most women have had exposure even if not remembered. Vaccine available prior to pregnancy if no immunity
Parvovirus B19 (Fifth Disease)	First 20 weeks especially Third trimester possible cause of stillbirth	Miscarriage and fetal haemolytic anaemia causing hydrops fetalis	Monitor with biweekly ultrasound; many will recover.

TABLE 6.1 continued

Teratogen	Timing	Result	Notes
Rubella	First 20 weeks	Congenital rubella syndrome includes cataracts, IUGR, thrombocytopenia, purpura, patent ductus arteriosus, osteitis and hearing impairment. Microcephaly and chorioretinitis are also common.	Immunity available through childhood vaccination program
Occupational hazards			
Radiation	First trimester	Miscarriage	Avoid procedures involving high doses if possible or use lead screening
Organic solvents	First trimester	Hydrocephalus, skeletal and cardiovascular malformations, neurodevelopmental defects	Exposure at normal safety levels not associated with increased risk
Drugs			
Isotretinoin	Prepregnancy and first trimester	Craniofacial, limb, ear, and cardiovascular defects	Used to treat severe acne
Anticonvulsants (phenytoin, carbamazepine, valproic acid)	Mainly first trimester	1–2% risk of neural tube defects Cardiac defects Interferes with maternal vitamin K production	Take 5 mg folic acid Consider supplement with vitamin K after 34 weeks
Warfarin	6–9 weeks	Nasal hypoplasia and stippled epiphyses	Later use may result in fetal CNS haemorrhage
Tetracyclines	After 16 weeks	Damage to developing teeth and bones	
Sulphonamides	Late pregnancy	Neonatal hyperbilirubinaemia	
Lithium	First trimester	Cardiac defect	Cardiac ultrasound of neonate Monitor Li levels carefully throughout pregnancy and also check thyroid function regularly
Vitamin A		Cardiac and ear defects, facial dysmorphism and oral facial clefting	Risky in doses higher than 30 000 IU/day
Alcohol	Pre-pregnancy and throughout	Fetal alcohol syndrome (growth restriction, facial dysmorphia, CNS impairment, skeletal and cardiac anomalies and ophthalmological effects) and fetal alcohol effects (neuro behavioural)	No safe level determined. Occasional light social drinks probably safe.

Although women must be cautioned against drug ingestion in pregnancy, few drugs have been shown to have serious teratogenic affects. Drug information databases are available in the major maternity or paediatric hospitals and should be consulted in cases of inadvertent drug exposure in pregnancy. It is important to carefully document both dosage and timing of the ingestion with respect to gestation.

Disruption/deformation

An insult event may occur to a normally developing fetus and result in birth defects. Loss of amniotic fluid from premature rupture of the membranes in the first trimester may result in multiple malformations. Rupture in later pregnancy may result in limb amputation defects. Careful examination of the fetus, or baby, and placenta is necessary to establish the diagnosis. Oligohydramnios may result in deformation in the facial appearance and causation of joint contractures. Positional deformities may also be secondary to neuromuscular defects in the fetus.

Pregnancy-associated tests

Couples need to be given detailed information about their options so they can make informed choices about future pregnancies. Screening tests are available to all pregnant women, and diagnostic tests for women of known increased risk for a specific disorder (Box 6.3). It needs to be made clear that none of the available tests for prenatal diagnosis can ensure that the baby is free of all birth defects. It should not be assumed that just because a test is available the family will choose to use it. There is a need for open discussion about the chances of problems in further pregnancies and how the couple would regard the diagnosis of the problem in the next pregnancy. In particular it needs to be established whether or not they would elect to interrupt the pregnancy. The family is made aware that in the course of testing for a particular condition other abnormalities may be diagnosed incidentally. In such instances they would be fully informed about the findings and their implications.

The single-gene disorders for which prenatal tests are most commonly requested include:

- cystic fibrosis
- Duchene/Becker muscular dystrophy (X-linked)
- beta-thalassaemia
- fragile X syndrome
- inborn errors of metabolism.

Where a disorder occurs frequently in a community or specific group, population antenatal carrier testing or targeted screening might be available (for example, Tay-Sachs' disease has a prevalence of 0.25 per 1000 births among Ashkenazi Jews—some 100 times higher than the general population).

Diagnostic tests in pregnancy

Chorionic villus sampling

Chorionic villus sampling (CVS) is performed for the diagnosis of chromosome abnormalities and biochemical disorders, and is the preferred DNA test in pregnancy.

BOX 6.3 **Antenatal tests for women**

Screening tests

These tests can identify a woman who is at a greater risk of having a baby with a birth defect but cannot diagnose the particular condition a baby may have.

<table>
<tr><th>Procedure</th><th>When?</th><th>Why?</th><th>What happens next?</th></tr>
<tr><td>Combined first trimester blood test and ultrasound scan</td><td>Blood test at 10 weeks, ultrasound at 11–13 weeks</td><td>Predicts the risk of the baby having trisomy 21 or trisomy 18 by combining a nuchal translucency measurement with serum screening</td><td rowspan="2">Women identified to be at increased risk may be offered the option of a diagnostic test (chorionic villus sampling or amniocentesis).</td></tr>
<tr><td>Nuchal translucency scan</td><td>At 11–14 weeks</td><td>Predicts the risk of the baby having trisomy 21 by measuring the pocket of fluid in the fetal nuchal region</td></tr>
<tr><td>Quadruple serum screening</td><td>At 14–20 weeks (optimal timing 15–17 weeks)</td><td>Predicts the risk of the baby having trisomy 21, trisomy 18 or a neural tube defect</td><td>If a high risk for neural tube defect is identified, a tertiary level ultrasound is recommended.</td></tr>
<tr><td>Second trimester ultrasound scan</td><td>At 18–20 weeks</td><td>To detect many structural problems, such as neural tube, heart and limb defects</td><td>If concern is raised, a further scan and a specialist referral may be offered.</td></tr>
</table>

Diagnostic tests

Invasive tests which allow direct analysis of fetal cells for definitive diagnosis. These tests are offered when there is increased risk indicated by a screening test, where there is a family history of an inherited condition and a specific test is available or when the mother will be 37 years or older at the time of delivery.

Procedure	When?	Why?
Chorionic villus sampling (CVS)	Usually 10–12 weeks	To diagnose chromosomal abnormalities or in specific cases single gene defects.
Amniocentesis	Usually 15–18 weeks	To diagnose chromosomal or biochemical abnormalities.

The procedure is performed at 10–11 weeks of pregnancy (Figure 6.2). A sample of chorionic villi is obtained under ultrasound guidance by either the trans-abdominal or trans-cervical route. The villi are checked to remove maternal tissue and cultured in the laboratory. Usually more than one culture is set up and the cells can be examined according to the condition being screened. Chorionic villus sampling carries a small risk of miscarriage—about 1 in 100. The pre-procedure risk is influenced by the gestation at which the procedure is performed, the maternal age, and the indication for sampling. The magnitude of the procedural risk is dependent on the expertise of the operator and the technical difficulties. Most test results are available within two weeks; aneuploidy screen by FISH (fluorescent in situ hybridisation for chromosomes 13, 16, 18, 21, 22) will produce results overnight. If the pregnancy needs to be interrupted for an abnormal result this can be by curettage.

If a CVS is performed before 10 weeks there is an increased risk of limb deformities in the fetus.

FIGURE 6.2 Chorionic villus sampling

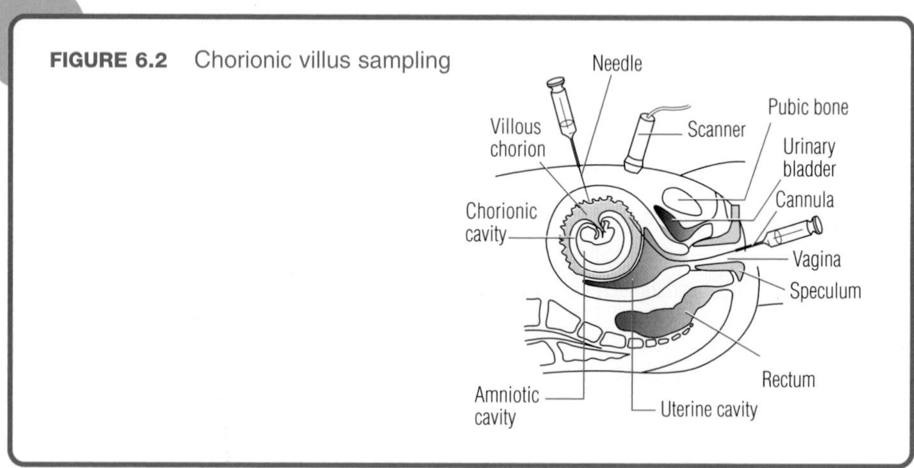

FIGURE 6.3 Amniocentesis

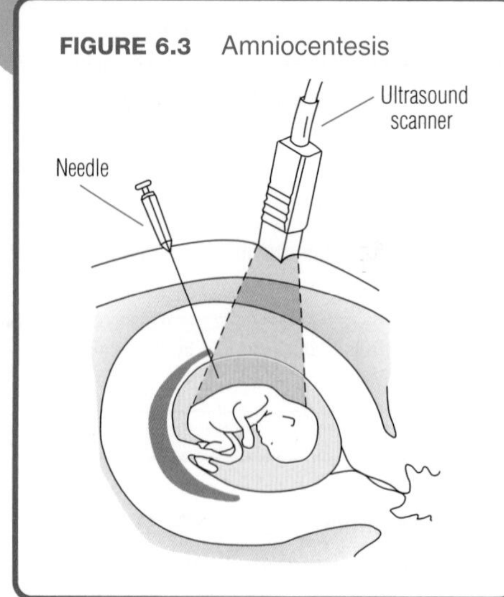

Amniocentesis

Amniocentesis is performed at 15–18 weeks of pregnancy (Figure 6.3). It involves removing some amniotic fluid with ultrasound guidance. The amniotic fluid may be tested for metabolites, or the amniocytes and ectodermal cells shed by the baby can be cultured and examined. A sufficient volume of cells needs to be cultured for biochemical or DNA tests. Cultured cells can be karyotyped. This procedure carries a smaller risk of miscarriage. The actual risk is operator-dependent (an experienced operator being one who performs at least 50 procedures per annum) and the average risk is 1 in 200. Being a second trimester test, interruption of pregnancy, when indicated, is undertaken by prostaglandin induction of labour.

Fetal blood sampling

This may be performed rarely for:

- Genetic diagnosis: for women at high risk who book late, a culture failure after amniocentesis, and a mosaic result requiring definitive diagnosis
- Fetal anaemia (also diagnosed with Doppler ultrasound) and severe fetal thrombocytopenia.

Tissue sampling

Fetal tissue sampling has been largely superseded by the availability of gene testing for rare disorders. For example, a more direct diagnosis than fetal skin biopsy for the diagnosis of lethal epidermolysis bullosa dystrophica may be available if the mutation has been identified in the index case. Tissue sampling is performed by trans-abdominal puncture under ultrasound guidance. In some instances this may still need to be performed using fetoscopy (inserting a very thin telescope into the amniotic cavity), which involves the mother in a spinal or general anaesthetic.

Pre-implantation genetic diagnosis

Pre-implantation genetic diagnosis (PGD) may be available in the context of assisted reproduction or in vitro fertilisation. Eggs are harvested and fertilised by intra-cytoplasmic sperm injection (ICSI), where one sperm is injected into each egg. The fertilised egg begins to divide and by day 3 it is 6–8 cells in size. Of these one or two can be removed safely for testing. An increasing number of gene tests can be performed on single cells. Fluorescent in situ hybridisation can identify whether one or more copies of specific chromosomes are present, identifying conditions such as trisomy 21. The apparently 'normal' embryo can then be selected for transfer to the uterus to achieve a pregnancy. These techniques are now well established. A couple may need to undergo more than one cycle of treatment to achieve a pregnancy.

Evaluation of the neonate/child

A geneticist should be consulted when a baby is born with multiple malformations, dysmorphism or disproportion. Evaluation of the baby may reveal a syndrome, a chromosome abnormality or an inborn error of metabolism. Many syndromes are recognised by the features in the baby, the so-called 'gestalt'. Confirmatory tests are available for chromosome and metabolic disorders and by gene testing for an increasing number of conditions.

Children may also present because of growth and/or developmental delay or dysmorphism. The family member with the most striking features presents and often other family members are incidentally diagnosed on more subtle features of the condition. When there is a known disorder in the family, parents may seek to clarify whether their child has inherited the condition or the gene. Predictive testing is offered only to minors if they are likely to benefit directly from the information—for example, if there is treatment available or benefit from early surveillance. Adolescents may wish to know their carrier status to clarify their reproductive risks. The timing of these tests needs individual consideration.

Postnatal genetic tests

Other indications for chromosomal analysis in childhood and adulthood include:

- recurrent abortions (at least three)
- primary amenorrhoea
- infertility
- familial chromosome rearrangement in a relative
- newborn with a birth defect, including ambiguous genitalia
- children with a learning disability
- premature menopause
- familial cancers (eg two or more members with endometrial cancer under 60 years or endometrial cancer and a family history of bowel cancer).

The cause of most cancers is unknown. Five to ten per cent of cancers of the breast, ovary and bowel are due to the presence of an inherited cancer-predisposing autosomal dominant mutation. People can be referred for risk assessment, genetic testing and surveillance advice to a family cancer genetic centre where genetic counselling is available. The finding of multiple family members with the same cancer, particularly at a young age or multiple cancers in the family or even in the one individual, indicate potential high risk for individuals in the same lineage and so genetic counselling is recommended. A carefully compiled family tree is necessary to help interpret the risks. For example, with ovarian cancer, having a first-degree relative under the age of 50 years with the disease confers a risk of 1 in 15 compared to 1 in 70 for the general population. There is an overall relative risk of seven in families with two or more cases of ovarian cancer. This gives an absolute risk of ovarian cancer by the age of 70 years of 11 per cent.

Breast cancer gene 1 and 2 (BRCA1 and BRCA2) testing is available to high-risk breast cancer families. An index case (a family member with breast cancer) needs to be tested to clarify the mutation present in the family. Having both breast and ovarian cancer in the family also constitutes a high chance of a BRCA mutation. Not all people who have inherited the mutation will develop breast or ovarian cancer. A surveillance regimen is recommended.

Familial endometrial cancer most often occurs as part of the hereditary non-polyposis colon cancer syndrome (HNPCC), due to mutations in mismatched repair genes. During their lifetime, female mutation carriers of HNPCC have a 60 per cent risk of uterine cancer, a 12 per cent risk of ovarian cancer, a 54 per cent risk of colorectal cancer and a 13 per cent risk of gastric cancer.

Referral of women for genetic counselling can be undertaken after a careful history has been taken and the wishes of the woman established. It is important that these be informed choices for these life-defining decisions. Predictive testing in particular needs to include counselling to carefully consider the potential benefit and harm of such knowledge.

Pre-pregnancy counselling

The opportunity to counsel a woman about her health before a pregnancy is the ideal. However, 50 per cent of pregnancies are unplanned, so this may be less easy to arrange. A health professional should be prepared to offer 'opportunistic advice' to any woman of childbearing years. Although not all problems can be prevented, good pre-conception and antenatal care can improve pregnancy outcomes. The consultation should include an assessment of individual risks, a discussion of health promotion and a plan of interventions (Box 6.4). A number of the conditions listed can be found under the specific section on that topic.

BOX 6.4 **Pre-pregnancy counselling**

- Assessing risks for discussion
  - Individual: age, ethnic background, family history
  - Social: support, economic status, work environment, access to health care
  - Health behaviours: smoking, alcohol, illicit drugs
  - Existing medical conditions: hypertension, CVD, renal disease, diabetes, thyroid disease, epilepsy
  - Psychological: depression, anxiety, stress, abuse
  - Reproductive history: all pregnancies and their outcomes
- Advice on promoting health
  - Nutrition: folic acid supplementation, balanced diet
  - Drugs: quit smoking programs, controlled alcohol intake, discuss illicit drug use
  - Sex: STI prevention, hepatitis and HIV counselling
  - Exercise: regular activity to improve general fitness
- Interventions
  - Cervical screening
  - Rubella and hepatitis immunisation
  - Weight control
  - Medication advice (change, cease, maintain)
  - Genetic counselling

Parental age and pregnancy

Women are choosing to wait for a pregnancy until they are in their late twenties or thirties. Monthly fecundity and cumulative pregnancy rates decline progressively at five-year increments beginning at age 30 years.[1] Much of this data has come from fertility clinics. In general terms, for women 30 years or younger the cycle fecundity is 20 per cent, compared to 10 per cent in women aged 36–40 years, and 5 per cent in women older than 40 years.

Women having their first birth in Australia have an average age of 29 years. Maternal age at conception in the late thirties is linked to an increased rate of fetal loss, a steep increase occurring after age 35, with more than one-fifth of all pregnancies in 35-year-old women resulting in fetal loss, and more than half in 42-year-olds. Spontaneous miscarriages, stillbirths and ectopic pregnancies are all more likely in older women. In addition, almost every complication of pregnancy is increased in nulliparous women who give birth beyond age 40, including pre-eclampsia, gestational diabetes, malpresentation, shoulder dystocia and placenta praevia. Paternal age is also correlated with increased morbidity rates—for example, achondroplasia and schizophrenia.[2,3] The biological disadvantages of being older parents may be balanced by social advantages—such as a better economic situation.[4] This is information that a couple may find relevant when planning to start a family.

Nutrition, weight and diet

In developed countries the standard of nutrition is good and maternal nutrition has only a small effect on the health of the infant.[5]

Infection from food

Listeria monocytogenes, a bacterial infection with the reservoir in animals, can contaminate foods. It can survive protected from host defences as an intracellular pathogen in macrophages and monocytes. It is destroyed by cooking but will grow in refrigerated foods (Box 6.5). Maternal infection with *Listeria* can lead to miscarriage, stillbirth, premature birth or neonatal septicaemia and pneumonia. However, it is uncommon; in one study the incidence of perinatal listeriosis was around 4.0 per 10 000 live births. Chorioamnionitis was the predominant clinical presentation. The overall neonatal mortality rate was 7.7 per cent among infected live births. Early antenatal treatment with ampicillin improved neonatal outcome and resulted in the birth of healthy babies.[6]

BOX 6.5 Avoiding *Listeria* infection

- Avoid raw meat contaminating other foods.
- Thaw frozen food in the refrigerator or microwave.
- Reheat food to steaming hot.
- Avoid:
  - chilled ready-to-eat foods
  - unpasteurised milk
  - ready-cooked take-away foods.

Weight

Evaluating a woman for overweight, underweight or particular dietary patterns pre pregnancy may be of value. Both extremes of weight are associated with increased risks for the mother and baby in a pregnancy. Obesity during pregnancy is associated with many acknowledged health risks, including a higher prevalence of caesarean section, hypertension, deep vein thrombosis and diabetes mellitus. Several epi-demiological studies have suggested that being overweight before pregnancy is a risk factor for neural tube defects (NTDs). A body mass index > 29 kg/m^2 doubles the risk of NTDs. This risk appears to be higher among female offspring and can be only partially reduced by folate supplementation.

Folic acid

Miscarriage

It is suggested that women with a low plasma folate (< 2.19 ng/ml or 4.9 nmol/l) may have an increased risk of miscarriage compared to women with folate concentrations > 5 nmol/l, although this is not confirmed in a Cochrane review.[7] Women with low plasma folate who miscarried were more likely to have been carrying a fetus with a chromosomal abnormality.[8] Folate is necesary for methyl group metabolism, including methylation of DNA, and therefore control of gene expression.[9]

Neural tube defects

It has been shown that taking folic acid supplements during early pregnancy reduces the risk of NTDs in babies (relative risk 0.28, 95% CI 0.13–0.58).[7] Folic acid is a B-group vitamin. Dietary intake of folic acid is seldom sufficient to meet the RDI for pregnancy; therefore supplementation is recommended. Neural tube defects occur 25–29 days after conception, before many women even realise they are pregnant, and therefore it is important for women to begin taking folic acid supplements before conception (ideally, when birth control measures are discontinued).[10] Most healthy women should take 0.4 mg of folic acid every day. Women should take 5 mg folic acid every day before and while pregnant if they have:

- diabetes or epilepsy
- a family history of neural tube defects
- given birth to a baby with neural tube defects.

Iron

The cause of any anaemia can be established and treatment instigated before pregnancy. Iron deficiency is common in women. It is often associated with heavy periods, frequent pregnancies and breastfeeding; some women also have a dietary component. A woman approaching pregnancy and delivery who is anaemic and iron deficient will have fewer reserves to call on in the event of an unexpected haemorrhage.

Pap test

A Pap test should be undertaken according to local recommendations, ideally before pregnancy. A test during pregnancy may provoke bleeding due to the increased vascularity of the cervix. This bleeding occurs outside the uterine cavity and is not harmful to the pregnancy, but it may cause concern for the woman.

Promoting an ideal intrauterine environment

Alcohol

It is now recognised that fetal alcohol syndrome (FAS) represents only a small part of a much larger clinical and social problem termed 'fetal alcohol effects' (FAE).

Alcohol-related fetal effects are among the most common causes of mental retardation, and they can be prevented completely at the primary level. Advising women about drug use before a pregnancy occurs is essential. However, a balance must be maintained as retrospective advice to 'not drink during pregnancy' becomes not only impractical but also unnecessarily alarming (Section 2).

Smoking

The prevalence of cigarette smoking among women of childbearing age continues to be an important health concern as most women who smoke regularly began smoking before 18 years of age. Advice from a health professional has been shown to be effective in moving women through the stages towards quitting (Section 2).

Managing existing conditions

The decision to discontinue medications during pregnancy should be based on scientific evidence. Not all chronic maternal conditions have an impact on pregnancy. However, some, such as poorly controlled diabetes mellitus, phenylketonuria, epilepsy and antiphospholipid syndrome, may be associated with significant fetal risks. Consideration of any medical condition should involve how the condition may affect a pregnancy and how the pregnancy affects the condition (Section 9).

Diabetes mellitus

Women with type 1 diabetes mellitus have 6.4 times the reported risk of a congenital malformation and 5.1 times the reported risk of perinatal mortality in the general population.[11] The importance of good blood glucose control before starting a pregnancy needs to be emphasised to diabetic women. Optimisation of care is often associated with improved outcome; there is good data to suggest that stabilisation of glycaemic control in diabetes reduces the number of malformations. Ideally all women with pre-existing diabetes and a past history of gestational diabetes should be seen before they embark on a pregnancy. At this consultation the objectives are to:

- Review her diabetes, in particular looking for microvascular complications (eg retinopathy and renal involvement)
- Help the woman achieve optimal blood glucose control which may mean starting insulin therapy for women with type 2 diabetes or altering the timing and dosage of insulin for type 1 diabetics
- Start folic acid therapy (5 mg daily) to reduce the risk of neural tube defects
- Evaluate her diet, including weight control particularly for overweight women with type 2 diabetes
- Address other lifestyle issues such as smoking and exercise
- Build a relationship with the team who will be caring for her during the pregnancy, including an obstetrician, an obstetric physician, a dietitian and a midwife.

Epilepsy

Approximately 3 in 1000 pregnant women have some form of seizure disorder. The reproductive hormones may affect the reproductive health of women with epilepsy[12]

(Box 6.6). Oestrogen enhances neuronal excitability and lowers seizure threshold, whereas progesterone enhances inhibition and increases the seizure threshold. Congenital malformation is the most commonly reported outcome among the offspring of women with epilepsy. Anti-epileptic drugs reduce the serum folate level and folic acid supplements are therefore recommended to women taking these drugs. In general, women with epilepsy should be counselled before becoming pregnant and should be controlled with a single drug at the lowest possible dose that will control the epilepsy.[13]

BOX 6.6 Reproductive health, hormones and women with epilepsy

- Increased anovulatory cycles
- Increased incidence of polycystic ovary disease
- Increased risk of seizures perimenstrually and around ovulation
- Onset or exacerbation of epilepsy at puberty

Checking for infections

Some infections can be identified and treated pre pregnancy; others might be avoided by giving appropriate information and advice (Table 6.2).

Sexually transmissible infections

Identifying and treating a sexually transmissible infection (STI) (Sections 9 and 12) before pregnancy can minimise the chance of the baby being infected and can allow for the safe use of antibiotics (Table 6.2).

TORCH syndrome

Numerous congenital infections of the fetus in utero can infect the central nervous system. The infectious agents causing the TORCH syndrome are: toxoplasmosis, rubella, cytomegalovirus and herpes simplex. The features of this syndrome are:

- low birth weight
- microcephaly
- congenital heart disease
- jaundice
- hepatosplenomegaly
- eye lesions
- petechiae and purpura
- late effects: developmental delay, deafness, visual defects and mental retardation.

Pre-pregnancy is a good opportunity to educate women about lifestyle issues, to minimise the chance of acquiring these infections.

TABLE 6.2 Pre-pregnancy testing for infection

Infection	Test	Reason	Action
Viruses			
Rubella	IgG antibody	Check immunity	If not immune arrange vaccination, delay conceiving for 1 month post vaccination.
Hepatitis B	HepBsAg	Baby at risk of infection	Arrange immunisation/administration of globulin at birth
Hepatitis C	Hep C Ab/RNA	Detect women infected/alert staff exposed	Check liver function, advise risks
Varicella	Varicella Ab	Identify non-immune women	Arrange antenatal vaccination if not immune
HIV	HIV antibody	Identify HIV +ve women	Counsel and discuss treatment
CMV	CMV IgG	Identify non-immune women	Advise high-risk women
Bacteria			
Treponema pallidum Syphilis	VDRL/RPR FT-Abs	Identify current infection	Treat appropriately
STIs: *Chlamydia trachomatis* *Gonorrhoea neisseria*	Genital swabs	Associated risk of miscarriage Neonatal conjunctivitis	Treat, contact trace
Protozoa			
Toxoplasma gondii	Toxoplasmosis IgG	Identify non-immune women	Advise about risk

The tests may vary according to the community, the epidemiology, cost, available treatment and local decisions.

Toxoplasmosis

Infection in humans can be minimised by simple precautions (Table 6.3). In immunocompetent people, infection is usually asymptomatic. Screening for the disease in pregnancy has been suggested. However, it is not clear whether antenatal treatment of presumed toxoplasmosis will reduce the congenital transmission of *Toxoplasma gondii*.

Rubella

Rubella virus is a human-specific ribonucleic acid virus that causes mild infection in children and adults with peak incidence in the late winter and early spring. Rubella (other than intrauterine) is transmitted through direct contact with nasopharyngeal

TABLE 6.3 Primary prevention of congenital toxoplasmosis for pregnant women[14]

Food	Environment
Eat well-cooked meat and avoid unpasteurised milk products	Empty cat litter daily (spores take 48 hrs to develop)
Wash hands, utensils and counters after handling raw meat and before eating	Wear gloves during and wash hands after handling cat litter
Avoid touching eyes and mucous membranes	Disinfect cat litter box with boiling water
Wash raw foods before eating	Avoid feeding cats uncooked meat
Wash hands after handling raw foods (fruit and vegetables)	Wear gloves while gardening

secretions. Immunity is usually prolonged, and reinfection adequate to cause transplacental infection is very rare. Some women may not have been vaccinated as a child or adolescent and other women may have emigrated from a country where vaccination is not available. Women should be tested pre pregnancy and vaccinated if they are not already immune. Prior to vaccination pregnancy needs to be excluded, and women should be advised not to become pregnant within one month of vaccination. Approximately 5 per cent of women will not develop high levels of circulating antibody in spite of repeated vaccination. These women will, however, have protection from congenital rubella syndrome and do not need repeated vaccinations.

Cytomegalovirus

Cytomegalovirus (CMV) infection, the most common congenital viral infection in humans, carries high risk of long-term morbidity and mortality. Women working in day-care centres and nurseries, where annual seroconversion rates range from 12 to 20 per cent, should determine their antibody status before conception. Seronegative women should ideally adhere to strict hygiene practices to reduce the risk of acquiring primary CMV.

Herpes simplex

Women with recent acquisition of herpes simplex virus (HSV) are more likely to have asymptomatic viral shedding from the cervix. If the infection occurred before pregnancy, it is uncommon to have associated problems for the baby. Neonates born to mothers with recurrent HSV-2 infection appear to acquire protective immunity from the mother and are at low risk of acquiring HSV infection.

Chickenpox (varicella)

A woman's immunity can be tested and, if she is susceptible, she can be offered vaccination. It is essential to ensure she is not pregnant at the time of vaccination, as the vaccine's safety for the fetus has not been proved.

Genetic counselling

Genetic counselling is often helpful to assist couples in making choices about whether or not to become pregnant or have antenatal testing during the pregnancy (see Genetics). It is important to emphasise to women who are counselled that no test has 100 per cent accuracy. The fetus may still have a birth defect, and some problems cannot be detected by testing.

Maintaining psychological health

Women with a depressive illness and those without adequate interpersonal and social supports are at increased risk for depression during pregnancy. Identifying these women before the pregnancy and discussing with them how they can obtain support may prevent exacerbation of any mental health problems during and after the pregnancy (Section 3).

Abuse

Abuse is controlling behaviour towards a woman without regard to her rights, body or health. Identifying an abusive relationship allows the problem to be acknowledged and information to be given (Section 3 and see Antenatal care).

Checking for past obstetric/gynaecological problems

The outcome of a previous pregnancy is predictive of future pregnancy outcomes. A history of any previous pregnancy should be obtained and details that might need to be conveyed to the woman sought (see history in Box 6.8). Many women report feeling more concerned about a second or subsequent pregnancy or birth, based on previous experiences. It may be possible to allay fears, correct misinformation and make a plan with a woman that can involve better management, avoid unnecessary stress, and make pregnancy and childbirth a positive experience for her.

Conclusion

An educational opportunity exists to provide advice on preventive activities to women considering a pregnancy.

Pregnancy

CLINICAL PRESENTATION

Many women know or suspect by the various symptoms and signs that they are pregnant and some wish for further confirmation of this (Box 6.7).

The most common presentation for pregnancy is a period of amenorrhoea. However, some women who are pregnant may have periodic vaginal bleeding, thus camouflaging the fact they are pregnant. These periodic vaginal bleeds can be repeated episodes of threatened miscarriage, and masquerade as 'periods'. Also women who ovulate irregularly and have infrequent periods (oligomenorrhoea) may not realise that they are pregnant, as they are not expecting regular bleeding.

BOX 6.7 Symptoms and signs of early pregnancy

- Amenorrhoea
- Nausea
- Irritation of the breasts
- Increased frequency of micturition
- Breast fullness
- Pigmentation of the areola and Montgomery's tubercles (enlarged sebaceous glands around the areola)

Nevertheless, a woman who usually menstruates regularly, but has experienced a period of amenorrhoea should always be considered pregnant unless proved otherwise.

Examination

There is usually little on examination that will aid the diagnosis of an early pregnancy. The uterus is not appreciably enlarged on bimanual examination until about 6–8 weeks of gestation. On speculum examination it is often suggested that the cervix has a bluish tinge, and on bimanual examination that it is 'soft'. However, neither of these signs is reliable.

Investigations

The first biochemical signal of a pregnancy is the secretion of β-HCG (beta human chorionic gonadotrophin hormone) by the blastocyst (early embryo) and then later by the syncytiotrophoblast cells of the placenta. Human chorionic gonadotrophin hormone has two subunits: α and β. The β subunit is specific to HCG, whereas the α subunit is also present in other gonadotrophins (eg luteinising hormone).

1 *Blood test.* The measurement of β-HCG in plasma is more accurate and pregnancy can be detected 6–7 days after ovulation (around the time of implantation). Quantitative measurement of β-HCG gives some indication of embryonic development.
2 *Urine test.* Many quantitative tests are available and most have a sensitivity equivalent to 50 IU/l in blood concentration. It is impossible to detect the presence of a very early pregnancy during the 'window period' of fertilisation until established implantation about 14 days later.
3 *Ultrasound.* Once the blood level of β-HCG > 1000 IU/l, about four weeks after ovulation, a transvaginal ultrasound should show the presence of a gestational sac. Viability is established by measuring the size of the sac, the length of the embryo, and the presence of a fetal heartbeat (Table 6.4 and Figure 6.4). To be sure that the embryo is at the correct milestones, the gestation must be verified. It may be clinically indicated to perform two ultrasonic examinations 7–10 days apart, and confirm that normal growth has taken place.

TABLE 6.4 Ultrasound findings in the presence of a positive pregnancy test

Gestational sac	Considerations
Present	Normal intrauterine pregnancy
Absent	Ectopic pregnancy
> 10 mm + embryo	Fetal heart detectable (if not, consider a missed miscarriage)
> 20 mm	Embryo should be present (if not, consider a blighted ovum)

FIGURE 6.4 A fetal pole of CRL (crown–rump length) of 1 mm (6 weeks) is present between the yolk sac and the gestation wall. The fetal heart pulsation may be observed in a fetal pole measuring 1 mm but is not always seen until the CRL measures over 4 mm (6 weeks 3 days).

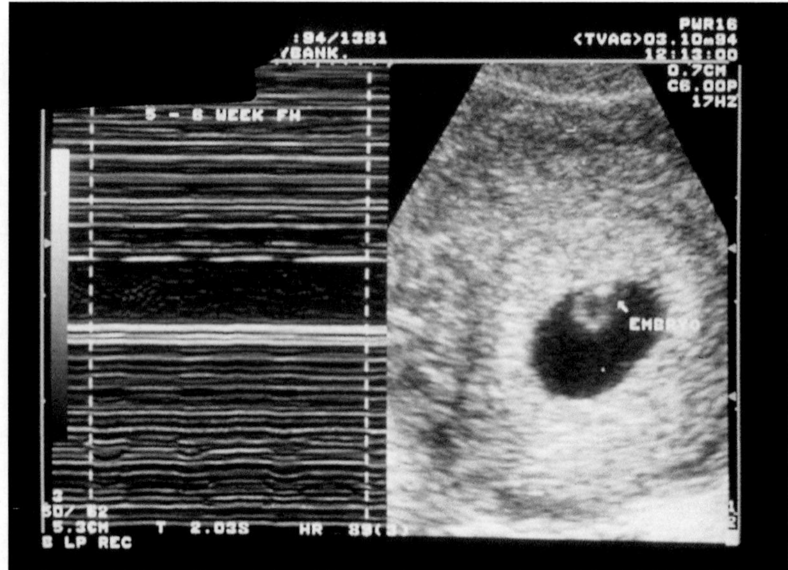

Changes and development during pregnancy

The fetus

The fetus changes in proportion and size as it develops (Table 6.5 and Figure 6.5). Normal fetal growth during pregnancy varies and studies using ultrasound measurements can provide the range of growth in a specific population—known as a normogram. This can be used to identify fetal growth outside the normal range—for example, a fetus with an abdominal circumference < 5th percentile indicates growth restriction, and one > 95th percentile indicates macrosomia.

Palpation is used clinically to estimate fetal size and growth in a normal pregnancy. However, this has not proved to be ideal in detecting a baby with intrauterine growth retardation. Although measurement of the symphysis–fundal height by tape measure is simple and inexpensive, there is not enough evidence to evaluate its effectiveness in detecting particularly small or large fetuses and improving fetal outcome.[15]

TABLE 6.5 Growth in length and weight during the fetal period

Age (weeks)	Crown–rump length (cm)	Weight (g)
8	2.5	4
12	9	20
24	30–35	600
30	40	1400
36	45	
40	50	2500–4500

FIGURE 6.5 Size of fetal head in relation to the body at different gestational ages

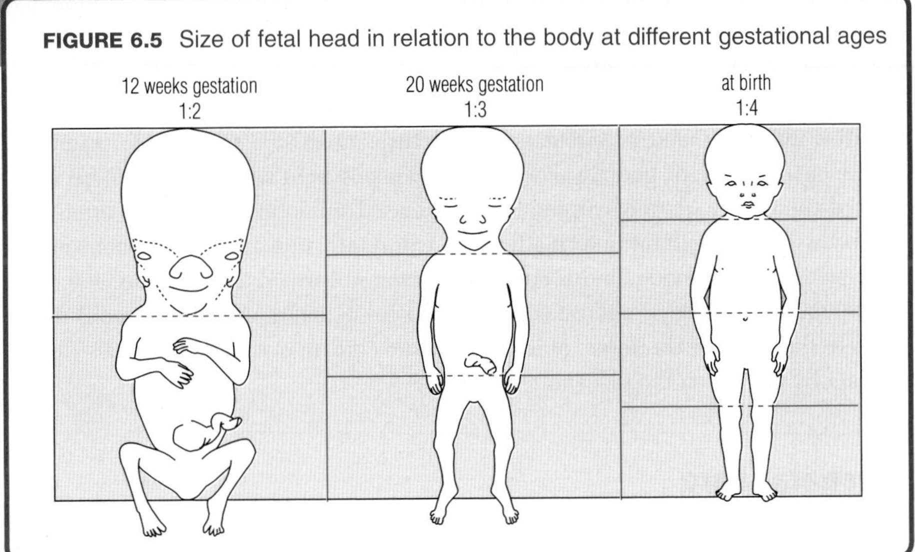

Placenta

At full term the placenta is 15–25 cm in diameter and approximately 3 cm thick, weighs one-sixth that of the baby, and covers 25–30 per cent of the internal surface of the uterus. The maternal surface consists of 12–20 compartments or cotyledons separated by decidual septa. The presence of intact cotyledons is part of the inspection of the placenta after its delivery to check that no part has been retained within the uterus. The fetal side of the placenta is smooth and covered entirely by the chorionic plate. Within this run arteries and veins that converge toward the umbilical cord, joining to form two umbilical arteries and one vein.

The placenta is implanted on the upper uterine segment in 95 per cent of women at term (Section 11). Identification of the site of implantation can be important clinically:

- For diagnosis of placenta praevia

- In a woman presenting with abdominal pain or vaginal bleeding in pregnancy (to determine if this might involve the placental site)
- Prior to caesarean section—particularly useful for a repeat caesarean section where the implantation site might be over the previous uterine scar and a morbidly adherent placenta may result. The latter occurs where the placental tissue invades the myometrium and there is no plane of cleavage. This may cause haemorrhage at the time of operation, and the possible need for a hysterectomy should be discussed with the woman beforehand.

Amniotic cavity and umbilical cord

The 'membranes' lining the intrauterine cavity consist of the amnion united by the end of pregnancy to the chorion. The amniotic cavity is filled with clear fluid formed from fluid produced by the amniotic cells and fetal urine. This acts as a cushion and protects the fetus in the early months and allows the fetus to move and grow during the pregnancy. From around the beginning of the fifth month the fetus swallows its own amniotic fluid, then this passes through the gut and into the bloodstream and thus into the maternal circulation. In fetuses unable to swallow (for example, oesophageal atresia, or poor swallowing mechanisms as in anencephaly) there is increased amniotic fluid (polyhydramnios). Decreased amniotic fluid (oligohydramnios) may be associated with intrauterine fetal growth retardation and/or fetal abnormality (Section 9). The amniotic fluid is constantly being re-formed and its volume at term is 1000 ml. At birth the umbilical cord is 50–60 cm in length. A very long cord might encircle the neck of the fetus, and a very short cord may cause difficulties during delivery by pulling on the placenta.

Antenatal care

Antenatal clinic care began in Adelaide, Australia in 1910 and Edinburgh, Scotland in 1915. Before this time, the pregnant woman usually had only one antenatal visit with a doctor, to estimate her date of delivery. She would only be seen again if a complication occurred during her labour. In developed countries, the majority of pregnant women today have a normal pregnancy and outcome, and require little formal medical intervention. The aim of modern antenatal care is to distinguish the 'high-risk' pregnancy with specific problems for monitoring and the 'low-risk' pregnancy for routine care. However, women assessed as 'low risk' at the first visit may later develop problems during the pregnancy.

Aims of antenatal care

The aims of antenatal care are:

- Prevention of maternal and fetal problems
- Treatment of problems if they arise
- Preparation of the parents for pregnancy, childbirth and parenting.

Attendance for antenatal care

Given these aims it would seem that most women would elect to attend for care. However, some do not. A number of factors may contribute to this:

- Waiting time at the clinic
- Transport
- Care of other children
- Cultural barriers: language, preference for a female doctor
- Financial constraints
- Concerns about reception from staff.

It is recommended that a woman have an antenatal visit every four weeks until 28 weeks, then every two weeks until 36 weeks, and then weekly until delivery. The number of visits recommended for a well woman has been questioned and other options are under investigation to reduce the number of visits for women with low-risk pregnancies.[16]

Models of care

A number of changes have been instigated in recent years. These include community-based clinics, home visits, special clinics (for example, a clinic for teenagers), midwife clinics, and various shared-care arrangements (between obstetricians, general practitioners and midwives). Communication between practitioners is assisted by patient-held records. Interestingly, the various 'models' of antenatal care have not been shown to improve maternal or perinatal mortality. Some women report increased satisfaction with community care and others with flexibility of care.[17] However, there have been few studies comparing different options for care, the outcomes and cost-effectiveness.

The development of day units, where women with a potential problem can be assessed without admission to hospital, has further decreased the need for women to attend hospital. There is currently insufficient evidence about the maternal, perinatal and psychosocial consequences for women and the cost-effectiveness of day care compared with in-patient care to confirm the perceived advantages.[18] In-patient care is often confined to specialist services such as ultrasonography, genetic investigations and obstetric medical care.

First antenatal visit

The first visit, or 'booking' visit, to an antenatal clinic should ideally occur early in the pregnancy. The aim of the first visit is to familiarise the woman with the hospital and clinic, allow her to meet both midwifery and medical staff, be assessed medically and decide on the model of care. In some traditional Indigenous communities, the 'quickening' or first fetal movement marks the moment of recognition of a spirit child, and therefore acceptance for the woman that she is pregnant. This is usually at around 16 weeks of pregnancy, and this may lead to a delay in the first visit to an antenatal clinic.

Risk assessment

In an attempt to improve the identification of problems a number of risk factor lists are often used to determine if the woman falls into a 'high risk' or 'low risk' category (Box 6.8). The options for antenatal care most suitable for the individual woman can then be discussed. A number of women may need to move between these categories and models as their circumstances change during the pregnancy. Good communication between services is essential. During the first visit, a midwife will usually take an initial history from the woman (Box 6.9).

BOX 6.8 Factors associated with potential 'high-risk' pregnancy

- Maternal risk factors in the present pregnancy
- Present pregnancy
  - Age < 16 years, > 35 years
  - Weight < 50 kg, > 100 kg
  - Smoking, alcohol, illicit drug use
  - Lack of social support
- Past obstetric history
  - Parity > 4
  - Preterm delivery
  - Congenital abnormality
  - Intrauterine growth retardation
  - Operative delivery
  - Third-stage complications
  - Medical complications: hypertension, diabetes
  - Depressive illness
- Family history
  - Medical problems: diabetes, hypertensive or heart disease
  - Congenital abnormality
- Booking examination
  - Blood pressure > 140/90 mmHg
  - Cardiac murmur
  - Discrepancy between uterine size and gestation
- Investigations
  - Abnormal blood test
  - Abnormal ultrasound assessment
- Factors arising in pregnancy
  - Vaginal bleeding
  - Malpresentation (presentation other than cephalic)
  - Preterm labour

BOX 6.9 History at the first antenatal clinic visit

- Gynaecological history
  - Menstrual history including first day of the last normal menstrual period, usual menstrual cycle
  - Previous contraceptive history, including when ceased
  - Last Pap smear and result
  - Possible date of conception, if known (note any ultrasound results)
- Obstetric history
  - Number of pregnancies
  - Pregnancy outcome (eg ectopic, miscarriage, termination, live birth, stillbirth or neonatal death)
  - Gestation of each pregnancy at the conclusion
  - Type of delivery and reason for instrumental or caesarean section, birth weight and length of labour
  - Any pregnancy complication, such as pre-eclampsia, diabetes, postpartum haemorrhage
- Medical history
  - Any previous medical conditions: hypertension, diabetes, renal disease, cardiovascular disease, epilepsy, asthma, previous blood transfusion
- Surgical history
  - Any previous surgery, especially gynaecological, pelvic surgery or injury
- Family history
  - Including: medical illness, congenital malformations, and multiple pregnancies
- Medications
  - Including prescribed medications, over-the-counter preparations and herbal or natural preparations used before pregnancy, ceased herself since discovering that she is pregnant or currently being taken
- Social circumstances
  - Work: nature, time
  - Housing: others at home, space, likelihood of change
  - Tobacco, alcohol, caffeine, and illicit drug use
  - Family structure
- Ethnic origins
  - Some ethnic groups are at higher risk of inherited diseases or infectious diseases such as hepatitis B. Some women may have undergone a genital mutilation procedure.

Examination

A routine general physical examination (Section 1) is performed. The aim is to assess gestational age, detect any previously unrecognised medical conditions, assess the severity of any known medical conditions and promote health awareness.

1 General examination

This should include height and weight, assessment of any major anomalies (such as skeletal abnormalities), condition of the teeth and gums, and palpation of the thyroid gland.

2 Cardiovascular examination

Check for heart sound, murmurs and oedema. Blood pressure measurement in the pregnant woman should be taken with the woman sitting and with both arms at the level of the heart. At the first visit, both arms should be used and the right arm at subsequent visits. Use a mercury sphygmomanometer, and measure blood pressure using the Korotkoff phase V (K5) for diastolic pressure. This is the level at which the sounds disappear completely. The K5 has been found to be more accurate and reflect the true diastolic pressure in pregnant women. It is also important to select the correct blood pressure cuff. A large cuff (15–33 cm bladder) should be used if the upper arm circumference is greater than 33 cm. If the cuff is too small the blood pressure reading will be falsely elevated.

3 Breasts

A routine breast examination should be performed, looking for inverted and abnormal nipples and breast lumps.

4 Abdomen

Examine the abdomen for surgical scars and signs of pregnancy. Check the fundal height. Auscultation for fetal heart sounds should be possible with a Doppler machine at 10–12 weeks gestation.

5 Pelvic examination

There is debate as to whether a routine pelvic examination is required. Some clinicians undertake a pelvic examination only if there are specific clinical indications to suggest a problem. Other clinicians recommend that a pelvic examination be performed to detect congenital abnormalities of the lower genital tract, signs of infection, the size and shape of the uterus, any abnormality of the cervix and adnexa, and the pelvic capacity. In general, most women have an ultrasound during the second trimester of pregnancy, to check the gestation and detect an adnexal mass.

Investigations

A number of tests are recommended; other tests may depend on specific places/populations and the prevalence of a specific disorder in that area (Box 6.10). It is important to ensure informed consent to any investigations. Women at low risk for a problem may not consider the possibility of an abnormal test result. This applies to both blood tests and ultrasound. The use of first trimester scanning as routine may identify a chromosomal or structural anomaly. Women may not be prepared for this result or have considered the possibility of having to make a decision about continuation of the pregnancy. Timely counselling may avoid later psychological morbidity.[19]

BOX 6.10 Antenatal blood tests

- Blood group
- Rhesus group and antibody screen
- Full blood count
- Rubella antibody level
- Syphilis test
- Hepatitis B and hepatitis C
- HIV serology

At present CMV and toxoplasmosis serology are not routinely recommended in Australia, as they are not clinically useful or cost effective. Some tests (eg HIV) are performed routinely in some countries or populations and based on risk factors in other groups.

Results of tests

Blood group and antibodies

If the blood group is already known it does not need to be repeated; however, the antibody screen is performed at the beginning of each pregnancy. The antibodies are tested again at 24 and 36 weeks (Section 9).

Full blood count

A full blood count is also usually performed at the beginning of pregnancy, and at 24 and 36 weeks. It is useful for detecting anaemia or a haemoglobinopathy (such as thalassaemia minor or sickle cell trait). Women with severe anaemia (haemoglobin < 10.5 g/dl) should be investigated for iron, B12 and folate deficiency. Women with mild anaemia, especially with a reduced mean cell volume, require iron supplementation. If they do not respond to iron therapy, further investigation is required. Routine supplementation with iron and folate prevents a low haemoglobin at delivery but there is little data on other outcomes for mother and baby.[20] A platelet count is also part of a full blood count, and tends to decline as the pregnancy progresses. The white cell count tends to be higher in normal pregnancy than in the non-pregnant state.

Rubella serology

Rubella serology should be performed with each pregnancy, as antibody levels can decline after immunisation, and the serology (immunoglobulin levels) can identify women at risk of contracting rubella (German measles) during pregnancy. If the IgG indicates low levels of immunity, the woman should be advised to avoid children with a possible infection, and a rubella immunisation performed post partum. An IgM should also be performed if recent infection is suspected (a history of a rash or contact with a rash). Rubella antibodies take 17 days to develop, and therefore the serology should be repeated 17 days after suspected contact. If there has been no antibody rise, then the risk of infection is low. The serology should be again repeated at four weeks after contact. Rubella-specific IgM may be present for a year or more, so there is a need to interpret the laboratory results in the light of the clinical details.[21]

Syphilis serology

Syphilis screening tests are the *Treponema pallidum* haemagglutination test and rapid plasma reagin test. Screening for syphilis should be done in every pregnancy because it is easily treated, and untreated syphilis in pregnancy causes potentially severe disease in both mother and fetus.[22]

Hepatitis B serology

Up to 30 per cent of women from Africa and Asia may be infected with hepatitis B (HBV), compared to < 1 per cent in the developed countries. It is transmitted by percutaneous, sexual, perinatal and 'horizontal' routes (transmission in the absence of the previous routes—exact mechanism unknown but probably the most common method of transmission to children worldwide). Risk factors include intravenous drug use, rectal intercourse, multiple sexual partners, history of other sexually transmitted diseases, and work in a health care field. Hepatitis B is a small RNA virus that has three main antigens: hepatitis B surface antigen (HBsAg), hepatitis B core antigen (HBcAg), which is only present in hepatocytes, and hepatitis Be antigen (HbeAg), which indicates active viral replication and infectiousness. Hepatitis B surface antigen test is used to screen for recent and chronic hepatitis B infection. Women with chronic HBV are potentially infectious to others in contact with their blood or other bodily fluids. Hospital staff caring for these women should take recommended precautions to avoid infection. The woman who is HBsAg positive should also have her liver enzymes checked, and her partner and other children checked for infection and vaccinated if not already infected. The main risk for the neonate is at the time of delivery. The combination of immune globulin and vaccination prevents the majority of perinatal transmissions (Section 9).

Hepatitis C serology

Women at risk of infection or exposure should be offered testing for hepatitis C (HCV). Risk factors include past or current use of IV drugs and tattoos; sexual transmission is inefficient but multiple partners and sexual behaviour may be important. The risk of hepatitis C transmission to the fetus is approximately 4 per cent but increased where the mother is infected with HIV. The mother should have liver enzyme testing and her partner and other children should be tested for infection.

HIV serology

Universal screening would be cost effective in the UK,[23] and testing of pooled antenatal sera would be valuable in monitoring any increase in cases in other countries with a lower prevalence. Screening should be offered to pregnant women after appropriate counselling is given as to the limitations of the testing and the implications of both positive and negative findings. HIV transmission to the fetus can be markedly reduced by a caesarean section delivery and the use of antiviral medications during the pregnancy; in developed countries, breastfeeding the infant should also be avoided.

Microscopy of urine

Asymptomatic bacteriuria occurs in up to 10 per cent of pregnant women. There is also an increased risk (10–15 per cent) of recurrence of bacteriuria. In pregnancy there is an increased risk of symptomatic urinary tract infection, and pyelonephritis can occur in up to 25 per cent of these women if untreated. Pyelonephritis in pregnant women can cause complications such as premature labour, transient renal failure and sepsis. Antibiotic treatment for pregnant women with asymptomatic bacteriuria found on antenatal screening can reduce the risk of pyelonephritis in pregnancy.[24] Midstream urine for microscopy and culture is the gold standard, but this may not be cost-effective in the antenatal population.

Cervical smear

This can be delayed until the end of pregnancy if there has been documented normal cervical cytology in the preceding 18 months and there is no clinical indication to check the cervix.

Screening for gestational diabetes

Population screening for gestational diabetes is controversial. Gestational diabetes is defined as the development of abnormal glucose tolerance during pregnancy in a woman who did not have diabetes prior to pregnancy. Testing may be based on risk factors or specific 'at-risk' groups within a community (Section 9).

Ultrasound in pregnancy

First trimester

Earlier scans may be performed:

- If there are pregnancy complications such as bleeding, abdominal pain, hyperemesis gravidarum.
- If an invasive procedure such as chorionic villus sampling is performed.
- To reassure a mother who has had a previous ectopic pregnancy or miscarriage. The presence of a viable fetus at 12 weeks is associated with a live birth in over 98 per cent of cases.[25]
- To check nuchal fold translucency: an ultrasound performed at 11–14 weeks of pregnancy can measure the nuchal fold (a skin fold measurement at the back of the neck). If the nuchal translucency is increased beyond 6 mm, there is a 10-fold increase in the risk of Down syndrome in the fetus. This test, in combination with maternal age, has a sensitivity of 75–80 per cent. Recently it has been found that if combining this test with biochemical markers (free β subunit of HCG, and pregnancy-associated plasma protein PAPPA), there may be an increase of sensitivity to 90 per cent.

Specialist transvaginal ultrasound can be used to visualise the fetal anatomy (Figure 6.6). Routine ultrasound in early pregnancy allows better gestational assessment, earlier detection of multiple pregnancy and earlier detection of unanticipated fetal abnormality.[26]

FIGURE 6.6 Earliest gestation when fetal structures are visualised using transvaginal sonography

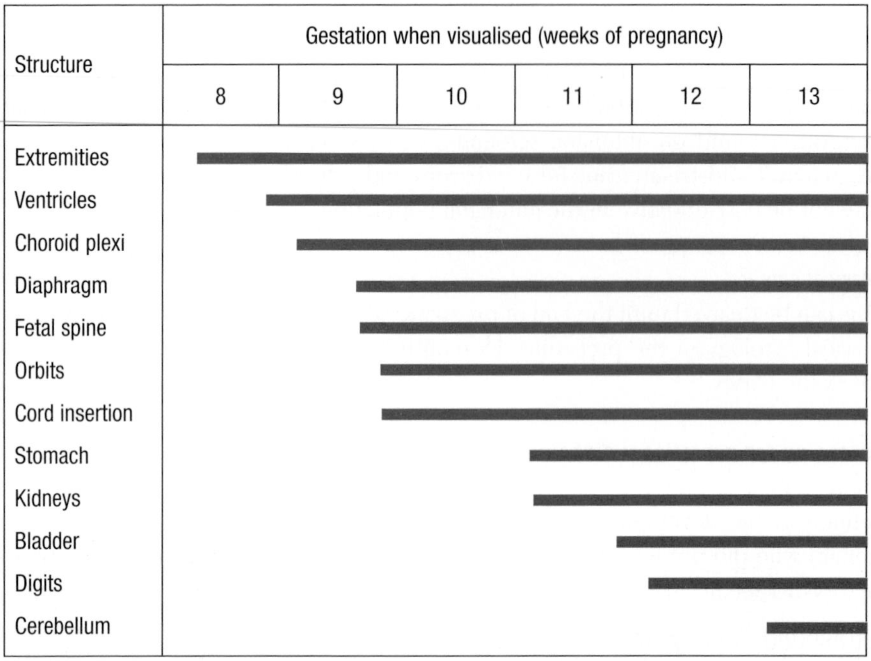

Structure	Gestation when visualised (weeks of pregnancy)					
	8	9	10	11	12	13
Extremities						
Ventricles						
Choroid plexi						
Diaphragm						
Fetal spine						
Orbits						
Cord insertion						
Stomach						
Kidneys						
Bladder						
Digits						
Cerebellum						

Later ultrasound

Most women have at least one ultrasound during the pregnancy. The most common time for an ultrasound is at 18–20 weeks. At this time the ultrasound is useful to confirm dates, assess fetal morphology, exclude a multiple pregnancy, and assess placental location (Figures 6.7–6.9).

Later in the pregnancy, additional scans may be requested if the fundal height is large or small for dates, for pregnancy complications such as diabetes, multiple pregnancy or hypertension, if there is bleeding, an unstable or abnormal fetal presentations, or to check the position of a low-lying placenta diagnosed on an earlier ultrasound examination.

Prenatal diagnosis

Chromosomal abnormalities

Testing for fetal abnormalities, especially chromosomal abnormalities, is rapidly changing. Women over the age of 35 are at increased risk for a chromosomal abnormality (Box 6.11). These women and women who have had a child with a neural tube defect or chromosomal abnormality are offered counselling and some form of prenatal diagnosis.[27]

Even women not considered at risk for chromosomal abnormalities should also be offered the screening tests available and their limitations. If there are

FIGURE 6.7 Fetal ultrasound showing measurement of biparietal diameter of fetal head, which can be related to the gestational age.

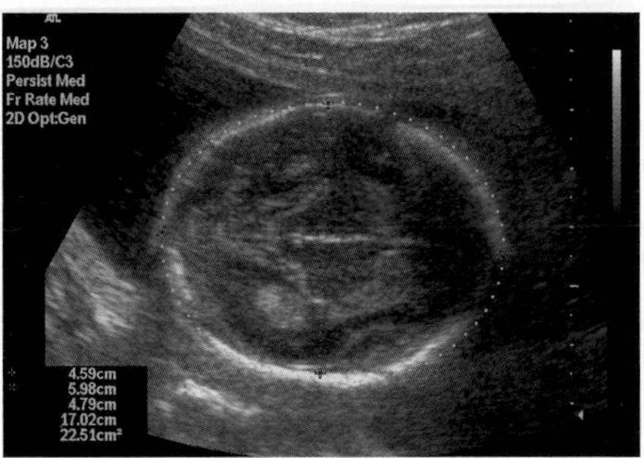

FIGURE 6.8 Fetal ultrasound showing measurement of femur length, also related to the gestational age

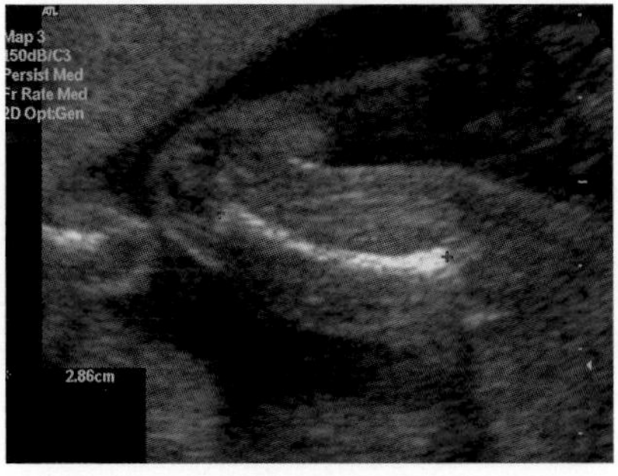

FIGURE 6.9 Fetal ultrasound showing fetal facial profile is an exciting and 'bonding' experience for the couple.

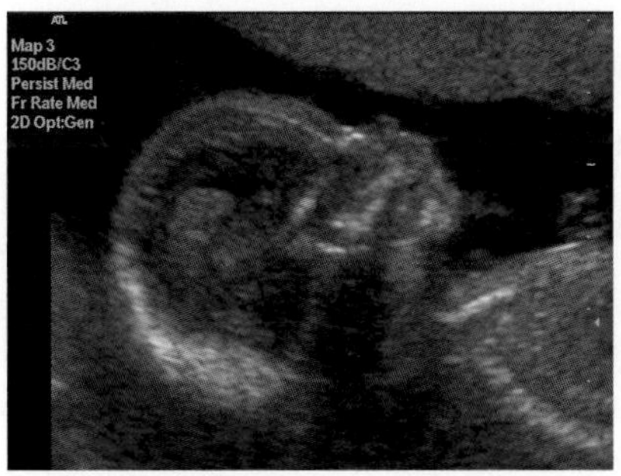

BOX 6.11 Trisomy 21 age-related risk at birth

Age	Age-related risk
20	1/1527
25	1/1352
30	1/895
35	1/356
40	1/79
44	1/30

abnormalities on an ultrasound, the woman may be counselled regarding amniocentesis or chorionic villus sampling. A routine 18-week ultrasound scan will detect only about 50 per cent of fetuses with trisomy 21. It is not a recommended primary screening test.

Structural abnormalities

Most fetal abnormalities are not anticipated. Fetal structural abnormalities are at least twice as common as chromosomal abnormalities. Neural tube defects are the most common serious anomaly for terminating a pregnancy.[28] The optimal age to examine fetal anatomy and measure nuchal translucency is 13 weeks.[25] Fetal abnormalities from all the major systems have been diagnosed in the first trimester, although spina bifida, heart anomalies and limb defects are more difficult to detect and require further scanning in the second trimester.[25]

Further management

The expected date of delivery (EDD) is calculated by adding 9 months and 7 days to the first day of the last menstrual period (LMP) (Section 1). Alternatively, the EDD can be calculated from an ultrasound examination performed before 20 weeks gestation. Where there is a difference of more than one week between these two estimates, the ultrasound EDD is taken as the correct EDD.

The model of care preferred or recommended can be discussed and decided. The antenatal shared care card will often list the expected examination and investigations for the woman during the pregnancy (Figure 6.10).

Antenatal visits

At each visit a brief history of events since the last visit is taken, and blood pressure measured. There is no evidence that routine urine dipstick testing or checking of maternal weight in a woman of average weight is of any clinical significance. An examination of the abdomen noting fundal height, fetal lie and position, liquor volume and fetal heartbeat is performed. The woman can be asked about fetal movements (usually noticed 10 times or more each day). If the woman reaches 41 weeks of pregnancy it is recommended that she be assessed by vaginal examination for induction of labour. Routine induction of labour after 41 weeks has been shown to be associated with decreased perinatal mortality.[29]

Birthplace

Approximately 10–15 per cent of women in the UK would prefer to give birth at home, although far fewer actually achieve this.[30] In Australia, home births carry a higher perinatal death rate than all Australian births and home births elsewhere.[31] There is no evidence that home birth is safer than hospital birth or associated with fewer interventions.[32] It may be that encouraging a home-like setting in conventional labour wards has some benefits for the mother, with lower use of analgesia, less augmentation of labour and operative delivery.[33] However, it is difficult to dissociate the surroundings from the benefits of caregiver support. Most women give birth in a hospital. A number of options now exist for the time spent in hospital: some women may go home within eight hours, others after 24 hours, and so on. Early hospital discharge needs to be supported by adequate community services such as home visits by a midwife for the mother and an early check of the baby by the doctor.

FIGURE 6.10 An example of an antenatal shared care card (to 32 weeks)

PREGNANCY HEALTH RECORD (ALWAYS CARRY THESE NOTES WITH YOU)

DATE	MODEL OF CARE (Indicate)	SIGNATURE

	RISK FACTORS	

ANTENATAL ADMISSION SUMMARY

DATE	DIAGNOSIS	SIGNATURE

ANTENATAL CARE PATHWAY (Please tick where appropriate)

FIRST GENERAL PRACTITIONER VISIT

	Discussed		**Discussed**	**Information Given**
Risk Assessment	☐	Alcohol	☐	☐
Social Factors	☐	Smoking	☐	☐
Physiotherapy/exercise	☐	Models of Care	☐	☐
Dietary Advice	☐	Genetic Screening (if > 35)	☐	☐
		Medication	☐	☐

Pathology Routine Screening Tests Sent to: ....

Results			
Blood Group		Full blood count	
Antibody screen		Rubella Titre	
Syphilis Serology		Hepatitis Bs Ag:	
Cervical smear	Date of last smear: / /	Normal ☐	Abnormal ☐

Other: ....

FIRST HOSPITAL VISIT *Standard Care as per protocol and Antenatal Sheet:*
Confirmed Model of Care ☐ Checked Pathology ☐
Checked Risk Factors ☐ Antenatal Classes Arranged ☐
16 WEEK VISIT *Standard Care as per protocol and Antenatal Sheet:*
Discussed morphology scan Result [ ]
20 WEEK VISIT *Standard Care as per protocol and Antenatal Sheet:*
Confirmed EDC ☐ Agreed EDC: ..../........../..........
24 WEEK VISIT *Standard Care as per protocol and Antenatal Sheet:*
Discussed Glucose Challenge Test if age ≥ 30 ☐ BMI > 27 ☐ FH Diabetes ☐
High risk ethnicity ☐ Past Obstetric History
Results if applicable: ☐ GCT: .... GTT: ....
Discussed Breast Feeding: ☐
28 WEEK VISIT *Standard Care as per protocol and Antenatal Sheet:*
30 WEEK VISIT *Standard Care as per protocol and Antenatal Sheet:*
Antibody Screen (if Rh Negative) ☐
32 WEEK VISIT *Standard Care as per protocol and Antenatal Sheet:*

Special situations

Pregnancy and abuse

Pregnancy is a time when abuse by partners can commence, continue or increase, with prevalence rates of 3.9–8.3 per cent (see Abuse in Section 3).[34] Young and disadvantaged women are most at risk of violence during pregnancy. Partner abuse can cause both chronic and acute mental and physical illness in mothers, such as sexually transmitted diseases (including HIV), urinary tract infections, substance abuse and depression.[35] Violence can result in low birth weight[36] and fetal death, miscarriage and elective pregnancy termination.[35] Many studies have noted associations of abuse with preterm delivery, fetal distress, antepartum haemorrhage, and pre-eclampsia, but the evidence is inconsistent across studies.

Women who have experienced childhood sexual abuse are more likely than non-abused youth to become pregnant before the age of eighteen. Childbirth often triggers memories of past sexual abuse and vaginal examinations may be difficult for these women.

Female genital mutilation

Female genital mutilation (FGM) constitutes all procedures involving partial or total removal of the external female genitalia, with the number of girls and women who have been subjected to FGM estimated at more than 130 million individuals worldwide.[37] It is a traditional cultural practice where it is believed necessary to ensure the self-respect of the girl and her family and increase her marriage opportunities. The practice constitutes a health risk to women that hinders their care. It is usually carried out between birth and puberty. The degree of mutilation varies and each case should be assessed individually. It has extremely negative consequences for women, with painful births and subsequent urogenital fistulae in many cases.

Complications of FGM:

- Psychosexual and psychological problems
- Acute shock, haemorrhage, sepsis. Mortality 1 in 10.
- Renal problems: problems with micturition, recurrent urinary tract infections, end-stage renal failure
- Genital tract problems: non-consummation, dyspareunia, vaginal infections.

Management

Ideally de-infibulation should be performed before the pregnancy. However, it may be only noticed or reported during the antenatal period. The optimum time is thought to be 20 weeks for a reversal operation, which can be done under regional anaesthesia. If the mutilation is noticed only once the woman is in labour then reversal can be carried out during the first stage.

The aim of a surgical reversal is to restore the anatomy to normality.

In the postnatal period these women and their families need careful discussion, hopefully to not have the procedure redone and to prevent FGM happening to any female offspring in the family.

Legal issues

Female genital mutilation constitutes violence against women under international law, United Nations General Assembly Declaration, 'Violence Against Women' 1993.

Advice and common complaints in pregnancy

Women often request advice about everyday activities and the effect on their pregnancy, and expect their health professional to be able to provide an answer. In addition, women may experience a number of symptoms or problems during pregnancy that can be regarded as normal events. It is important to provide an explanation and the prognosis, especially where these will resolve during the post-partum period. It is essential that these 'normal' symptoms be distinguished from potential problems that may present similarly.

Antenatal classes

Antenatal classes and education are offered to pregnant women. These classes are usually held over a number of weeks and may be held in community centres. Topics covered include general health and dietary advice, changes during pregnancy, labour and delivery, postnatal care and breastfeeding, parenting and contraception. Most classes will also offer a tour of the labour ward. They are designed to be interactive, and questions and discussions are encouraged. They can also offer the new parents a chance to meet others in the same situation and often the friendships formed continue after the pregnancy. Although classes are intended to educate and empower women, there is little more than anecdotal evidence to support their effectiveness.[38]

Back and pelvic pain

Most women report back pain in pregnancy, particularly in the last trimester. The causes suggested are the altered posture (increasing lumbar lordosis) due to the need to balance the enlarging uterus, laxity of ligaments caused by the hormone relaxin, and fluid retention in the connective tissues.[39] The pain leads to daytime discomfort with activity and contributes to nighttime insomnia. At two years post partum most women are fully recovered.[40] Pelvic pain (from the pubic symphysis or sacro-iliac joints) also causes morbidity that may continue into the postpartum period for a small percentage of women.[41] These problems may recur earlier in the pregnancy for subsequent pregnancies. Pubic symphysis diastasis (pelvic osteoarthropathy) occurs when the relaxation of the ligaments around the pubic joint allows the pubic bones to move on each other. This results in severe pubic and back pain on walking. The problem continues during the pregnancy and for a few weeks after the birth. Treatment consists of analgesia and rest if necessary.

Breast changes

The changes which occur in pregnancy are characterised by extensive proliferation of the ducts and glandular elements provoked by a combination of hormonal effects.

Initially there may be heaviness and discomfort in the breasts with associated tingling in the nipples. Darkening of the nipples and areola (hyperpigmentation) is characteristic of a first pregnancy.

Carpal tunnel syndrome

Tingling (paraesthesiae) and numbness in the fingers (particularly the thumb and first fingers) results from oedema in the carpal tunnel of the wrist causing pressure on the median nerve. This can be especially troublesome at night and can contribute to insomnia. It is relieved by moving the fingers. There is no place for the use of diuretics. It most often resolves post partum.

Contractions

The uterus contracts intermittently from early pregnancy (Braxton Hicks contractions). These become stronger and more frequent from about 30 weeks gestation and are especially noticeable on movement and sexual activity. For some women these cause marked discomfort and, as the uterine activity increases further after 36 weeks, can be difficult to distinguish from the onset of labour. The latter, by definition, is associated with progressive thinning and dilatation of the cervix.

Exercise

Women are encouraged to follow all normal activities during pregnancy. Regular aerobic exercise improves physical fitness and body image. There is insufficient data to ascertain fully the risks and benefits for mother and baby.[42]

Exocrine gland secretion

A common complaint is increase in salivation, nasal discharge, sweating and vaginal secretions. No particular management is useful except reassurance about this normal variant.

Fainting

This may occur when the woman lies on her back in the latter half of pregnancy (due to the weight of the uterus impeding the venous return to the heart—supine hypotension). It may also occur after prolonged standing or on sudden rising from a sitting or lying position (due to the altered cardiovascular dynamics). Management is based on awareness and avoidance of these activities.

Hair and nail changes

Scalp hair growth often increases during pregnancy. However, the hairs often go into an arresting phase around the time of delivery and this may result in some noticeable hair loss around two months post partum. Nail growth also increases towards the end of pregnancy and a variety of nail problems can occur, including splitting and the development of grooves, but they usually resolve post partum.

Heartburn

This is more frequent with advancing pregnancy. It is caused by the relaxation of the lower oesophageal sphincter allowing the regurgitation of gastric contents. The pyloric sphincter may also relax and allow bile into the stomach. Raising the head of the bed at night may be helpful.

Leg cramps

These are experienced by many women and may become more troublesome as the pregnancy progresses, especially at night. The underlying mechanism is unclear. It is helpful to walk around, stretch and massage the muscle. The evidence that calcium or other supplements are of benefit is weak. The best evidence is for magnesium lactate or citrate 5 mmol in the morning and 10 mmol at night.[43]

Oedema

This is common in the lower limbs towards the end of pregnancy. It is probably hormone-related and, in the absence of hypertension, can be regarded as a normal adaptation of pregnancy. There is no place for the use of diuretics. Oedema of the lower limbs, face and hands with a rise in blood pressure needs further management (Section 9). If the oedema is only in one leg then the possibility of venous thrombosis should be considered.

Palpitations and headaches

Both of these complaints are the result of changes in the cardiovascular dynamics. Examination should be undertaken to exclude an organic cause before the woman is reassured.

Sexual activity

Women can be advised to continue normal sexual activity during pregnancy, unless there is vaginal bleeding or the possibility of ruptured membranes. On average, female sexual interest and coital activity decline slightly in the first trimester, are variable in the second trimester and decline further in the third trimester. Women may report marked uterine contraction at the time of orgasm. In the later months of pregnancy changes in position need to be adopted for the mother's comfort.

Skin changes

Stretch marks

Stretch marks (striae gravidarum) develop in most pregnancies due to stretching of the elastic fibres of the skin. In women who have previously suffered with stretch marks in pregnancy one cream appears to be useful in preventing these recurring.[44] There is no particular treatment that can help most women but their prominence tends to fade post partum. Whether these are related to an increased cortisol level in pregnancy has not yet been determined.

Skin pigmentation

Hyperpigmentation of the nipples, areola, genitalia and axilli occur in 90 per cent of pregnant women, probably due to melanocyte-stimulating hormone (MSH) from the pituitary gland. Darker-skinned women develop more darkening of the affected areas than lighter-skinned women. It is thought that oestrogen and progesterone increase melanocyte activity. A good proportion of the hyperpigmentation fades post partum but some always remains.

Chloasma

Chloasma is commonly termed 'the mask of pregnancy' and can be seen in up to 50 per cent of women. It sometimes also occurs in women taking oral contraceptive pills. It presents as hyperpigmented patches on the cheeks, forehead or upper lip. Treatment usually involves sunscreens and, after pregnancy, avoidance of oestrogen therapy.

Oily skin

There is increased activity in the endocrine glands during pregnancy, particularly towards the end of pregnancy. Sebaceous gland activity also increases, giving many pregnant women oily skin.

Blood vessel changes

The increase in blood volume and vasodilatation often leads to several phenomena: palmar erythema develops in many pregnant women; superficial and deep varicose veins occur because of increased venous pressure; and small spider angiomata commonly appear on the hands and face.

Skin diseases

Some skin conditions improve in pregnancy and some may worsen. Psoriasis improves in about a third of women, whereas the other conditions stay the same in all women. Skin tags, keloids and naevi may become more prominent. There are a number of diseases that occur only in pregnancy.

- Pruritic urticarial papules and plaques of pregnancy (PUPPP) is the most common skin disease appearing only in pregnancy. It usually begins in the third trimester and starts as a rash around the umbilicus and spreads onto the abdomen and extremities. Pruritus can be minimal or severe and treatment is symptomatic with antihistamines.
- Generalised itching without a specific rash has been reported in up to 20 per cent of pregnancies. In the third trimester intense itching can be related to bile cholestasis. Liver function tests should be checked.
- Two potentially serious skin conditions for mother and fetus are the blistering diseases of pregnancy, herpes gestationalis and impetigo herpetiformis.

Tiredness

Many women feel tired when pregnant, particularly if they are working or have other children. Sometimes this may be due to anaemia. A 'physiological' anaemia occurs

(Hb > 10.5 Gm) commonly due to a diluting effect from the increased plasma volume. A true anaemia (Hb < 10.5 Gm) is more common in multigravida, where pregnancies/lactation are close together, and there is a previous history of menorrhagia. Anaemia in pregnancy is associated with an increased maternal mortality and stillbirth rate. A haemoglobinopathy may be present in women from Mediterranean countries, and a haemoglobin electrophoresis (HbA2 > 3.5 indicates a B-thalassaemia trait). Sickle cell anaemia should always be considered and investigated in women from African countries. Women with this disorder require prophylactic folic acid, regular haemoglobin estimation, prompt treatment of infections and antibiotic prophylaxis during childbirth.

Urinary frequency

This is particularly common in the first trimester and the last few weeks of pregnancy. It may also suggest a urinary tract infection as dysuria is an uncommon complaint in the pregnant woman.

Urinary incontinence

This is common in pregnancy. It may be difficult for a woman to differentiate between urinary incontinence and leaking amniotic fluid.

Vaginal discharge

Many women notice an increase in the amount of normal vaginal secretions in pregnancy. This may be heavy enough to discolour underwear or necessitate wearing a pad.

Varicose veins

These may be noticeable in the legs, around the anus ('piles' or haemorrhoids), and sometimes in the vulval area. They can cause aching in the area concerned and those around the anus and vulva may become more troublesome after delivery.

Vomiting

Nausea and vomiting affect up to 70 per cent of pregnant women. It is mostly mild but is occasionally severe (termed 'hyperemesis gravidarum'). It is attributed to the rapid rise in beta-HCG and oestriol and the differential diagnosis includes: urinary tract infection (more common throughout pregnancy); multiple pregnancy and hydatidiform mole in early pregnancy; liver disease and pre-eclampsia in the last trimester of pregnancy.

Weight gain

Pregnant women may be concerned about too little or too much weight gain. The average weight gain in a normal pregnancy in an average-sized woman is 10–14 kg overall. The pattern of weight gain may vary in different women, many women gaining little in the first trimester and the last month of pregnancy.

SECTION

7

Labour and childbirth

Women's experiences in labour

Most women are satisfied with their care in labour. Women are less concerned about the gender of the carer than about the carer's personal qualities, particularly their communication skills and technical expertise.[1] Continuity of care seemed important to many women randomised to team midwife care and standard clinic care. However, this applied mainly to the antenatal period, less so intra partum and post partum, with no difference in emotional well-being at two months post partum.[2] Women in different 'shared care' programs reported higher satisfaction with midwife-led programs, again citing information transfer, decision making, choice and the relationship with the health carer as important issues.[3] The 2844 women in a study that randomised between midwife-managed delivery and consultant-led labour ward in a 2:1 ratio reported similar satisfaction in both groups, although the midwife-led group were more likely to report being given more choice with mobility, positions for delivery, and pain relief.[4] The fact that women in a birth centre had high levels of satisfaction was thought to be related to the carer's attitude, the philosophy of care, and the environment.[5]

The factors that women express as areas of dissatisfaction are: lack of involvement in decision making, insufficient information, where an obstetric intervention was undertaken, and a perception that caregivers were unhelpful.[6]

It would appear overall that, as in other areas of health care, the important issues for pregnant women at all stages of their care revolve around their personal interactions and communication with health care personnel. A caring attitude, willingness to provide information for women, allowing them to exercise choice and make their own decisions seem to be the key to greater satisfaction with their birthing experience.

Women with disabilities

Women with a disability may need to overcome not only the obstacle of the disability but also those posed by able-bodied professionals.[7] Consulting the woman herself about her specific needs will aid communication and prevent misunderstandings. Women with a disability, like all other women, require information that will enable them to make informed choices during pregnancy, childbirth and parenting.[8]

Women from different ethnic backgrounds

Differences in ethnic background between caregiver and woman may influence the woman's experience of labour. For example, this may affect the pain experienced, the expression of that pain by the woman and the interpretation of that pain by the caregiver.

Different cultural groups may have specific needs and birth practices. However, personal expectations, the amount of support from caregivers, the quality of the caregiver–patient relationship, and involvement in the decision making are so important that they mostly override the influences of other factors including cultural background.[9]

Progress of labour

Most labours represent a normal physiological process and a normal vaginal delivery is achieved. In a few situations there are serious problems, the progress of the labour becomes obstructed and operative delivery is required. In the remainder the progress may be variable and the mode of delivery, and outcome for mother and baby, will depend on the factors that have influenced the progress. A method that is used to consider these factors comes under the areas of:

1 passages
2 powers
3 passenger
4 placenta.

1 Passages

The pelvic bones and soft tissues (the pelvic floor, cervix, and perineum) provide the passage through which the fetus travels. These features need to be assessed in relation to the features of the presenting part (most often the fetal head) rather than as independent factors. The pelvis is not routinely assessed for size and shape during a first pregnancy unless the mother's history anticipates a particular problem with the pelvis (eg previous pelvic fracture).

The pelvic inlet is smallest in the anterior–posterior diameter and largest in the transverse diameter. The ischial spines are the narrowest part of the pelvis. The outlet is represented by the ischial tuberosities and the sub-pubic arch. The transverse diameter is the smallest outlet diameter (Figure 7.1).

During labour the presenting part of the fetus moves down and rotates through the pelvis—from the largest diameter of the pelvis at the inlet (pelvic brim) through 90 degrees to the outlet. As it rotates it also changes direction by 90 degrees from down to forward in the sagittal plane to permit the presenting part of the fetus to pass under the pubic symphysis (see Mechanism of normal labour). The pelvic floor consists of the levator ani, the pubococcygeus and the coccygeus muscles. These form a muscular sling through which the urethra, vagina and rectum pass (Figure 7.2).

2 Powers

The myometrium of the uterus contracts at regular intervals, resulting in an intrauterine pressure of 50–75 mmHg during a contraction. The wave of excitation, and hence the resulting contraction, normally passes downwards from the fundus of the uterus. As the muscle contracts, it also retracts: the muscle does not relax to its original length but stays at a shorter length. This has the effect of reducing the size of the uterine cavity and pushing the presenting part forward.

A pattern of well-coordinated regular contractions lasting up to 90 seconds with good uterine relaxation in between is necessary for the progress of labour. More frequent or intense contractions increase the uterine tone and decrease the oxygen exchange in the placental bed, which can lead to fetal distress. In clinical practice, if an oxytocic drug is used to stimulate the contractions, careful monitoring of the uterine response to the drug is essential to avoid a tonic (continuous) contraction of the uterus.

FIGURE 7.1 The female pelvis (a) The pelvic brim: the largest diameter is in the transverse. (b) The pelvic outlet has its largest diameter in the anteroposterior. (c) The pelvic planes

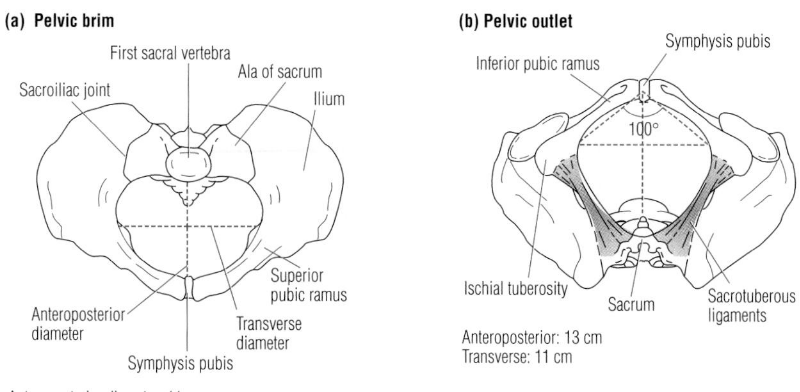

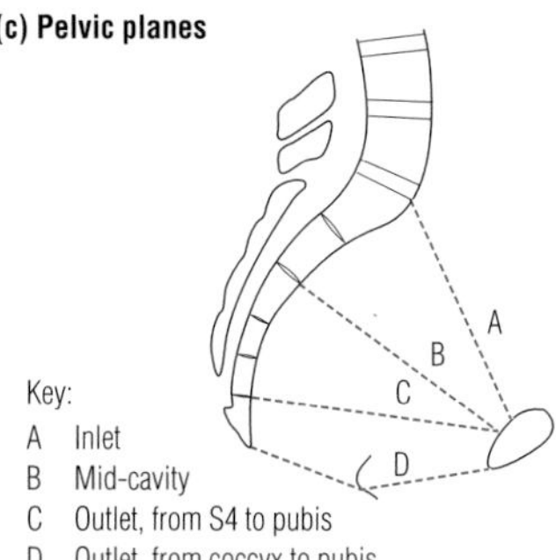

FIGURE 7.2 Pelvic muscles (a) Levator ani from above, pelvic aspect. (b) Levator ani from below, perineal aspect

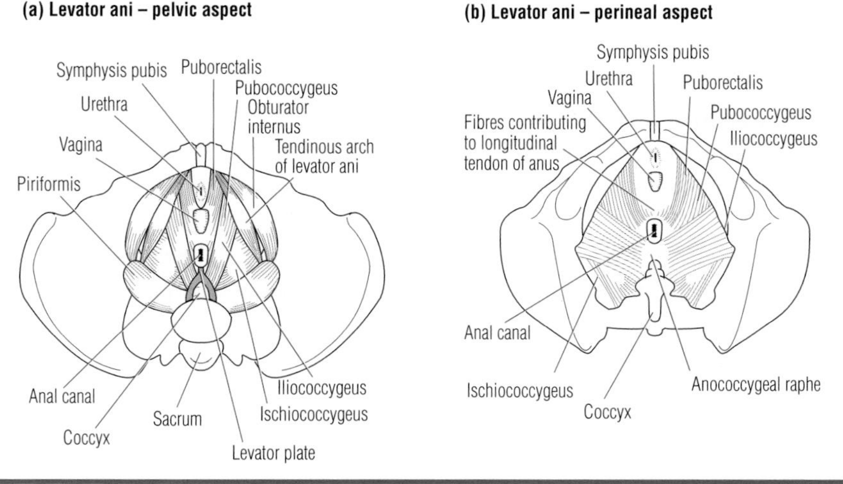

In the second stage of labour the woman uses the contraction of the diaphragm and the abdominal muscles, in addition to the uterine contractions, to aid delivery. Uterine activity continues after the birth of the baby and the placenta is expelled in 2–6 minutes. The uterine contractions then decrease over the next 48 hours. However, they may be painful for some women during the immediate postpartum period.

3 Passenger

The three parameters that are an important influence on the outcome of labour are the size, position and attitude (degree of flexion) of the fetal head. A well-flexed head presents the smallest diameter to the pelvis. The position and flexion of the head can be assessed in labour by vaginal examination to identify the sutures and fontanelles. The head may change in shape in labour to reduce its size in one plane to fit the pelvic shape. This is achieved by the parietal bones overriding the occipital bone (moulding). Pressure on the head impedes the venous and lymphatic return and causes serum to collect under the fetal scalp (caput succedaneum) (Figure 7.3).

Mechanism of normal labour

This refers to the steps or movements that the presenting part (fetal head) undergoes to negotiate the pelvis and deliver vaginally (Figure 7.4). The following movements may occur in sequence or simultaneously.

- *Descent.* The head of the fetus in the primigravida most often moves into the pelvis during the last weeks of pregnancy. However, in the multigravida this may not occur until the onset of labour.
- *Engagement* is said to occur when the maximum diameter of the head has passed through the pelvic brim. The head usually engages in the occipito-transverse position (the maximum diameter of the pelvic inlet).
- *Flexion* occurs continuously during labour. When the head is fully flexed the posterior fontanelle is easily palpable on vaginal examination. The fully flexed head presents the smallest diameter of the fetal head to the pelvis.
- *Internal rotation.* This is the rotation of the head inside the pelvis that occurs due to the natural shape of the birth canal.
- *Extension.* Once the head reaches the perineum, it 'crowns' (distends the introitus and does not move back between contractions) and extends for the head to deliver.
- *External rotation (restitution).* The head reverts back to its normal position (perpendicular) on the shoulders, held before the internal rotation occurred.
- *Lateral flexion.* The anterior shoulder appears under the pubis symphysis, followed by the posterior shoulder riding up the perineum, and the trunk is delivered by lateral flexion. The baby is lifted onto the mother's abdomen.

FIGURE 7.3 The fetal head. (a) Fetal skull from above anterior fontanelle (bregma), a large diamond-shaped depression where the frontal coronal and sagittal sutures meet. Closes at 18 months. The posterior fontanelle is a smaller, triangular-shaped depression where the sagittal suture meets the lamboidal sutures. (b) Fetal skull from the side. (c) Fetal skull showing the caput succedaneum, seen at birth causing the misshapen head—resolves over a number of hours. (d) Moulding of the fetal skull.

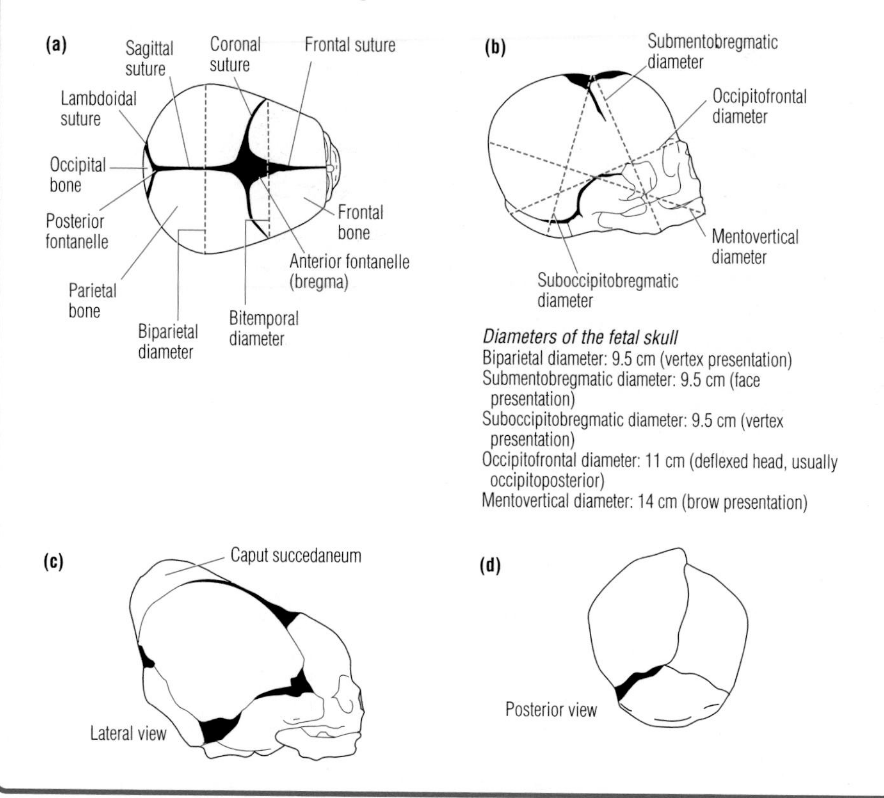

4 Placenta

Once the baby is delivered, the cord is clamped and divided, and the baby is dried and given to the mother to hold. Delivery of the placenta and control of bleeding complete a safe birth. At term the uterine blood flow is 500–800 ml/minute. A tonic contraction of the uterine muscle that occludes the spiral arteries as they pass through the myometrium controls the bleeding. Continued contraction of the muscle is essential to avoid a serious haemorrhage (see Third stage of labour).

After delivery of the placenta, it is checked to ensure that it is complete. Some variations of placentation can occur that might cause bleeding during the pregnancy or after birth, or lead to retained placental tissue (Figure 7.5).

FIGURE 7.4 Mechanism of labour. 1 Descent of the head onto the pelvic floor and flexion of the head to decrease the diameter of the presenting part. 2 Internal rotation as the head moves from an occipito-lateral to an occipito-anterior position. 3 & 4 The head moves down the birth canal to the perineum and delivers by extension. 5 As the head delivers, the shoulders have entered the pelvic brim in its largest transverse diameter. The delivered head moves through 45° to line up perpendicular to the shoulders (restitution). The shoulders undergo internal rotation and the head is seen to move through a further 45° as the shoulders align in the AP diameter of the outlet ready for delivery.

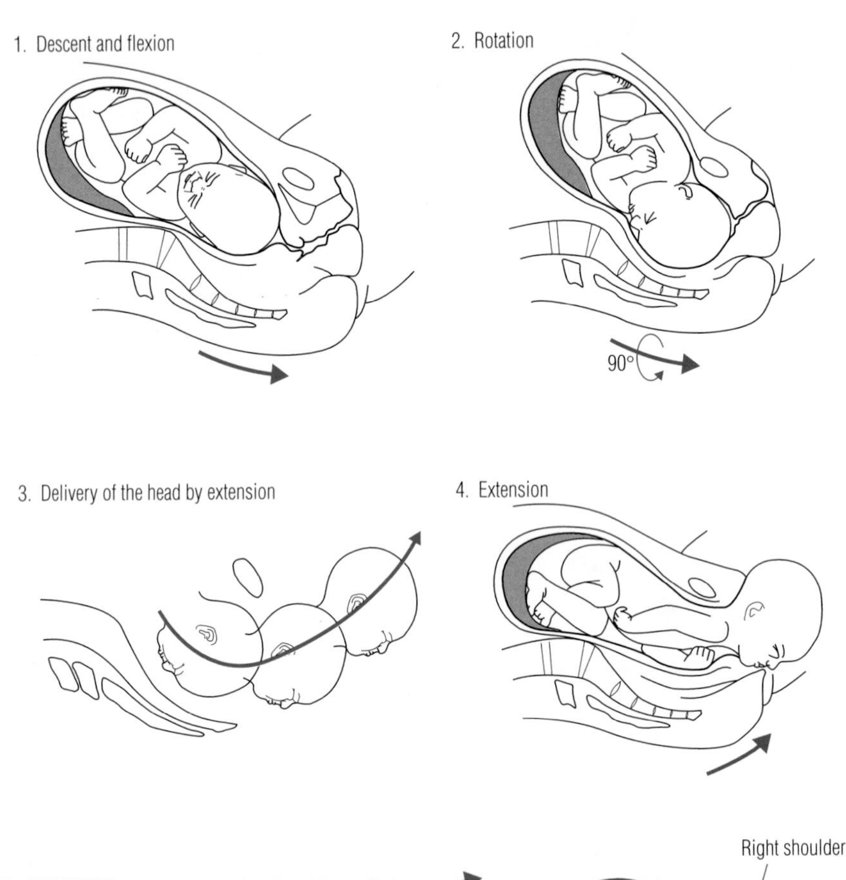

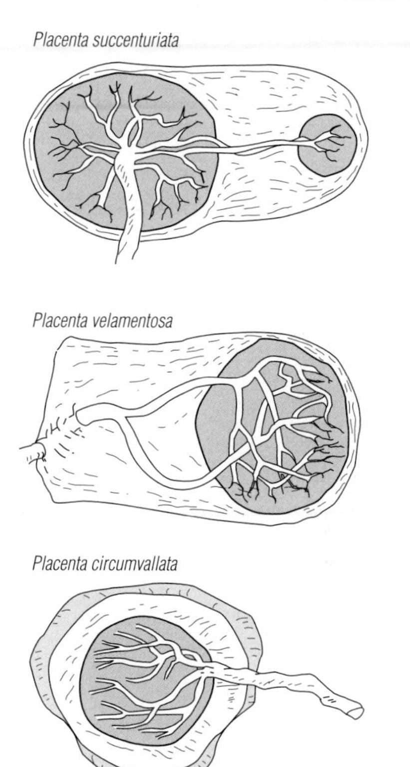

FIGURE 7.5 Clinically relevant abnormalities of the placenta. Succenturiate lobe: There is a vascular connection between the main and an accessory lobe. This may be torn at delivery and/or the accessory lobe may be retained in utero. Placenta velamentosa: the placenta is some distance away from the attachment of the cord and vessels. If the vessels cross the lower pole of the chorion (vasa praevia) fetal haemorrhage may occur on rupture of the membranes. Placenta circumvallata: The membranes appear to be attached internally to the placental edge, and on the periphery is a ring of whitish tissue (a fold of infarcted chorion). This abnormality may be associated with ante- and postpartum haemorrhage.

Phases of labour

Labour is divided into two phases (latent and active) and the active phase is divided into three stages. These divisions have been useful for studying the progress of labour and for comparing labour in different populations.

Latent phase

During the final weeks of pregnancy in many women the cervix starts to change; the hormonal control of these processes is not understood. The changes are termed 'cervical ripening' and consist of progressive softening, thinning and shortening of the cervix as it is incorporated into the lower uterine segment (effacement) (Figure 7.6). Some women are aware of the change and experience suprapubic discomfort and a 'pulling or stretching' sensation. For some women these changes do not occur until the onset of uterine contractions. The time taken for the cervix to become thin, completely effaced and dilated to 3 cm varies with the individual woman and may take many hours or days; this time is termed the latent phase. The woman who starts regular contractions with a cervix that is thin, short and three or more centimetres dilated has a delineated time to labour. Women who report being in labour for a

FIGURE 7.6 Changes in the cervix at the end of pregnancy and during labour (a) Latent stage of labour. Changes in cervix occurring prior to active labour: the muscular upper uterine segment pulls on the thinner lower uterine segment and cervix. The cervix becomes progressively shorter until it is flush with the vaginal vault (termed effacement). Dilatation may occur at the same time, particularly in the multiparous woman. (b) During the first stage of labour the head moves progressively down and the cervix is completely 'taken up'.

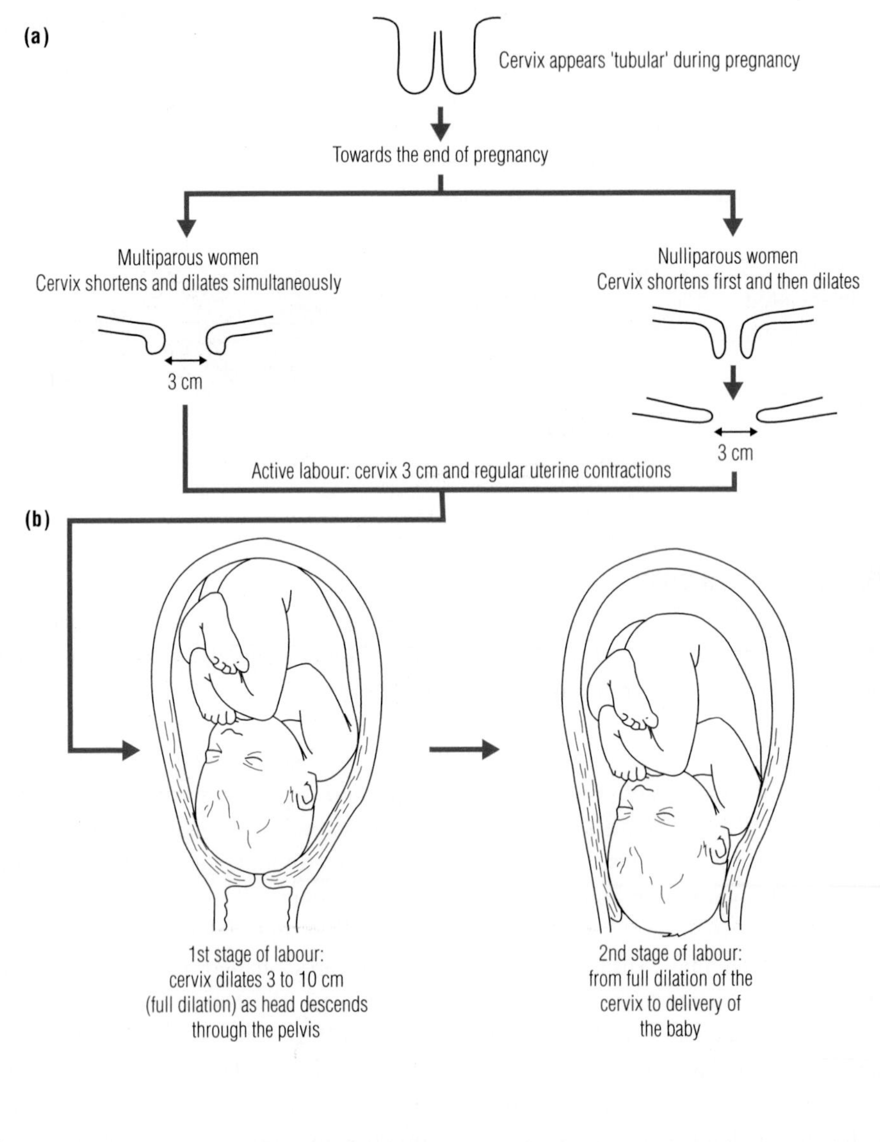

prolonged period may have started labour with an uneffaced cervix. Programs which delay the admission of women to birth suites until the active phase of labour may reduce the incidence of subsequent interventions for poor progress in labour.[10]

Active phase

The definition of active labour is dilatation of the uterine cervix from 3 cm or more in the presence of regular uterine contractions. The minimum rate of cervical dilatation accepted in a primigravida is 1 cm/hour. The active phase of labour to reach full dilatation therefore takes on average seven hours for nulliparous women and 5–6 hours for multiparous women.[11] A *partogram* is a graphic record of the progress of labour that allows efficient and effective communication between the health professionals (Figure 7.7). This should be commenced as soon as the onset of active labour has been diagnosed, unless delivery is imminent. Routine observations are undertaken in a normal labour and entered on the partogram, in addition to any drugs or intravenous fluid administered (Table 7.1). Cervical dilatation lagging two hours behind that expected from the normal graph suggests the need for reassessment.[12] The rate of progress in labour may vary between populations and different graphs may need to be developed for a particular population.

TABLE 7.1 Routine observations in a normal labour

Observation	Frequency
Temperature	4-hourly if normal
Blood pressure	2-hourly if normal
Pulse	2-hourly
Fetal heart	Auscultation with a fetal stethoscope or Doppler every 15–30 minutes in the first stage or 5 minutes in the second stage
Colour of the liquor	At each vaginal examination once the membranes have ruptured
Urine	Encourage to empty her bladder every 2–4 hours and urine analysis performed on admission unless indicated otherwise
Uterine contractions	Duration and frequency ½- to 1-hourly
Abdominal palpation	4-hourly
Vaginal examination	4-hourly

First stage of labour

(from the onset of regular contractions and cervix > 3 cm to full dilatation of the cervix)

After the initial examination a vaginal examination should be performed at least every four hours. If the progress of cervical dilatation is 0.5 cm/hour or less then medical staff should be notified. Once the cervix is more than 3 cm dilated the membranes can be ruptured to check the colour of the liquor if there is any concern about fetal well-being. Rupture of the membranes will reduce the duration of the labour, but a trend is suggested towards an increase in caesarean section and therefore perhaps

FIGURE 7.7 Partogram: this is a pictorial representation of the progress of labour (dilatation of the cervix and descent of the fetal head). It also records all the maternal vital signs, fluid balance, drug administration and fetal heart. Any particular problem for the mother and baby noted in the antenatal period must also be recorded. Any health professional reviewing the chart must be able to see the stage of labour and all the important information related to mother and baby.

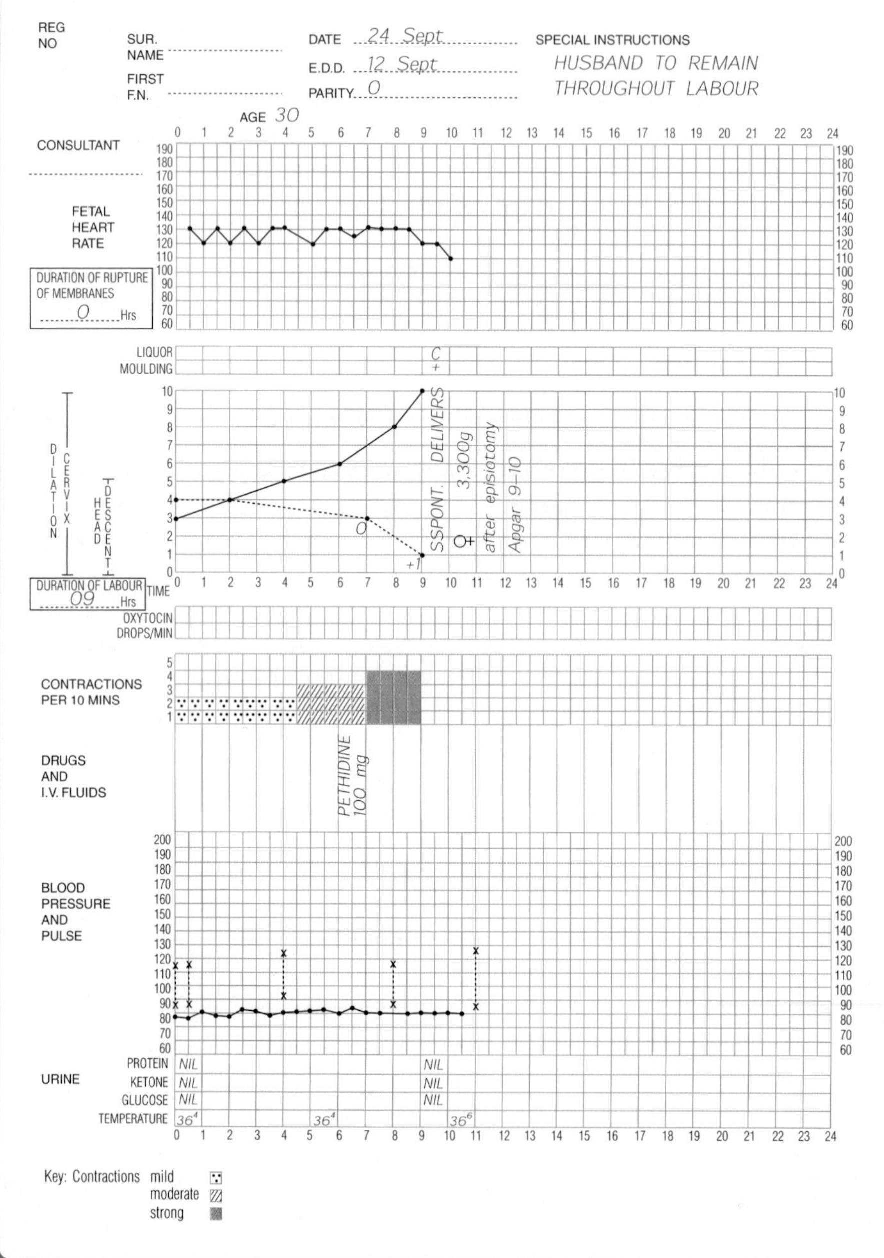

amniotomy should be reserved for women with abnormal labour progress.[13] If there is a delay in the progress of labour then intravenous syntocinon is often commenced to increase the frequency, strength and efficiency of the uterine contractions and a vaginal examination is usually undertaken two hours later.

Second stage of labour

(from full dilatation of the cervix to delivery of the baby, Figure 7.8)

This is diagnosed when the woman has an overwhelming urge to push, the cervix is found to be fully dilated on examination, or a presenting part is visible at the introitus. Once the cervix is fully dilated, if the woman has a desire to push, she should commence pushing and if not delivered after an hour she should be reassessed.

If at full dilatation there is no desire to push she should be allowed a further two hours for presenting part to descend. At this stage if she still has no desire to push she should be reassessed.

It is not unusual for a small tear at the introitus to occur during delivery. Asking the mother to 'pant' rather than push as the head is delivered will slow the delivery of the head and minimise tearing. Once the head is delivered, the baby's neck is checked for the presence of the cord. This can be divided at this stage if it is tight and the delivery expedited.

Third stage of labour

(from delivery of the baby to delivery of the placenta and control of bleeding)

The three signs of separation of the placenta should be observed. These are a trickle of blood at the introitus, the uterus becoming smaller and rounder and appearing to lift up in the abdomen, and lengthening of the cord. The third stage may be managed physiologically or actively. Physiological management exposes the mother to three times the risk of postpartum haemorrhage and a blood loss of over 1000 ml.[14] Using an oxytocic drug to contract the uterus reduces the risk of postpartum haemorrhage.[15] An ergometrine-containing oxytocic is most effective but may cause transient hypertension, and nausea with vomiting in 21–28 per cent of women. An oxytocic alone has fewer side effects but a slightly increased risk of postpartum haemorrhage.[16]

Active management of third stage

As the anterior shoulder of the baby is delivered an intramuscular injection of syntometrine 1 ml or syntocinon 10 IU (to avoid an increase in the maternal blood pressure) should be given, usually into the mother's thigh. The cord is clamped and divided once the baby is delivered. After signs of placental separation the placenta is delivered by continuous cord contraction: the left hand is placed on the lower abdomen above the pubic symphysis, to support the body of the uterus and ensure that it is contracted, and the cord is pulled downwards with the right hand in a continuous fashion. If the uterus is not contracted and supported with the left hand, traction on the cord may cause partial separation of the placenta with haemorrhage and/or inversion of the uterus. The fundus of the uterus should be checked and rubbed to ensure a firm contraction. The placenta should be checked by holding it on two cupped hands and checking that the cotyledons are intact.

FIGURE 7.8 Delivery of the baby. 1 The perineum bulges and the anus dilates as the head pushes down. 2 If an episiotomy is required then infiltration with local anaesthetic in area a, b or c can be made at this stage. 3 & 4 The head should be delivered gently and slowly to protect the maternal tissues. 5 The head delivers by extension. 6 The neck is examined for the presence of a cord. 7 If this is tight it may be divided at this stage. 8 The head rotates through 45° to align itself on the shoulders. 9 A further 45° rotation occurs as the shoulders undergo internal rotation to the AP diameter of the outlet. 10 Pressure on the head by the accoucher downwards delivers the anterior shoulder from under the pubic symphysis. 11 Quickly the accoucher lifts the head upwards to deliver the posterior shoulder, taking care of the mother's perineum.

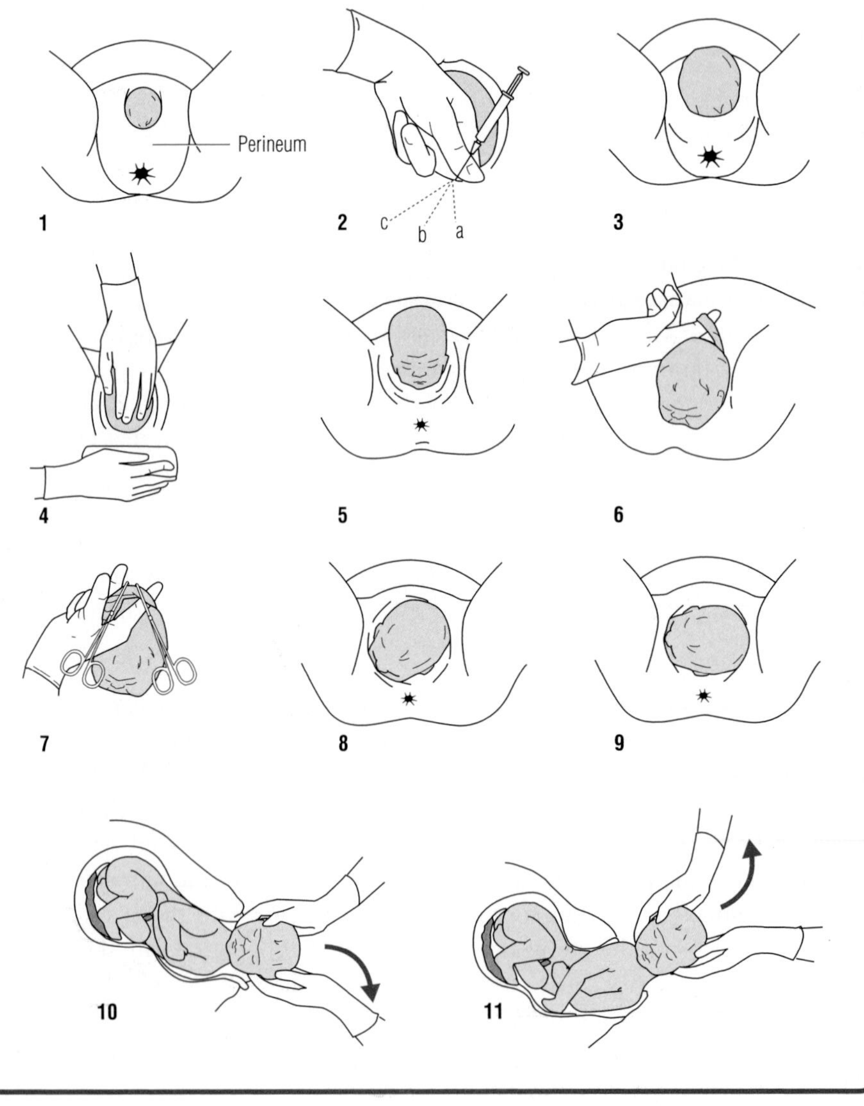

Retained placenta

A retained placenta may be associated with haemorrhage if the placenta has partly separated or the uterus is atonic. There is some evidence that umbilical vein injection of saline solution plus oxytocin is effective in the management of a retained placenta.[17] If the placenta remains undelivered after an hour, or if there is bleeding, a manual removal with appropriate analgesia for the mother is organised (Section 11). Sometimes the placenta is morbidly adherent to the uterine myometrium and is unable to be removed. This occurs where the trophoblast has invaded the decidua and myometrium partially (placenta accreta) or through to the serosal surface (placenta percreta).

Normal labour

CLINICAL PRESENTATION

1 Regular uterine contractions: this is the most frequent presentation.
2 Ruptured membranes: this may occur at any time with and without contractions. If the pregnancy is < 37 weeks duration then a specific policy may be suggested (Section 9).
3 The presence of a 'show' (cervical mucus streaked with blood) can occur some days before any other sign of labour.

Definition: labour is defined as the progressive dilatation of the uterine cervix as a result of regular uterine contractions that leads to delivery of the baby. Active labour has started when the cervix has dilated to 3 cm or more in the presence of regular uterine contractions.

History

1 Time of onset of contractions.
2 Current pattern of contractions:
   - Frequency—expressed as the number of contractions in 10 minutes (usually 1–4).
   - Duration and strength expressed as mild: 20–40 seconds, moderate: 40–60 seconds, strong: > 60 seconds.
3 Ask whether the membranes have ruptured or a show has been noticed.
4 Ask for any other symptoms or problems the woman or the couple may have.

Record check

1 Antenatal notes: any risk factors during the pregnancy or expected in labour.
2 Dates: LMP and ultrasound results. Estimate the gestation.
3 Results of any investigations during the pregnancy.
4 Support during labour. This will reduce the need for analgesia and operative delivery, and improve fetal outcome.[18]

Examination

Mother

1 *Routine observations:* pulse rate, blood pressure and temperature (Table 7.1).
2 *Abdominal palpation:*
   - *Fetus:* fundal height, lie, presentation and engagement of the presenting part.
   - *Contractions:* frequency, strength and duration.
   - *Tenderness between contractions* (may suggest antepartum haemorrhage, dehiscence of uterine scar, inflammation).
3 *Vaginal examination:* performed in the presence of active labour in a woman whose gestation is 37 weeks or more. This examination assesses a number of important features:
   - *Cervix:* dilatation recorded in centimetres
   - *Membranes* (ruptured or intact)
   - *Liquor* (clear, blood-stained, meconium-stained). Meconium-stained liquor should be recorded in the notes at each vaginal examination. At delivery meconium should be aspirated from the oropharynx as soon as possible. It is advisable to have a neonatal paediatrician present at the delivery.
   - *Presenting part* (most commonly the fetal head) is assessed for:
     - Application of the cervix to the presenting part
     - Level of the head, which is related to the mother's ischial spines, usually in centimetres above the spines (recorded in minus centimetres) or below the spines (recorded in plus centimetres)
     - Position by palpation of the fontanelles and sutures
     - Signs of adaptation to the birth canal: moulding and caput succedaneum.

Fetus

The fetal heart should be auscultated every 15–30 minutes in the first stage, every five minutes or around every contraction in the second stage of labour. The heart should be listened to during and after a contraction for a minimum of 60 seconds (Table 7.2).

Cardiotocography (CTG) (Figures 7.9, 7.10): intrapartum fetal heart rate monitoring is used in an attempt to identify fetal signs warning of potentially adverse events in time to permit appropriate intervention. When electronic fetal heart rate monitoring was introduced it was initially thought to be superior to intermittent auscultation, but studies have failed to support this; it has not been shown to be more effective than auscultation in preventing intrapartum stillbirth.

An admission CTG need not be performed in women who have had a normal pregnancy, who have no risk factors and in whom the fetus is appropriately grown. There is some evidence that in such low-risk women an admission CTG increases the risk of operative delivery without fetal or maternal benefit.[19]

Continuous electronic fetal monitoring should be offered or recommended for an 'at-risk' pregnancy or where the labour is not progressing normally. It can be undertaken with an external or internal monitor (a scalp electrode). If the CTG is normal, it may be repeated at 3–4 hourly intervals.

TABLE 7.2 Fetal heart rate characteristics

Characteristic	Normal	Suspicious	Abnormal
Baseline	110–160 bpm	100–109 or 161–180 bpm	< 100 or > 180 bpm
Variability	> 5 bpm	< 5 bpm for 40–90 sec	< 5 bpm for > 90 min
Decelerations	None	Early. Variable. Single prolonged for up to 3 min	Late. Single prolonged for > 3 min
Accelerations	Reactive: 2 or more in 20 min		

FIGURE 7.9 Fetal monitoring using a scalp electrode. An electrode can be applied to the fetal scalp during vaginal examination.

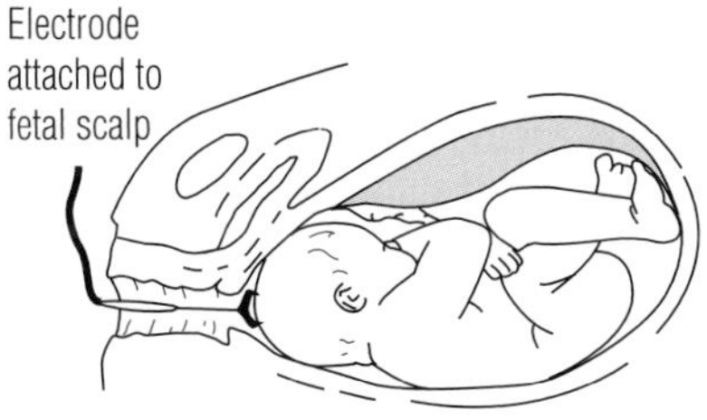

FIGURE 7.10 Representation of fetal heart rate changes to indicate a normal pattern and the variants

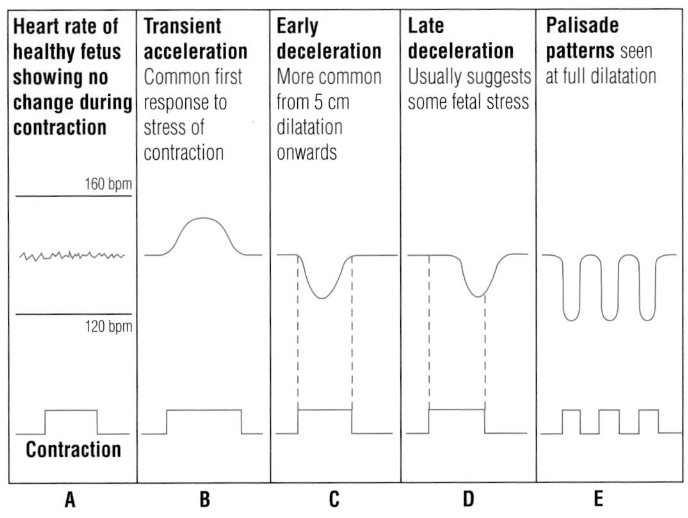

Progress in labour

The progress of labour is recorded on the partogram (Figure 7.7). This pictorial representation of the labour is used to monitor progress and detect any deviation from the expected norm. This can indicate a potential problem that might be averted with the appropriate action (Section 10).

A prolonged labour is dangerous to mother and baby and may lead to undesirable consequences of fetal and maternal exhaustion, fetal hypoxia and infection. Active management of labour is an approach to ensure that women in their first pregnancy deliver a healthy baby after an active labour of less than 12 hours. The caesarean section rate can be reduced by applying correct active management. The first labour will determine the woman's childbirth future both physically and emotionally. The principles of active management are:

- antenatal education
- regular assessment of the progress in labour
- the presence of a support person in labour
- early correction of abnormal progress
- suitable analgesia as requested.

Management during labour

A variety of options exist for women in labour. Some units have specific policies. Most units offer women choice, particularly where there is no evidence for the procedure altering the outcome for mother and baby.

Enema and pubic hair shave

At one time it was routine to perform both these procedures on all women in early labour. However, their value has not been adequately evaluated, and whether or not they are used depends on the inclination of the staff and the wishes of the woman.[20]

Ambulation

Women should be encouraged to mobilise, but to find positions in which they feel most comfortable during labour. Changing position can often help to alleviate the pain.

Caregiver support

During labour, a woman who has continuous support may have both psychological benefits and benefits for the labour (eg reduced medication for pain relief).[21]

Oral intake

It is important for the woman to be comfortable and to be allowed to drink as she feels necessary. She should also be encouraged to empty her bladder at regular intervals.

Pain relief

All women should be made aware in the antenatal period of the options for pain relief in labour. A woman's choice will depend on her own attitude towards analgesics, the degree of pain she experiences and the length and progress of the labour. Some women prefer to try to do without the assistance of any drugs, whereas other women prefer to make use of available methods. Each method of pain relief has benefits and risks (Table 7.3). Pain sensations enter the spinal cord at the level of T10 and L1 and are referred to the corresponding dermatomes (Figure 7.11).

TABLE 7.3 Pain relief in labour

Women should be given as much information as possible during the pregnancy about options that will be available to them for management of pain during labour. For the individual woman many factors will influence the way she is able to cope with the pain of labour.

Method	Use	Efficacy	Side effects and complications
Transcutaneous electrical nerve stimulation (TENS)	Self-administered	Pain scores lower during TENS. Relief rarely complete and some women find no benefit.	None
Entonox (50% nitrous oxide and 50% oxygen)	Self-administered with mouthpiece or face-mask. Takes 45–60 seconds to reach maximum analgesic effect. Begin inhaling at the start of a contraction.	75% of women find it helpful. May be used in all stages of labour.	Safe for mother and baby. Prolonged use in the first stage causes dry mouth and dizziness. Can cause some light-headedness, confusion, nausea. Also tends to make women hyperventilate.
Pethidine	Intramuscular injections 75–150 mg 3-hourly.	Good sedation but suggested poor analgesic in labour	*Mother:* CNS (sedation, confusion and respiratory depression) GIT (nausea, vomiting and delayed gastric emptying.) No effect on progress of labour. *Neonate:* Can cause respiratory depression especially if delivery less than two to three hours after administration. Counteract with Lanoxone. May cause sleepiness and delayed establishment of breastfeeding. *Contraindications:* Absolute contraindication: MAOIs. Severe pregnancy-induced hypertension also prohibits use (norpethidine, an active metabolite, is proconvulsant)

(continued overleaf)

TABLE 7.3 continued

Method	Use	Efficacy	Side effects and complications
Epidural anaesthesia	Administered by an obstetric anaesthetist. Initial bolus injection and subsequent top-up or continuous low-dose infusion.	Reliable, effective pain relief	Headache less than 1% Hypotension Ineffective Local back tenderness, itching or shivering Risk of nerve damage low (less than 1 in 13 000) Dural puncture *Contraindications:* Absolute (sepsis, coagulopathy) Relative (spinal abnormality, severe fetal distress, cardiac disease, hypovolaemia)

MAOIs: monoamine oxidase inhibitors

FIGURE 7.11 Pathways and dermatomes of labour pain and the effect of epidural anaesthetic

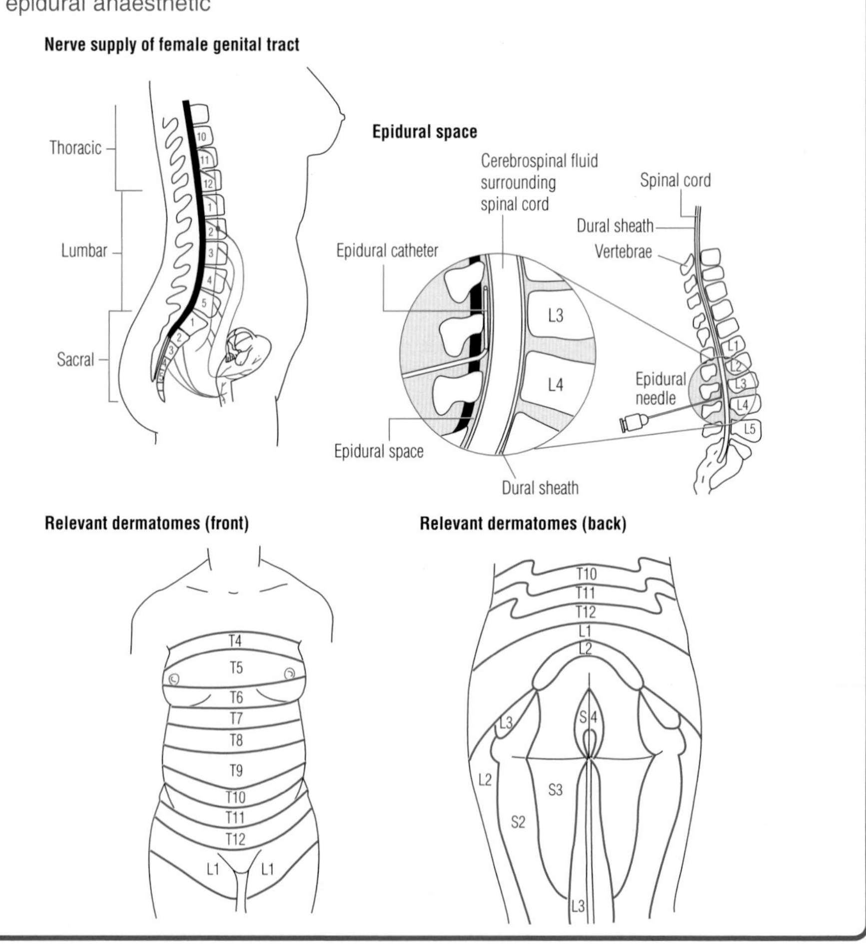

Birth position

There is no data that suggests that one particular birth position (Figure 7.12) has advantages over another for mother and baby.[22] The mother should be encouraged to deliver the baby in the position that is most comfortable for her. If she lies on her back, a wedge should tilt her towards the side to avoid pressure of the pregnant uterus on the vena cava, which can result in hypotension and faintness.

Some women request immersion in warm water during labour and delivery. The benefits (eg assist relaxation, pain relief) and the possible harms (decreased mobility, infection) have not been adequately evaluated.[23]

FIGURE 7.12 Birth positions: a number of different positions may suit individual women. Where the labour progresses normally, the mother should be allowed to choose the position for delivery in which she feels most comfortable.

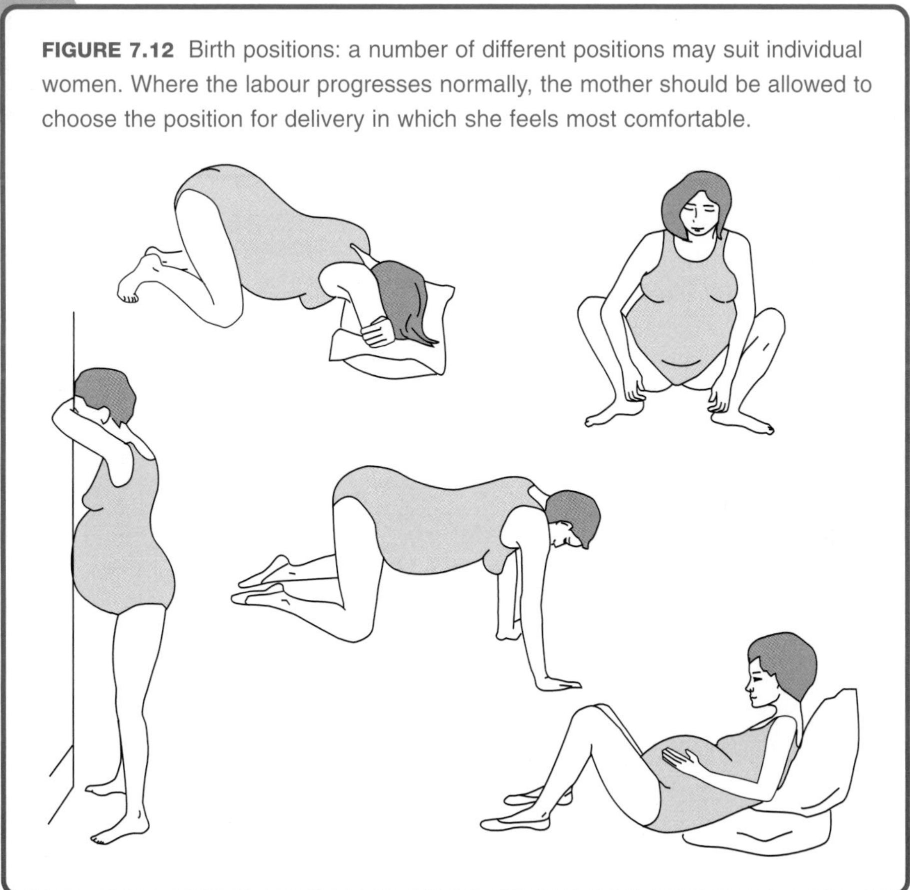

Episiotomy

This is a posterior or medio-lateral incision through the perineum to enlarge the outlet. Some labour ward units perform routine episiotomy and others use a restrictive policy. The indications include: if the tissues are very tight and in danger of tearing or to expedite delivery (where the baby is distressed).[24] This restrictive use is associated with less perineal trauma, less suturing and fewer complications, although there is an increased risk of anterior perineal trauma.[25] The perineal tissues are best repaired in their anatomical layers under local anaesthesia using a continuous subcuticular technique.[26]

Birth attendant

An attendant during delivery can work with the mother and her support person to achieve a controlled, safe delivery. This can be assisted by doing the following:

1. Ensure gradual descent of the head onto the perineum to allow time for the maternal tissues to stretch and thin.
2. Ensure slow, controlled delivery of the fetal head to protect the perineum.
3. Assist delivery of the baby's shoulders, allowing first the anterior shoulder to deliver under the pubic arch and then the posterior shoulder to deliver, thus preventing a tear at the posterior introitus.
4. Clamp and divide the umbilical cord, check for the presence of one artery and two veins in the cord.
5. Suck out the mucus from the baby's mouth and ensure that breathing is established (Section 8).
6. Actively manage the third stage to minimise the risk of haemorrhage.
7. Check that the placenta is complete.
8. Control the bleeding from the uterus after the placenta has delivered by rubbing the uterine fundus to maintain muscle contraction.
9. Check and repair any incisions or tears in the maternal tissues.
10. Encourage the mother to initiate breastfeeding.
11. Answer any queries from the mother or her support person.

After birth

Immediately after the delivery the baby may be placed on the mother's abdomen. If the baby needs resuscitation, the cord should be cut and the baby taken to the resuscitation trolley for management (Section 8). As soon as possible, according to the baby's response, the baby should be dried and wrapped in a warm towel and offered to the mother or father to hold. If it is necessary for the baby to receive special care in the nursery this should be explained immediately to the parents, who would be encouraged to visit the baby as soon as possible.

SECTION

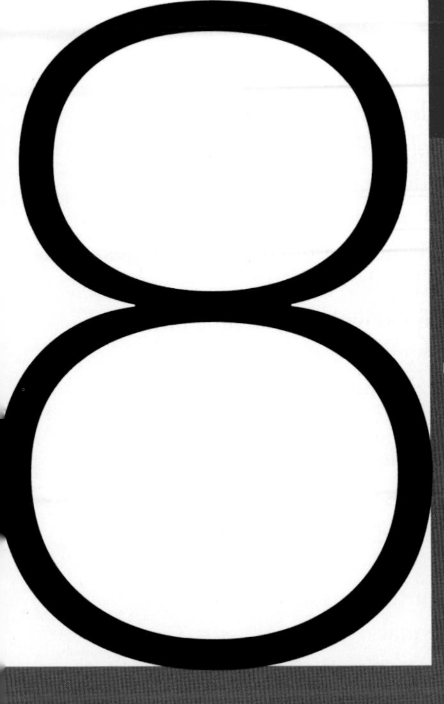

The newborn infant and postnatal care

The newborn infant

Adaptation at birth

At birth the fetus undergoes a transition from an environment in which the gas exchanges, nutrition and thermoregulation are provided by the placenta to one in which it is self-sufficient for these functions. The physiological processes which permit this transition begin well before birth and include reabsorption of lung liquid, synthesis and release of pulmonary surfactant, and dramatic changes in hormonal milieu which alter the function of nearly every fetal tissue and organ. The changes that occur at birth are sudden and dramatic, and include:

- The onset of respiration when the lungs become filled with air and lung fluid is absorbed
- The falling of the right ventricular pressure as the lungs expand and the pulmonary arterial pressure is reduced
- An increase in the systemic vascular resistance and left ventricular pressure when the placental circulation is removed and surface cooling occurs
- Flow of blood now from left to right through the foramen ovale—this will cause its closure (Figure 8.1)
- Decrease in the blood flow through the ductus arteriosus as the pressures on the left and right sides of the heart become equal
- Closure of the ductus arteriosus as a result of constriction of the ductal smooth muscle (Figure 8.1)

FIGURE 8.1 Changes in the heart at birth. With the first breath the lungs expand and the pulmonary vessels increase in size, the ductus arteriosus closes by muscular spasm and the amount of blood flowing through the lung vessels rapidly increases. The pressure in the left atrium rises, and the pressure in the right atrium decreases. The septum primum is then apposed to the septum secundum and the ovale foramen closes functionally.

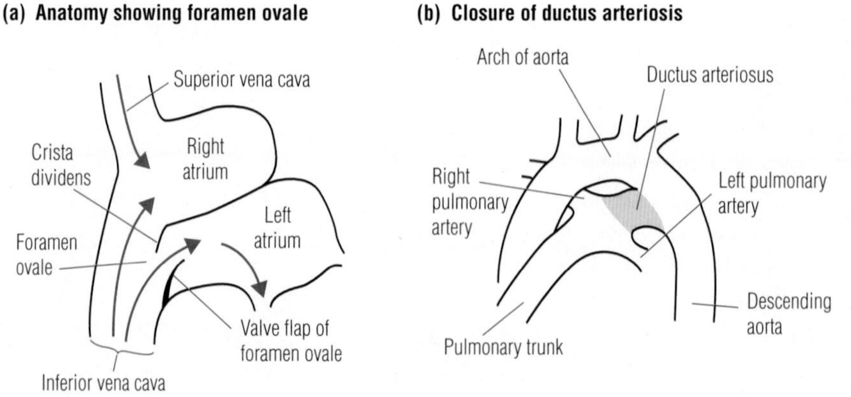

(a) Anatomy showing foramen ovale

(b) Closure of ductus arteriosis

- Increase in glycogenolysis
- Onset of thermoregulation
- Activation of gut motility.

Maladaptation of this process has important implications and may result in a variety of clinical conditions, including:

- neonatal depression/perinatal asphyxia
- meconium aspiration syndrome (MAS)
- transient tachypnoea of newborn (TTN)
- respiratory distress syndrome (RDS)
- persistent pulmonary hypertension of newborn (PPHN)
- patent ductus arteriosus (PDA)
- polycythaemia/hypervolaemia.

Neonatal depression and resuscitation: perinatal asphyxia

Perinatal asphyxia is the most frequent and serious preventable problem of the fetus and newborn infant. Severe, inadequately treated perinatal asphyxia may lead to problems after birth, with major long-term sequelae such as mental retardation, spasticity and epilepsy. Good perinatal care can prevent or minimise fetal and neonatal hypoxia. Approximately 10 per cent of all newborn infants require active resuscitation, with 1–2 per cent needing advanced resuscitation. The following principles should govern obstetric hospital resuscitation practice.

- Every newborn has a right to a resuscitation performed at a high level of competence.
- At least one person skilled in neonatal resuscitation should be in attendance at every delivery.
- An additional skilled person should be readily available.
- Appropriate equipment must be immediately available, well maintained and clinical staff must be familiar with its function.
- Clinical staff must be capable of working smoothly as a team.

Assessment of birth depression

Most newborns establish spontaneous respirations by one minute after delivery. If this does not occur, active intervention is required; the degree of intervention depends on the severity of the depression. The Apgar score, usually recorded at 1 and 5 minutes after birth, provides a useful guide to the extent of intervention required. The Apgar score uses five clinical observations which receive a score between 0 and 2. The maximum possible score is 10, representing the most vigorous response at birth (Table 8.1). The major components of the Apgar score that determine the extent of resuscitation are colour, respiratory effort and heart rate.

Resuscitation

A rapid and skilled assessment of the baby is needed in order to determine what actions are necessary. As these actions are undertaken their effectiveness needs to be assessed and further decisions made. Thus, resuscitation is undertaken in stages, with

TABLE 8.1 The Apgar score

Sign	0	1	2
Heart rate	Absent	< 100/min	> 100/min
Respiratory effort	Absent	Weak cry	Strong cry
Muscle tone	Limp	Some motion	Cry
Reflex irritability (suctioning pharynx)	No response	Some motion	Cry
Colour	Pale Overall cyanosis	Centrally pink Otherwise blue	Pink

cycles of reassessment and decision making. The key to successful neonatal resuscitation is establishment of adequate ventilation. Reversal of hypoxia, acidosis and bradycardia depends on adequate inflation of the fluid-filled lungs with air or oxygen.

1 Prepare for the delivery
   - Turn on the radiant warmer on the neonatal resuscitation trolley.
   - Ensure that all equipment is present, clean and in working order.
   - If advanced resuscitation is anticipated, start the oxygen and low suction flow and ensure that the equipment for suction and intubation is in immediate reach.
   - Call for assistance if needed.

2 Receive the baby
   - Transfer the baby to the preheated neonatal resuscitation trolley, note the time and turn the timer clock on.
   - Dry the baby and remove wet blankets.
   - Place the baby on dry warm blankets to prevent heat loss.

3 Assess the baby's condition
   - Apgar score—see Table 8.1.

4 Airway (A)
   - Position the baby flat on his/her back with the head slightly extended in the sniffing position to ensure a patent airway.
   - Suction the airway for secretions as required.
   - Provide tactile stimulation by rubbing the soles and slapping the heels of the feet or rubbing the infant's back.
   - Administer facial oxygen at the same time.

5 Breathing (B)
   - If the baby is cyanosed but breathing, suction the airway, oropharynx then nasopharynx (15–20 kPa) with a No 8 suction catheter to 5 cm.
   - Administer facial oxygen (5 lpm) through the corrugated end of the Laerdal bagging system or oxygen tubing with a cupped hand.

- If there are no respirations, suction the airway as above and position the baby in the sniffing position. Create a tight seal over the nose and mouth with the face mask. Initiate positive pressure ventilation via a bag and mask at a rate of 40–60 bpm. Oxygen should be administered at 10 lpm with a Laerdal bag or 5 lpm with an anaesthetic bag.
- If there is not adequate chest wall movement, no air entry and no improvement in colour with ventilation, check the mask fit, airway patency and head position. Consider inserting a pharyngeal (Guedel's) airway and recommence bag and mask ventilation. On arrival of a neonatal registrar/consultant or other team member skilled at intubation, endotracheal intubation and intermittent positive pressure ventilation will be commenced if necessary.

6 Circulation (C)

After 15–30 seconds of effective mask ventilation:

- Assess brachial/umbilical or apical heart rate (6 seconds) to determine the need for external cardiac massage.
- If the heart rate is greater than 80–100 bpm continue appropriate respiratory support.
- If heart rate is less than 60 bpm and not increasing with adequate ventilation, initiate external cardiac massage at a rate of 90 compressions per minute. Find the position for compression by drawing an imaginary line across the nipples—just below that line is the lower sternum. Either the two-finger or thumb technique may be used (Figure 8.2). The sternum should be compressed to a depth of 1–2 cm. The compression-to-ventilation ratio is approximately 1 breath to 3 compressions (120 events per minute) with two operators.

FIGURE 8.2 External cardiac massage, two-thumb technique: the sternum should be compressed by about 1–2 cm in a term baby at a rate of about two compressions per second, and the lungs should be reinflated with oxygen after every three compressions.

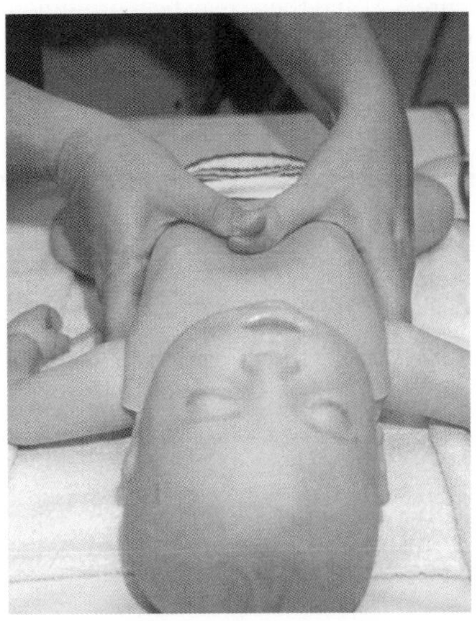

- Assess the heart rate at 30 seconds and if greater than 60–100 bpm and increasing with a good pulse and improving perfusion, cease external cardiac massage; otherwise continue the resuscitation.

7 Continued assessment
- Assess brachial/apical pulse at 30 seconds and then at 1-minute intervals during cardiopulmonary resuscitation to ascertain effectiveness of external cardiac compression.
- Do not interrupt the cardiopulmonary resuscitation cycle for more than 10 seconds, to ensure maintenance of oxygenation and circulation.

Meconium aspiration syndrome

Meconium aspiration syndrome (MAS) is a serious and potentially preventable cause of respiratory distress in the newborn. Meconium staining of the amniotic fluid occurs in about 13 per cent of deliveries and might indicate fetal distress, breech presentation or post-term delivery. The possibility of aspiration into the lungs must be taken seriously whether or not it is a sign of fetal distress. Meconium aspiration may occur during labour or at the onset of neonatal respiration. The response of the infant to intrapartum asphyxia is to gasp, and if meconium is present it will be aspirated deep into the bronchi. Once respiration begins, distal migration of the meconium into small airways occurs (Figure 8.3).

CLINICAL PRESENTATION

There is a wide spectrum of presentations ranging from severe birth asphyxia requiring active resuscitation, to early onset of respiratory distress, to a vigorous baby with no major problems. The clinical and pathological features interact (Table 8.2). Typically, the infant is born covered in meconium-stained liquor and has meconium staining of the umbilical cord, skin and nails. The chest appears to be hyperinflated (Figure 8.4) and there may be a prominent sternum. Respiratory distress may be mild initially, becoming rapidly more severe after several hours. The baby may also show signs of cerebral irritability.

TABLE 8.2 Interaction of the clinical and pathological features of MAS

Fetal compromise	Neonate	Pathological effects	Complications/possible outcomes
FHR irregularity Meconium passage	Meconium-stained liquor Asphyxia Aspiration Retained lung fluid	Plugging → collapse Ball valve → pulmonary air leaks Irritant → pneumonitis, bacterial contamination	Pulmonary hypertension Encephalopathy

Morbidity and mortality for MAS can be prevented or minimised by optimal perinatal management.

FIGURE 8.3 Meconium-stained liquor flow chart

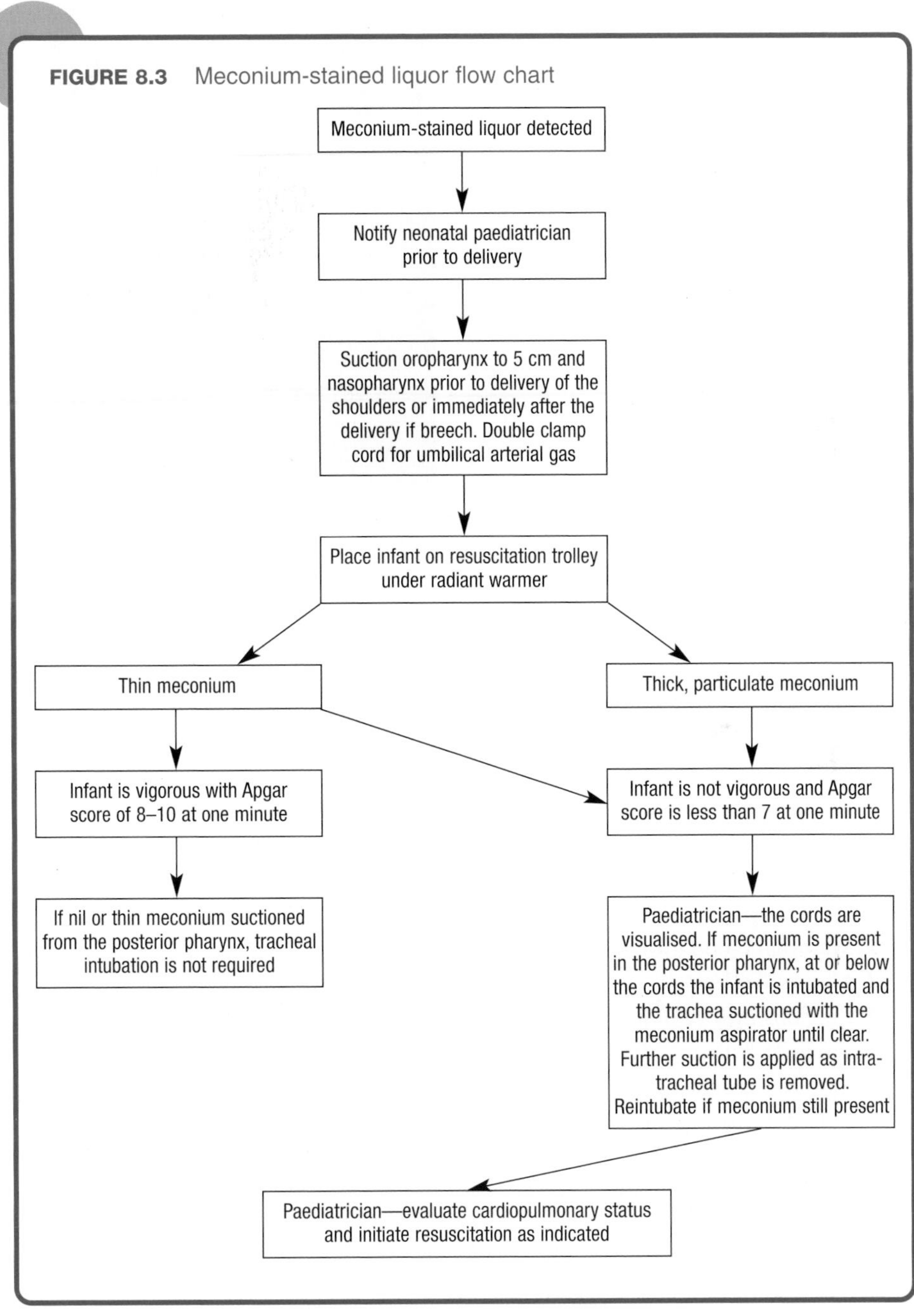

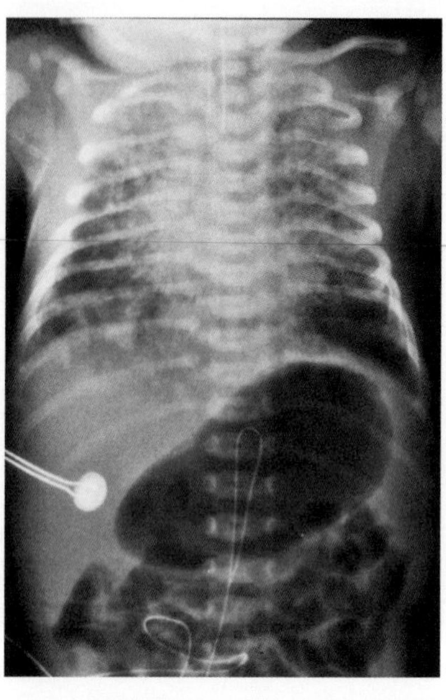

FIGURE 8.4 Chest X-ray of meconium aspiration syndrome reveals hyperinflated lungs with widespread, coarse pulmonary infiltrate and collapse.

CLINICAL PRESENTATION: Jaundice

Although 50–60 per cent of all full-term and 80 per cent of preterm infants develop jaundice, it cannot be assumed that it is mild or physiological unless examination, evaluation and investigation have excluded a pathological cause (Table 8.3). Jaundice is important because it may cause kernicterus, bilirubin-induced neurological dysfunction, or sensorineural hearing loss, or be a presenting sign of another condition.

Management of neonatal jaundice involves perinatal history, physical examination, investigations and treatment.

Perinatal history

- Maternal blood group and serological testing
- Maternal ethnic group
- Previous history of jaundiced infants, familial gallstones
- Mode of delivery, birth weight, gestational age
- Maternal drugs
- Feeding history—breastfeeding, frequency of bowel actions and wet nappies
- Day of onset of jaundice

Physical examination

- Assessment of infant's general health
  - Unwell, sick, lethargic, sleepy
  - Hydration status, weight loss

TABLE 8.3 Possible causes of jaundice presenting at different times in the neonatal period

Day	Unconjugated jaundice	Conjugated jaundice
1	Haemolytic disease assumed until proven otherwise	Neonatal hepatitis Rubella CMV Syphilis
2–5	Haemolysis Physiological Jaundice of prematurity Sepsis Extravascular blood Polycythaemia G6P dehydrogenase deficient Spherocytosis	As above
5–10	Sepsis Breast milk jaundice Galactosaemia Hypothyroidism Drugs	As above
10+	Sepsis Urinary tract infection	Biliary atresia Neonatal hepatitis Choledochal cyst Pyloric stenosis

- Severity of jaundice (Kramer's rule—see below)
- Cause of jaundice
  - Polycythaemia, anaemia, extravascular blood, purpura, cataracts, hepatosplenomegaly
- Abdominal distension
- Obstructive jaundice—khaki skin colour, bile-stained urine, pale stools
- Encephalopathy or kernicterus

Clinical assessment

Jaundice can be detected in the newborn period when the serum level is approximately 100 μmol/l. As jaundice is common, it is essential to have a clinical method for determining its severity.

Kramer's rule depends on blanching the infant's skin with the examiner's finger at standard zones (1–5) and observing the colour in the blanched area. The zones of jaundice reflect the downward progression of dermal icterus (Table 8.4).

TABLE 8.4 Clinical assessment of the jaundiced infant

Zone	Jaundice	Serum indirect bilirubin (per μmol), average
1	Limited to head and neck	100
2	Over upper trunk	150
3	Over lower trunk, thighs	200
4	Over arms, legs, below knee	250
5	Hands and feet	> 50

In assessing the significance of jaundice in a newborn infant, the guidelines in Boxes 8.1 and 8.2 may be useful.

BOX 8.1 Investigating jaundice

- Investigations should be carried out under the following circumstances:
  - Any infant who is visibly jaundiced in the first 24 hours of life
  - Any jaundiced infant whose mother has Rhesus antibodies
  - A preterm infant whose estimated serum bilirubin is greater than 150 μmol/l
  - A term infant whose estimated serum bilirubin exceeds 200 μmol/l
  - Any infant who has the clinical signs of obstructive jaundice
  - Prolonged hyperbilirubinaemia beyond one week in term infants, and two weeks in preterm infants.

BOX 8.2 Management of jaundice prevention

- Appropriate detection and management of Rhesus immunised pregnancy
- Avoidance of traumatic births, general anaesthesia
- Adequate fluid intake on days 1–2
- Frequent breastfeeding in first 72 hours of life
- Supplementary feeding/fluids for at-risk infants
- Treatment (Figure 8.5):
  - Phototherapy
  - Exchange transfusion

FIGURE 8.5 Nomogram for management of jaundice in the term infant > 2500 g birth weight

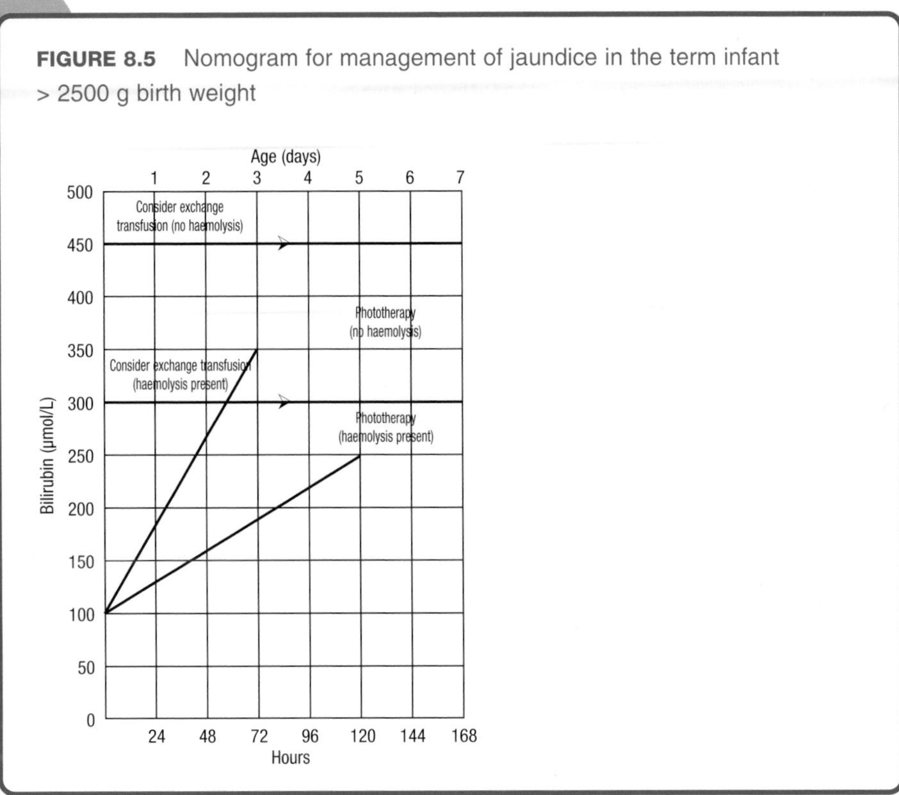

Classification of newborn infants

Newborn infants may be classified according to birth weight, gestational age, or size (large or small) for gestational age (Table 8.5).

Assessment of gestational age

The assessment of a child as SGA or preterm depends on an accurate assessment of gestational age. Gestational age is determined from a combination of maternal dates and antenatal parameters, including ultrasound examination. When antenatal dating is not reliable, neonatal assessment of gestational age is obtained from a combination of assessment of physical and neurological characteristics.[1,2]

The low birth weight (LBW) infant (< 2500 g birth weight) may be preterm, small for gestational age (SGA), or both. The anticipated neonatal problems and subsequent management depend on whether the LBW infant was born too early or too small.

TABLE 8.5 Classification of newborn infants according to birth weight, gestational age, or size for gestational age

	Incidence in Australia
Birth weight	
< 2500 = low birth weight (LBW)	6.5%
< 1500 g = very low birth weight (VLBW)	1.3%
< 1000 g = extremely low birth weight (ELBW)	0.6%
Gestation age	
(completed weeks after last normal menstrual period)	
< 37 weeks = pre term	7.0%
> 42 weeks = post term	0.4%
Size for gestational age	
Weight between 3rd and 97th percentiles for gestational age (AGA)	95.0%
Weight less than 3rd percentile	
= small for gestational age (SGA)	2.5%
Weight greater than 97th percentile	
= large for gestational age (LGA)	2.5%

The preterm infant

The following survival and disability figures quoted can only be achieved when infants are born in a tertiary perinatal centre or are transferred after birth by an expert neonatal emergency transport team (Table 8.6). The figures are therefore not generalisable to births occurring in other environments.

TABLE 8.6 Survival and disability rates for preterm infants

Completed weeks of gestation at birth	Survival	Birth weight (g)	Survival	Completed weeks of gestation at birth	Major disability among survivors
≤ 22	0%	< 500	< 10%		
23	< 10%	500–749	60%	23	50%
24	50%	750–999	85%	24	30%
25	75%	1000–1499	> 95%	25–27	15%
26	85%	≥ 1500	> 95%		
27	90%				
28 & 29	> 95%			28	10%
≥ 30	> 98%				

Specific problems of the preterm infant

During the last three months of intrauterine life organ systems are undergoing continued structural and functional development. Preterm birth requires rapid adaptation to extrauterine life before these organ systems are adequately developed. Preterm infants are at risk for a number of problems as a result of the early birth. These include:

- birth asphyxia
- thermal instability
- lack of the primitive survival reflexes of suck, swallow, cough and gag, with high incidence of milk aspiration
- jaundice
- pulmonary disease
- metabolic disturbances
- patent ductus arteriosus—congestive heart failure
- intracranial lesions
- infection—perinatal and nosocomial
- gastrointestinal intolerance and necrotising enterocolitis
- ophthalmic lesions
- surgical lesions
- haematological disorders
- renal immaturity.

Supportive care

For the preterm infant this involves close attention to:

- resuscitation
- monitoring
- oxygen therapy
- maintenance of BP
- thermoregulation
- nutrition: parenteral fluids, enteral feeding
- fluid balance chart.

Problems unique to the preterm infant

Respiratory distress syndrome

Respiratory distress syndrome (RDS), also known as hyaline membrane disease, is a specific entity in preterm infants caused by a lack of surfactant (a surface tension lowering agent) in the alveoli. It has a characteristic clinical picture, and chest X-ray shows hypo-aeration, a diffuse granulo-reticular pattern, air bronchograms and, in its most severe form, a diffuse 'white out' (Figure 8.6).

CLINICAL PRESENTATION

- Diagnosed at birth or first 4 hours
- Signs of respiratory distress: tachypnoea, cyanosis, nasal flaring, expiratory grunt

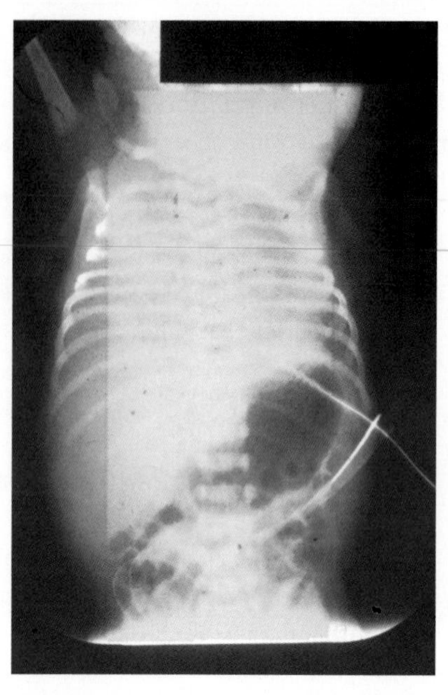

FIGURE 8.6 Radiological appearance of respiratory distress syndrome (hyaline membrane disease) showing diffuse 'frosted glass' appearance throughout both lungs, 'air bronchogram' effect and loss of cardiac outline

- Breath sounds: harsh, diminished
- Oedema
- Apnoea

Course

- Classically RDS increases for 24–72 hours, then diuresis and recovery occurs over 48–96 hours.
- If severe and requiring mechanical ventilation, a slow recovery over weeks to months is more likely

Epidemiology

- Common condition occurring in 1 per cent of all newborn infants
- Incidence relates to degree of prematurity
- Predisposing factors: maternal diabetes mellitus, antepartum haemorrhage, second twin, hypoxia/acidosis at birth, male gender, caesarean section not in labour, positive family history
- RDS, including extreme prematurity, and its complications contributes 37 per cent to all causes of neonatal death.

Pathophysiology

Surfactant is a phospholipid secreted by the type II alveolar cells of the fetal lung from about 28 to 32 weeks gestation. The major phospholipid is lecithin but other phospholipids and surfactant proteins A, B and C must be present for full activity.

Prognosis

Acute, subacute and chronic complications are shown in Table 8.7. The prognosis for RDS relates to severity and gestational age, but has improved since the availability of exogenous surfactant.

TABLE 8.7 Complications of respiratory distress syndrome

Acute	Subacute	Chronic
Cardiopulmonary		
Perinatal asphyxia	Encephalopathy	Neurosensory disability
Pulmonary air leak	Consolidation/collapse	Bronchopulmonary dysplasia
Patent ductus arteriosus	Lung oedema	SIDS
Pulmonary hypertension	Opportunistic infection	Subglottic stenosis
Pulmonary haemorrhage		Chronic obstructive pulmonary disease
Cerebral		
Cerebroventricular haemorrhage	Ventricular dilatation	Hydrocephalus
Periventricular leucomalacia	Cysts	Porencephaly
		Cerebral atrophy
Gastrointestinal tract		
Necrotising enterocolitis	Bowel obstruction	Malabsorption

Necrotising enterocolitis

Necrotising enterocolitis (NEC) is an inflammatory bowel disease most commonly affecting the terminal ileum or sigmoid colon.

CLINICAL PRESENTATION

The clinical signs and symptoms of bile-stained aspirates, bloody stools and abdominal distension are often associated with systemic features of apnoea, bradycardia, shock, oliguria and acidosis. Diagnosis is confirmed by pneumatosis intestinalis, portal vein gas or pneumoperitoneum on supine and cross table lateral abdominal X-rays (Figure 8.7), a toxic pattern on the full blood count (FBC), and positive faeces and blood cultures for pathogens. Predisposing factors other than prematurity are direct bowel mucosal injury, hypoxia and ischaemia.

FIGURE 8.7 Radiological appearance of necrotising enterocolitis, showing distended bowel loops and intramural gas

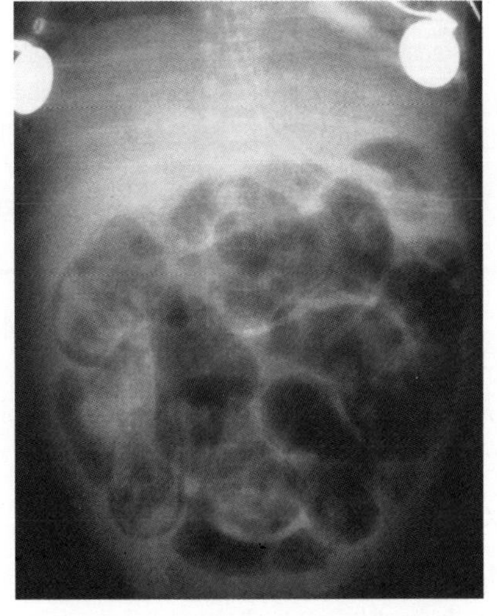

Retinopathy of prematurity

Retinopathy of prematurity (ROP) is a fibrovascular disease of extreme prematurity with additional risk factors being prolonged mechanical ventilation and O_2 usage, episodes of sepsis, frequent blood transfusions, severe apnoea and intraventricular haemorrhage. All infants < 1250 g birth weight and/or < 30 weeks gestation should be screened by an ophthalmologist for ROP commencing at 32 weeks post menstrual age. A baby who has reached a specified critical threshold will require laser retinal surgery to minimise risk of loss of visual acuity.

The small for gestational age infant

Although several synonyms have been used to describe the growth-retarded infant, the preferred term based on common usage is now 'small for gestational age' (SGA). There has been no such uniformity in the definition of SGA. From a statistical viewpoint, infants born at any gestational age, and weighing more than two standard deviations below the mean, can be defined as SGA. Some larger babies who have suffered growth-retarding influences in utero, such as poor placental function, may have some problems such as hypoglycaemia in common with this group.

From an obstetric viewpoint, it is important to identify the fetus starved of nutrition as a result of intrauterine growth restriction. These babies show growth failure greatest for weight, then length, with head circumference the least affected. Typically these SGA infants have little subcutaneous fat, the skin may be loose and thin, muscle mass is decreased, especially buttocks and thighs, and the infant often exhibits a wide-eyed and anxious face. This extrinsic type can be distinguished from the uniformly growth-retarded type, which implies either a fetal cause (eg chromosomal) or a very early insult (Table 8.8).

TABLE 8.8 Causes of intrauterine growth restriction

Fetal	Placental	Maternal
Chromosomal abnormalities	Toxaemia of pregnancy	Maternal disease
Prenatal viral infection	Multiple pregnancy	Alcohol
Dysmorphic syndromes	Small placental size	Smoking
X-rays	Site of implantation	Malnutrition
	Vascular transfusion in monochorionic twin placentas	

When considering the specific problems of SGA infants it is more appropriate to compare them with their gestational-age peers rather than with preterm infants of similar birth weight. A number of problems can be anticipated for the SGA fetus or neonate (Table 8.9).

Examination of the newborn

The newborn infant is examined by a variety of people at different times in the first few days of life. The birth attendant assesses condition at birth by ascribing the Apgar

TABLE 8.9 Anticipated problems in the fetus/neonate who is SGA

Fetus	Newborn	Subsequent outcome
Stillbirth	Asphyxia	Impaired growth
Fetal distress	Hypoglycaemia	Intellectual deficit
Meconium aspiration	Meconium aspiration syndrome	Cerebral palsy (due to asphyxia)
Oligohydramnios	Polycythaemia	
Congenital malformation	Hyperviscosity	
Deformations	Hypothermia	
Cord compression	Hypocalcaemia	
Premature rupture of membranes	Infection (impaired immune system)	
Preterm delivery	Pulmonary haemorrhage Transient neonatal hyperglycaemia	

score at 1 and 5 minutes, and performs an external examination for overt congenital abnormalities. The mother will closely scrutinise her baby for birth defects. A medical officer should perform a full physical examination either shortly after birth in the delivery suite or operating room, or on admission to the postnatal ward or within the first 24 hours after birth. All babies should have a full physical examination by a skilled medical officer prior to hospital discharge.

The newborn physical examination is the most valuable screening test performed at any time during life, as the early detection of various occult abnormalities (eg congenital heart disease, developmental dysplasia of hip, cataract, cleft soft palate) may allow early and effective treatment before morbidity occurs. It can also identify changes that are not serious and allow discussion and reassurance for the parents (Tables 8.10–8.12).

TABLE 8.10 Common conditions in the newborn (photo section 2)

These may be of little clinical importance but may be a cause of anxiety for the parents.

Condition	Cause/outcome
Skin lesions: haemangiomas, capillary (strawberry)	Appear after a few days or weeks and gradually increase during the first five months. Static for a few months and then starts to involute. The initial soft, raised, bright red capillary haemangioma begins to turn a grey colour and usually disappears completely by age three.
'Stork' marks	Flat, pink capillary haemangioma at nape of neck, middle of forehead or upper eyelids. Those at the nape of the neck persist throughout life; facial lesions fade during first two to three years.

(continued overleaf)

TABLE 8.10 continued

Condition	Cause/outcome
Port wine stain	Flat capillary haemangioma. Does not fade but darkens as time goes by to form a flat, purple patch of skin. Treated with laser therapy. Those over the skin innervated by ophthalmic division of trigeminal nerve may be associated with intracranial haemangioma (Sturge-Weber syndrome).
'Mongolian' blue spots	Large grey to blue-black macules resembling bruises. Found in infants of Asian or African origin. Commonly over buttocks and lower back. They are collections of melanocytes within the dermis. Gradually fade and rarely visible after five years.
Erythema neonatorum (toxic erythema)	Erythematous rash during the first week of life. Small, pale papule commonly evolves into a vesicle. Each papule surrounded by bright erythema. Comes and goes over several days. Cause unknown.
Epithelial 'pearls' in mouth	On back of hard palate. Related to birth and fades in one to two weeks.
Cephalohaematoma	Occurs when bleeding over outer surface of a skull bone elevates the periosteum, causing a fluctuant swelling confined to limits of bone.
Positional talipes	Minor degrees common from mechanical pressures in utero. Commonly plantar flexion (equinus) and foot adduction (varus) at mid tarsal joint. If the foot can be fully dorsi-flexed and everted it will correct spontaneously. Otherwise orthopaedic referral required.
Tongue-tie	Is due to a short frenulum with limited protrusion of tongue. Rarely causes speech problems.
Natal teeth	Mostly lower incisors, are quite common and if loose should be removed to prevent aspiration.
Traumatic cyanosis	Petechiae over head and neck related to difficult delivery of head, eg breech, nuchal cord, face presentation.
Breast engorgement	Breast engorgement is commonly seen after birth and relating to withdrawal of maternal hormones – breasts must not be expressed.
Vulval mucosal tags	Hymenal skin tags are common and are associated with protrusion of redundant vaginal mucosa. Usually regresses spontaneously in first few weeks.
Sacral dimple	In lower part of sacrum at upper end of natal cleft. Not associated with underlying spinal abnormalities. (However, any sinus, naevus or superficial lesion higher up in the spine may be associated with underlying defect. Needs evaluation.)
Eyelid oedema	Mild lid oedema may be present following a long labour, particularly with face or brow presentation.
Hydrocele	A fluid collection in scrotum may be present at birth and transilluminates brilliantly. It may extend up spermatic cord.
Skin tags and diminutive accessory digits	Particularly pre auricular and on fingers are common and may be removed with silk tie or surgically.
Sticky eye	Common in the newborn. Requires bathing with warm sterile saline. If inflammation (conjunctivitis), a swab should be taken. Common organisms: staphylococci, streptococci, *E. coli* and *Haemophilus*. Beware *Chlamydia* and *Neisseria*, which can cause corneal scarring.

TABLE 8.11 Incidence of some common major malformations

These figures may vary according to local prevalence. Incidence figures for congenital abnormalities are confounded by antenatal diagnosis and termination of some major anomalies.

Condition	Incidence
Anencephaly	1:2500
Spina bifida	1:1750
Hydrocephalus	1:2600
Cleft palate	1:1850
Cleft lip and palate	1:1250
Oesophageal atresia	1:3000
Anorectal atresia	1:2500
Polydactyly	1:1000
Syndactyly	1:2000
Reduction deformity of the limbs	1:1300
Club foot	1:700
Exomphalos/gastroschisis	1:2800
Diaphragmatic hernia	1:3500

TABLE 8.12 Prevalence of some common birth defects*

These figures may vary according to local prevalence. Incidence figures for congenital abnormalities are confounded by antenatal diagnosis and termination of some major anomalies.

Condition	Incidence
Malformations of heart and great vessels	11.1
Developmental dysplasia of hip	7.5
Hypospadias	3.2
Talipes equino-varus	2.2
Hypertrophic pyloric stenosis	1.9
Down syndrome	1.4
Cleft lip with or without cleft palate	1.0
Spina bifida	1.0
Anencephaly	0.8
Renal agenesis and dysgenesis	0.7
Oesophageal atresia, tracheo-oesophageal fistula	0.5
Abdominal wall defects: omphalocele, gastroschisis	0.6
Diaphragmatic hernia	0.3

* Rate per 1000 births including terminations of pregnancy, stillbirths and live births

Preparation for physical examination after hospital discharge

- Review maternal history, mode of delivery, condition at birth.
- Provide a safe, warm, well-lit environment with a flat surface.
- Review history of passage of urine, meconium/stools, and feeding history.
- Examine in the presence of at least one parent.
- Wash and scrub hands and arms using antiseptic.
- Prepare equipment: tape measure, stethoscope, baby scales, ophthalmoscope, tongue depressor.

Anthropometric parameters

- Birth weight (BWt) is measured to the nearest gram.
- Head circumference (HC) is measured with a non-stretchable tape, and measured to the nearest 0.1 cm as the maximum occipito-frontal circumference.
- Length is the crown heel measurement taken by two people with the aid of a measuring board.

Birth weight, head circumference and length are plotted on gender-specific growth curves appropriate to the hospital of birth and population base.

Neurological examination

The behavioural state of the newborn will severely affect the neurological signs elicited, and needs to be described. The assessment consists of observations, examination, and recording of the following:

- Abnormal movement—tremors or convulsions
- Spontaneous movement—quality and quantity. Observe monoplegia, hemiplegia, diplegia.
- Posture—depends on gestational age. Observe for hypotonia, hypertonia, or intrauterine crowding.
- Tone—limb, head and truncal tone is assessed, especially for symmetry
- Deep tendon reflexes—usually easily elicited
- Ankle clonus—sustained clonus is abnormal
- Primitive reflexes—reflexes are assessed for maturity, symmetry, and neurological function
- Cranial nerves—always assess the VIIth. Others when impaired neurological function is suspected.

Physical examination

A thorough systematic neonatal assessment is assisted by the use of a neonatal examination chart from a neonatal unit.

Specific tests:

1 *Barlow's test* assesses whether or not a hip is dislocatable. The flexed hips are adducted while gentle posterior pressure is applied. The examiner feels for the femoral head slipping backwards out of the acetabulum.

2 *Ortolani's reduction test* detects a hip that cannot be abducted because of dislocation. The hips and knees are flexed and the knees brought together. The hips are then abducted while the examiner feels for the femoral head slipping forward into the acetabulum.
3 *Moro reflex* is elicited by suddenly dropping the infant's head onto an examining hand and assessing the limb response.
4 *Stepping reflex* examines the infant in the upright position when weight is taken through the feet.
5 *Plantar response* tests the reaction of toes and feet when the sole of the foot is stimulated.

Issues for discussion with new parents

The following issues should be addressed by clinicians before or at hospital discharge of newborn infant and mother.

- Anthropometric parameters—height, weight, HC at birth, measured and serially plotted on growth curves
- Vitamin K administration
- Physical examination of newborn:
  - Birth
  - At hospital discharge
  - At 5–10 days by the general practitioner (GP)
- Advocacy, promotion and support of breastfeeding
- Reduce the risk of SIDS by providing advice and an information pamphlet
- Assess the family for risk of child abuse
- Immunisation: provide advice and promotion
- Accident/injury counselling
- Anticipatory guidance:
  - Cigarette smoke avoidance
  - Circumcision advice
- Support role of GP, child health clinic and other community services
- Assess development, hearing, vision, speech
- Personal health record.

Advocacy, promotion and support of breastfeeding

Perinatal data units in Australia currently report rates of breastfeeding at hospital discharge of approximately 80 per cent. If breastfeeding is not established at time of early discharge, the GP needs to provide support, advice and assistance with feeds, such as positioning and attachment. The GP needs to be aware of the community resources available to assist lactating mothers, which include Nursing Mothers' Association, lactation consultants and child health clinics.

Vitamin K

Classic haemorrhagic disease of the newborn is caused by a deficiency of the Vitamin K-dependent clotting factors, and its decline in incidence is due to the routine administration of Vitamin K 1 mg (Konakion IMI) at birth. A small percentage of parents elect for their infants to have three oral doses (at birth, at time of newborn screening, and again in the fourth week if breastfed). The GP must administer the third dose to prevent late-onset vitamin K-deficient haemorrhage.

SIDS prevention advice

One of the most successful public health strategies in recent years has been the campaign to reduce the risk of SIDS. Advice such as supine sleeping, feet to foot of cot, avoidance of over-wrapping and inhalation of cigarette smoke, and promotion of breastfeeding, have reduced the incidence of SIDS from approximately 1.5 to 0.5 per thousand live births in Australia and the UK.

Child protection issues

Ask about any parental distress that may result from situations such as crying and colic. Anticipatory guidance can then be provided and follow-up arranged to reduce the risk of maltreatment. Awareness of the risk factors for maltreatment (eg parental history of abuse, poor social support, low socio-economic status, young mother, or substance abuse) is important, particularly given the effectiveness of home visiting by a child health team.

The new models of midwifery care (community and home visits) provide less opportunity for social work input and evaluation in the antenatal period. Any early discharge program (where the mother and her baby leave the hospital within 24 hours of delivery) means at-risk infants are likely to have been discharged before being identified as such. The role of the GP and community services therefore include an awareness and identification of risk factors, recognition, and management of infants with evidence of withdrawal from maternal drugs (neonatal abstinence syndrome), and assessment of home care and parental interaction with the infant.

Accident/injury counselling

Injury prevention counselling during child health visits (eg child restraints in cars, avoidance of baby walkers, locked cupboards for medicines, and fenced swimming pools) has been shown to be effective in reducing childhood accidents.

Parental advice

Immunisation, circumcision, and nutritional advice are important components of the parental postnatal education program.

Umbilical cord care

Parents should be instructed on routine care of the umbilicus, consisting of cleansing with water or saline. When there is reddening or cellulitis of the skin around the umbilicus, swabs are taken of any discharge for bacteriological culture, and the baby may be treated with oral flucloxacillin and 1 per cent chlorhexidine baths. An umbilical granuloma should be treated by application of a silver nitrate stick on one or two occasions.

Newborn metabolic screening

In many countries all newborn infants are screened for phenylketonuria (1 in 15 000), hypothyroidism (1 in 3500) and galactosaemia (1 in 22 000), and in some with predominance of Caucasians, cystic fibrosis (1 in 2500). With the progressive availability of mass spectrometry, it is also possible to screen for a wide variety of rarer metabolic diseases. If the baby is discharged before 72 hours of age, blood is taken by a community midwife on day 4 or 5; otherwise, heel stick blood will be taken at discharge. Follow-up testing may rarely involve a repeat blood spot or venous blood for more specialised metabolic tests.

The postnatal period

The postnatal period begins following the birth of the baby and by tradition ends at six weeks. The time period of 40 days for the postnatal period is found in many cultures throughout the world from the Asia-Pacific region to Africa and parts of Europe. It may be linked to the time taken for lochial discharge to cease, or it could signify deeper religious and cultural roots. The six-week postnatal check-up is a common feature of Western maternity care, despite the lack of evidence that the check-up improves health outcomes for women.[3,4] The time period is of little clinical significance nowadays—it is just as valid to think in terms of the first 24 hours, the first week, the first month or the first year.

What happens after pregnancy?

The pregnant woman is now a mother. But what happens to her body and psyche after she has given birth? There is a lack of carefully conducted studies of the normal changes that occur following childbirth and a lack of longitudinal studies of representative samples of women. There is little evidence to support routine practice or information about effective interventions for many of the common postnatal problems. Hytten provides the first systematic review of knowledge about the normal puerperium and many of the findings are at odds with 'current clinical opinion'.[5]

Despite lack of evidence, postnatal care has followed many rigorous protocols; from the period of strict 'lying-in', the four-hourly breastfeeding regimen, to the current practice of early return to normal duties.[6]

A woman experiences major physiological, anatomical and psychological changes during pregnancy. Externally, her body shape and appearance change, and she faces, particularly following the first pregnancy, a complete redefinition of her role within society.

Physical changes

The uterus

The transformation of the 1 kg pregnant uterus back to a pre-pregnant state is an amazing physiological feat that is poorly understood. The 1 kg uterus contracts within minutes after expulsion of the placenta, and yet, contrary to popular belief, it does not return to its pre-pregnant state. The length of the uterus decreases by about 1 cm per day for the first 3 or 4 days and then 6 mm per day up to about nine days. A study undertaken in 1995 found that the uterus was still palpable above the symphysis at 14 days post partum.[5]

The cervix usually sustains some damage during a vaginal birth, and the os remains slightly open for a few days, closing around seven days after giving birth. However, the shape of the os is no longer round as in the nulliparous state but is a flattened horizontal oval shape.

The vagina

The vagina is a smooth-walled passage for the first few days after childbirth, after which it begins to reduce in size. Vaginal rugae begin to redevelop around week 3, and by week 6 the vagina has established the post-pregnancy state as a larger organ with less rugae than before pregnancy.

The pelvic floor

Pelvic floor damage is common after childbirth. It is more common in women who have experienced a prolonged second stage of labour or given birth to a larger baby (especially >4 kg). Older maternal age, obesity and multiparity are also associated with increased risk of damage. Pelvic floor damage increases the likelihood of urinary incontinence, faecal incontinence and prolapse of pelvic organs, and it may be linked to sexual dysfunction. At present there is little information to recommend specific antenatal or postpartum management strategies to improve these outcomes for women.[7]

The lochia

Women experience some vaginal loss for some days after giving birth. Lochia refers to the bloody vaginal discharge consisting of blood from the placental site, and the debris from necrotic decidua and any trophoblastic remains. This was described in the past as: 'lochia rubra' (frank blood), for 2 and 6 days, then 'lochia serosa' (brownish pink) for 16–35 days and finally 'lochia alba' (yellowish white) for 10–14 days. These descriptions may not be supported by women's experience. More recent studies suggest that the loss lasts on average 21 days (10th to 90th percentiles: 10–42 days) and the colour is predominantly red/brown.[8]

Gastrointestinal system

The tone of the lower oesophageal sphincter returns to the pre-pregnant state by about six weeks post partum and the reduced gastric motility of pregnancy returns to normal in the early days following the birth. A study of 411 women found that 60 per cent of women have a normal bowel motion by six days post partum.[5] This figure is probably higher today as women are no longer confined to bed after childbirth.

Cardiovascular system

In pregnancy the plasma volume has increased by about 50 per cent and the red cell mass by 20–25 per cent. Some blood loss is a normal part of childbirth but does not account for loss of the excess accumulated during pregnancy. The exact mechanism of how a woman's body manages to deal with the increased blood volume of pregnancy is not clearly understood; within 24–48 hours the red cell mass returns to normal levels and by the end of the first week the blood volume is at the pre-pregnant state.[5] Haemoglobin levels reach their lowest point on the fourth postpartum day and then rise progressively to reach normal non-pregnant levels between four and six weeks post partum.[5]

Sexuality

Studies on sexuality following childbirth have found that around 40 per cent of postpartum women report a decreased interest in sex, yet some women report an increase in sexual desire and satisfaction. A UK study found that 90 per cent of women reported having sex by 10 weeks postpartum, but 2 per cent of women had still not attempted intercourse one year after giving birth.[9] Women who have an instrumental delivery, experience perineal trauma, and report depression or tiredness are more likely to experience problems with sex.[9,10] Women who breastfeed are more likely to report loss of interest in sex, although this did not persist long term.[11] Only 15 per cent of women who had a postnatal sexual health problem reported discussing it with a health professional.[12]

Return of fertility

After childbirth and delivery of the placenta the levels of circulating sex steroids drop rapidly. Initially there is a period of pituitary gonadotroph recovery related to the suppressive effect of the high steroid levels in pregnancy. In a woman who is breastfeeding, the sucking stimulus reduces the pulsatile GnRH/LH secretion which drives the follicular growth, although the mechanism is not clear. As the suckling stimulus falls, an organised pulsatile LH secretion resumes, with some steroid secretion and follicle development. When suckling is further reduced, positive feedback of oestradiol triggers the pre-ovulatory surge and ovulation occurs.[13] It is suggested that to suppress ovulation, suckling should occur at least five times a day for more than 10 minutes per feed.[14] In breastfeeding women the mean duration of amenorrhoea is 8.5 months.[15] In women who are not breastfeeding the mean time to resumption of menstruation is variable. However, research suggests that ovulation could occur as early as the 28th day.

Psychological changes

Changes in mood (see Section 3) are universally accepted as a normal part of the puerperium. Elation is experienced by many women following childbirth. A feeling of elation, often on day 2–3, can be replaced by lowered mood and teariness on day 5–6. Anxiety and irritability are common in early puerperium. Post partum women experience less sleep and a dramatic change in role, both of which contribute to the mood changes they experience.

Transition to motherhood

The transition to motherhood is a major milestone in a woman's life and if she has an uncomplicated birth, is adequately supported (emotionally, financially, practically) and has a healthy baby she will make this transition with ease. For many women, however, these requirements are not met, and they experience difficulty in making this transition. Current research points to the importance of ensuring that a woman has an active say in her pregnancy and intrapartum care to ensure psychological well-being post partum. In addition, a woman requires adequate social support, someone to talk to and someone to share the work of caring for her baby. These three simple things are often the most neglected in postnatal care. Her relationship with her partner (if present) is also of major importance. The birth of a baby introduces new dimensions to their relationship and they will need to readjust many aspects (from work habits to sexual habits).[16]

Health and ill health after childbirth

In developed countries maternal mortality is low (around 1 in 30 000 pregnancies) yet maternal morbidity is under-recognised and poorly managed. It takes longer for a woman to return to full functional status compared to physiological recovery after childbirth.[17] Tables 8.13 and 8.14 list the common problems, their frequency and guidelines for management.[18] Despite these problems being common, many women are extremely reluctant to mention their problem to a health professional, even though they would like advice and assistance in dealing with them.[10] On average, a mother and her baby will visit a GP eight times in the six months after birth, providing many opportunities for these problems to be addressed.[19]

Before the woman and her baby leave for home it is important to undertake a thorough interview for problems and concerns. In addition to covering information relevant to the baby it is essential to listen carefully to the woman, demonstrate active listening skills, and allow this to guide the interview. Listening is therapeutic in itself and most diagnoses are made on the history alone.[20] It is important that sufficient time is allowed for this major event in the life of a family. The emotional, social, physical (ESP) model can be used as a guide:[20]

- *Emotional*—Ask how the woman is feeling since the birth of her baby and how she is finding the role of 'mother'. Let her know that is important to talk about how she is feeling and that some women may experience depression after giving birth. Encourage her to talk to a health professional she trusts if she begins to feel depressed or unable to cope.
- *Social*—Who is going home with her today? Who will be there to share in the work of caring for the baby? What else will she be expected to do once at home? Is she returning to work?
  Ask her whether she has or anticipates any problems with her relationship. What interests does she have apart from caring for the baby? And how will she arrange to have time for herself?
- *Physical*
  - Pain—perineal, wound, breasts, nipple, back.
  - Haemorrhoids—ensure adequately treated if present.

TABLE 8.13 Common problems experienced by mothers in the first six months after birth

Problem	Prevalence of problem in the six months after birth	Associated factors	Management
Exhaustion	69% at six months[10]	Not related to parity or method of delivery Tiredness is common, even among women who are not depressed Sleep pattern of baby	Offer time to talk Encourage time out Encourage sharing of work Encourage acceptance of invitations to help Discuss other potentially linked problems: haemorrhoids, back pain, perineal pain, problems with sex, relationship problems, breastfeeding problems, baby sleep pattern, uncommon problems (anaemia, thyroid)
Backache	44%	Higher birth weight Epidural anaesthesia	Avoid bed rest, resume normal activities NSAIDs (eg ibuprofen) for short-term use Provide emotional support Suggest practical help Encourage socialisation Back care advice (carrying, lifting) Exercise programs using cognitive behavioural principles led by experienced physiotherapist have been effective
Sexual problems	26%	Instrumental delivery Perineal trauma/pain Depression/exhaustion Breastfeeding	Avoid unnecessary instrumental deliveries If appropriately skilled use vacuum extraction rather than forceps Encourage time out from mothering Encourage practical and social support Offer time to talk—acknowledge the problem, reassure her that problems are common and discuss changes in relationship Establish referral networks for ongoing problems

- Check on infant feeding.
- Sex—allow her to ask questions about her concerns, mention the use of lubricant if she experiences vaginal dryness, address her contraceptive needs.
- Incontinence—mention urinary and faecal incontinence, encourage regular pelvic floor exercises, encourage her to seek help if she experiences problems once at home.

TABLE 8.14 Common problems experienced by mothers 6–9 months after birth

Problem	Prevalence of problem in the 6–9 months after birth	Associated factors	Management
Perineal pain	21%	Instrumental delivery Long second stage of labour Higher birth weight Perineal trauma	As for sexual problems Restricted use of episiotomy Perineal repair with continuous sub-cuticular Dexon or Vicryl throughout all layers results in less short-term pain than other methods NSAIDs provide effective analgesia Pelvic floor exercises may reduce pain Insufficient evidence to recommend therapeutic ultrasound
Depression	17%	Perceived lack of social, emotional and practical support Negative life events Past history Infant factors—unsettled baby Exhaustion Physical health problems	Support and encourage women to speak about their own emotional well-being Suggest sharing the work of caring for children and taking time out for oneself Active listening and non-directive counselling, cognitive behaviour therapy and anti-depressants are effective. Choice of treatment should be offered to women
Mastitis	17%	Oversupply of milk Exhaustion/tiredness Poorly fitting breast support Rough handling of the breast	Improve breast drainage Anti-inflammatory (ibuprofen) or analgesic If very unwell or symptoms > 24 hours: antibiotics—dicloxacillin or cephalexin 500 mg qid
Haemorrhoids	21%	Instrumental delivery Long second stage of labour Higher birth weight History of constipation	There are no trials of treatment in postnatal women Avoid constipation—dietary advice Topical creams—some contain steroids Rubber band ligation is most effective treatment for grade 1–3 haemorrhoids but can be very painful and infrared coagulation may be the preferred treatment[21]
Faecal incontinence[22]	6%	Forceps/vacuum extraction Nerve injury/structural damage Ageing	Inconclusive evidence regarding management Pelvic floor exercises, electrical stimulation with or without biofeedback may be useful—further research is required

- Colds and coughs—let her know that she will need to take care of herself and that in order to avoid getting 'run down' she should have some time away from her baby and as much rest as she can manage.
- Anaemia and other medical problems—check her notes. Is there something that should be followed up: low haemoglobin, hypertension, gestational diabetes, cervical abnormality?
- Lack of energy—take time to encourage her to ensure adequate nutrition, rest and activity.

This is a useful approach that can be used at subsequent visits.

The postnatal check-up

Traditionally women are encouraged to attend for a postnatal check-up at around six weeks postpartum. There is no evidence that a postnatal check-up improves health outcomes for women, yet it is generally accepted that a postnatal check-up provides the opportunity to ensure that women have no ongoing problems. The IMPACT trial in the UK showed that midwife-led postnatal care that was woman-centred did result in improved health outcomes for women.[23]

The length of hospital stay after childbirth can vary from 1–2 days up to five days or more. This has resulted from both the attempt to increase consumer satisfaction and provide choice, and the pressure on service providers to reduce costs.[24] There was some concern about the possible adverse effects of an early discharge on mother and baby, but these have not been borne out and an early postnatal visit after discharge from hospital did not seem to add any benefit.[25–27] Even though women report increased morbidity postpartum, the postnatal visit in general does not always meet women's needs.[28]

Postnatal effects of operative delivery

Operative delivery is a cornerstone of modern obstetrics and is responsible for saving many lives and preventing morbidity for the woman and her baby. Nevertheless, operative delivery may have the potential for negative health outcomes for women and babies. Women reported more exhaustion, lack of sleep, and bowel problems after a caesarean section and more perineal pain and sexual problems after an operative vaginal delivery.[29]

The decision to undertake operative delivery should always be discussed clearly with the woman and her partner. This should include the reasons that delivery is advised by an operative method, an assessment of the benefits and potential harms that can be incurred from both delivering and waiting, and reassurance for the woman that the situation is not related to her performance. Good communication can avoid misconceptions and ensure that birthing by whatever route is a positive experience.

Being there

One of the most important and rewarding parts of caring for women in the weeks and months after giving birth is the beneficial effect of 'being there' for the woman and her family. Never underestimate the importance of listening to concerns and acknowledging difficulties. It will not always be possible to solve the problems and issues that confront women at this time, and when this occurs remember that 'being there' is beneficial.

Giving birth is a major event in the life of a woman and her family. While this is a normal event, a woman faces many challenges—emotional, physical and social. Women and those who care for them need to work towards achieving evidence-based postnatal care. This will not be easy, as firmly held beliefs may impede the progress of putting evidence into practice.

Lactation and feeding

Breastfeeding rates are relatively high in Australia in comparison to other developed countries such as the UK or in comparison to the low rates of the 1970s. Today, most new mothers initiate breastfeeding: about 80 per cent of women are breastfeeding on discharge from hospital, 60 per cent at 3 months, 45 per cent at 6 months and 20 per cent at 1 year.[30] In the UK in 2000, 69 per cent of women initiated breastfeeding, 42 per cent were continuing at 6 weeks and 21 per cent at 6 months.[31]

Breastfeeding and health

Breastfeeding provides infants with optimal nutrition and milk specific for human babies. Infants who are not breastfed may be more likely to experience gastrointestinal and respiratory infections, asthma, otitis media, urinary tract infections, necrotising enterocolitis, insulin-dependent diabetes, inflammatory bowel disease, lymphoma and atopy.

Women who breastfeed have the benefits of:

- less postpartum bleeding
- delayed resumption of ovulation
- improved bone remineralisation post partum
- less ovarian and premenopausal breast cancer.[32]

Intended duration of breastfeeding is probably the strongest predictor of actual breastfeeding duration. Younger, less-educated women in Australia are currently less likely to maintain breastfeeding.[33] Fathers play an important role in the breastfeeding decision and have a strong influence on duration of breastfeeding. Researchers have found that low levels of community support for breastfeeding in a low socio-economic community may also be influential.[34]

Onset of lactation

After delivery of the placenta, the rapid drop in maternal levels of progesterone triggers lactogenesis. Early skin-to-skin contact after birth facilitates successful breastfeeding and the first feed should be initiated as soon as mother and baby show they are ready.[35]

As the mother starts to feed her infant, nipple stimulation leads to a release of oxytocin from the posterior pituitary gland. Oxytocin travels in the bloodstream to the breasts and leads to contraction of the myoepithelial cells around the milk-producing alveoli and dilatation of the milk ducts. This is known as the 'let-down' or milk ejection reflex, and mothers may notice a leaking of milk from the other breast, a tingling feeling in the breasts or a sudden thirst. In the early postpartum period, she will also notice a contraction of the uterus, which may be painful for a few minutes.

The first milk, known as colostrum, is thick and contains high levels of protein, immunoglobulins and carotenoids (which give it the yellow colour). Small amounts of colostrum are produced (2–20 ml per feed), but after about four days the breasts will be producing about 600 ml of milk per day.[36]

Although prolactin is necessary for milk secretion, the volume of milk is regulated by local mechanisms within the breast. After approximately five days, control of lactation changes from hormonal to local, or autocrine, control. The removal of a protein in the milk (the feedback inhibitor of lactation, FIL) stimulates the breasts to continue to produce milk.[36]

Maintenance of lactation

Feeding patterns should be flexible; frequent feeds of unrestricted length will ensure adequate milk removal and prevent engorgement (Box 8.3).[35] Young babies usually feed regularly day and night: often 10–12 times in 24 hours. If the baby is unable to feed, the mother should express her milk every three hours or so in order to maintain her milk supply.

After the rapid increase in milk production in the first week, milk volume slowly increases to about 750 ml/day during the third to fifth months and to about 800 ml/day at six months.[37]

BOX 8.3 Promoting successful breastfeeding

- To promote successful breastfeeding:
  - Offer the breast early
  - Ensure the baby is well attached to the breast
  - Feed freely.

Correct attachment to the breast

The basis of pain-free breastfeeding is making sure the baby is well attached at the breast. First, the mother should be comfortable, either sitting upright with her feet supported or lying on her side. The baby's body should be facing the mother and held close. She lines up the baby so that the baby's nose is opposite the nipple. She waits for the baby to open the mouth wide, and then quickly brings the baby to the breast so that the lower gum is 3–4 cm below the nipple . This ensures that the baby takes a large amount of breast into the mouth. Inside the baby's mouth, the tip of the nipple should be at the junction of the hard and soft palates. A wave of compression by the baby's tongue moves along the underside of the nipple in a posterior direction, directing milk into the baby's throat (Figure 8.8).

FIGURE 8.8 Make sure the baby is well attached at the breast

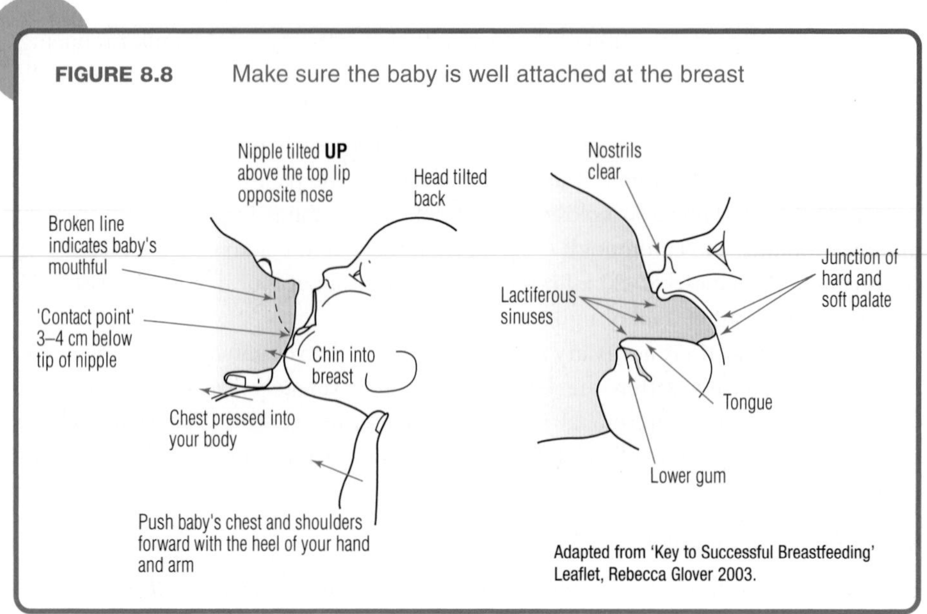

Adapted from 'Key to Successful Breastfeeding' Leaflet, Rebecca Glover 2003.

Expression of milk

New mothers should be taught hand expression so that they can remove milk if their breasts become overfull. After washing her hands, the mother usually massages the breasts gently from the periphery to the areolae. Then she positions her thumb on top of the breast and one finger below, about 3–4 cm from the nipple base. First she presses in towards the chest wall and then compresses the thumb and finger together, in a 'milking' action towards the nipple.[36] She continues in a rhythmic motion, and gradually rotates her hand around the breast to drain all quadrants.

An electric breast pump may be used if the mother needs to express frequently, for example for a premature infant or if she returns to paid work. Women who express less frequently may choose to use a hand pump.

Protecting, promoting and supporting breastfeeding

The WHO and UNICEF jointly launched the Baby Friendly Hospital Initiative in 1991 to improve maternity services support for breastfeeding initiation. Hospitals that fulfil the Ten Steps to Successful Breastfeeding (Box 8.4) may be designated as Baby Friendly. Thousands of maternity services around the world have achieved these global criteria.

The WHO Code for marketing breast milk substitutes includes:[38]

- No advertising of these products to the public
- No free samples to mothers
- No promotion of products in health care facilities
- No gifts of personal samples to health workers
- No words or pictures idealising artificial feeding, including pictures of infants, on the products.

BOX 8.4 The Ten Steps to Successful Breastfeeding[38]

Every facility providing maternity services and care for newborn infants should:

Step 1 Have a written breastfeeding policy that is routinely communicated to all health care staff.

Step 2 Train all health care staff in the skills necessary to implement this policy.

Step 3 Inform all women (face to face and leaflets) about the benefits and management of breastfeeding.

Step 4 Help mothers initiate breastfeeding within half an hour of delivery.

Step 5 Show mothers how to breastfeed and maintain lactation (by expressing milk) even if they should be separated from their infants.

Step 6 Give newborn infants no food or drink unless 'medically' indicated. No promotion of formula milks.

Step 7 Practise 'rooming-in'. All mothers should have their infant cots next to them 24 hours a day.

Step 8 Encourage breastfeeding on demand.

Step 9 Give no artificial teats or pacifiers to breastfeeding infants.

Step 10 Foster the establishment of breastfeeding support groups and refer mothers to them.

2 Neonate to adolescent

A Strawberry naevus

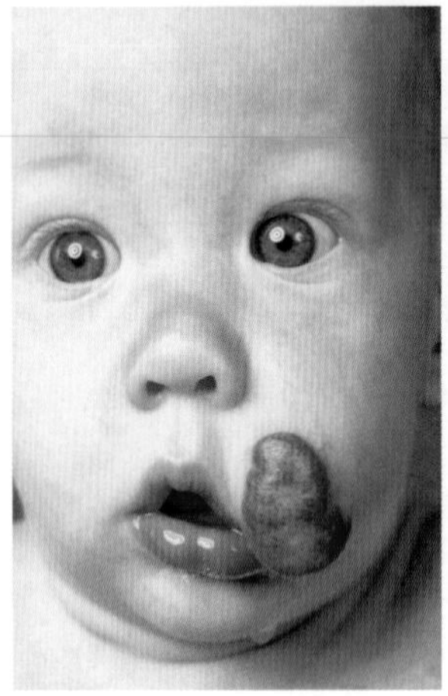

B Port wine stain

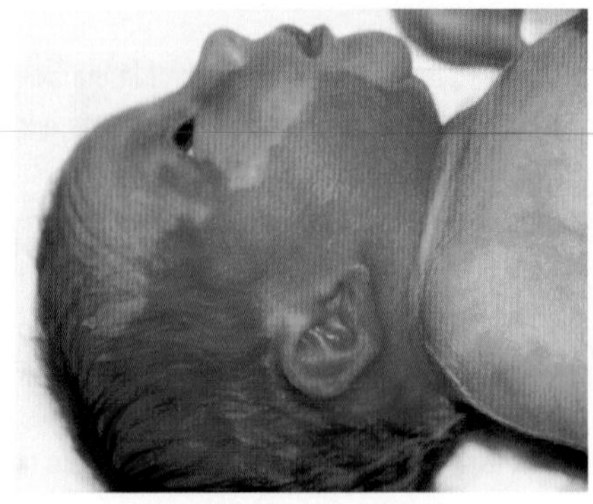

C Mongolian spot

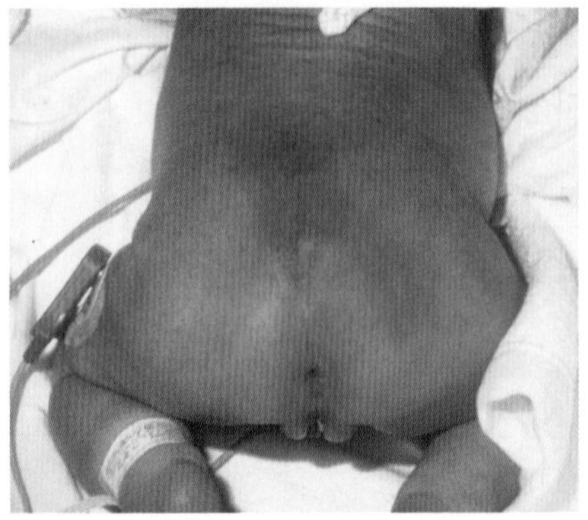

D Talipes equines varus

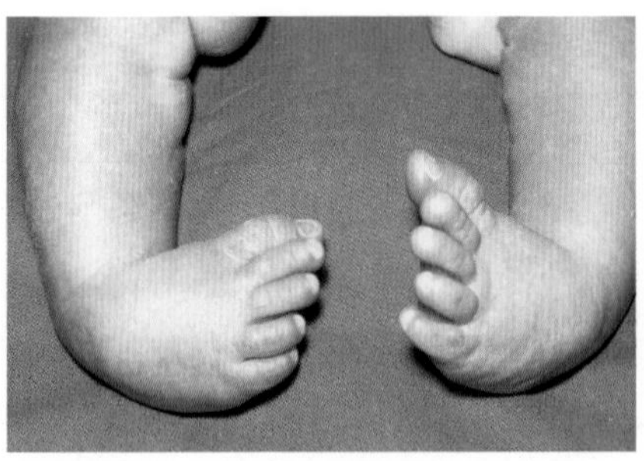

E Meningiomyelocele

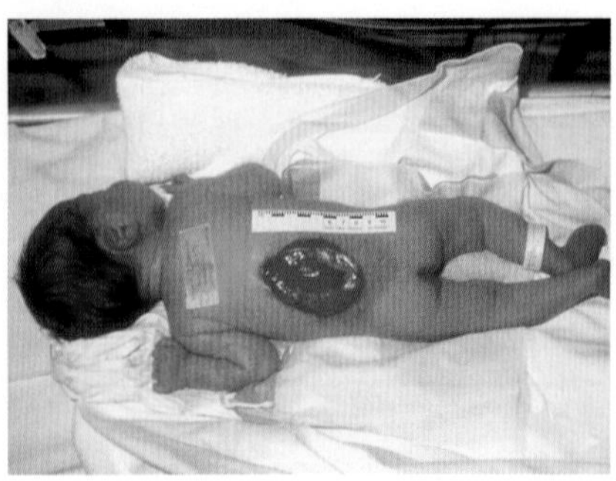

F Cystic hygroma

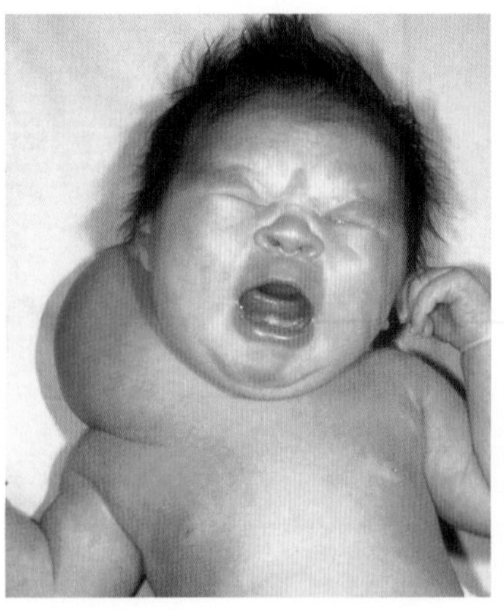

A Congenital teeth

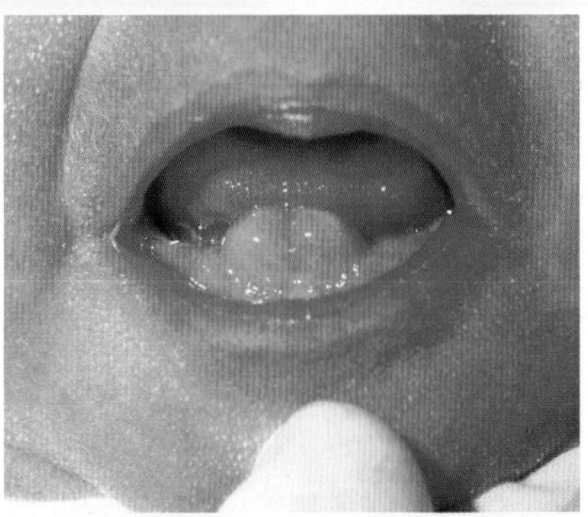

B Extra digit

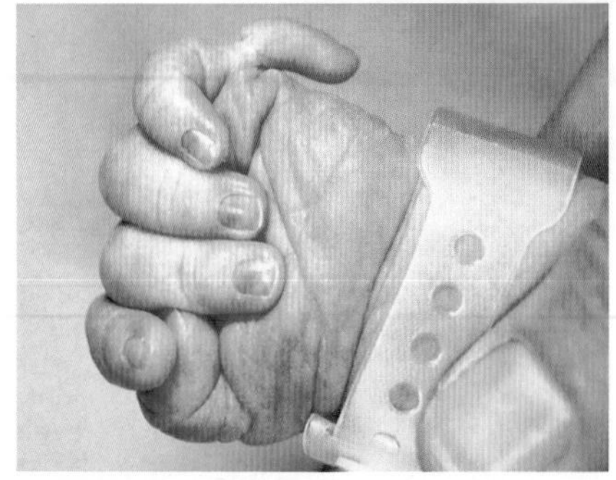

C Bilateral cleft lip and palate

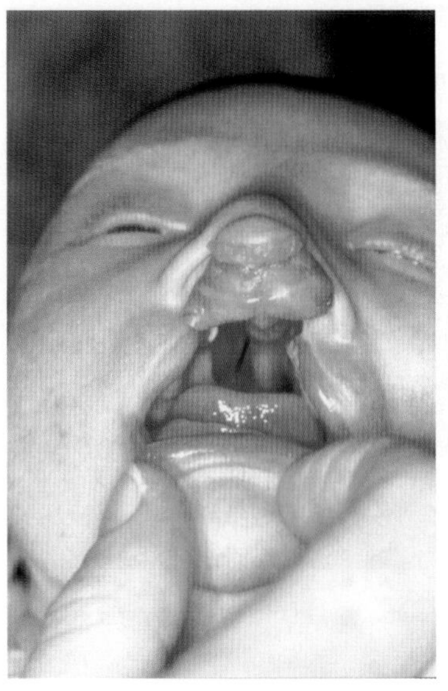

D Sacral teratoma

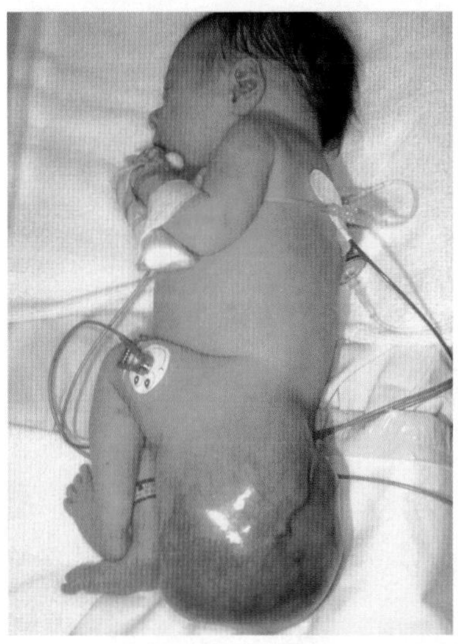

E Exomphalus

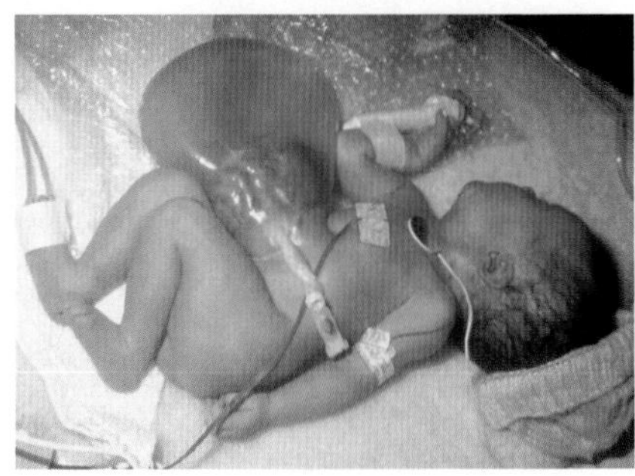

F Macrosomic baby of diabetic mother on left

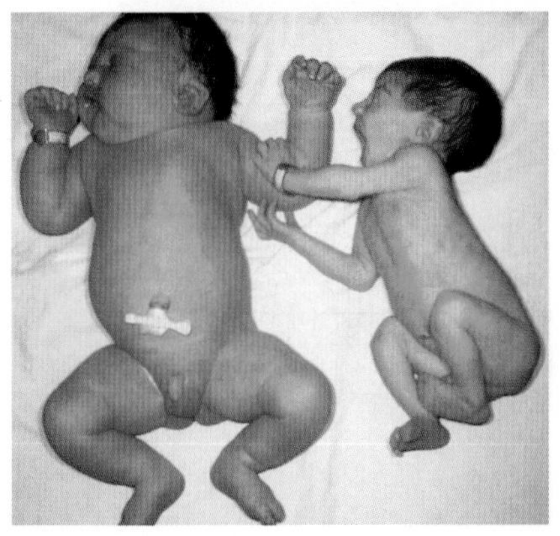

A Congenital absence of vagina

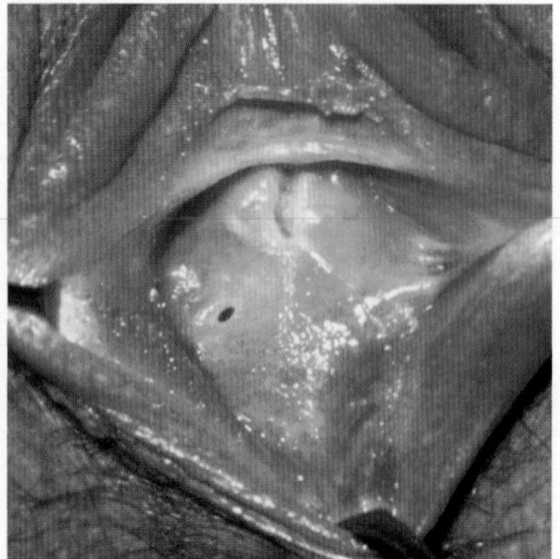

B Paraurethral cyst

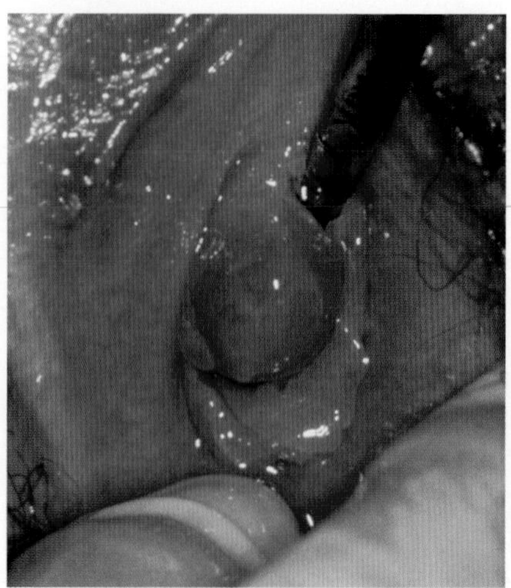

C Turner syndrome

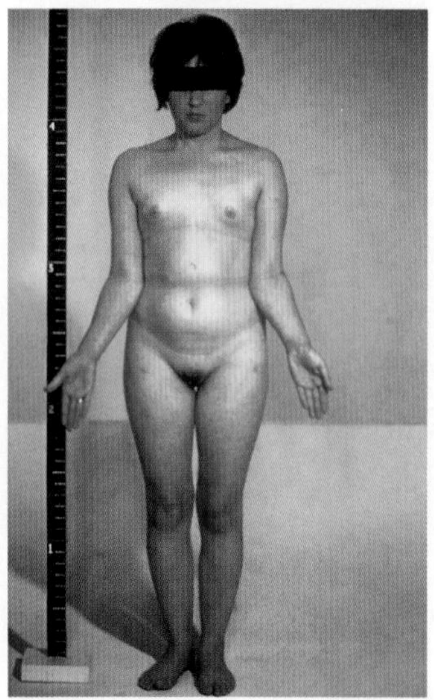

D Streak ovary

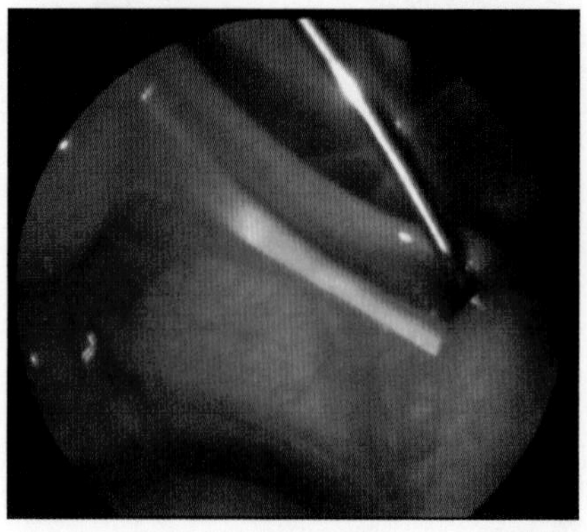

E Imperforate hymen

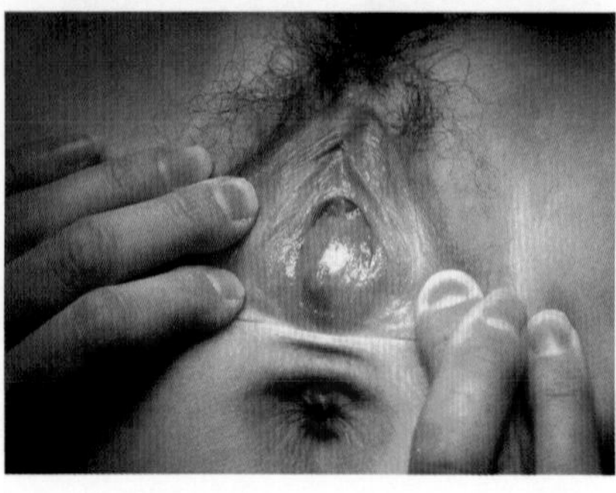

F Clitoromegaly in the masculinised 46XX female baby

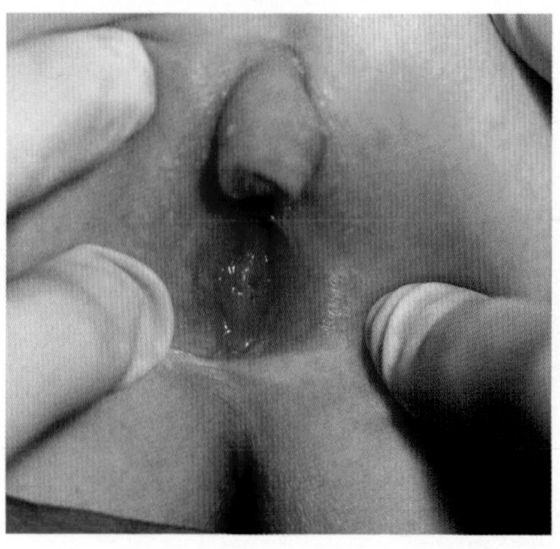

SECTION

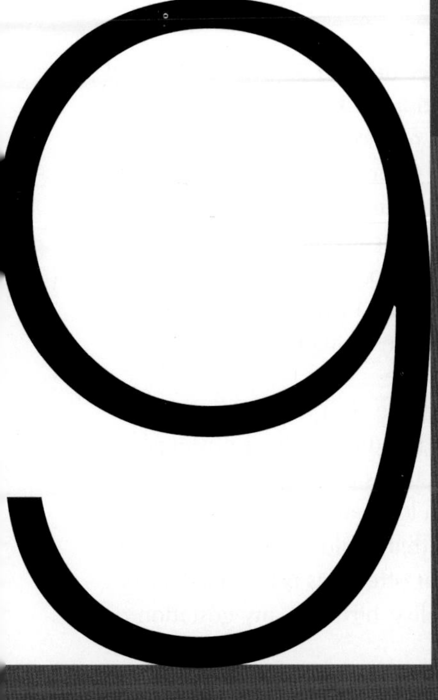

Pregnancy problems

Maternal and perinatal mortality and morbidity

Maternal mortality

Maternal mortality is uncommon in developed countries but still occurs and some of these may be avoidable. The International Classification of Diseases, Injuries and Causes of Death defines a maternal death as 'the death of a woman while pregnant or within 42 days of delivery, miscarriage or termination of pregnancy, from any cause related to or aggravated by the pregnancy or its management, but not from incidental or accidental causes'.[1] A new category of Late Maternal Death has the same criteria but extends to one year. The deaths are further divided into groups including:

- *Direct:* an obstetric complication of the pregnant state from interventions, omissions, incorrect treatment or a chain of events resulting from any of the above.
- *Indirect:* resulting from a previously existing disease or a disease that has developed during the pregnancy and which was not due to direct obstetric causes, but was aggravated by the physiological effects of pregnancy.

A triennial report issued in the UK and in Australia looks at these deaths and any factors that could have contributed to them or actions that could have avoided them. The maternal mortality denominator used may vary but often this is the deaths from obstetric causes per 100 000 maternities (number of live births at any gestation or stillbirths of 24 weeks or later).

The most recent report in the UK (1997–99) included the following findings:

- Twenty per cent of women who died had booked for care after 24 weeks or had missed more than four antenatal visits.
- Other factors associated with an increased risk of death included: woman aged less than 18 years, obesity, increasing maternal age and parity.
- Diagnoses being missed included ectopic pregnancy, sepsis and pulmonary embolism.

Lack of communication and teamwork, missed diagnoses, and lack of clear unit policy or guidelines were identified as factors involved in substandard care.

The main causes of maternal death were:

- thromboembolism
- cardiac disease (cardiomyopathy, dissecting aneurysm of the thoracic aorta and myocardial infarction)
- suicide
- sepsis (this has increased since the previous report)
- ectopic pregnancy
- hypertension
- amniotic fluid embolism
- haemorrhage.

In Australia, the *Report on Maternal Deaths in Australia 1994–96* included the following key findings:[2]

- The 1994–96 Australian maternal mortality ratio was 13.0 per 100 000 confinements, compared with the 1991–93 ratio of 10.9 per 100 000 confinements.

- The increase in deaths occurred almost exclusively in the direct deaths category and indicated factors which were considered to be possibly or certainly avoidable.
- The principal causes of direct maternal deaths remained pulmonary embolism (8 deaths [17%]), amniotic fluid embolism (8 deaths [17%]) and pre-eclampsia (6 deaths [13%]).
- Cardiorespiratory disease was the most common cause of indirect maternal death.
- The Indigenous maternal mortality ratio (34.8 deaths per 100 000 confinements) remains about three times that of the non-Indigenous maternal mortality ratio (10.1 deaths per 100 000 confinements).

Many problems are rarely seen by an individual health professional, but can be highlighted by appropriate collection of data.

Perinatal mortality and morbidity

The main causes of perinatal loss include: fetal abnormality, preterm birth, unexplained intrauterine death, infection and maternal disease. Preterm delivery is a major cause of neonatal mortality and long-term neurological and neonatal morbidity. It accounts for 60 per cent of perinatal mortalities in developed countries and 50 per cent of childhood neurological disabilities, although this varies within populations. Improved neonatal care has reduced the incidence and severity of handicap and improved survival. Intrauterine growth restriction (IUGR) is a major cause of antepartum stillbirths. Most IUGR fetuses are not identified and are of uncertain aetiology.

Figure 9.1 outlines definitions used for events during pregnancy.

FIGURE 9.1 Definitions used to describe pregnancy events, fetal and neonatal loss

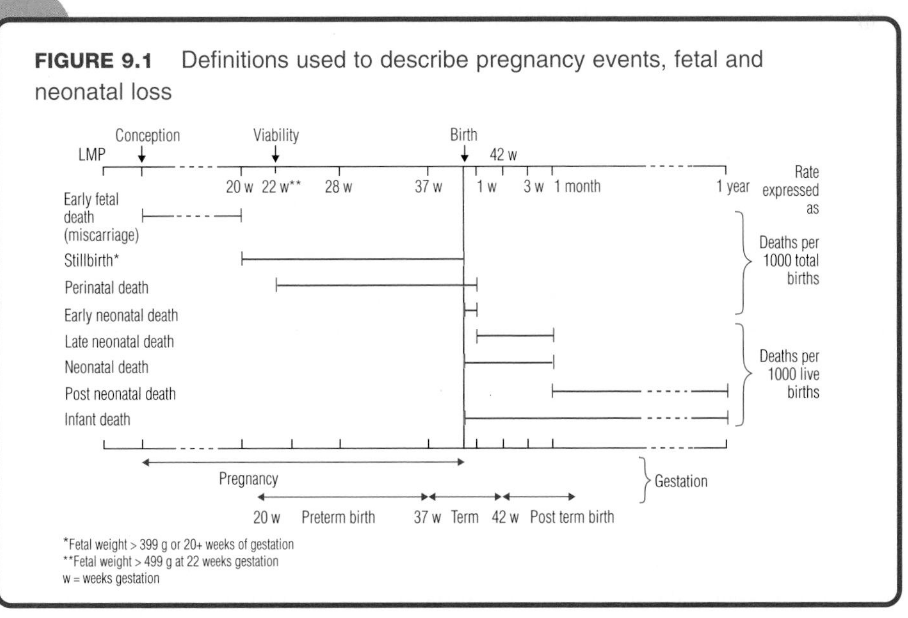

*Fetal weight > 399 g or 20+ weeks of gestation
**Fetal weight > 499 g at 22 weeks gestation
w = weeks gestation

Common presentations in early pregnancy

Infections in pregnancy

Throughout normal pregnancy the fetus is in a sterile environment. This is maintained by the properties of the placenta, cervix, membranes and amniotic fluid to prevent the spread of infections.

- The cervix provides both a mechanical barrier to ascending infection and a chemical barrier due to the antimicrobial action of cervical mucus.
- Amniotic fluid also has both bacteriostatic and bacteriocidal activity due to the presence of immunocompetent cells, immunoglobulins, and factors such as transferrin and zinc.
- The placenta selectively transfers maternal IgG across the placenta to provide passive immunity to the fetus.

The fetus is at risk of becoming infected by transplacental haematogenous transmission of pathogens and ascending infection of pathogens from the lower genital tract either during pregnancy or at the time of delivery. Pathogens can also be transmitted to the neonate in breast milk (Table 9.1). Good antenatal care identifies women who are at high risk of infection on the basis of history, examination or general screening. In some cases there are effective strategies that reduce the risk to the fetus significantly. Infection is recognised as an important cause of preterm delivery.

TABLE 9.1 Transmission of infections during pregnancy, labour and delivery

Transmission: intrauterine	Perinatal (labour/delivery)		Postnatal
Haematogenous	**Haematogenous**	**Genital**	**Breastfeeding**
Rubella	GBS	GBS	Rubella
Treponema pallidum	Herpes	Herpes	
Cytomegalovirus	Cytomegalovirus	Cytomegalovirus	Cytomegalovirus
Toxoplasma gondii	Hepatitis B & C	Chlamydia	Hepatitis B
Parvovirus	HIV	*N. gonorrhoeae*	HIV
Varicella	Varicella		
	Listeria	Listeria	

GBS: Group B streptococci. HIV: human immunodeficiency virus.

CLINICAL PRESENTATION

The most frequent presentations are either from a laboratory test result, specific symptoms, or reported contact with an infection. Outcomes and possible presentations in pregnancy include:

1 Laboratory findings of an existing infection

Routine prepregnancy and pregnancy screening or contact with another infected person may elicit a positive test that should be investigated further and the appropriate action taken. In general, serological testing should be repeated three weeks after exposure to check for seroconversion (from negative to positive). Confirmatory laboratory results include IgG immunoglobulin (IgG) seroconversion, with a significant increase in IgG level; IgM detection, or detection of the pathogen. In other cases the diagnosis might be based on the clinical picture if it is too late for other tests.

2 Mild symptoms with positive laboratory test

A woman may report non-specific symptoms that might indicate an infection with consequences for the pregnancy. These symptoms may include: fever, skin rash, malaise, lymphadenopathy or reduced fetal movement. Infections to be considered are rubella (German measles), parvovirus infection, varicella (chicken pox), primary toxoplasmosis and primary CMV.

3 Serious illness in the mother leading to miscarriage, premature labour, and risks to the fetus

Examples of maternal infections and their consequences for the fetus are listed in Table 9.2.

Specific infections

(See also Sections 6 and 12.)

Cytomegalovirus

Cytomegalovirus (CMV) is the most common congenital and perinatal infection worldwide. Approximately 1 per cent of newborns are infected in utero and around 10 per cent of these will have signs and symptoms at birth and develop sequelae including deafness and mental retardation.

A primary maternal infection in the first half of pregnancy is more likely to be associated with clinically apparent CMV infection during the neonatal period. If primary maternal infection occurs in pregnancy the risk of transplacental infection is 50 per cent. There is a 94 per cent certainty of in utero CMV infection with positive isolation of the virus and positive PCR values in the amniotic fluid, but this cannot predict fetal outcome.[3,4] The overall risk of delivering an infant with serious handicap after a primary infection is estimated at between 10 and 20 per cent.[5] Primary CMV infection is more common among younger (15–23 years) primigravida than other pregnant women and the majority of these are asymptomatic.

Close proximity to young children, a child care environment and sexual activity are associated with acquisition of CMV. An IgM test can be used to detect infection in a woman whose previous pre-pregnant status is unknown. If the IgM is positive, further tests are required to determine whether or not this is due to a primary infection. Congenital disease can also occur with recurrent infection in about 0.2 to 1 per cent of immune women but is less severe, and less than 10 per cent of affected infants have long-term sequelae.[6] There is no current effective treatment for CMV infection although clinical trials of treatment in late pregnancy are in progress.[7]

TABLE 9.2 Examples of the consequences of maternal infection for the fetus

Infection	Maternal facts	Fetal infection	Neonatal effects	Sequelae
CMV	At risk: young, contact with children, sexual activity. Viral illness, lymphocytosis, mild hepatitis	50% risk of transplacental infection from primary infection	1% infected 10% of these have sequelae	Deafness, Mental retardation Overall risk of serious problem after primary infection is 10–20%
Toxoplasmosis	Contact with soil, cat litter, under-cooked meat. Mostly asymptomatic or viral illness with arthralgia and lymphadenopathy		1 to 10 in 10 000 with congenital toxoplasmosis	Chorioretinitis, intracranial calcification and hydrocephalus
Group B streptococcus	Asymptomatic carriage in 10%	10% colonised	1% risk of meningitis	Death, neurological damage
Varicella	70% of women immune Rash, viral illness	Highest risk of fetal infection if maternal infection between 13 and 20 weeks		Central nervous system, eye and limb malformations
Parvovirus	33% of women asymptomatic or maculopapular rash, viral illness	1 in 10 fetal loss if infection before 20 weeks. Stillbirth in third trimester		Sometimes: anaemia and hydrops fetalis
HSV	Sexually acquired	Fetal infection more common if primary attack at the time of delivery		Encephalitis
Rubella	Maculopapular rash, mild viral illness	In first 3 months of pregnancy		Deafness, cataracts, heart defects, mental retardation

Rubella

Rubella is a human-specific ribonucleic acid virus that may cause serious birth defects. Rubella infection is spread by aerosol or direct contact with nasal or salivary secretions of infected people. People are infectious up to seven days before and four days after the appearance of the rash. Infection within the first three months of pregnancy is especially likely to result in congenital infection.

Toxoplasmosis

Congenital toxoplasmosis affects 1 to 10 in 10 000 newborn babies. Toxoplasmosis is a parasitic disease caused by a protozoan, *Toxoplasma gondii*. Infection is confirmed by serological testing. Diagnosis in the pregnant woman is made by detecting IgM antibody to toxoplasmosis and significant changes in IgG antibody titre. The IgM can remain positive for several months. False-positive tests occur frequently and the diagnosis should be confirmed with a reference laboratory.[8] Fetal infection can be confirmed by detecting toxoplasma DNA in the amniotic fluid by PCR and cordocentesis for the detection of IgM-specific antibody in the blood; ultrasound may be useful.[9] It is unclear whether or not antenatal treatment for women with presumed toxoplasmosis reduces congenital transmission of disease.[10] Treatment is with a combination of pyrimethamin, sulfadiazin, folinic acid and spiramycin.

Hepatitis B

Maternal hepatitis B (HBV) may be asymptomatic (chronic disease) or present acutely in pregnancy. Both passive and active forms of immunisation against HBV are safe in pregnancy. A non-immune woman at high risk or a woman exposed to HBV should be offered vaccination.

Chronic HBV infection is the more common presentation. In pregnancy, 85–95 per cent of cases of perinatal transmission of HBV are related to intrapartum exposure. It is standard practice to screen all pregnant women for HBV because the risk of infection to the baby can be effectively prevented with appropriate treatment. The risk of vertical infection to the baby is related to the maternal hepatitis B viral load. Initial screening involves checking for the presence of hepatitis B surface antigen (HBsAg). If positive, hepatitis Be antigen (HBeAg) then helps ascertain risk. The risk is 10 per cent in HbeAg-negative mothers compared with 90 per cent with HbeAg-positive mothers. The risk of chronic HBV infection in a neonate who does not receive immunoprophylaxis and vaccination for HBV is 40 per cent. Babies born to mothers who are HbsAg-positive should receive, at different sites, hepatitis B immune globulin (0.5 ml) and their first dose of hepatitis B vaccine (0.5 ml) at birth. The vaccine is repeated at one month and six months of age. Breastfeeding is not contraindicated. Such a policy reduces the risk of vertical transmission to close to zero.

The acute presentation is similar to that of the non-pregnant individual (malaise, anorexia, nausea, right upper quadrant abdominal pain with signs of jaundice, hepatosplenomegaly and dark urine). The differential diagnosis would include pre-eclampsia and acute fatty liver of pregnancy. The diagnosis of acute viral hepatitis B is confirmed with the presence of HBsAg and anti-HBc IgM antibody in the serum. The risk of perinatal transmission depends on the stage of gestation at the time of infection: first trimester infection is associated with a 10 per cent risk and third trimester with an 85–90 per cent risk.

Hepatitis C

Most hepatitis C (HCV) infections are associated with minimal symptoms and only rarely with identifiable jaundice. At present it is usual that only high-risk women (history of IV drug use, blood transfusion, abnormal liver function tests and high-risk sexual behaviour) are screened for hepatitis C by checking for the presence of HCV antibodies. Those women who are positive should have regular liver function tests and be counselled about the long-term sequelae. In time, 90 per cent of infected individuals develop chronic hepatitis and approximately 20 per cent will develop cirrhosis of the liver.

Babies born to mothers with detectable RNA in the bloodstream are at increased risk of vertical transmission of the virus. Confirmation of HCV infection in the baby requires waiting several months to ensure that the HCV antibody has not been passively acquired from the mother. The risk is about 4 per cent. No therapy has been proved effective in preventing vertical transmission. The long-term consequences for the baby are uncertain.

Varicella

Congenital varicella syndrome is characterised by serious central nervous system, eye and limb malformations. In the Western world, most women are immune to varicella and varicella during pregnancy is rare (0.7/1000);[11] most had chickenpox during childhood even if they do not remember having it. A study by Motherisk showed that 70 per cent of those with a 'negative history' were in fact immune.[12] Women from some countries have lower rates of immunity (eg in the West Indies it is 50 per cent).

Maternal varicella before 13 weeks gestation had an observed risk of 0.4 per cent for congenital varicella syndrome; the highest risk is between 13 and 20 weeks, with an observed risk of 2 per cent.[13] Women who are not immune and are in contact with chickenpox should receive varicella immunoglobulin up to 10 days after exposure. A pregnant woman presenting with chickenpox should be prescribed acyclovir if it is within 24 hours of the rash appearing. Acyclovir reduces the severity of the maternal symptoms. If maternal infection occurs at term, there is a significant risk of varicella of the newborn. The neonate should receive varicella immunoglobulin (VZIG) if delivery occurs within five days of maternal infection, or if the mother develops chickenpox within two days of giving birth.

Parvovirus

Parvovirus 19 is a common infection among preschoolers and schoolchildren. Infection is associated with a characteristic erythematous rash on the cheeks, termed 'slapped cheek' disease. Infection is associated with fever and generalised joint pains. In adults the rash is less commonly seen and up to 33 per cent of women are asymptomatic.[14] Infection is confirmed by the presence of Parvovirus 19 IgM. If infection occurs early in pregnancy, miscarriage can occur. Around 1 in 10 women infected before 20 weeks gestation will suffer a fetal loss.[15] If infection occurs in the third trimester it may cause stillbirth.[16] Sometimes parvovirus can suppress the bone marrow of the fetus, the baby becomes anaemic and can develop hydrops fetalis.

If infection in pregnancy is confirmed the baby should be monitored for signs of anaemia. The findings of ascites, pleural or pericardial effusion and skin oedema on ultrasound suggest severe fetal anaemia. If anaemia is suspected, fetal blood sampling is indicated and intrauterine transfusion can reduce the mortality rate. There is insufficient evidence to support routine screening in pregnancy.[17]

Listeriosis

Listeriosis is the disease caused by *Listeria monocytogenes*, which is a Gram-positive rod (Section 6). Symptoms of listeriosis are of a mild, flu-like illness. In the absence of an epidemic listeriosis is rare, affecting about 1/10 000 births. Infection is blood-borne across the placenta and leads to stillbirth, chorioamnionitis and early delivery. Listeria is difficult to culture in the laboratory. Suspected infection is treated with penicillin and gentamicin.

Herpes simplex virus

Herpes simplex virus type 2 (HSV-2) is responsible for genital herpes. Infection, characterised by painful vesicular lesions around the labia, may be primary or recurrent in pregnancy. The risk of acquisition of the virus in pregnancy varies between Western communities from approximately 0.34 to 3.7 per cent per year.[18] Congenital infection from a transplacental route appears rare. A primary infection in the first 20 weeks of pregnancy may cause a spontaneous abortion in half of women. Other effects from primary infection during pregnancy include preterm birth, growth retardation and neonatal infection. The risk of neonatal herpes in the UK is less than 2 per 100 000 live births. Primary infections in pregnancy are treated with acyclovir. There is no evidence of an association between HSV-2 infection during pregnancy and fetal death.[19] The acquisition of the infection with seroconversion completed before labour commences does not appear to affect the outcome of pregnancy.[20] Neonatal herpes occurs as a result of direct contact with maternal lesions at the time of delivery. Neonatal herpes has a high morbidity and mortality. The greatest risk occurs when the mother acquires a primary HSV infection towards the end of pregnancy. In these women a normal delivery carries a transmission risk of up to 40 per cent and a caesarean section is recommended if the woman is in labour or her membranes rupture.

Group B streptococcus

Approximately 10 per cent of women will be demonstrated to have asymptomatic group B streptococcus (GBS) in the genital tract in pregnancy. Group B streptococcus may be pathogenic, causing septicaemia and meningitis in the neonate. The mode of transmission is most frequently via direct contact between vaginal secretions and the mucosa of the infant's nose and mouth during birth. Babies born to mothers with GBS carry a 1 per cent risk of developing life-threatening sepsis. The administration of intrapartum antibiotics (most commonly penicillin) is effective in preventing neonatal infection. Different strategies are employed to prevent neonatal GBS infection. Universal screening of all pregnant women at 36 weeks has strong proponents. An alternative approach is to administer antibiotics in high-risk situations such as preterm labour or when urinary infection with GBS has been detected antenatally. Neonates can sometimes acquire GBS sepsis beyond seven days of age (late-onset disease)—this is not associated with maternal GBS colonisation.

Chlamydia

Chlamydia infection may present as dysuria or vaginal discharge, or be asymptomatic. Mother-to-fetus infection can occur at the time of birth by direct transmission. The infant may develop conjunctivitis or pneumonitis. The risks are thought to be up to 25 per cent and 15 per cent respectively. If a mother is positive for *Chlamydia* in pregnancy the risk to the neonate is reduced by a course of antibiotics. Erythromycin is considered the first drug of choice. Azithromycin or amoxicillin are indicated if erythromycin is not tolerated.

Bacterial vaginosis in pregnancy

This is a common cause of vaginal discharge and is characterised by an imbalance in the normal vaginal flora, with a decrease in *Lactobacillus* spp and an increase in *Gardnerella* spp, *Mycoplasma* spp and anaerobic bacteria. Epidemiological studies suggest an increased risk of miscarriage, preterm delivery and low birth weight infants among women with bacterial vaginosis. However, the mechanisms are not completely understood and intervention studies have not been shown to be effective in reducing preterm birth.[21] There is insufficient evidence to recommend routine screening in average-risk pregnant women.

Chorioamnionitis

Chorioamnionitis is the term used to describe inflammation of the chorion and amnion that is usually the result of ascending infection from the vagina. It is often associated with preterm premature rupture of the membranes and is responsible for approximately 50 per cent of spontaneous preterm births. Infection may involve the amniotic fluid, which is then swallowed by the fetus to cause fetal infection. Organisms may also ascend via the umbilical cord. Histologically, inflammation of the umbilical cord is termed funisitis. Common organisms responsible for chorioamnionitis are group B streptococcus, *Ureaplasma urealyticum* and *Escherichia coli*.

CLINICAL PRESENTATION: Recurrent early pregnancy loss

About 12–15 per cent of pregnancies end in spontaneous abortion; therefore, one in six women will have one miscarriage, and 1 in 36 women will experience two in a row. When a woman has had three miscarriages she is said to have 'recurrent pregnancy loss'. It is usual to investigate a couple who have had three recurrent abortions, but some couples request investigation after two miscarriages.

History

There is little specific in the history. The miscarriages can have presented as missed abortions or incomplete miscarriages. It is of some interest whether the fetus stopped growing during the first trimester or the abortion occurred during the second trimester, which is more likely to be caused by mechanical factors.

Examination

This is usually unrewarding.

Investigations

In over 50 per cent of women with recurrent pregnancy loss the cause remains uncertain even after investigation.

Serology

Blood group, Rhesus (Rh) and atypical antibodies is undertaken to determine the Rh-negative woman who requires anti-D immunoglobulin.

Special tests

See Table 9.3.

- *Cytogenetics*
  - *Parents:* karyotype on both partners indicate that 3–5 per cent of couples with recurrent abortion have a chromosomal abnormality. The most common abnormality is balanced Robertsonian translocation.[22]
  - *Aborted products:* this may be of more value. Women < 36 years with recurrent miscarriage have a higher frequency of euploid miscarriage.

TABLE 9.3 Summary of results of investigations in women after recurrent pregnancy loss

Investigations	Diagnosing	Incidence in RPL
Karyotyping both partners	Chromosome abnormality	3–5%
Pelvic ultrasound	Polycystic ovary syndrome	> 50%
Midfollicular raised LH	Raised LH	10%
Anticardiolipin (aCL), antiphospholipid antibodies (aPL), and lupus anticoagulant (LA)	Antiphospholipid syndrome	15%
Activated protein C resistance (APCR), antithrombin III, and Factor XII deficiency, Protein C, Protein S	Thrombophilia	20%
Vaginal swab	Bacterial vaginosis	20%

RPL: recurrent pregnancy loss; LH: luteinising hormone

Adapted from Rai & Regan[23]

- *Infection screening.* This is an unlikely cause of recurrent pregnancy loss. Bacterial vaginosis has been suggested as a possible cause of recurrent pregnancy loss, but further studies are needed.
- *Thrombophilia screening.* It has been suggested that increased tendency for blood clotting may result in placental vascular damage and early pregnancy loss, and may affect trophoblast function.
- *Immunological screening* (see Red cell iso-immunisation page 341). A proposed allo-immune factor has not been confirmed. Autoimmune factors (antiphospholipid and antithyroid antibodies) are described. Antiphospholipid syndrome is fetal wastage in the presence of significant anticardiolipin antibody levels: it associated with a 50 per cent rate of fetal loss, intrauterine growth retardation in 30 per cent and pre-eclampsia in 50 per cent of pregnancies.
- *Anatomical.* Hysteroscopy or ultrasound examination of the uterus can detect intrauterine pathology such as submucous fibroids, or anatomic anomalies such as intrauterine septa. It is sometimes difficult to determine whether these findings are 'causative' or 'co-incident'.

Treatment

In most cases of recurrent abortion, no abnormality is detected on investigations (idiopathic recurrent pregnancy loss). These women need no specific treatment, but are best followed in a specialised clinic, where supportive treatment and serial ultrasound examinations are undertaken.[24] Two out of three women will have a successful pregnancy with this supportive care. Treatment that has no proven value (such as progesterone support in early pregnancy) should not be offered.

If thrombophilia or antiphospholipid syndrome is diagnosed, the use of low-dose aspirin at 75 mg per day pre conception followed by low-dose heparin post conception (5000 units 12-hourly) can be effective.

CLINICAL PRESENTATION: Bleeding in early pregnancy

Many pregnancies are complicated by bleeding during the first trimester. This can be insignificant, due to an incidental cause, or may signify that the pregnancy will not progress.

Differential diagnosis

The least serious cause of bleeding in early pregnancy is painless bleeding indicating a 'threatened abortion'. Usually the bleeding settles and the pregnancy progresses normally. In other situations the pregnancy does not continue.

Examination

In order to differentiate between the various forms of abortion (Table 9.4), consider the symptoms, amount of bleeding, degree of pain, and the status of the cervix.

TABLE 9.4 Symptoms and signs for differential diagnosis of miscarriage

Miscarriage	Pain	Bleeding	Internal os Uterus
Threatened	Nil	Slight	Closed Uterus = dates
Inevitable	Significant	Moderate/heavy	Open Uterus = dates
Incomplete	Yes	Moderate/heavy	Open/tissue passed Uterus < dates
Complete	Yes Settling	May have stopped	Open or closed Uterus < dates
Missed	No	Slight or none Brown discharge	Closed Uterus < dates
Septic	Yes	Slight to heavy Infected discharge	Open or closed Uterus =/< dates, tender++

Investigations

1 *Haemoglobin:* to determine blood loss—sometimes substantial.
2 *Blood group:* important to offer anti-D immunoglobulin for the Rhesus-negative woman.
3 *Human chorionic gonadotrophin and progesterone levels* have been used as markers of early pregnancy failure. A serum progesterone 20 nmol/l or more has a positive predictive value of 97 per cent.[25]
4 *Ultrasound:* this will determine whether:
   - there is a pregnancy in the uterus (if the uterus is empty, consider an ectopic pregnancy)
   - the pregnancy is viable (presence of a fetal heart)
   - there are retained products where the pregnancy is non-continuing
   - the diagnosis is a hydatidiform mole.

Expectant management

Threatened miscarriage

There is no specific treatment, including bedrest, that can alter the outcome. The woman should be advised to continue normal activities unless the bleeding becomes heavy or pain develops, when she should be clinically reviewed.

Incomplete miscarriage

Expectant management can be safely offered to women without heavy bleeding with an incomplete miscarriage. Over 90 per cent of women can be expected to complete the miscarriage without intervention.[26] Women undergoing expectant management should be reviewed fortnightly and an ultrasound examination made to check that the miscarriage is complete.

Operative management

If some of the placenta is retained within the uterus or there is heavy bleeding, curettage needs to be undertaken (also called ERPC—evacuation of retained products of conception). If an evacuation is required then vacuum aspiration is safe, quick to perform and associated with less blood loss than a curettage.[27] For a missed abortion (a non-continuing pregnancy that has failed to abort), evacuation of the uterus is usually required.

Counselling

It is important to reassure women that none of their normal activities will have contributed to bleeding in early pregnancy, whether or not the pregnancy continues. Women are also concerned that any bleeding may indicate an abnormality in the pregnancy. There is no association between a threatened abortion in a continuing pregnancy and an abnormality of the fetus. The loss of an early pregnancy has similar psychological effects to a loss at other times (see Section 3).

Hydatidiform mole

Gestational trophoblastic disease includes a range of disorders of the trophoblast, interesting from the aspect of their different origins, pathological variants, clinical presentations and differential responses to treatment. Classification may be based on pathology or clinical presentation.

CLINICAL PRESENTATION

1 Bleeding in early pregnancy
2 Uterus larger than the expected gestation by dates
3 Passage of 'vesicular tissue'
4 Less commonly, hyperthyroidism and early-onset pre-eclampsia
5 Ultrasound: a characteristic appearance
6 Pathology: whenever tissue is obtained from products of conception, it should be examined histologically to exclude the presence of trophoblast disease.

Diagnosis

1 With the use of ultrasound, this is often diagnosed before curettage, as it gives a characteristic appearance.
2 HCG: the most useful marker remains the β-subunit HCG, its usefulness being greatly enhanced by improved assay sensitivity and specificity. Initial HCG levels are not diagnostic; however, they represent trophoblastic activity and determine clearance time and risk of persistence.
3 Histology and karyotype: classification (Figure 9.2).

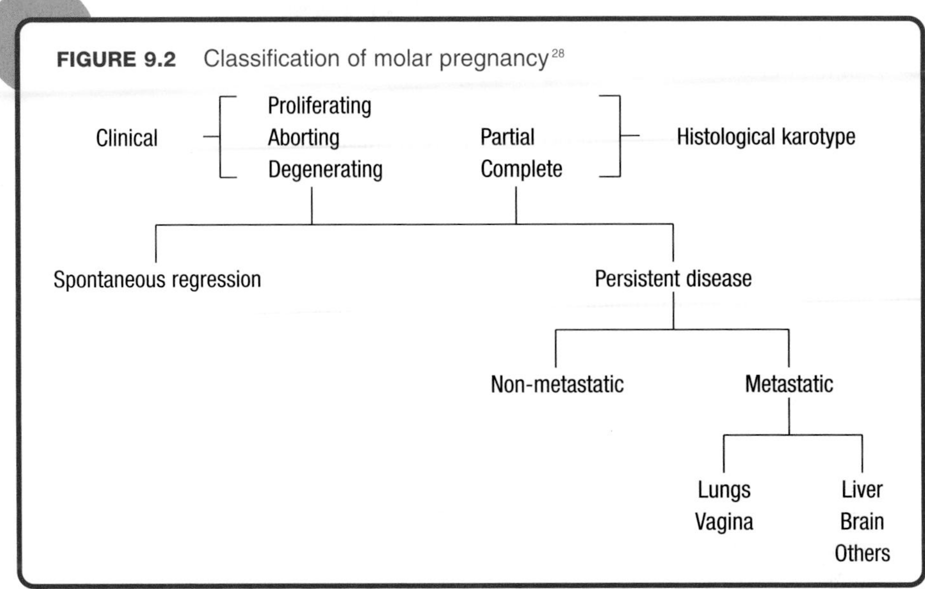

FIGURE 9.2 Classification of molar pregnancy[28]

Protocol of management

- Removal of molar gestation (by uterine evacuation or hysterectomy)
- Weekly serum β-HCG until two consecutive negative results (< –2U/l)
- Then monthly for six months, second-monthly for next six months (six months in low activity or partial mole)
- Effective contraception from evacuation
- Review:
  - β-HCG levels stationary or elevated for more than two consecutive weeks
  - exclude metastases by CT scan (chest, abdomen, pelvis, head).

The duration of follow-up after 'negativity' is debatable; monthly intervals for 6–12 months are reasonable and should be sufficient to detect persisting disease and late recurrence. A clearly defined set of criteria for treatment is important.

Cytotoxic chemotherapy is the mainstay of treatment for persisting and metastatic disease. There are a variety of treatment regimens, ranging from one to multiple drugs, given in several schedules.

- For 'low-risk' disease, methotrexate is the drug of choice, given in conjunction with folinic acid rescue; side effects are negligible and response rates are very good.
- For 'high-risk' disease, a variety of regimens are described. The two groups of metastases relatively resistant to treatment are those in the liver and in the central nervous system; in particular, the development of 'new' metastases during treatment has a very poor prognosis.

Criteria for treatment

- The place of prophylactic chemotherapy is limited but may be used in the non-compliant patient or the patient unable to access HCG testing, especially in 'high-risk' disease.

- Increased or stationary β-HCG levels on three consecutive weeks at any time after evacuation.
- > 20 U/l β-HCG level more than 12 weeks after evacuation
- Evidence of metastases, in presence of detectable β-HCG level
- Continuation of abnormal uterine bleeding, after curettage, and in presence of detectable β-HCG level
- Histological evidence of choriocarcinoma.

Risk factors for chemoresistance

- Delay in treatment (> 4 months)
- Previous failed chemotherapy
- Metastases other than in lung/vagina (especially in liver/brain)
- Diagnosis of choriocarcinoma.

There are two rare but interesting variants of the disease, which require a different approach to management: the mole with coexisting fetus, and the placental-site tumour. In the former variant, the mole can be associated with a normal or an abnormal fetus (triploidy) but fetal survival is not good; the latter variant is less responsive to chemotherapy and surgery is the primary treatment for localised disease.

Future outlook

Collated data support an increased risk of recurrent mole. The reproductive performance after a mole with or without treatment compares well with the general population.[29]

CLINICAL PRESENTATION: Acute abdominal pain in early pregnancy

History

Abdominal pain in pregnancy can be divided into causes associated with the pregnancy, or coincidental causes.

Differential diagnosis

This includes:

- Pregnancy-related:
  - Inevitable incomplete abortion
  - Ectopic pregnancy
  - Red degeneration of a fibroid
  - Urinary tract infection
  - Ovarian cyst (corpus luteum cyst) complication
- Coincidental:
  - Appendicitis
  - Cholecystitis
  - Sickle cell disease crises (more common in pregnancy).

Examination

Has the patient got an acute abdomen?

- If signs of guarding and rebound tenderness are present there is a surgical emergency, and urgent treatment is required.

Has the patient lost significant blood?

- If signs of shock due to haemorrhage are present, resuscitation with intravenous fluids and possibly blood is required.

Are there any products of conception in the cervix?

- Retained products in the cervix can cause severe pain, shock and profuse bleeding. Their gentle removal with polyp forceps can quickly control the situation.

Are there symptoms suggesting that the pain is not related to pregnancy?

- Urinary tract infection, which is more common in pregnancy, always has to be considered.
- Appendicitis can occur during pregnancy also. It is important to note that structures such as the appendix or ovary are displaced upwards and laterally by the growing uterus.

Investigations

1. *Pregnancy test:* essential.
2. *Ultrasound:* this will show the presence and viability of intrauterine pregnancy. The presence of a positive pregnancy test and an 'empty uterus' is a very strong suggestive diagnosis for an ectopic pregnancy. Sometimes the presence of a pregnancy outside the uterus is also visible. Ultrasound will also detect the presence of ovarian cysts.
3. *Full blood examination:* looking for signs of infection and blood loss.
4. *Urine examination* (dip stick test and mid-stream specimen) may be indicated.

Diagnosis

The presence of an abortion complication is easily diagnosed on ultrasound, whereas an ectopic pregnancy is usually a presumptive diagnosis, although sometimes it can be clearly seen on ultrasound. Ovarian cyst complications are usually a clinical diagnosis in conjunction with an ovarian cyst on ultrasound (often a corpus luteum cyst). Similarly, red degeneration of a fibroid would be diagnosed on clinical features in conjunction with ultrasound appearance.

The non-pregnancy causes always have to be considered, and it must be remembered that pregnancy may alter the usual presentation due to disturbed anatomy.

Ectopic pregnancy

A most important cause of bleeding in early pregnancy, often associated with pain, is ectopic pregnancy. This is a pregnancy that implants outside the uterine cavity. The most common site is in the uterine tube (previously damaged or obstructed).

CLINICAL PRESENTATION

The classical diagnostic triad to arouse suspicion of the possibility of an ectopic pregnancy is:

1. An episode of amenorrhoea
2. Vaginal bleeding
3. Abdominal pain.

However, the diagnosis should be considered in any woman presenting with lower abdominal pain or vaginal bleeding for whom pregnancy is a possibility.

History

1 Symptoms and signs of early pregnancy should be sought.
2 Menstrual history (amenorrhoea or irregular bleeding) and contraceptive history.
3 Risk factors associated with ectopic pregnancy: assisted reproductive treatment (ART), previous ectopic pregnancy, pelvic inflammatory disease, sexually transmissible infection, intrauterine contraceptive device.

Examination

1 *Vital signs:* these can range from normal, where there has been little intra-abdominal blood loss, to shock requiring urgent resuscitation and management.
2 *Abdominal examination:* there may be abdominal tenderness, rebound tenderness, or even abdominal guarding if a significant amount of bleeding within the abdominal cavity has taken place.
3 *Vaginal examination:* this may elicit tenderness on the side of adnexal involvement or the presence of an adnexal mass (more likely where the ectopic pregnancy has been 'walled off' with omentum). Where there is significant bleeding, the pain may be too great for any specific findings.

Investigations

The presumptive diagnosis of ectopic pregnancy is made when there is a positive pregnancy test (> 1500 IU/l) with:

- a lower than expected progesterone, in conjunction with
- a lower than expected quantitative β-HCG at presentation or a lower increase over time
- an empty uterus on ultrasonic examination
- laparoscopy—this is the definitive investigation for diagnosis.

Treatment

If the woman's observations are stable

1 *Medical.* The use of intramuscular methotrexate is sometimes used to treat an early ectopic pregnancy. It is administered in a single dose of 50 mg/m^2 of body surface area. Methotrexate is an inhibitor of folic acid reductase and results in degeneration of the rapidly growing trophoblast. Reported studies have found success rates of over 90 per cent. The treatment is most effective when β-HCG level is less than 5000 IU/l. Side effects are rare and may include nausea and diarrhoea.
2 *Surgical.* At the time of the laparoscopy, it is often possible to surgically remove the tubal ectopic pregnancy.
   - *Salpingostomy* is the simplest procedure, where the antimesenteric aspect of the Fallopian tube overlying the ectopic pregnancy is incised

longitudinally, usually using unipolar diathermy. The ectopic pregnancy, usually mainly trophoblastic tissue, is then removed with forceps and its base cleaned using suction and irrigation. Any bleeding points on the edge of the fallopian tube are then cauterised using diathermy.

- *Partial salpingectomy* using operative laparoscopy is ideal in women not wanting a future pregnancy. In this procedure, the section of the tube containing the ectopic pregnancy is removed.

If the woman has an acute abdomen or is in shock

Resuscitation and arranging surgical intervention are organised in parallel. The most immediate action is to establish an intravenous line and give appropriate fluids. Then proceed to a formal laparotomy, secure the bleeding points and carry out a partial salpingectomy.

Follow-up

After methotrexate treatment or laparoscopic removal of an ectopic pregnancy, it is advisable to perform serial β-HCG blood levels to confirm that the level is falling and that all trophoblast tissue has been removed.

Future outcome

Future fertility is more dependent on the condition of the contralateral fallopian tube than on the specific type of therapy used to treat the affected tube. There is no consensus on which treatment is most effective or influences future fertility.

Second and third trimester presentations

Small for dates

Intrauterine growth restriction is a major cause of perinatal morbidity and mortality. It places the fetus at risk in the antenatal, intrapartum and postnatal period. The growth-restricted infant is more likely to die than an appropriately grown premature baby of the same birth weight. Between 30 and 60 per cent of these deaths are related to underlying problems such as chromosomal abnormalities or congenital infections.

Intrauterine growth restriction (IUGR) can be difficult to detect antenatally with clinical examination alone, and can be missed in up to 60 per cent of affected pregnancies. Antenatal detection is improved when the examination is performed by an experienced clinician, and when the same observer examines the same patient repeatedly. Diagnosis is especially difficult in multiple pregnancies or in an obese patient. Hence, women at high risk for a growth-restricted fetus (Box 9.1) should be monitored carefully and ultrasound estimation of fetal growth should be performed when there is a suspicion of growth restriction. Undetected IUGR means a lost opportunity for increased fetal surveillance, which may have affected the timing and mode of delivery.

There is no universal definition for intrauterine growth restriction ('growth restriction' is a preferable term to 'growth retardation'). It can be defined as a failure to reach the genetic potential for birth weight. However, an individual baby's genetic potential is not usually known. A common definition used is birth weight less than the 10th centile for gestational age. When using this definition, one must be aware that smaller women, primiparous women and women from some ethnic groups can have small but healthy babies.

Intrauterine growth restriction can be classified into symmetrical or asymmetrical. Asymmetrical growth, where the growth of the abdominal circumference lags further behind than the head circumference (head sparing effect), is more suggestive of placental insufficiency. Symmetrical growth restriction, where all parameters are proportionally reduced, is more often associated with genetically small babies, or early-onset growth restriction (causes include congenital fetal anomalies, congenital infections, severe maternal disease).

BOX 9.1 Alerts to possible fetal growth restriction

- Past obstetric history: previous
  - Small baby < 2500 g
  - Stillbirth
  - Neonatal death
- Lifestyle factors
  - Maternal weight < 50 kg or obesity
  - Smoking, other drugs
- Maternal disease
- Present pregnancy
  - Clinically small uterus
  - Bleeding in pregnancy
  - Multiple pregnancy

CLINICAL PRESENTATION

1 SFD at antenatal clinic visit
2 Suspected SFD on alert

Differential diagnosis

1 *Incorrect dates:* identification of the small for gestational age fetus requires an accurate knowledge of gestational age. Gestational age can be determined from menstrual dates or ultrasound. Where menstrual dates are unknown or uncertain, an ultrasound scan performed before 20 weeks can provide gestational age estimation to within 10 days of accuracy. With an early ultrasound, up to 19 per cent of patients with regular cycles, and 51 per cent with irregular cycles, can have their EDC revised by more than seven days.[30,31] When the gestational age is unknown and the patient is already beyond 20 weeks,

assessment of growth adequacy can be made by checking for growth velocity on serial ultrasound examinations.

2 *Fetal causes:*
   - Fetal abnormality—an abnormal fetus is frequently growth restricted. When a diagnosis of early onset IUGR is made, chromosomal abnormality can be present in approximately 25 per cent of fetuses. Karyotyping should be considered. This is especially important if trisomy 13 or 18 is a concern, as they are lethal conditions. If lethal abnormalities are confirmed, obstetric interventions with maternal risks (such as caesarean sections) should be avoided.
   - Congenital infections
   - Single umbilical artery
   - Multiple pregnancy—where this is uncomplicated, impaired fetal growth is thought to be related to inadequate placental supply. The risk of growth restriction increases with each additional fetus in a multiple pregnancy. Growth rates are commonly slow from 32 weeks in twins and from 28 weeks in triplets compared to singleton growth curves. The mean weight for triplets at 38 weeks is the same as the 10th centile for twins.

3 *Maternal causes:* the maternal environment is a major determinant of fetal growth (Box 9.2). Maternal medical conditions that cause growth restriction are those that affect uteroplacental perfusion and so affect fetal nutrition and oxygenation, or are associated with abnormal placentation in early pregnancy.

4 *Idiopathic:* often no cause can be found for growth restriction, particularly when the changes are mild.

BOX 9.2 Environmental factors affecting fetal growth

- Pre-eclampsia
- Cardiovascular—hypertension, diabetes mellitus, renal disease, SLE, cyanotic heart disease, antiphospholipid syndrome, thrombophilias
- Respiratory—severe asthma, cystic fibrosis, smoking
- Anaemia—nutritional, sickle cell
- Infections—CMV, rubella, toxoplasmosis, malaria, HIV, varicella zoster
- Drugs—cigarettes, narcotics, alcohol

Identification of the growth-restricted fetus

Ultrasound is the accepted method of diagnosing inadequate fetal growth when there is a clinical suspicion. Fetal weight estimation is performed by ultrasound using a formula which combines standardised measurements of abdominal circumference, biparietal diameter/head circumference and femur length. This gives an accuracy of plus or minus 15 per cent. Eighty-five per cent of growth-restricted fetuses can be detected by ultrasound. Ultrasound also enables assessment of other markers of fetal well-being such as amniotic fluid volume, biophysical profile and Doppler assessment of blood flow. In conjunction, these parameters enable the clinician to assess the severity of the growth restriction and so plan management.

Investigation

Depending on the severity of growth restriction and the clinical picture, a cause for the IUGR should be sought where possible. This may involve detailed ultrasound examination for anomalies, investigations for maternal disease, karyotype and serology for infectious causes (Box 9.3).

BOX 9.3 Possible investigations for intrauterine growth restriction

- Ultrasound for anomalies
- Maternal:
  - Blood pressure, urinalysis for protein, glucose
  - Urea and electrolytes, urate
  - Antiphospholipid and thrombophilia screen
  - CMV, rubella, toxoplasmosis, HIV serology
- Karyotype—amniocentesis

Treatment of fetal growth restriction

There are few effective interventions to prevent or improve fetal growth apart from quitting smoking. Other treatment strategies such as hyperalimentation and bed rest have not proved effective. In some women with recurrent miscarriages and IUGR because of antiphospholipid antibodies, early use of heparin can reduce the incidence of growth restriction.

Management

The aim of management is to balance the risk of continuation of the pregnancy versus the risk of delivery (preterm). The timing of delivery depends on gestational age, underlying aetiology, availability of neonatal facilities and fetal condition. Because of the variations in measurements, growth parameters of the fetus should in general not be examined more often than once every two weeks. The frequency of other fetal well-being assessments should be performed according to the severity of the growth restriction; for example, CTG (cardiotocography), AFI (amniotic fluid index) and Doppler examinations can be performed twice a week in moderately severe cases of IUGR. Indications for delivery may include absent end diastolic flow on umbilical Doppler, abnormal CTG, or absence of fetal growth (Figure 9.3).

The mode of delivery will depend on the severity of growth restriction, fetal presentation, cervical ripeness, parity, and ready access to emergency caesarean section. A mildly growth-restricted fetus usually tolerates labour well, but a severely growth-restricted fetus who is already hypoxic or acidotic will usually tolerate labour poorly. Continuous CTG monitoring in labour is mandatory for the growth-restricted fetus.

FIGURE 9.3 Investigation of suspected intrauterine growth retardation

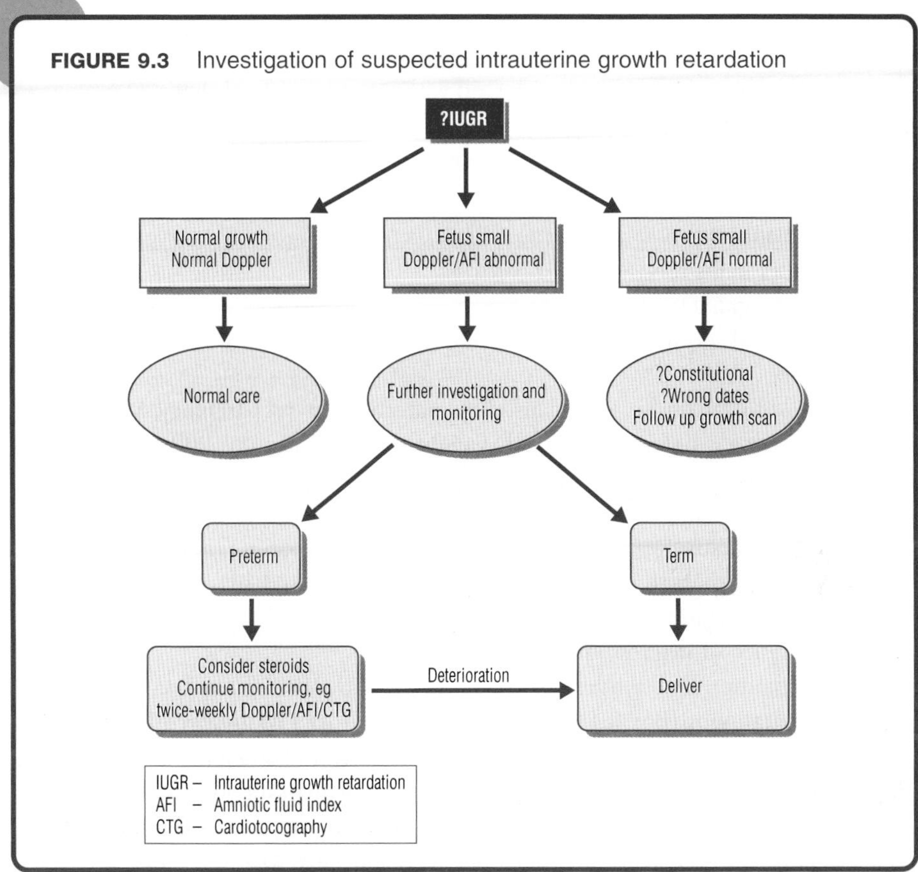

Outcomes of fetal growth restriction

The majority of growth-restricted fetuses will have no underlying abnormality and will exhibit catch-up growth during the first year of life. Recent research has shown that fetal growth restriction may have a long-term effect on the future, with increased rates of adult diseases such as ischaemic heart disease, hypertension, diabetes and cerebrovascular accident (CVA).[32]

Large for dates

A fundus larger than expected for dates may be a marker for many significant obstetric conditions. As with other aspects of antenatal care, early detection of problems may enable appropriate antenatal and intrapartum management.

CLINICAL PRESENTATION

Large for dates on examination.

Symptoms

1 Usually none
2 Breathlessness and abdominal discomfort (hydramnios)
3 Excessive vomiting (multiple pregnancy, hydatidiform mole)

Examination

- *Observation:* the uterus appears larger than expected for the gestation and the shape may be uniformly enlarged without obvious fetal shape
- *Palpation:* the uterus may be tensely distended, often with a fluid thrill (hydramnios); more than one fetal pole can be felt (multiple pregnancy).

Differential diagnosis

1 Incorrect dates (See Small for dates)
2 Molar pregnancy
3 Accelerated growth. The underlying mechanisms for a macrosomic fetus include:
   - Constitutionally large, or caused by maternal or fetal pathology. Macrosomia is variously defined as a birth weight greater than the 90th centile, over 4000 g or over 4500 g. Approximately 10 per cent of babies are over 4000 g and 2 per cent over 4500 g. Birth weight is higher in male babies (mean 3421 g versus 3286 g in females) and in obese or parous women.
   - Maternal diabetes—macrosomia can also be caused by maternal diabetes, either gestational or pre-existing. Good diabetic control reduces the incidence of macrosomia.
   - Uncommon fetal syndromes (such as Beckwith-Weidelman syndrome).
4 Polyhydramnios (Box 9.4). This is defined as an AFI of greater than 20 cm or maximum pocket depth of greater than 8 cm on ultrasound (see Fetal assessment below for definitions). Investigation of polyhydramnios involves detailed ultrasound of the fetus and a maternal glucose tolerance test. The more severe the polyhydramnios, the more likely it is that a cause will be found.

BOX 9.4 Causes of polyhydramnios

- Idiopathic
- Maternal—diabetes mellitus
- Fetal
  - Fetal abnormalities:
    - Gastrointestinal—eg duodenal atresia, oesophageal compression
    - Neurological—eg CNS lesions, neuromuscular disorders
    - Hydrops—eg isoimmunisation, sacrococcygeal teratoma
    - Infection—eg syphilis
    - Twin-to-twin transfusion syndrome
- Placental
  - Chorioangioma

Complications of polyhydramnios

1 Premature labour (related to overdistension of the uterus)
2 Unstable lie

3 Cord prolapse
4 Abruptio placentae (accidental haemorrhage) if the membranes rupture, releasing large amounts of fluid suddenly

Management of polyhydramnios

Treatment may be necessary for maternal comfort and to reduce the risk of obstetric complications. Specific treatment of the underlying cause is only possible in a few conditions, eg hydrops caused by anaemia, twin-to-twin transfusion. In all other cases, amnioreduction, which involves removing amniotic fluid transabdominally under ultrasound guidance, is the mainstay of treatment. The volume of liquor removed depends on the severity of the polyhydramnios, but may be many litres. Unfortunately, polyhydramnios usually reaccumulates and repeated drainage is often required. Medical treatment with prostaglandin synthetase inhibitors has caused fetal complications and has a limited role in treatment.

Diagnosis of macrosomia

Unfortunately, it is extremely difficult to accurately predict macrosomia antenatally. Ultrasound estimation of fetal weight has an error rate of up to 22 per cent in large babies, with a tendency to overestimate. The sensitivity and specificity to detect a fetus of over 4000 g by ultrasound is 75 per cent.

Complications of macrosomia

1 Obstructed labour
2 Birth trauma
3 Shoulder dystocia and its associated complications such as fetal hypoxia and Erb's palsy can be as high as 15 per cent in a 4500 g infant of a non-diabetic mother, and 50 per cent in an infant of a diabetic mother. For fetuses over 4000 g, the risks are 7 per cent and 14 per cent respectively.[33] Shoulder dystocia might be anticipated during delivery as the large head fails to completely clear the introitus—the neck is not easily visible.

Assessment of fetal well-being

Fetal movements

The simplest way to assess fetal well-being is by maternal perception of fetal movements and this should be assessed at every antenatal encounter in all patients. This can be formalised with various tools such as a kick chart where the patient records fetal movements over a specified time and contacts her caregivers if the number of movements is less than specified. Unfortunately, this simple method of fetal assessment has not been shown to reduce perinatal mortality, although it may provide maternal reassurance.

Cardiotocography

Cardiotocograph (CTG) monitoring can be used antenatally or in labour. Antenatal CTG has not been shown in randomised trials to reduce perinatal mortality. The most common role in the antenatal period is in the patient with decreased fetal movements or a fetus at risk of acute hypoxia, such as antepartum haemorrhage. A CTG records fetal heart rate and uterine contractions. A reactive CTG is defined as a baseline between 110 and 160, short-term variability of at least five beats per minute and two accelerations of at least 15 bpm lasting 15 seconds in a 20-minute period. Signs of fetal compromise are reduced variability and decelerations. Interpretation of the CTG needs to take into account the fact that the normal fetus can have periods of reduced variability as part of the sleep–wake cycle, and that variability can also be affected by maternal medications or preterm gestation. The main problem with CTG is the variability in interpretation, and the high false positive rate.

Doppler ultrasound

Doppler ultrasound of umbilical arterial flow is the fetal surveillance test that has been subjected to the most randomised controlled trials, and meta-analysis of these randomised controlled trials has shown that its use can reduce perinatal mortality in normally formed high-risk fetuses, without increasing maternal intervention.[34] The umbilical arterial flow shows decreased flow in diastole in response to increased placental resistance. This can be quantified as a ratio of velocity in systole-to-diastole (S/D ratio), where increasing S/D ratio reflects worsening placental resistance. As the placental resistance increases, the umbilical flow can demonstrate absent flow in diastole, and then eventually reversed flow. Perinatal mortality is markedly increased in these circumstances.

The hypoxic fetus may also display abnormalities of the circulation in the ductus venosus, middle cerebral artery and other vessels. The role of these vessels in the monitoring of the high-risk fetus is still under investigation. It is important to note that Doppler assessment is not helpful in the low-risk population.

Liquor volume

Abnormalities of liquor volume are a strong predictor of fetal compromise and poor perinatal outcome. Normal amniotic fluid volume is either expressed as AFI (amniotic fluid index), which is measured as the maximum pocket depth in the four quadrants of the uterus, with a normal range at term of 7–20 cm (5th to 95th centile). An alternative measure is of a single maximum pocket depth, with a normal range of 2–8 cm. Decreased liquor volume in the uterus is due to decreased placental perfusion, leading to decreased fetal renal perfusion and subsequently decreased urine output. Reduced liquor can also be due to ruptured membranes or fetal genitourinary abnormalities.

Biophysical profile

The biophysical profile (BPP) is a composite score given for liquor volume, reactive CTG and the presence of fetal breathing movements, gross body movements and tone. Each parameter scores 0 or 2. A score of 8–10 is reassuring of fetal well-being; less than 8 suggests fetal hypoxia. The test requires ultrasound scanning of the fetus for at least 30 minutes to ensure that reduced activity is not due to a sleep state.

Biophysical profile scores show a good correlation with umbilical vein pH and poor outcomes such as cerebral palsy and perinatal mortality in high-risk patients. Unfortunately, randomised controlled trials have failed to show reductions in perinatal mortality with its use. The BPP is relatively time consuming to perform and requires a trained sonographer.

CLINICAL PRESENTATION: Onset of labour before 37 weeks

Preterm labour (PTL) is defined as labour from 20 completed weeks gestation to 36 weeks and 6 days gestation. Delivery prior to 20 weeks is classified as a miscarriage. Preterm delivery (PTD) remains one of the major causes of perinatal morbidity and mortality. Six per cent of babies are born before 37 weeks and two per cent of these before 32 weeks.

Common associations with PTL include:[35]

- Lower socio-economic status
- Previous preterm birth (odds ratio (OR) three after one PTL and delivery, or six after two PTL)
- Pyelonephritis (15 per cent PTL and PTD)
- Uterine structural anomalies and cervical incompetence
- Multiple pregnancy (10 per cent PTL and PTD with twins)
- Infection and premature prelabour rupture of membranes (PPROM)—up to 20 per cent of PTL may be caused by beta-haemolytic streptococcal infection
- Antepartum haemorrhage
- Polyhydramnios.

Major risks of preterm delivery include perinatal death and neonatal morbidity (Box 9.5). There is increasing evidence demonstrating a relationship between intrauterine infection and the development of neonatal intraventricular haemorrhage and periventricular leucomalacia (permanent cortical damage), with the subsequent occurrence of cerebral palsy. This is thought to be mediated through the generation of pro-inflammatory cytokines by the fetus.[36]

BOX 9.5 Causes of mortality and morbidity in preterm babies

- Respiratory distress syndrome
- Hypothermia
- Hypoglycaemia
- Necrotising enterocolitis
- Jaundice
- Infection
- Retinopathy of prematurity

Assessment

Mother

Specific information should be sought for precipitating factors to the premature labour, including:

- A history of vaginal bleeding, fluid leakage or discharge

- Previous preterm delivery or uterine abnormality
- Polyhydramnios—may be indicated by a history of rapidly increasing abdominal girth in the setting of maternal diabetes or fetal abnormality
- Previous investigations and procedures—important, particularly the presence of multiple pregnancies or insertion of cervical suture
- Systematic questioning may reveal urinary symptoms suggestive of pyelonephritis.

Diagnosis of PTL relies on a history of regular painful uterine contraction plus effacement and/or dilatation of the cervix on sterile speculum/vaginal examination (although vaginal examination is contraindicated if PPROM to avoid introduction of infection).

Chorioamnionitis may be diagnosed by elevated temperature (> 37.5°C), abdominal/ uterine tenderness, fetal tachycardia, maternal tachycardia and offensive vaginal discharge. This may result in serious morbidity and/or mortality for mother and baby, so prompt attention is required.

Fetus

A history of fetal movements is sought, and examination to ascertain the lie and presentation of the fetus.

Investigations

- High vaginal and endocervical swabs for bacterial infection and *Chlamydia*
- Elevated C-reactive protein and white cell count on maternal blood as an indicator of infection, although be aware that steroids may increase maternal white cell count
- Fetal fibronectin screening, performed on cervical swab, may indicate probability of PTL and PTD; a negative result means that delivery is unlikely
- Assessment of fetal well-being by cardiotocography and ultrasound, including biophysical profile and fetal morphology.

Management options

Management options for preterm labour are summarised in Figure 9.4.

1 Promotion of fetal lung maturity

Corticosteroids between 24 and 34 weeks gestation stimulate fetal production of surfactant by Type 2 pneumocytes and reduce perinatal morbidity and mortality. They take 24 hours for optimal effect and are given by two injections 12 hours apart. Steroids do not increase the risk of infection.

2 Tocolysis

Tocolysis for 24 hours to enable administration of corticosteroids has been shown to reduce perinatal morbidity and mortality. Many different agents have been used:

- *Nifedipine* (a calcium channel blocker) may cause maternal headache and hypotension. Randomised controlled trial evidence has revealed that nifedipine is as effective in preventing preterm delivery as ritodrine but with fewer maternal side effects, making this a preferred tocolytic.[37] It is more effective if the cervical dilatation is < 5 cm.
- *Beta-adrenergic agents*, including ritodrine or salbutamol, have side effects of maternal tachycardia, tremor, anxiety, hypokalaemia, ketoacidosis in diabetics (particularly when administered with corticosteroids), and pulmonary oedema.
- *Magnesium sulfate* has been associated with adverse outcomes in the fetus and neonate (hypokalaemia, hypotension and fetal heart changes).
- *NSAIDs* (indomethacin, a prostaglandin H synthase (PGHS) inhibitor) are known to cause premature closure of ductus arteriosus, necrotising enterocolitis, intracranial haemorrhage, and oligohydramnios.

FIGURE 9.4 Summary of the management of preterm labour

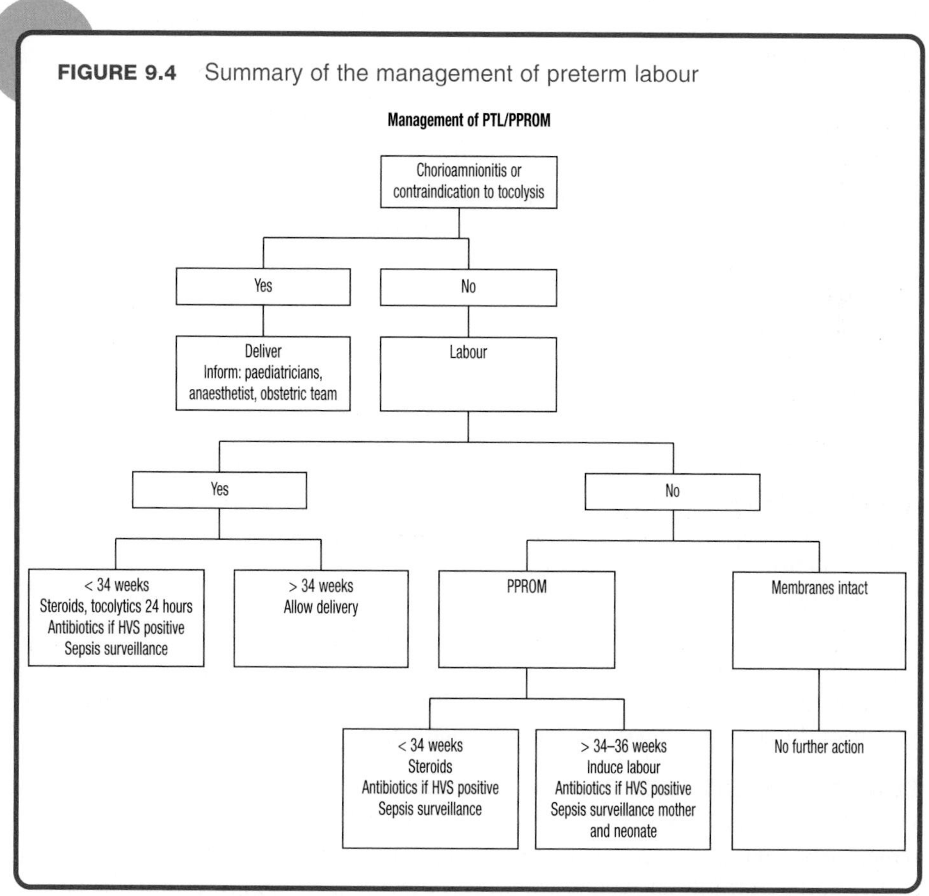

Contraindications to tocolysis

- Fetal
  - Suspected intrauterine infection
  - Labour in the setting of placenta praevia
  - Placental abruption/undiagnosed significant vaginal bleeding
  - Severe fetal growth restriction
  - Lethal fetal anomalies
- Maternal
  - Hypotension
  - Previous adverse reaction to calcium channel blockers.

Delivery

Labour may ensue despite attempts to stop it. Apart from the usual indications, a caesarean section is often considered if the fetus is < 32 weeks gestation, a breech presentation, or if there are other complications. However, there is no evidence that caesarean section will improve fetal survival.

Prevention

Prevention of PTL involves:

1. Counselling regarding the risk of recurrence and checking for causes/precipitating factors
2. Advising against cigarette smoking (associated with fetal growth retardation)
3. Infection:
   - Vaginal bacteriology screening if recurrent PTL
   - Treatment of GBS and bacterial vaginosis in high-risk population useful
   - The use of antibiotics for preterm premature rupture of membranes shows health benefits for the neonate with the use of erythromycin, whereas antibiotics do not seem to play a beneficial role in spontaneous preterm labour without evidence of clinical infection.[38,39]
   - Inflammatory cytokine measurement may be useful.
4. Prediction of PTL:
   - Fetal fibronectin status to predict high-risk cases may be helpful[40]
   - Transvaginal ultrasound assessment of cervical length and funnelling in recurrent PTL may lead to improvement when combined with fibronectin status.
5. Corticosteroids—undisputed benefit in improving neonatal outcome. A single course appears to have benefit for about 10 days. The risk-benefit effect of multiple courses has yet to be proved.
6. Cervical cerclage—a surgical intervention involving a suture placed aroud the cervix (the role is limited and controversial).

CLINICAL PRESENTATION: Rupture of membranes before the onset of labour

Preterm prelabour rupture of the membranes (PPROM) is defined as rupture of the membranes from 20 completed weeks gestation to 36 weeks and 6 days gestation. It occurs in one-third of all preterm deliveries. All the associations of preterm labour and delivery apply, although in many circumstances the cause is unknown.

Complications include:

- Preterm delivery: > 50 per cent of cases, within 48 hours
- Ascending infection of the genital tract, resulting in chorioamnionitis
- Umbilical cord prolapse
- Complications of prematurity as above
- Oligohydramnios resulting in pulmonary hypoplasia and compression deformities, particularly if PPROM < 25 weeks gestation.

Assessment

(See Preterm labour.) Check for a history of gush of fluid, followed by continued leaking, and symptoms and signs of chorioamnionitis. Confirmation of diagnosis is sought by speculum examination, searching for pooling of fluid in the posterior vaginal fornix and/or cough impulse of fluid through the cervix.

Investigations

- High vaginal and endocervical swabs for bacterial infection and chlamydia
- Elevated C-reactive protein and white cell count on maternal blood, although note that steroids may increase maternal white cell count
- Assessment of fetal well-being by cardiotocography and ultrasound, including biophysical profile and fetal morphology. Liquor volume may still be normal. Fetal lung lengths are of limited benefit in prediction of pulmonary hypoplasia.

Management

As for preterm labour (see Figure 9.4). The principle of management is to balance the risks of delivery and prematurity against the risk of infection to mother and baby. Early identification of infection is a key feature. The use of antibiotics for PPROM shows health benefits for the neonate with the use of erythromycin.

Medical disorders and pregnancy

Haematological system

Normal haematological system changes in pregnancy

A hypercoagulable state occurs in pregnancy predisposing to thrombosis. There are alterations in the thrombotic and fibrinolytic mechanisms. In the first trimester there are increases in prothrombin, fibrinogen, and Factors VII, VIII, IX and X. In the first few days after delivery there is an increase in Factors V, VII and X. Antithrombin III levels decrease throughout pregnancy and return to normal a few hours after delivery. There is also venous stasis in pregnancy from the gravid uterus reducing the venous return from the lower limbs, and an oestrogen effect on smooth muscle, leading to venous dilatation.

Thromboembolic disease

Pulmonary embolus is a significant cause of maternal mortality, with a risk of death of 1 in 100 000 after spontaneous vaginal delivery and 7 in 100 000 after caesarean section.

Risk factors include:

- Immobilisation: bed rest during pregnancy, prolonged labour, after operative delivery
- Multiparity: > 4 deliveries
- Age: > 30 years
- Obesity
- Operative delivery
- Anaemia, dehydration, sickle cell disease
- Antiphospholipid antibodies
- Inherited deficiencies of natural inhibitors of coagulation (protein C, protein S and antithrombin III, factor V Leiden and Prothrombin gene mutations, and hyperhomocysteinaemia).

The following facts are of interest:

- Frequency of deep vein thrombosis (DVT) is 0.5–3 per 1000 pregnancies
- Incidence of DVT is equally distributed through three trimesters
- Greatest risk is in first few weeks after delivery
- Investigation as in the non-pregnant woman: ultrasound for DVT, computed tomographic pulmonary angiography (CTPA) if suspect pulmonary embolus
- Prothrombotic screen indicates falling free protein S levels
- Treatment: low molecular weight heparin (LMWH), eg clexane 1 mg/kg twice daily subcutaneously with an aim four-hour post injection for anti-Xa level 0.5–1.2
- Change to warfarin post partum: mother can continue breastfeeding if < 12 mg/day.

Prophylactic doses of LMWH can be used to reduce the risk of recurrent thromboembolic events in pregnancy. The regimen used will depend on the previous history, the family history and the presence of risk factors, including the genetic and acquired causes of thrombophilia.[41]

Anticoagulation and regional anaesthesia: therapeutic dose LMWH—should be ceased at least 24 hours before regional anaesthesia; prophylactic dose LMWH—an interval of more than 20 hours from the last dose should allow for regional anaesthesia. Intravenous unfractionated heparin (UH) should be discontinued at least six hours and preferably 12 hours before regional anaesthesia.

Thrombocytopenia

Thrombocytopenia complicates approximately 5 per cent of pregnancies with a platelet count < 150 000. Provided underlying causes are excluded, isolated maternal thrombocytopenia in the latter half of pregnancy is not associated with adverse consequences for mother or neonate.

Differential diagnosis includes:

- Idiopathic thrombocytopenic purpura (ITP)
- Systemic lupus erythematosis (SLE)
- Severe pre-eclampsia
- Thrombotic thrombocytopenic purpura (TTP)

These are differentiated by review of the blood film for microangiopathic haemolysis, checking the renal and liver function, and looking for antiplatelet antibodies, ANA and anticardiolipin antibodies.

Pregnancy is said to have little effect on the course of ITP, and treatment with glucocorticoids or intragam is indicated if the platelet count is less than 30 000. No maternal characteristic reliably predicts the fetal platelet count, and it is controversial as to whether fetal scalp sampling should be used to decide on mode of delivery.

Red cell iso-immunisation

Antibodies of the IgG class (but *not* IgM) can cross the placenta from the mother to the fetus. This assists both the fetus in utero and the neonate in the battle against infection. There is, however, the capacity for maternal antibodies directed against fetal tissues to cross the placenta and cause problems for the fetus.

Autoimmune diseases

In autoimmune disease, antibodies are made against antigens expressed by the individual's own cells. Autoantibodies causing conditions like SLE, thyroid disease and ITP can produce similar conditions in the fetus and newborn. Sometimes the fetal condition is quite different to that in the mother. For example, anti-Ro antibodies are associated with salivary and lacrimal gland malfunction in the adult but may produce heart block in the fetus.

Iso-immune diseases

In 'iso-immunity' (or 'allo-immunity'), the immune response is directed against an antigen that the mother does not normally possess—'individual-specific' antigens. Transplant rejection and an incompatible blood transfusion are examples of iso-immunity.

The fetus represents a source of 'foreign' antigens against which the mother could initiate an antibody response. Predictably, conditions are recognised where the mother can make antibodies against the red cells, white cells or platelets of the fetus, thereby potentially causing anaemia, neutropenia or thrombocytopenia respectively. Allo-immune neutropenia and thrombocytopenia are relatively uncommon and beyond the scope of this section, but have many similarities with red cell iso-immunisation.

CLINICAL PRESENTATION

1. Routine antenatal screening: antibody detection

Although only about 1 per cent of women have anti-red cell antibodies of some type in pregnancy, 15 per cent of women do not have the 'D' antigen (so-called 'Rh-negative' women) and are therefore at risk of making anti-D antibodies. All women are capable of making antibodies against fetal red cell antigens and all women (Rh-negative and Rh-positive) are screened for the common iso-antibodies at the first antenatal visit.

2. Anticipated: history of previous pregnancy with antibodies/affected baby

In addition to the routine management at the first visit, a woman with antibodies will require:

1 *Partner test for phenotype.* The red cell antigen inheritance is simple Mendelian. The partner may therefore be homozygous positive (all children will be affected), heterozygous positive (50 per cent affected) or negative (no children can be affected). If the partner is heterozygous, consideration should be given to typing the fetus for the relevant antigen through amniocentesis at 15 weeks gestation and DNA analysis. This should only be performed if a negative result would avoid more invasive testing.

2 *Risk allocation.* It is important to estimate the risk of severe disease in all women based on their obstetric history and the antibody level (Table 9.5). As a general rule, antibody type is less important although anti-Kell antibodies are particularly serious as they affect the erythroblast as well as erythrocyte.

3 *Counselling.* Discussion with the couple should involve an estimate of the possible outcomes, and risks and benefits of any tests or procedures.

TABLE 9.5 Disease risk based on history and antibody level

Risk group	Antibody titre and past history
Nil	Partner homozygous negative for the antigen
Low	< 16 (titre) or < 4 IU/ml
Medium	64–256 (titre)
High	> 512 (titre)
	Previous hydrops or transfusions

Management during pregnancy of a woman with antibodies

Low risk

1 *Antibody titre each visit.* Relatively small feto-maternal haemorrhages are capable of causing large rises in antibody levels in women who are already immunised, and they should be checked frequently for such an occurrence.

2 *Deliver 38–40 weeks.* Progressively more antibody crosses the placenta in the last weeks of pregnancy but with earlier gestations the neonatal impact of jaundice is greater. The optimal gestation for delivery is usually between 38 and 40 weeks gestation.

Medium risk

1 *Antibody titre two-weekly from 20 weeks gestation*

2 *Ultrasound from 20 weeks gestation.* Although this group is not expected to become seriously anaemic before 28 weeks gestation, this can occur and close non-invasive surveillance is recommended.

3 *Amniocentesis at 28 weeks gestation.* Subsequent management is based on the level of the bilirubin which can be assessed using a validated zone chart.[42,43]

For example:

- *Zone 1 (mild):* little bilirubin is present. The baby is unlikely to be significantly affected and may well be 'negative' for the affecting antigen if the partner is heterozygous.
- *Zone 2 (moderate):* moderate amounts of bilirubin are present and the fetus is likely to be significantly affected, possibly needing exchange transfusions after birth. The amniocentesis will usually be repeated two or three times and delivery is likely to be necessary at around 35 weeks gestation.
- *Zone 3 (severe):* large amounts of bilirubin are present and the fetus is likely to be seriously affected—probably already anaemic. Corticosteroids should be administered, cardiotocographic monitoring commenced and the management team will need to decide between delivering the baby or performing a fetal blood sampling with possible intrauterine transfusion.

High risk

1. *Ultrasound scan weekly from 17 weeks.* The fetus is at risk of early anaemia, the first signs of which may be detectable on ultrasound. Possible signs of early anaemia include fluid accumulation or abnormal Doppler ultrasound of fetal vessels.
2. *Fetal blood sampling at 18–24 weeks.* Although attempts have been made to use amniocentesis bilirubin at early gestations in the more severe cases, there are many reports of this being unreliable. Direct sampling of fetal blood (usually via the umbilical cord) provides accurate information on the fetal haemoglobin and fetal blood type. Decisions can then be made with respect to:
   - *No further intervention needed:* this will be the case if the fetus proves to be antigen-negative by virtue of a heterozygous partner.
   - *Repeat fetal blood sampling at a later gestation:* if the fetal red cells have maternal antibody attached (a 'positive Direct Coombs' Test') but the fetus is not as yet seriously anaemic, intrauterine transfusion is likely to be necessary at a later date.
   - *Intrauterine transfusion:* antigen-negative blood can be transfused directly into a fetal vein, while the fetus remains in utero. This is not without significant risks, particularly if the fetus is already seriously compromised by anaemia. In these cases, repeated intrauterine transfusions will be necessary until approximately 34 weeks gestation. Beyond this time, the risks of further intrauterine transfusions become greater than the risks of prematurity.

Pathophysiology: antigens involved

Fetal red cells express a number of antigens on their surface against which antibodies could be made by the mother. The most important of these is the 'D' antigen, which is by far the most common antigen involved in cases of red cell iso-immunisation. Other potentially 'haemolytic' antigens at the Rhesus locus include c, C and E. There are many other antigens, some of which are very rare, but the more common include the Kell, Kidd and Duffy antigens. Kell is particularly important because it is expressed by the erythroblast and anti-Kell antibodies have an impact on erythropoiesis as well as causing haemolysis.

Fortunately, antibodies against some antigens are largely IgM and almost never cause in utero problems, although they can still be responsible for quite severe neonatal jaundice. This group of antibodies includes anti-A and anti-B—the most so-called 'naturally occurring' antibodies.

The primary immune stimulus

Any woman not possessing an antigen (eg a D-negative woman) has the capacity to make antibodies against that antigen (eg anti-D antibodies). She will, however, only do this if she is first exposed to the D-antigen. This exposure can occur at the time of a D-positive blood transfusion or when some D-positive fetal blood crosses the placenta ('feto-maternal haemorrhage') allowing her immune system to interact with the D-antigen.

Consequences of red cell iso-immunisation

When anti-red cell antibodies cross the placenta, they bind to the antigen on the surface of the red cell and have the capacity to cause haemolysis. At low levels of haemolysis, there are no problems.

As the antibody levels rise and more fetal red cells are destroyed, the rate of bilirubin production can exceed the ability of the newborn to cope, resulting in neonatal jaundice. When this is severe, it has the capacity to cause damage to the basal ganglia of the brain (kernicterus). Jaundice is *not* a problem for the fetus in utero because the mother removes and processes the bilirubin on behalf of the fetus.

With further rises in antibody levels and larger degrees of haemolysis, the rate of fetal erythropoiesis can no longer match the rate of red cell destruction, and anaemia ensues. This can be so severe as to cause high-output cardiac failure ('fetal hydrops') or even fetal death.

Prevention of iso-immunisation

D-negative women needing a blood transfusion should obviously only ever be given D-negative blood. To prevent immunisation by feto-maternal haemorrhage, 'passive' anti-D can be administered to bind to the fetal red cell D-antigen and prevent the maternal immune system 'seeing' it. Passive anti-D administration is therefore indicated at times of likely feto-maternal haemorrhage as follows:

- Bleeding in pregnancy (abortion (any type), ectopic pregnancy, APH)
- Trauma (chorionic villous sampling, amniocentesis, fetal blood sampling, external cephalic version, car accident)
- Delivery
- Routine at 28 and 34 weeks recommended if local anti-D stocks are sufficient.

There is no benefit of anti-D administration if the woman is already immunised or the fetus/neonate is D-negative, as there would be no D-antigen present to initiate the immune response. Therefore, the mother is usually checked to ensure that she has not already been immunised and, at delivery, the neonatal blood group is ascertained before anti-D is administered to a D-negative woman.

It is possible to estimate the amount of feto-maternal haemorrhage by doing a Kleihauer test on a maternal blood sample. If there is little or no feto-maternal haemorrhage detected, a low volume of anti-D can be administered. If a large volume is detected, larger doses of anti-D can be administered to neutralise all the fetal D-antigen in the maternal blood. This test is unnecessary very early in pregnancy when the fetal blood volume is low.

Summary

The presence of maternal anti-red cell antibodies may be innocuous but also has the potential to cause life-threatening neonatal jaundice or severe anaemia in the unborn fetus. Prevention of anti-D antibodies by the administration of passive anti-D at appropriate times has reduced the incidence of iso-immunisation. Early diagnosis of red cell iso-immunisation is essential and necessitates screening of all women for anti-red cell antibodies in pregnancy. If antibodies are found, the pregnancy should be managed by a unit experienced in this uncommon complication of pregnancy.

Respiratory system

Normal respiratory system changes in pregnancy

- Normal value for P_{O_2} in pregnancy is 100 mmHg and for P_{CO_2} is 28–32 mmHg
- Fetus requires maternal $P_{O_2} > 70$ mmHg, therefore aim to keep maternal oxygen saturation > 95 per cent.

Asthma

This affects approximately 7 per cent of pregnant women. During pregnancy one-third get better, one-third remain stable and one-third get worse, with the latter tending to be those with the worst disease pre conception.[44] Asthma is associated with preterm labour, low birth weight, pre-eclampsia and hyperemesis gravidarum. Approximately 10 per cent of asthmatic women will have an attack during labour, hence it is important that they keep up their usual medications. Inhaled β-antagonists, inhaled, oral and intravenous glucocorticoids, theophylline and sodium cromoglycate are all safe to use in pregnancy (Table 9.6).

TABLE 9.6 Pharmacological step therapy of chronic asthma during pregnancy

Category	Step therapy
Mild intermittent	Inhaled β-agonists prn
Mild persistent	Inhaled sodium chromoglycate Substitute inhaled corticosteroids* if above inadequate
Moderate persistent	Inhaled corticosteroids Continue inhaled salbutamol if good response prior to pregnancy Add oral theophylline and/or inhaled salmeterol if inadequately controlled by medium-dose inhaled corticostroids
Severe persistent	Above + oral corticosteroids

*Beclomethasone or budesonide if inhaled corticosteroids initiated during pregnancy.
Consider montelukast if recalcitrant asthma + favourable response in past.

Neurological system

Epilepsy

Epilepsy affects 1 in 200 pregnant women. It is important to reassure mothers that over 90 per cent of women can expect a favourable outcome of pregnancy.

Medication

Congenital anomalies/malformations are 1.5–2.5 times more frequent in children born to epileptic mothers taking anticonvulsants. The risk is higher in women taking a combination therapy, so an attempt should be made to stabilise women on mono-therapy prior to starting pregnancy (Table 9.7). If a women has been seizure-free for 2–5 years and has a normal EEG, consideration to attempting weaning and withdrawing therapy should be made. However, the risk of adverse maternal and fetal outcomes from recurrent seizures is greater than the risk of teratogenicity with anticonvulsants.

TABLE 9.7 ADEC drug classifications for anti-epileptic drugs

Drug	Level of risk
Carbamazepine	D
Phenobarbitone, primidone	D
Phenytoin	D
Sodium valproate	D
Benzodiazepines	C
Lamotrigine, tiagabine, topiramate	B3
Gabapentin	B1
Vigabatrin	D

ADEC: see Box 1.17.

For pregnant women with epilepsy:

- Folic acid 5 mg day from three months pre-conception
- Maternal serum alphafetoprotein levels at 15–18 weeks (if taking valproate or carbamazepine)
- Normal ultrasound at 18 weeks to exclude open NTD in 95 per cent
- Vitamin K 10 mg daily in last four weeks of pregnancy if mother taking phenytoin, carbamazepine, barbiturates to reduce the risk of postpartum and neonatal haemorrhage
- Approximately 15–30 per cent of women have increased frequency seizures during pregnancy—usually seen in first trimester and in women with higher pre-conception seizure frequency
- Reduced drug levels and bioavailability phenytoin, phenobarbitone, carbamazepine—monitor levels every 4–6 weeks
- Risk of seizure during labour approximately 1 per cent
- Infant should be given vitamin K

- Breastfeeding encouraged:
  - Phenytoin, valproate highly protein bound—minimal amount in breast milk
  - Carbamazepine and phenobarbitone present in high concentrations—watch for infant sedation
- Risk of epilepsy in offspring of epileptic mothers is approximately 2 per cent
- Contraception: 50 μg oestrogen OCP (especially if taking phenytoin/phenobarbitone more than carbamazepine; there is no effect with valproate).

Renal system

Normal renal system changes in pregnancy

Major renal physiological changes in pregnancy are:

1. Renal plasma flow rises by 60–80 per cent.
2. Glomerular filtration rate rises by 50 per cent.
3. Urine protein excretion may increase markedly in pregnancy without progression of underlying renal disease.

Renal function

- Glomerular filtration rate (GFR) begins to increase within one month of conception, reaching a peak 50 per cent above pre-pregnancy levels by the end of first trimester, decreases by approximately 20 per cent during last trimester, and returns to pre-pregnancy levels within three months of delivery.
- Up to 50 per cent of normal women will have glycosuria at some time during pregnancy, as the increased GFR exceeds the tubular capacity to reabsorb glucose.

Renal structure

- Renal volume increases by approximately 30 per cent.
- In 80 per cent of pregnant women there is dilation of the urine-collecting system, more pronounced on the right side. It is uncertain as to whether this is due to compression of the ureters by the enlarging uterus or ovarian vein plexus, or whether progesterone plays a role through ureteral smooth muscle relaxation. These changes may persist for 3–4 months post partum.

Renal disease in pregnancy

With the exceptions of renal polyarteritis nodosa, scleroderma, SLE and membrano-proliferative glomerulonephritis, the prognosis of pregnancy in women with renal disease is determined by the pre-conception serum creatinine function and the presence or absence of hypertension (Table 9.8).

Proteinuria may increase dramatically during pregnancy without reflecting any deterioration in renal function or superimposed pre-eclampsia. Pre-eclampsia may be difficult to differentiate from flares of lupus nephritis though an active urine sediment and low complements favour the latter.

TABLE 9.8 Renal dysfunction and the impact of pregnancy

Pre-conception creatinine (mmol/L)	Live birth	Prematurity	Worse renal function	Permanent
< 0.13	96%	< 10%	Rare	
0.13–0.22	90%	59%	43%	20–50%
> 0.22	51%	73–86%	> 50%	53%

Management

General principles of managing women with renal disease during pregnancy include optimisation of blood pressure aiming for diastolic BP 80–90 mmHg, correction of anaemia recognising that requirements for erythropoietin are greater during pregnancy, prevention of metabolic acidosis and hypocalcaemia, adequate protein and calorie supply and intensified fetal monitoring from the time of viability.

Dialysis

Where there is deterioration in renal function, dialysis should be initiated once serum creatinine is greater than 0.35 mmol/l, or urea is greater than 20 mmol/l.

Gastrointestinal system

Normal gastrointestinal system changes in pregnancy

Liver function tests in normal pregnancy show normal serum bilirubin and transaminase levels, but reduced total protein and albumin levels. An increase in serum alkaline phosphatase is secondary to placental production.

Vomiting in pregnancy

History

The tendency of early pregnancy to induce nausea is well recognised. It may be worse in the mornings and is often referred to as ‘morning sickness’, although many women experience nausea for the whole day. Hyperemesis gravidarum refers to intractable vomiting resulting in dehydration, electrolyte disturbance and weight loss that requires admission to hospital with the administration of intravenous fluid.

Examination

The woman’s state of hydration should be assessed.

Differential diagnosis

Consider other causes such as appendicitis, cholecystitis, pyelonephritis and bowel obstruction, peptic ulcer disease, hyperparathyroidism, molar pregnancy.

Investigations

1 Fluid and electrolyte balance
2 Renal function, and excluding urinary tract infection that may dispose to vomiting
3 Associated with elevated transaminases, biochemical hyperthyroidism

Treatment

- Most women can manage with conservative treatment. Meals should be of small volume and administered frequently. Sufficient fluids should be taken to prevent dehydration.
- The use of antinauseants may need to be considered and include prochlorperazine maleate (Stemetil) 5 mg orally 4–6 hourly or by suppository, or metoclopramide hydrochloride (Maxolon) 10 mg orally 6-hourly.
- Also pyridoxine, ondansetron and glucocorticoids.
- Supplement thiamine replacement should be considered with prolonged vomiting because of the risk of Wernicke's encephalopathy.

Prognosis

The symptoms usually disappear by the second trimester, but occasionally persist throughout pregnancy, requiring repeated admissions to hospital for intravenous infusions.

Liver disease

Intrahepatic cholestasis of pregnancy

Intrahepatic cholestasis of pregnancy complicates 0.2–0.8 per cent of pregnancies in Australia, with higher prevalence in Scandinavia and Chile. It is characterised by pruritus, elevated bile salts and transaminases. Symptoms may precede biochemical changes by weeks. There are no sequelae for the mother but the fetus is at risk of prematurity, fetal distress and intrauterine death. Ursodeoxycholic acid improves maternal symptoms and biochemical changes. It is not known as to whether it influences fetal prognosis. Antihistamines, cholestyramine and methionine have a variable effect with respect to the maternal pruritus. Delivery should not be delayed beyond 38 weeks gestation. Vitamin K should be considered if the disorder has been present for more than two weeks prior to delivery. It recurs in about 70 per cent of subsequent pregnancies and can also be precipitated by the oral contraceptive pill and hormone replacement therapy in susceptible women.

Acute fatty liver of pregnancy

Acute fatty liver of pregnancy is a rare disorder complicating approximately 1:10 000 pregnancies. It may be found incidentally as a result of abnormal liver function tests, or symptoms may include nausea, vomiting, right upper quadrant pain, jaundice or deterioration in mental state due to fulminant hepatic failure. Investigations reveal elevated transaminases, coagulopathy, hypoglycaemia, neutrophil leucocytosis, low antithrombin III levels and renal failure (acute tubular necrosis) in 60 per cent. Preeclampsia may occur at presentation or at some time during course in 50 per cent and in severe cases infection and intra-abdominal bleeding are common. Treatment is delivery, and supportive care with prevention of hypoglycaemia, fresh frozen plasma if bleeding, prophylactic H2-blockade, dialysis for renal failure, and consideration of liver transplantation. The maternal mortality is 12.5 per cent. Mothers who recover do so fully with no long-term sequelae of the hepatic injury.

HELLP syndrome

HELLP syndrome refers to 20 per cent of patients with severe pre-eclampsia who develop features of microangiopathic haemolytic anaemia, thrombocytopenia and elevated liver enzymes. Other complications include pulmonary oedema, acute renal failure, hepatic infarction or rupture. Treatment is delivery, although several case series and reports have described the use of glucocorticoids ante partum to prolong gestation, as well as post partum to hasten recovery in laboratory parameters.

Endocrine system

Normal thyroid changes in pregnancy

The thyroid gland increases in size due to hyperplasia and increased vascularity. Normal changes to the blood tests:

- total T3 and T4 increase due to increased levels of thyroid-binding globulin (an oestrogen effect)
- reduction in free T3 and T4. (TSH levels required to diagnose hypothyroidism)
- TSH levels decrease in first trimester, with an inverse relationship to HCG.

The fetal thyroid commences function around 10–12 weeks gestation. The placenta acts as a barrier to maternal TSH, T4 and T3 but freely transports iodine and thyrotrophin-releasing hormone and TSH binding/inhibiting immunoglobulin in Graves.

Thyroid disease

Hypothyroidism in pregnancy:

- Fifty per cent of women will need a 50 per cent increase in thyroxine dose during course of pregnancy.
- If TFTs are normal, measure at 6–8 weeks, 16–20 weeks and 28–32 weeks.
- Measure six weeks after any change in dose.
- Iron and calcium supplements may interfere with thyroxine absorption.
- Approximately 3 per cent of women with Hashimoto's disease will have coexistent coeliac disease, which should be excluded given the latter's association with adverse pregnancy outcomes.
- Hyperthyroidism affects 2 in 1000 pregnant women. Antithyroid drugs are safe during pregnancy and breastfeeding.
- Ninety per cent of cases are due to Graves' disease, less commonly toxic adenoma, toxic multinodular goitre, hyperemesis gravidarum, gestational trophoblastic neoplasia.
- Treat with the aim of maintaining free T4 and T3 at the upper end of the normal range.
- Propylthiouracil is preferred to carbimazole during pregnancy and when breastfeeding.
- In approximately 50 per cent of patients the disease will remit during pregnancy, allowing cessation of drug therapy, but there is a need to watch for postpartum relapse.

In women with active Graves', or in those who have previously undergone surgical or radioiodine ablation, the titre of TSH binding/inhibiting immunoglobulin should be checked, as titres greater than five times the reference range are associated with risk of fetal and neonatal thyrotoxicosis.

Diabetes

Diabetes complicating pregnancy can either pre-date the pregnancy (pre-gestational diabetes) or be detected for the first time during the pregnancy (gestational diabetes, GDM). As the epidemic of diabetes escalates, there are increasing numbers of women with type 2 diabetes presenting during pregnancy. The prevalence of both pre-gestational diabetes and GDM depends on the ethnic mix of the patient population—the former complicates around 0.5 per cent and the latter about 3–9 per cent of pregnancies in Australia.

Screening in pregnancy

The diagnosis of gestational diabetes is controversial, especially the question of whether to screen all pregnant women or only those who have specific 'risk factors'.

- The current criteria used in Australia are the ADIPS criteria—fasting blood glucose of ≥ 5.5 mmol/l and/or a two-hour post 75 g glucose load of ≥ 8.0 mmol/l.[45] In Europe a one-step procedure using a two-hour 75 g tolerance test is used.[46] The test used mostly in North America has two steps: screening of a one-hour 50 g glucose challenge test at 24–28 weeks, followed, if positive, by a 100 g three-hour or a 75 g two-hour test.[47]
- Screening is usually performed around 26–28 weeks gestation either by testing all women or if there are one or more risk factors:
  - age ≥ 30 years
  - BMI ≥ 25
  - a family history of diabetes in a first degree relative
  - past history of GDM
  - ethnicity from a group with a high prevalence of type 2 diabetes (eg Aboriginal or Torres Strait Islander, Chinese, Vietnamese, Pacific Islander, Hispanic)
  - previous birth weight of > 4000 g
  - poor obstetric history (eg late intrauterine fetal death).

If there is a high degree of concern then ideally these women should be also tested early in pregnancy to exclude hyperglycaemia during the time of organogenesis.

Pathophysiology

A number of factors increase insulin resistance in pregnancy. Human placental lactogen in early pregnancy increases lipolysis, providing energy for the mother and thus sparing carbohydrates as a nutrient for the fetus. Progesterone, prolactin and cortisol individually and synergistically decrease insulin-mediated glucose uptake. If the woman has a potential degree of impairment of insulin secretion, this pregnancy induced resistance can tip the balance and hyperglycaemia results.

Glucose readily crosses the placenta but maternal insulin cannot so the fetus has to produce excess insulin, which can be demonstrated as early as 19 weeks gestation. The effects of this hyperinsulinism are to stimulate fetal growth (macrosomia 20%) interfere with lung maturation, cause polycythaemia (10–25%) and after delivery neonatal hypoglycaemia (20–40%), jaundice, hypocalcaemia (20–30%), hypomagnesaemia (10–15%) and respiratory distress (1–3%). In the long term the offspring are more likely to develop abnormal glucose tolerance at an early age and to become obese. Good control of maternal blood glucose can reduce these complications. In early pregnancy poorly controlled diabetes can lead to fetal anomalies (neural tube defects, cardiac, bowel and urinary tract anomalies and the rare but characteristic sacral dysgenesis) and also to an increased rate of spontaneous miscarriage. Thus the principal objective of the management of women with diabetes is to normalise the maternal blood glucose levels.[48]

Antenatal

1 *Blood glucose control.* The targets are a fasting BSL < 5.5 mmol/l, 1-hour postprandial < 7.8 mmol/l or 2-hour postprandial < 6.7 mmol/l. For women with pregestational diabetes this usually requires insulin therapy. Women with GDM may achieve the BSL targets with diet and exercise; otherwise insulin therapy, commonly three doses of regular insulin before meals and an intermediate insulin dose prior to bed (four times daily regimen).
2 *Investigations.* A first-trimester ultrasound to confirm gestation, then a detailed morphology scan at 18 weeks to exclude fetal anomalies, and a growth scan around 34 weeks to detect macrosomia or growth restriction, which may occur if there is maternal microvascular disease (diabetic retinopathy or nephropathy). Close observation for other complications such as pre-eclampsia (increased particularly with microvascular disease).
3 *Timing of delivery.* The objective is to deliver at 38 weeks if there is macrosomia, polyhydramnios or sub-optimal diabetic control; otherwise take to full term. Delivery is by elective caesarean section if the estimated birth weight > 4250 g because of the risk of shoulder dystocia. This risk rises from 2 per cent if birth weight < 4000 g, to 14 per cent for birth weight 4000–4500 g, to 55 per cent for birth weight > 4500 g.

Post partum

After delivery the baby needs careful assessment, particularly for neonatal hypoglycaemia. Glucose tolerance returns to pre-pregnancy status within hours of delivery of the fetus and placenta, so most women with GDM return to normal. In the long term 50 per cent will develop type 2 diabetes, so it is very important that they have a postnatal GTT repeated every 2–3 years if normal or annually if impaired.

Cardiovascular system

Normal cardiovascular system changes in pregnancy

There is profound cardiovascular adaptation to support the 'low pressure–high flow' uteroplacental circuit. The major physiological changes are a rise in the cardiac output and blood volume by about 40–50 per cent above pre-conception values by 24 weeks gestation, and a significant reduction in systemic vascular resistance. This reduction in peripheral resistance is offset by an increase in stroke volume and heart rate, and results in a fall in systolic and diastolic blood pressure in second trimester, with a rise back towards pre-conception values at the end of third trimester.

- Rise in cardiac output and blood volume by approximately 50 per cent by 24–28 weeks gestation
- Significant drop in systemic vascular resistance
- Periods of high risk for cardiac decompensation:
  - At the end of second trimester when the blood volume peaks
  - During normal labour
  - Post partum with the shift of fluid into the circulation.

Cardiac disease

Valvular heart disease

Pregnant women with stenotic valve lesions tend to have worsening symptoms during pregnancy and greater potential for morbidity, whereas those with incompetent valves tend to have an improvement in symptoms during pregnancy. In women with mechanical replacement valves, warfarin needs to be replaced with heparin in first trimester because of the 4–8 per cent risk of embryopathy (Box 9.6). It is controversial as to whether warfarin should be recommended after first trimester until 36 weeks gestation, as use in second and third trimester may be associated with late fetal loss, CNS abnormalities and internal fetal bleeding.

Another area of controversy relates as to whether to use antibiotic prophylaxis for uncomplicated vaginal delivery or caesarean section in the setting of abnormal valves. Women who have undergone successful repair of congenital heart disease tolerate pregnancy well.

BOX 9.6 Management of women with prosthetic heart valves

- Anticoagulation:
  - Warfarin: 4–8% incidence first trimester embryopathy, increased incidence miscarriage, late fetal loss, internal fetal bleeding, CNS abnormalities in later trimesters
  - Unfractionated heparin associated with serious thrombosis in approximately 10%
  - LMW heparin until 16 weeks gestation, then warfarin until 36 weeks, then LMW heparin until delivery.

Congenital heart disease

Pregnancy in the setting of severe pulmonary hypertension or Eisenmenger's syndrome is contraindicated given the 50 per cent maternal mortality.

- Women who have undergone successful repair tolerate pregnancy very well.
- Higher risk of maternal/fetal complications with:
  - The New York Heart Association (NYHA) functional classification of heart failure Class III (symptomatic on ordinary exertion) or Class IV (symptomatic at rest)

- Maternal cyanosis or erythrocytosis
- Stenotic lesions
- Presence of a right-to-left shunt.

Ischaemic heart disease

Ischaemic heart disease is uncommon in pregnancy. Myocardial infarction during the course of pregnancy is associated with a 25 per cent maternal mortality. The best non-invasive investigation for suspected myocardial ischaemia during pregnancy is a stress echocardiogram, although coronary angiography, angioplasty and even bypass grafting have been performed safely during pregnancy.

Marfan's syndrome

Marfan's syndrome is an autosomal-dominant connective tissue disorder involving the ocular, musculoskeletal and cardiovascular systems. Its importance in pregnancy relates to the risk of aortic dilatation and dissection.

- Prevalence 4–6/10 000
- Cardiac manifestations—mitral or tricuspid valve prolapse, aortic dilatation, dissection and regurgitation
- Favourable maternal and fetal outcomes where aortic root diameter < 40 mm
- Echocardiography each trimester
- Prophylactic beta-blockers lifelong.

Hypertension

Hypertensive disorders of pregnancy affect 5–10 per cent of all pregnancies and are major contributors to maternal and perinatal morbidity and mortality. The hypertensive disorders of pregnancy account for 15 per cent of maternal deaths.

Chronic hypertension

Chronic hypertension is defined as a blood pressure of equal to or greater than 140/90 mmHg prior to the 20th week of gestation. Chronic hypertension:

- affects 2 per cent women of child-bearing age
- has a 20 per cent risk of superimposed pre-eclampsia.

Investigation

Although very rare, phaeochromocytoma should always be excluded because of its grave maternal and fetal prognosis if undiagnosed. Baseline proteinuria and serum urate should be measured early in pregnancy for comparison later in pregnancy if there is a suspicion of superimposed pre-eclampsia.

Baseline investigations:

- 24-hour urine vanillyl–mandelic acid (VMA)/catecholamines
- Serum urate
- 24-hr urine protein/protein : creatinine ratio
- Check and document reflexes.

Outcomes

Chronic hypertension is also associated with placental abruption and intrauterine fetal growth restriction.

Management

The antihypertensives commonly used in pregnancy are alphamethyldopa, labetalol and nifedipine (Box 9.7). Target blood pressures should be 120–140 mmHg systolic and 80–90 mmHg diastolic.

BOX 9.7 Antihypertensives: ADEC classification

Methyldopa	A	Clonidine	B3
Labetalol	C	Prazosin	B2
Nifedipine	C	Hydralazine	C
Oxprenolol	C		

ADEC: see Box 1.17.

Pre-eclampsia

The incidence of eclampsia is approximately 1:2000, with a mortality rate of 2 per cent. Hypertensive disorders of pregnancy are the leading cause of antenatal hospitalisation in Australia, and are the leading cause of indicated premature delivery. As a result, hypertension in pregnancy is responsible for at least 10 per cent of perinatal deaths, and accounts for 25 per cent of low birth weight infants.

The classification of hypertension in pregnancy is based on that of the Australasian Society for the Study of Hypertension in Pregnancy (Box 9.8). The distinction between gestational hypertension and a mild degree of pre-eclampsia is not shared by all, and inconsistency of terminology is commonplace, unfortunately.

The booking and subsequent antenatal visits may reveal risk factors that suggest vigilance for pre-eclampsia (Box 9.9).

CLINICAL PRESENTATION: Pre-eclampsia

Pre-eclampsia (PET) is a multi-system disorder. Each system may produce specific signs or symptoms of the disease (Box 9.10). Clinical presentation commonly occurs in the antenatal clinic. Early and milder cases may be manifested by only hypertension and oedema, with proteinuria and other manifestations developing subsequently. However, in more fulminant cases it may also be during or after labour with hypertension or one of the complications of PET.

- Signs:
  - Hypertension confirmed on repeated measurements in the antenatal clinic. This is the most frequent presentation.
  - Proteinuria on routine testing

BOX 9.8 Classification of hypertension in pregnancy

Definition of hypertension in pregnancy

A systolic blood pressure (BP) ≥ 140 mmHg and/or a diastolic BP ≥ 90 mmHg

Classification of the hypertensive disorders of pregnancy

A Gestational hypertension

De novo hypertension alone, appearing after gestational week 20

B Pre-eclampsia

De novo hypertension after gestational week 20 (and resolving by three months post partum), and new onset of one or more of the following:

- Proteinuria (≥ 300 mg/day or a spot urine protein/creatinine ratio ≥ 30 mg/mmol)
- Renal insufficiency: creatinine ≥ 0.09 mmol/l or oliguria
- Liver disease: raised transaminases and/or severe right upper quadrant or epigastric pain
- Neurological sequelae: convulsions (eclampsia), hyperreflexia with clonus, severe headaches with hyperreflexia, persistent visual disturbances (scotoma)
- Haematological disturbances: thrombocytopenia, disseminated intravascular coagulation, haemolysis
- Fetal growth restriction

C Chronic hypertension

Presence or history of hypertension preconception or in the first half of pregnancy.

- Essential (90%)
- Secondary (10%): renal, endocrine (phaeochromocytoma, Conn's, Cushing's, coarctation, collagen vascular disease

D Pre-eclampsia superimposed on chronic hypertension

Development of new signs and/or symptoms associated with pre-eclampsia after gestational week 20, as above, in a woman with chronic hypertension.

Based on RANZCOG 2000.[49]

BOX 9.9 Risk factors for pre-eclampsia

- Past history of pre-eclampsia or eclampsia
- First pregnancy (or first pregnancy with a new partner)
- Conditions associated with a large placenta:
  - Multiple pregnancy
  - Molar pregnancy
  - Fetal hydrops
  - Diabetes mellitus
- Maternal vascular disease:
  - Thrombophilia
  - Hypertension
  - Renal disease
  - Collagen vascular disease

- Symptoms:
  - Swelling of lower limbs, fingers, face
  - Headache or visual disturbance
  - Upper abdominal pain (resembling indigestion, right hypochondrial pain from oedema of the liver capsule)
- Complications:
  - Bleeding (ante, intra or post partum) due to thrombocytopenia or coagulopathy
  - Eclampsia
  - Cerebrovascular accident
  - Placental abruption (accidental haemorrhage).

BOX 9.10 Body systems, related signs and symptoms involved in pre-eclampsia

- *Cardiovascular:* hypertension, oedema
- *Renal:* proteinuria, renal impairment
- *Haematological:* thrombocytopenia, coagulopathy
- *Neurological:* headache, visual disturbance, hyperreflexia, eclampsia, cerebrovascular accident
- *Alimentary:* upper abdominal pain, hepatic impairment
- *Respiratory:* pulmonary oedema
- *Uteroplacental:* IUGR, placental abruption, fetal compromise or death

Pathophysiology

The aetiology of pre-eclampsia is complex, multifactorial and not fully understood. It is perhaps best understood as a variety of influences resulting in placenta ischaemia, which in turn releases factor or factors unknown that mediate vasoconstriction, increased capillary permeability and platelet aggregation and microthrombus formation. These changes in physiology are responsible for the widespread symptoms and signs we clinically recognise as pre-eclampsia (Figure 9.5). This model demonstrates why, once developed, pre-eclampsia will progress inexorably until the fetus, and its 'toxic' placenta, are delivered. The rate of progression from hypertension to proteinuria and then widespread systemic disease varies, however, and this is the basis of outpatient or inpatient observation to allow advancement of gestation.

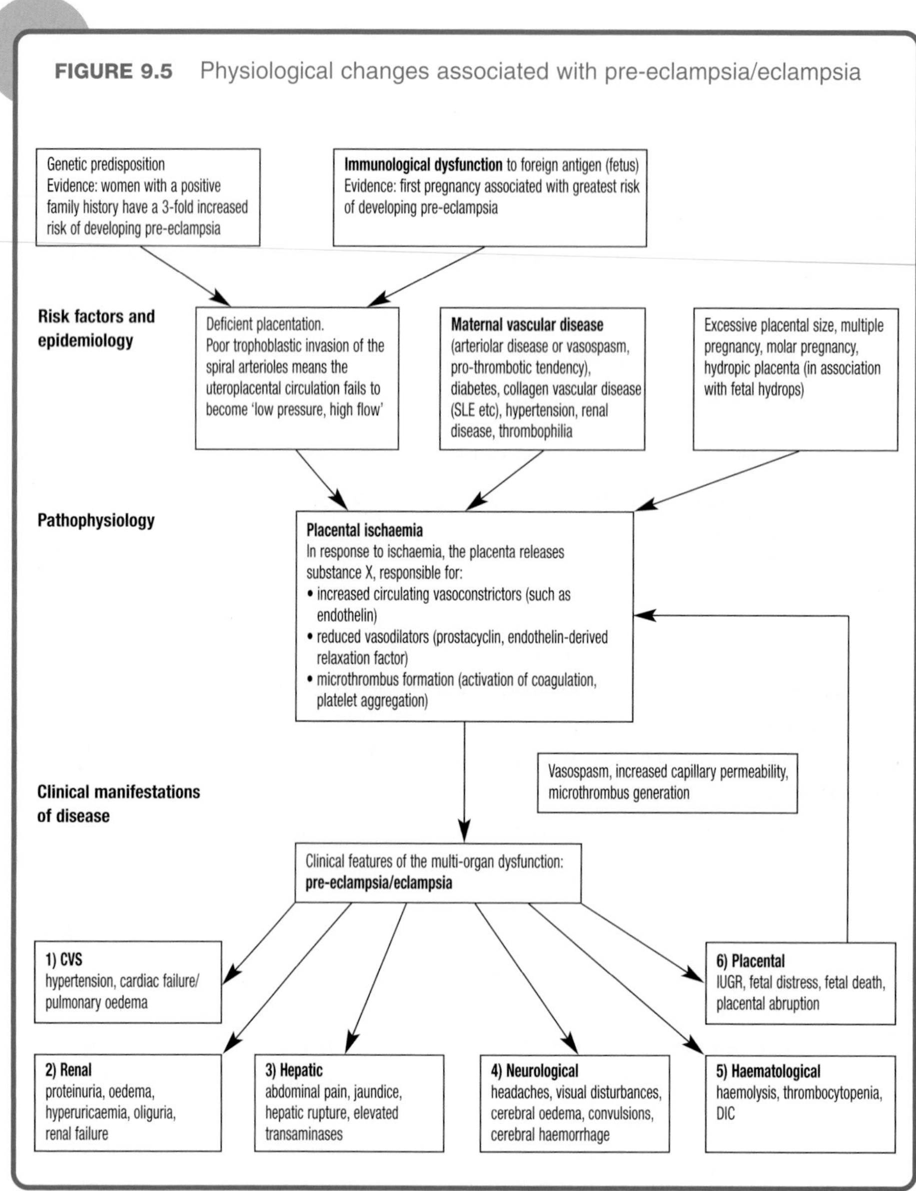

FIGURE 9.5 Physiological changes associated with pre-eclampsia/eclampsia

Investigation

1. Mother:
   - 24-hour urinary protein
   - Uric acid, urea, creatinine, electrolytes
   - Liver function tests
   - Full blood count, coagulation profile
2. Fetus:
   - Cardiotocography
   - Check biophysical profile.

Management

Like many conditions in obstetrics, management of pre-eclampsia will vary according to the severity of the illness and the gestation at diagnosis.

1 *Illness severity.* Delivery is indicated at any gestation if there is evidence of severe pre-eclampsia, ie:
   - uncontrollable blood pressure
   - severe neurological symptoms: eclampsia, cerebral haemorrhage, severe unremitting headache/visual disturbances
   - progressive disturbance of renal or liver function
   - progressive severe thrombocytopenia
   - clear evidence of fetal compromise: critical CTG, reversed end diastolic flow on umbilical artery Doppler, static fetal growth on serial ultrasound examinations.

2 *Fetal maturity.* The earlier the gestation, the more there is to be gained from delaying delivery, assuming fetal well-being has been confirmed. The length of delay will depend on the rate of disease progression, either short term (48 hours to gain steroids) or longer term (days to weeks) to effect a meaningful increase in birth weight and gestation. By contrast, at or around term there is little to be gained from the fetal point of view in delaying delivery, which unnecessarily exposes the mother to the risks of disease progression.

Figure 9.6 represents an algorithm for the management of women with hypertension detected in the antenatal clinic. In general, management consists of increased surveillance of both mother and fetus, with inpatient care as needed and timely delivery.

Severe pre-eclampsia

A diagnosis of severe pre-eclampsia starts a train of measures culminating in the delivery of the baby. The woman with severe pre-eclampsia should be managed and monitored in a high-dependency area such as the delivery suite or high-dependency unit for the immediate peripartum period, involving a team of both obstetricians and anaesthetists. Principles of management of a patient with severe pre-eclampsia are to confirm the diagnosis with maternal and fetal investigations, stabilise and deliver.

1 Stabilisation: prevention and treatment of complications

- *Eclampsia prophylaxis.* The prophylactic anticonvulsant of choice is magnesium sulphate.

  Protocol: Magnesium sulphate 50 per cent is administered via a syringe pump through the peripheral IV line. A 4 g loading dose (8 ml of 50% solution) is given over 30 min (16 ml/hr for 30 min). Patients should be advised of possible transient hot flushing on commencement. $MgSO_4$ is continued at 2–3 g/hr (4–6 ml/hr) until at least 24 hours post delivery. The therapeutic range for Mg (monitored 6-hourly) is 1.7–3.5 mmol/l. The dose is reduced if the knee jerks are abolished, respiratory rate is less than 10/min, urine output is less than 30 ml/hr or levels greater than 3.5 mmol/l

FIGURE 9.6 Management of hypertension detected in the antenatal clinic

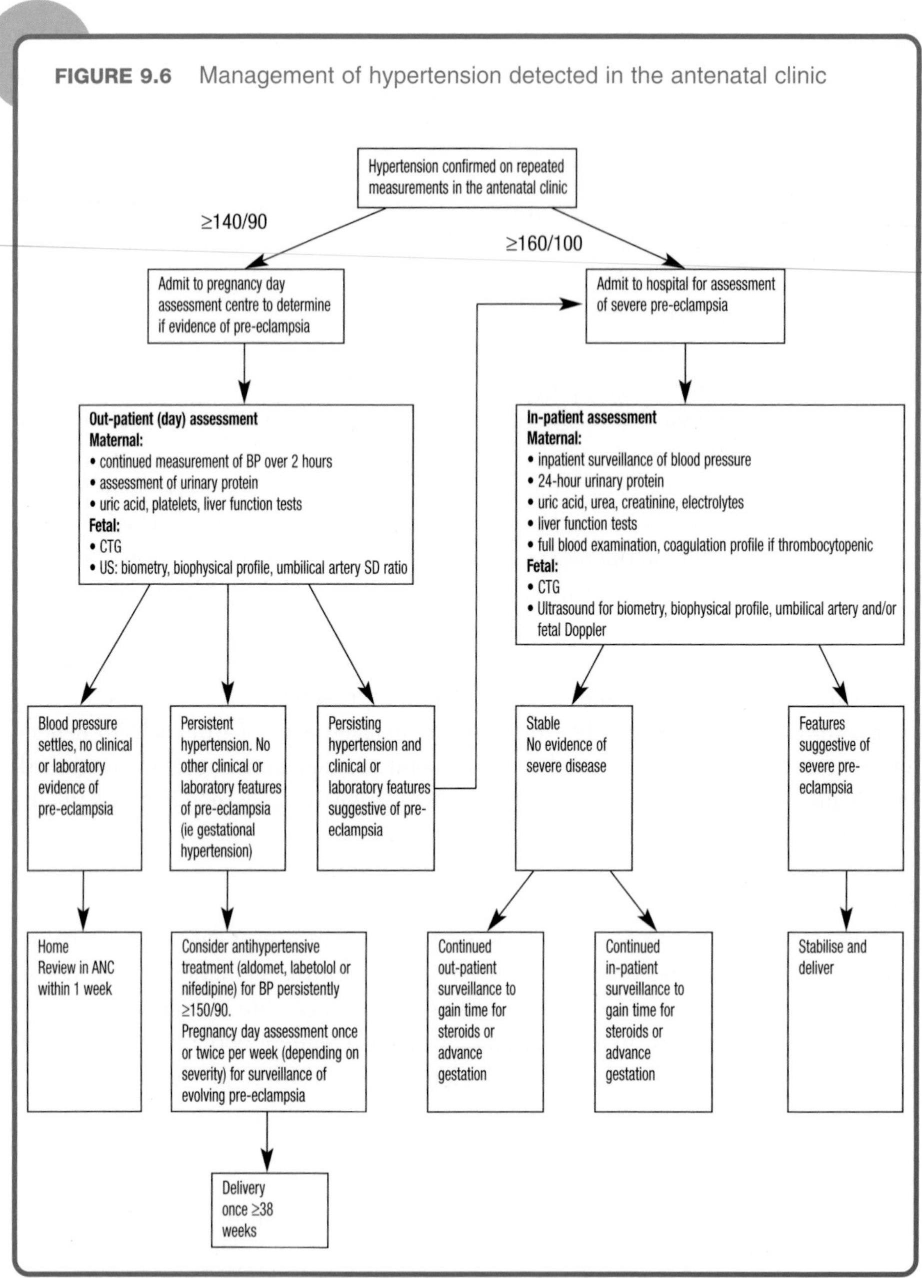

are obtained. The CVP line should not be used for $MgSO_4$ infusion because of marked side effects with sudden bolus doses. Adequate renal throughput is essential as magnesium is excreted renally. In the presence of oliguria, magnesium toxicity may quickly develop. Cardiac arrhythmias and respiratory depression may occur with overdose. Calcium chloride (5 ml of 10% solution) may be given IV slowly as an antidote if an accidental overdose occurs.

- *Blood pressure control.* The limits of autoregulation occur at blood pressures ≥ 170/110, with the attendant risk of cerebral haemorrhage. Therefore, antihypertensive should be instituted at or slightly below this level with parenteral antihypertensive, such as hydralazine. An epidural anaesthetic is often a useful adjunct. It should be noted that nifedipine should not be administered to women receiving magnesium sulphate, due to the possible synergistic effect on calcium metabolism. Hydralazine should be administered by syringe pump with 60 mg of hydralazine diluted to 60 ml with normal saline to produce a 1 mg/ml solution. Initially, hydralazine is given as a 5–10 mg bolus over 5–10 min via the peripheral IV line and then by continuous infusion starting at 5 mg/hr. The rate of infusion should be adjusted according to blood pressure response, aiming for 140/90 to 160/100 mmHg. Lower is undesirable, as it may threaten uteroplacental perfusion.
- *Intravascular volume depletion.* Patients with severe pre-eclampsia are intravascularly deplete, as evidenced by oliguria. If adequate renal throughput is not maintained, acute tubular necrosis and renal failure may ensue. For this reason, a urinary catheter should be inserted on admission, and hourly urinary output measured.
  In the presence of oliguria, intravenous replacement should be cautious, bearing in mind that patients with severe pre-eclampsia also have 'leaky capillaries' and low oncotic pressure, so are at risk of pulmonary oedema with over-zealous volume loading. To assist in these situations of difficult volume control, a central venous catheter should be inserted, and fluid replaced to a maximum of 8 mmHg to ensure a urinary output of > 0.5 ml/kg/hr. If facilities for a CVP are unavailable, a pulse oximeter should be kept on continuously to observe for any early signs of desaturation, suggesting pulmonary oedema.
- *Haematological abnormalities.* Platelets (minimum of six units) should be given for severe thrombocytopenia (< 30×10^9) where delivery is imminent. Platelet infusion may be indicated even with a higher platelet count (eg 40×10^9) in the presence of active bleeding. Epidural anaesthesia is generally contraindicated with a platelet count < 80×10^9.
  Fresh frozen plasma should be administered for clotting abnormalities, and occasionally cryoprecipitate (a more concentrated preparation of clotting factors) is chosen to minimise the volume given intravenously.
- *Other complications.* Pulmonary oedema should be avoided by judicious fluid management. If it occurs, oxygen should be administered to maintain oxygen saturations > 95 per cent, and diuretics may occasionally be required.

2 Regular reassessment of maternal and fetal condition

- *Maternal:* clinical assessment involves regular review for the onset of new symptoms, blood pressure measurements at least hourly, respiratory rate

and ongoing assessment of volume status by hourly urinary output measurement ± central venous pressure line. Laboratory reassessment should include: 6-hourly magnesium levels and repeat assessment of renal, liver and coagulation status as determined by the patient's condition (often 6–12 hourly).
- *Fetal:* assuming a viable gestation, fetal well-being should be confirmed with continuous fetal heart rate monitoring until delivery.

3 Delivery

The timing and mode of delivery will depend on gestation, disease severity, and the likely induction-to-delivery interval. Delivery is indicated immediately after stabilisation by caesarean section in the presence of fulminating disease (neurological complications, hepatic rupture, progressively deteriorating coagulopathy, renal or liver function or acute fetal compromise).

In the absence of these features, the patient may be sufficiently stable to briefly delay delivery. This may enable the administration of corticosteroids (allowing 24–48 hours to maximise fetal lung maturity) and/or the administration of prostaglandin gel, with the view to achieving a vaginal delivery in 12–24 hours. Vaginal delivery in a patient with severe pre-eclampsia is safe, but in the presence of significant hypertension, prolonged pushing should be avoided and oxytocin rather than ergometrine used for third stage management

4 Management of eclamptic fit

The principles of management of an eclamptic fit are as follows:
- Protect the patient.
- Protect the airway (position on left side).
- Administer oxygen.
- Secure intravenous access.
- Terminate convulsion with intravenous diazepam (5–10 mg).
- Monitor blood pressure every five minutes until controlled, then every 15 minutes.

Thereafter, the maternal and fetal condition should be reassessed and subsequent management should be as for severe pre-eclampsia.

5 Postpartum care

The patient should continue to be managed as for severe pre-eclampsia in the immediate postpartum period, and magnesium sulphate is continued until there are signs of resolution. This generally occurs within 24–48 hours of delivery, and is often heralded by a significant diuresis, as fluid from the third space re-enters the intravascular space, and renal perfusion improves. Blood pressure control improves, and laboratory indices start to normalise. The platelet count nadir is about 27 hours post delivery. Hypertension generally resolves as quickly as it came on; if continuing antihypertensives are required, the patient should be switched from hydralazine back to labetolol or nifedipine.

6 Counselling

Women should be counselled postnatally that:

- The recurrence risk in a subsequent pregnancy is about 50 per cent, although the disease is generally less severe and comes on later in gestation.
- Pre-eclampsia does not predispose to the development of essential hypertension later in life.
- The combined oral contraceptive pill is safe.
- Investigations should be directed towards an underlying cause (particularly if severe, early onset disease), ie 24-hour urinary protein/creatinine clearance, renal function tests, thrombophilia screen.
- Prevention with aspirin in a subsequent pregnancy should be considered if severe early-onset disease, or associated with severe intrauterine growth restriction.

SECTION 10

Induction of labour, assisted deliveries and postnatal problems

Choice for women

It is generally agreed that the woman should be part of any decision-making process and that her views and choice must be taken into account. There is evidence that where women are part of the decision-making process, a successful outcome and psychological well-being are more likely to occur. Now that women are having fewer babies and the chance of dying in childbirth is low, how much choice should women have in the mode of their delivery? The ideal for most women would be an uneventful pregnancy, labour and a normal vaginal delivery. This is more likely to be achieved for the woman who has spontaneous onset of labour, no interventions and one-to-one support.[1] However, even for a woman without any factors indicating an increased risk for a problem, there is no guarantee that the ideal will be attained. Risk selection during pregnancy may predict a lower risk during delivery, but major risks (placental abruption or the need for emergency caesarean section) cannot be reduced to zero.

Elective caesarean section

Given the choice, not all women would choose an elective caesarean section. At present a woman has no legal right to request a caesarean section. A number of arguments are given to women who make this request.

- Childbirth is a natural event.
- There is increased risk of morbidity and mortality from operative delivery (although higher from an emergency procedure than a planned one: it has been observed in the UK that there has yet to be a death reported of a previously well woman who has undergone an elective section under epidural anaesthetic with thrombo-prophylaxis and antibiotic cover.[2])
- Hospital care for caesarean sections costs more than for vaginal deliveries.

There are additional factors that need to be considered:

- Long-term costs of pelvic floor damage: anal incontinence and urinary incontinence.
- Medico-legal costs that may be involved in the case of an injured baby.
- Time saved off work by the woman and her partner by planning the date.
- Reduction of staff and equipment costs when used in a more efficient manner.
- Greater satisfaction from being given a choice.

The future

Encouraging women to view vaginal birth positively would promote satisfaction.[3] Both planned caesarean sections and vaginal delivery are not without risks (Boxes 10.1 and 10.2). It is suggested that a woman should be able to ask for a caesarean provided she is fully informed.[4] At present there is inadequate information on 'intention to treat' benefits and risks—a comparison of women of low risk choosing an elective caesarean compared to those choosing to attempt a vaginal delivery.[5] Both women and their medical practitioners need more information on this issue for an informed decision to be agreed upon.[6]

BOX 10.1 Elective caesarean versus vaginal delivery: maternal factors to consider

Operative risks

- Immediate morbidity and mortality from:
  - Haemorrhage
  - Infection
  - Bladder/ureter damage
  - Thromboembolic disease
  - Anaesthetic problems
- Long term:
  - Adhesions
  - Increased risk of placenta praevia[7] (repeat caesarean section more likely)
  - Increased risk of placenta accreta (added risk of hysterectomy)

Operative benefits

- Immediate:
  - Elective surgery has lower risks than emergency surgery

Vaginal risks

- Immediate:
  - Assisted vaginal delivery may be necessary—damage to maternal tissues
  - Failed vaginal delivery—emergency C/S
- Long term:
  - Urinary incontinence increased (up to a third of women after vaginal delivery and it is suggested that the lifetime risk for requiring surgery for incontinence or prolapse is 11%)
  - Faecal incontinence increased (anal sphincter is ruptured in 35% of women with their first vaginal delivery[8])

Vaginal benefits

  - Speedier recovery
  - Earlier discharge home
  - Increased satisfaction

BOX 10.2 Elective caesarean versus vaginal delivery: fetal factors to consider

Operative risks

- Fetal morbidity due to:
  - Compromised respiratory function—transient tachypnoea and respiratory distress syndrome
  - Prematurity if dates miscalculated

Vaginal risks

- Fetal death:
  - Unexpected antepartum stillbirth increases from 37 to 42 weeks
- Fetal morbidity:
  - Shoulder dystocia
  - Instrumentation problems: laceration, nerve palsies, cephalohaematoma or retinal haemorrhage
  - Neonatal encephalopathy (possibly 15% due to intrapartum causes)

Induction of labour

Induction of labour is an intervention to initiate labour. Ideally it should be associated with one or more specific evidence-based indications. It should be performed with the informed consent of the woman following a detailed explanation of the indications, methods, possible outcomes and complications.

CLINICAL PRESENTATIONS

- Post dates: the slight reduction in perinatal mortality that this intervention produces is such that approximately 500 inductions of labour may be necessary to prevent one perinatal death.[9]
- Continuation of the pregnancy threatens the health of the mother (eg the threats of cerebrovascular damage from uncontrolled pre-eclampsia, risk of genital tract sepsis with premature rupture of membranes).
- A perceived threat to the life or health of the unborn infant (eg maternal diabetes mellitus, iso-immunisation, placental abruption, intrauterine fetal growth restriction).
- Induction of labour may be requested by the woman on social grounds. This produces an ethical dilemma between a woman's choice and an intervention that is not medically indicated. Discussion of the risks and benefits is essential to the decision making.

Contraindications

Absolute contraindications are few: transverse lie and low-lying placenta. Relative contraindications include unstable lie, hydramnios.

Clinical assessment

1. *History:* induction of labour should only occur with the knowledge that the gestation is correct.
2. *Examination:*
   - *Abdominal*—check lie, position, and engagement of presenting part, volume of amniotic fluid
   - *Vaginal*—check 'favourability' or 'ripeness' of the cervix; pre-labour cervical changes of dilatation and shortening (effacement) may be assessed using the Bishop score (Table 10.1).

Methods

- *Amniotomy* (ARM or artificial rupture of the membranes): it is unclear why amniotomy causes labour to occur in most instances, but it is most successful when the cervix is 'ripe'.
- *Prostaglandins* are hormones naturally present in the uterus that cause contractions during labour. The local action of prostaglandins may be used to soften and ripen the cervix. Prostaglandin E2α, as a vaginally administered gel, is the most popular method of undertaking 'cervical ripening'.

TABLE 10.1 Assessing the cervix (based on the Bishop score)

Score	0	1	2	3
Cervix				
Cervical dilatation (cm)	< 1	1–2	2–3	> 4
Effacement (cervical length in cm)	> 4	2–4	1–2	< 1
Consistency	Firm	Medium	Soft	
Position (in relation to the pelvic axis)	Posterior		Mid/Anterior	
Fetal head				
Station (position in relation to ischial spines)	−3	−2	−1 to 0	+1

A high score (8 or more) makes successful induction likely. A low score makes successful induction by artificial rupture of the membranes unlikely unless some cervical preparation is undertaken first.[10]

- *Membrane 'sweeping'* at digital vaginal examination detaches the membranes from the lower uterine segment and may initiate labour by the local production of prostaglandins. Sweeping of the membranes, performed as a general policy in women at term, is associated with reduced frequency of pregnancy continuing beyond 41 weeks and 42 weeks. The number needed to treat (NNT) to avoid one formal induction of labour is seven.[9] This procedure may be uncomfortable for many women. Whether or not this method is appropriate is the source of current debate.[9]
- *Intravenous oxytocin* (syntocinon). This may be administered alone or used to supplement the effect of an ARM or prostaglandins. It should not be started for six hours following administration of vaginal prostaglandins. A recommended regimen should be followed, increasing the dose at intervals of 20–30 minutes until a maximum of 3–4 contractions occur every 10 minutes or to the maximum recommended rate.
- *Misoprostol* (unlicensed) is a prostaglandin E1 analogue. It has the advantages of being inexpensive, easily stored at room temperature, with few systemic side effects, and is rapidly absorbed orally and vaginally. Vaginal misoprostol is effective, although the occasional but serious adverse events of uterine hyperstimulation and uterine rupture are of concern. This needs further evaluation before it is introduced into regular practice.[11]

Management

Induction of labour is a positive experience for most women where there has been involvement in the decision making and adequate information provided.[12]

A primigravida suitable for prostaglandin induction can be admitted to a day ward. After insertion of prostaglandin gel the mother and fetus are monitored for six hours. If the cervix is unchanged, the prostaglandin can be repeated or the mother allowed home overnight to return the next day for a repeat dose. If the second dose fails to induce cervical changes, the reason for the induction should be reassessed and the management discussed with the woman. Postponement for a day or two in the non-urgent situation is feasible but may be difficult for the woman to accept. A woman who is a multigravida is most often monitored on the labour ward from the beginning of the induction, as the uterus can be expected to be more responsive to prostaglandin. Once the membranes are ruptured there is a commitment to deliver the woman within 24 hours.

Complications

Complications of induction of labour are rare, but they should be balanced by a specific reason for intervention. Potential complications of induction include:

- General complications:
  - *Failure of induction.* Where induction is necessary in the presence of an unripe cervix, the likelihood of caesarean section is approximately 35 per cent.
  - *Unexpected prematurity* if an error has occurred in the calculated dates.
  - *Postpartum haemorrhage* (RR 2.0 compared to spontaneous labour).
  - *Infection* if the induction–delivery interval is prolonged (> 24 hours) after the membranes rupture.
- Specific to the method used:
  - *Amniotomy:* rupture of a vasa praevia or prolapse of the umbilical cord.
  - *Oxytocin:* excessive uterine activity that might lead to a prolonged uterine contraction, rupture or increase the risk of amniotic fluid embolus. Neonatal hyperbilirubinaemia may be related to the dose and duration of oxytocic use.
  - *Prostaglandins:* the added risk of scar dehiscence needs consideration for a woman with a previous lower uterine segment scar. The risk is slightly increased with the use of an oxytocin infusion, and significantly increased with the use of prostaglandins. Amniotomy alone or repeat caesarean section are the safest available choices in such circumstances.

Abnormal labour

Progress in labour will be achieved if the baby progressively moves through the pelvis. The appropriate response to poor progress in labour depends on the stage of labour, the well-being of the fetus, the presence or absence of complicating factors in the pregnancy, and the wishes of the woman.

Delay in the first stage of labour

If cervical dilatation is less than 3–4 cm the woman is, by definition, not in the active phase of labour. Programs which delay the admission of women to birth suites until the active phase of labour may reduce the incidence of subsequent interventions for poor progress in labour.[13]

Partogram

Once in active labour, the progress and observations are recorded on the partogram (Section 7). Average progress may vary between populations. Primigravida are expected to progress at 0.5–1 cm/hour and multigravida at > 1 cm/hour. An 'alert line' is marked on the partogram at two hours to the right of the expected normal. An 'action line' is added two hours to the right of this. Delay in labour is suggested when the warning line is crossed, and diagnosed by the crossing of the action line (Figure 10.1).

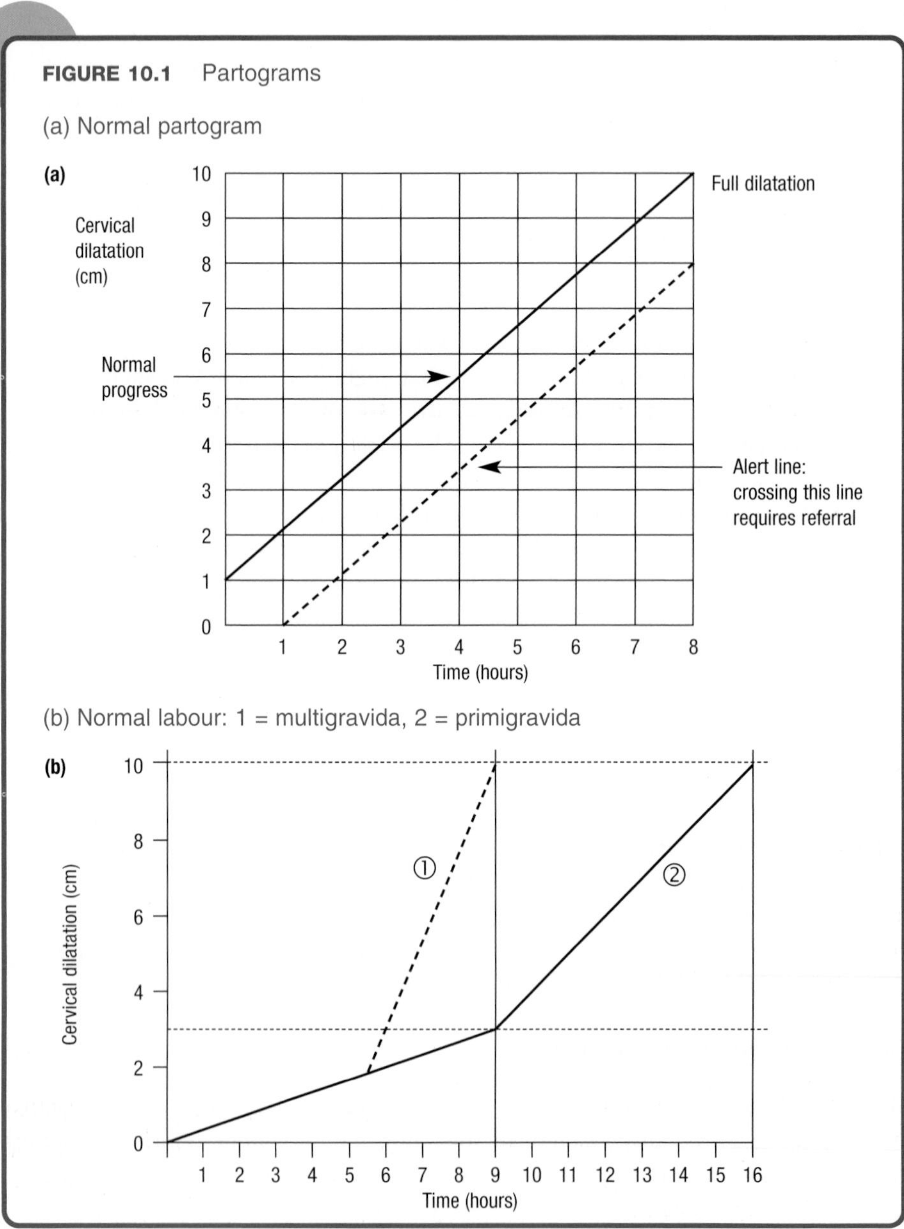

FIGURE 10.1 Partograms

(a) Normal partogram

(b) Normal labour: 1 = multigravida, 2 = primigravida

FIGURE 10.1 continued (c) Active management of labour: 1 = expected dilatation, 2 = actual dilatation (slow progress), 3 = syntocinon commenced and membranes ruptured, 4 = delivery achieved

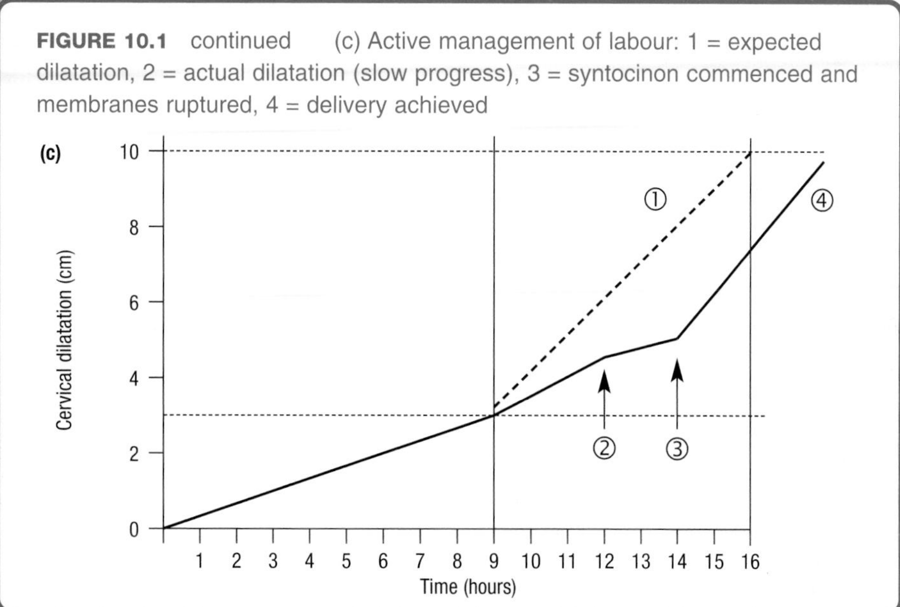

Differential diagnosis

Reasons for the delay in the first stage of labour to be considered:

1 Maternal:
   - Pelvis: size and shape (in relation to the presenting part)
   - Uterus: inefficient uterine action
   - Other: exhaustion

2 Fetal:
   - Position: occipito-transverse, occipito-posterior
   - Presentation: face, brow, shoulder
   - Other: macrosomia, fetal abnormality

The baby

The fetal head enters the pelvis in the occipito-tranverse position, rotating in most cases to the occipito-anterior position for delivery (Section 7). The degree of extension and malrotation of the head will influence the diameter of the fetal head and the progress through the pelvis (Figure 10.2).

Management of delayed labour

1 Review mother and baby: assess contractions, fetal heart, abdominal and vaginal examination.

2 Ambulation: encourage the labouring woman to move around, as this has been shown to improve progress in labour.

3 Augmentation of labour to improve the contractions by amniotomy, followed by the use of an intravenous infusion of oxytocin may be considered and may improve progress if this is the cause for the delay. This form of management is primarily indicated in primigravidae and is often used in conjunction with

epidural anaesthesia. Augmentation techniques should be used with caution in parous women, as poor-quality labour is more likely to be due to undiagnosed obstructed labour, and the use of an oxytocin infusion may lead to uterine rupture.

4 Once the uterine activity has been satisfactory, cessation of progress during the first stage of labour can be said to be due to feto-maternal disproportion (cephalo-pelvic disproportion, CPD). In such a circumstance, with the cervix less than fully dilated, caesarean section is the only safe available mode of delivery of the baby.

FIGURE 10.2 The fetal head (a) Flexion of the fetal head (b) Examination of fetal head to determine position (c) Outcomes of an occipito-posterior position

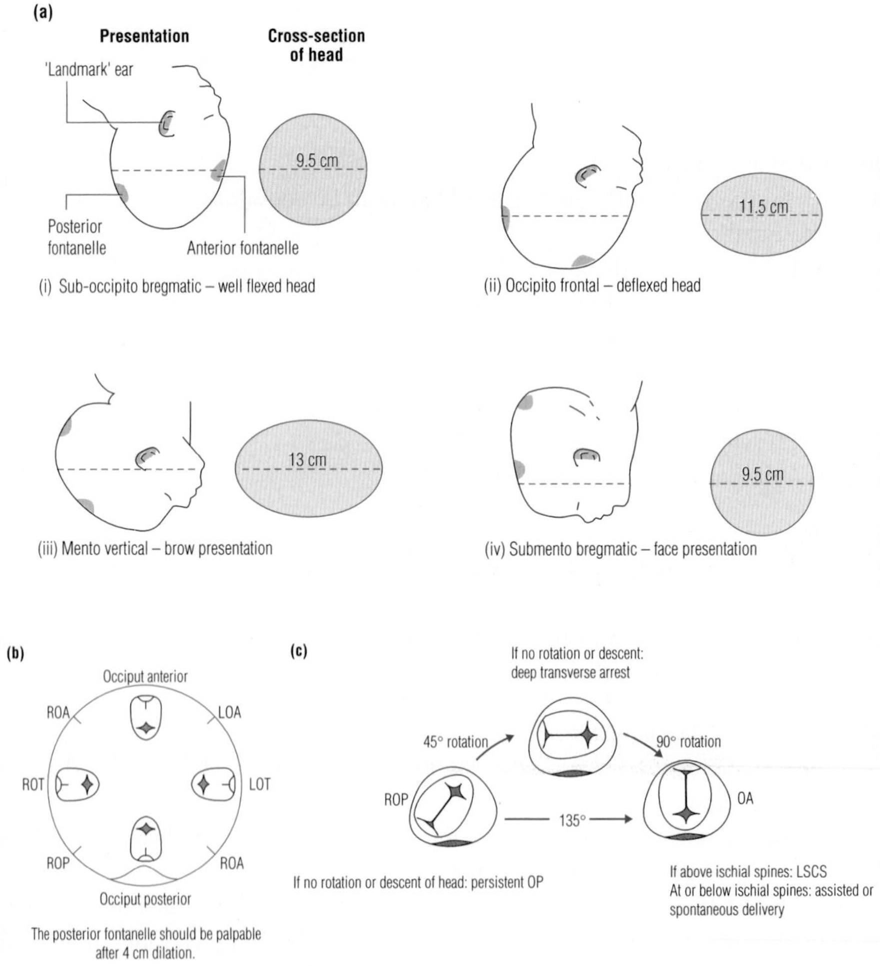

Delay in the second stage of labour

It was traditionally taught that the second stage of labour should not last more than two hours in a primigravida, and one hour in a multigravida. This is now modified to include only the phase of active pushing, and longer second stages may be acceptable in the presence of epidural analgesia.

Engagement means that the largest diameter of the fetal head has passed through the plane of the true pelvic brim. Any suggestion that the head is not engaged, after a period of appropriate augmentation, should lead to a caesarean section birth.

If the head is engaged the options available to assist the birth are vacuum extraction, forceps and the simple expedient of performing an episiotomy (Figure 10.3). The decision to use these techniques or perform a caesarean section will

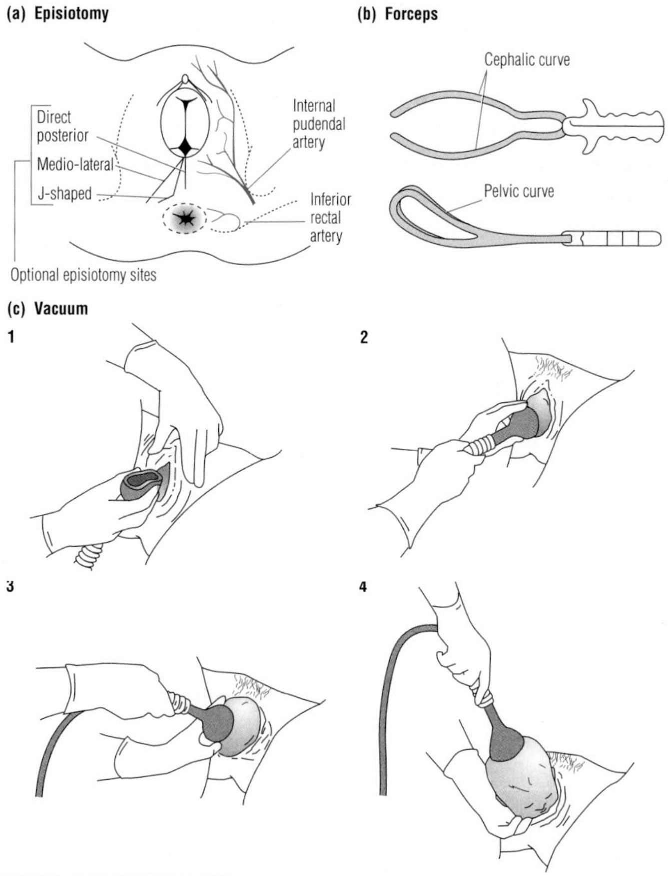

FIGURE 10.3 Methods to assist delivery (a) Episiotomy can be made in a direct posterior, mediolateral and in between in a J-shaped position.The direct episiotomy is associated with more third degree extensions. (b) Forceps have two curves: a cephalic one to fit around the baby's head, and a pelvic one to fit the shape of the birth canal. (c) The vacuum extractor can be used to assist the mother to expedite vaginal delivery

depend on the station (level), position, and degree of flexion of the head, and on the expertise and training of the operator. Vacuum extraction is primarily effective because its appropriate use assists flexion and rotation of the head, and hence the presentation of a smaller and more appropriate fetal head diameter to the maternal pelvic outlet. Forceps-assisted birth adds traction to the maternal pushing effort, and in some circumstances also rotates the head into a more advantageous position. Poor progress with the use of either of these techniques should lead to caesarean section (Section 18). The woman will require adequate analgesia or anaesthesia for an assisted delivery.

Abnormal fetal presentations

Cephalic presentations

The position and degree of flexion are verified on vaginal examination. The landmarks on the fetal head to determine this are the anterior and posterior fontanelles and the ear (Figure 10.2).

1 *Occipito-posterior position* is more common in primigravidae than in multigravidae. The outcomes may be: a longer labour associated with marked backache but with full rotation to an occipito anterior position and vaginal delivery; a partial or no rotation so that the head remains in the occipito-tranverse diameter (requiring an instrumental/operative delivery); or a persistent posterior position that may deliver spontaneously or require medical assistance (Figure 10.2).
2 *Face presentation* is uncommon, and more usually occurs in a multigravid woman. In this circumstance, the fetal neck is fully extended and the presenting submento bregmatic diameter is no greater than the sub-occipito bregmatic diameter that presents with a fully flexed head. If the fetal chin is anterior in the mother's pelvis, labour will progress normally, and this malposition may not be diagnosed until the head appears at the introitus; if the fetal chin is posterior, obstructed labour will usually result.
3 *Brow presentation* is rare and presents the largest of all the fetal cephalic diameters to the maternal pelvis. If labour is significantly preterm, spontaneous vaginal birth may occur, but virtually all term labours with a true brow presentation will end in caesarean section for obstructed labour.

Breech presentation

The fetus commonly lies in the breech position during the pregnancy: at 30 weeks 15 per cent, at 36 weeks 6 per cent and by term 3 per cent. External cephalic version at term can reduce non-cephalic births by 60 per cent.[14] However, this may carry a number of rare risks—fetal bradycardia, placental abruption.[15]

The Term Breech Trial showed a 1 per cent increased risk of perinatal death and a 2.4 per cent increased risk of serious neonatal morbidity when vaginal birth was planned.[16] These results cannot be extrapolated to premature babies or a twin pregnancy. The maternal morbidity was not increased in the Term Breech Trial but was significant in another meta-analysis.[17] The risks and benefits may need to be balanced in individual cases. Management of breech delivery may vary, with some obstetricians recommending an elective caesarean for all, others selecting appropriate term breech babies for whom to recommend a vaginal delivery.

Multiple pregnancy

The number of multiple pregnancies is increasing as a result of infertility treatment. Many are diagnosed early by ultrasound and, in some of these, one twin will die and be absorbed before 20 weeks gestation. The main risk to a twin pregnancy is that of prematurity. Most twin pregnancies will complete 37 weeks and can anticipate a normal vaginal delivery if the first twin is lying longitudinally. The position of the second twin is assessed after the delivery of the first and the lie can be made longitudinal by external or internal cephalic version.

Assisted and operative delivery

Of all deliveries between and within countries, forceps and vacuum (Ventouse) delivery account for between 10–30 per cent and caesarean section 15–20 per cent.

Forceps delivery

Indications

These include:

- Second stage problems—fetal distress, delay, maternal distress
- Control of the head in a breech delivery

Complications

These can include:

- Maternal—damage to vagina and rectum, bleeding from lacerations and episiotomy
- Fetal—scalp haematoma, temporary facial palsy.

Vacuum delivery

Vacuum delivery is becoming increasingly popular. It can be used to expedite delivery, flex the fetal head and for an occipito-posterior or occipito-transverse position. It is associated with less maternal morbidity than forceps delivery.[18]

Complications

- Maternal—damage to the cervix or vaginal wall if this is inadvertently caught under the vacuum cup
- Fetal—scalp haematoma, which usually resolves uneventfully.

Caesarean section

This may be elective (planned with the woman not in labour) or emergency. A repeat caesarean section is performed when the indication for the initial one is considered to be a recurrent or persisting problem (such as a small pelvis). In general about two-thirds of women try for a vaginal delivery after a previous caesarean section (vaginal birth after caesarean—VBAC) and approximately 60–70 per cent of these are successful.

Indications

Indications for caesarean section include:

- Relative cephalo-pelvic disproportion (CPD)—cervical dilatation and descent of the fetal head are arrested during labour. This may be related to the degree of flexion and position of the head and may not necessarily be recurrent.
- Absolute CPD—a reduced pelvic size
- Placenta praevia
- Fetal distress—intrapartum hypoxia occurs in about 1 per cent of labours. Once the decision to proceed to caesarean section has been made, this should be expedited as quickly and safely as possible.[19]
- Fetal malposition/malpresentation
- Maternal request.

Complications

See Section 18.

Postpartum problems

Morbidity in the postpartum period has been shown to be common, with 85 per cent of 1249 women surveyed reporting a health problem while still in hospital and 76 per cent still reporting a health problem six weeks later.[20] Severe maternal morbidity has a reported incidence of 12.0/1000 deliveries and most events were related to obstetric haemorrhage, severe pre-eclampsia and sepsis.[21] The factors independently associated with severe morbidity were:

- Age > 34 years
- Non-white ethnic group
- Past or current hypertension
- Previous postpartum haemorrhage
- Delivery by emergency caesarean section
- Antenatal admission to hospital
- Multiple pregnancy
- Social exclusion
- Taking iron or antidepressant medication at booking.

It is suggested that severe maternal morbidity may be an additional measure of obstetric care in developed countries where the maternal mortality rate is low. Other conditions, although less severe, can cause immediate morbidity and some long-term health effects.

CLINICAL PRESENTATION: Maternal fever

Postpartum or puerperal fever is defined as an increase in temperature to 380°C within 14 days of delivery or miscarriage and is a notifiable disease.

Differential diagnosis

The specific diagnosis will be determined from the history with confirmation on examination, supported by investigation.

- *Genital tract infection.* Associated pain, vaginal discharge and/or bleeding may be present. Increased risk after prolonged rupture of membranes, long labour, operative delivery, trauma or incision of perineum. In addition, the possibility of retained placental tissue or a haematoma should be considered. After cervical swabs, blood culture and blood count, an ultrasound might detect retained products or haematoma. Evacuation of the uterus or a haematoma may be required after commencing intravenous antibiotics.
- *Breast infection.*
- *Urinary tract infection.* Symptoms of urinary frequency, dysuria and/or loin pain will be supported by a raised white cell count in the urine and the culture of a specific organism. More likely after catheterisation and trauma to the bladder during labour.
- *Wound infection.* Either abdominal or perineal. Treat with antibiotics after taking appropriate swabs for culture. Evacuate any haematoma, drain and local toilet with either closure once clean or healing by secondary intent.
- *Intercurrent.* Any other infections may occur. Diarrhoea may suggest puerperal sepsis.

CLINICAL PRESENTATION: Mother complaining of pain

Abdominal pain

Urinary retention is more likely to occur in nulliparous women after a long labour, epidural anaesthetic, instrumental delivery and perineal damage.[22] After initial catheterisation and management of any local problems, normal function can be restored and there is resolution of the problem.

Abdominal pain may also be a feature of endometritis, wound infection or other abdominal conditions (eg acute appendicitis, gastroenteritis).

Chest pain

Pleuritic pain should alert to the possibility of pulmonary or amniotic fluid embolus. In addition, chest infections may occur subsequent to general anaesthesia.

Perineal pain

Discomfort from an episiotomy or lacerations is common post partum. Pain in the area should warrant careful inspection to exclude an infection or haematoma—remember that the latter may track along the vagina and pelvic side-wall, so the extent may not be immediately apparent. Drainage or conservative management will depend on the individual situation. The continuous subcuticular technique of perineal repair may be associated with less pain in the immediate postpartum period than the interrupted suture technique.[23]

Leg pain

Pregnancy and post partum are hypercoagulable states (Section 9). Calf pain and/or tenderness associated with swelling, pitting oedema, increased skin temperature and superficial venous dilatation suggests a deep venous thrombosis. Diagnosis can be confirmed with compression ultrasonography and D-dimer concentrations (a by-product of fibrin production). Deep venous thrombosis occurs during pregnancy in 0.6/1000 women < 35 years and 1.2/1000 women > 35 years; post partum in 0.3/1000 women < 35 years and 0.7/1000 women > 35 years. Rapid effective anticoagulation should be started and continued according to the woman's risk profile.[24] There is insufficient evidence to suggest routine benefit from thromboprophylaxis during pregnancy and post partum.[25]

CLINICAL PRESENTATION: Vaginal bleeding

Primary postpartum haemorrhage is defined as bleeding from the genital tract in the first 24 hours after delivery (Section 11); secondary postpartum haemorrhage occurs from 24 hours to 12 weeks post partum. Problems with vaginal bleeding between 28 days and 3 months post partum are reported in 20 per cent of women in the community, the most common being excessive or prolonged bleeding.[26] There has been limited research in this area to determine cause, management or outcome. In developed countries 2 per cent of women are admitted to hospital with secondary postpartum haemorrhage. Fifty per cent of these undergo uterine evacuation for possible retained products of pregnancy and most are treated with antibiotics for a proven or presumed endometritis. Possible long-term sequelae may be similar for other forms of pelvic inflammatory disease (Section 13).

CLINICAL PRESENTATION: Incontinence

Urinary incontinence

Urinary incontinence is a problem seen in one in three women after childbirth. It is probably multifactorial in origin including: first childbirth, genetic predisposition (tissue factors), instrumental delivery, long second labour stage.[27] The risk is reduced but not eliminated with abdominal delivery. There has been little research in the area and the value of prenatal assessment and pelvic floor exercise has not been fully evaluated.[28] Pelvic floor exercise post partum has limited benefit.[29]

Anal incontinence

Midline episiotomy predisposes to the development of incontinence of flatus and faeces during the first six months post partum compared to women who had spontaneous perineal tearing or did not have an episiotomy. Perineal massage in labour has not been shown to reduce the incidence of perineal, urinary or faecal problems.[30] Midline episiotomy is associated with higher rates of faecal and flatus incontinence.

CLINICAL PRESENTATION: Psychological problems

Whether psychological debriefing is beneficial to women after childbirth events is under debate.[31] Some obstetric events may be more traumatic than others, some women may find events more traumatic than other women, and some women may have more difficulty in dealing with these events than others. Psychological counselling in other traumatic situations may not have long-term benefits.[32] Further research is needed in the area of childbirth to determine whether debriefing has a preventative role, the nature of 'debriefing',[33] and the women who might benefit most (Section 3).

CLINICAL PRESENTATION: Detection of a breast lump during pregnancy or lactation

Any mass in a pregnant or lactating woman should be thoroughly evaluated (Section 15). About 1–2 per cent of all breast cancers occur during pregnancy or lactation, and a quarter of women who develop breast cancer under the age of 35 do so either during or within one year of pregnancy. Presentation may be delayed because of difficulty in identifying a mass in the enlarging breast of pregnancy.

- Ultrasound is the imaging modality of first choice
- Fine needle aspiration biopsy (FNAB) performed on any definite abnormality
- Close clinical and ultrasound review and consider mammogram once baby weaned.
- Any suspicious lesion will need surgical evaluation

CLINICAL PRESENTATION: Breastfeeding difficulties

Nipple pain is a common problem for breastfeeding women; the most likely cause is incorrect attachment of the baby at the breast. Other causes of nipple and breast pain can be seen in Tables 10.2 and 10.3.

'Not enough milk'

The most common reason that women give up breastfeeding is the belief that they don't have enough breast milk. Most of the time, women are lacking in confidence, not in milk supply. The breastfeeding kinetics table gives a schematic representation of the relationship between infant growth and milk and factors that may interfere with successful breastfeeding (Table 10.4).

Conclusion

The importance of accurate, consistent support for breastfeeding problems should not be underestimated. While some postpartum problems may seem minor to health professionals, they are likely to have a significant impact on the experience of early motherhood and long-term health and quality of life.

TABLE 10.2 Nipple pain

Cause	Assessment	Management
Incorrect attachment	Observe positioning and attachment of baby at the breast. After feeding, the nipple should not be flattened or misshaped.	Correct or refer for expert help. Ultrapure modified lanolin may help resolve nipple damage and reduce pain.
Nipple thrush	Nipples sensitive all the time, burning pain after feeds. Nipples look pink.	Antifungal treatment for mother and baby.
Eczema/dermatitis	Itchy, painful nipples. Rash on nipples/areolae, with well-demarcated edge.	Avoid precipitating factors. Steroid ointment sparingly for less than 7 days.
Bacterial infection	Nipple damage with yellow discharge, or non-healing crack.	Antibacterial ointment for 5 days, or less. Mother may need to express by hand to rest the nipple.
Vasospasm	Mother may have history of Raynaud's phenomenon. Nipple blanches at time of pain.	Keep nipples warm. Magnesium supplement or vasodilator (eg calcium channel blocker) may be needed.
Tongue tie	Baby has short/tight frenulum, tip of tongue is unable to reach past lower lip or reach halfway if mouth is open.	Assessment needed.
Incorrect sucking action	For example, baby has weak suck, not swallowing, slips off breast or sucks cheeks in.	Refer for expert help.
Herpes (rare)	Obvious sores on areola, extremely painful.	Avoid feeding in neonate, otherwise feed or express and consider anti-viral treatment.

TABLE 10.3 Breast problems

Cause	Assessment	Management
Blocked duct	Tender lump, afebrile	Improve breast drainage, massage, heat before feeds, cold after feeds
Mastitis	Red, painful lump, may be febrile	Improve breast drainage Antiinflammatory (ibuprofen) or analgesic If very unwell or symptoms > 24 hours: antistaphylococcal antibiotics—flucloxacillin, dicloxacillin or cephalexin 500 mg qid
Abscess	Usually following mastitis: localised red, painful lump. Can be confirmed with diagnostic ultrasound	Drainage by needle aspiration or referral to breast surgeon
Breast thrush	Breast looks normal Pain is burning, radiating into breast, especially after feeds	See nipple thrush

TABLE 10.4 Breastfeeding kinetics

	Factors impeding successful breastfeeding
Maternal health	Smoking (more than 10 cigarettes/day) Anaemia (eg postpartum haemorrhage)
↓	
Mammogenesis	Breast hypoplasia (eg tubular, wide-spaced breasts) Breast surgery (eg reduction mammoplasty)
↓	
Lactogenesis	Retained placental remnants Delayed breastfeeding
↓	
Galactopoiesis (ongoing production of milk)	Inadequate breast drainage
↓	
Milk transfer	Incorrect positioning of baby on breast Inadequate sucking of baby
↓	
Milk intake	Restriction of frequency or duration of feeds
↓	
Infant growth	Ill health in infant (eg UTI, congenital heart disease)

Adapted from Livingstone 1990.[34]

SECTION 11

Obstetric emergencies

Bleeding during and after pregnancy

Maternal death from haemorrhage is becoming less common in the developed world but is still an important cause of mortality in developing countries.

CLINICAL PRESENTATION: Antepartum haemorrhage

Bleeding from the genital tract after 24 weeks gestation is referred to as an antepartum haemorrhage (APH). The most common causes of APH are placenta praevia and placental abruption (Figure 11.1). However, a third of cases have no apparent cause found. Rarer causes are local lesions in the vagina or cervix, such as cancer of the cervix, vasa praevia—where a blood vessel in the membranes ruptures—and blood disorders. Sometimes a show at the beginning of labour can be confused with an APH.

Management

The rapid clinical assessment of a woman with bleeding initially involves checking the basic observations of maternal pulse and blood pressure, the amount of bleeding and the presence of the fetal heart.

History

- Duration and volume of bleeding, together with whether clots are present, as an assessment of quantity.
- The presence of precipitating factors such as trauma or intercourse should be sought.
- The presence or absence of pain can help distinguish the cause of the bleeding. If pain is present, the duration, intensity, nature and site of the pain are important. Constant pain tends to suggest a placental abruption whereas intermittent colicky pain could be labour triggered by the bleeding or labour leading to a show.
- The obstetric history needs to establish gestation, whether a singleton or multiple pregnancy, whether ultrasound has been performed in the pregnancy (to establish the gestation and placental site) and the history of cervical screening.

Clinical examination

The uterus should be palpated. Classically placental abruption presents with pain, a tender, woody hard uterus and an absent fetal heart, with fetal parts difficult to feel, whereas with placenta praevia the uterus is soft and the fetal heart satisfactory. With placenta praevia the presenting part will be free or there may be a malpresentation.

Investigations

- Haemoglobin
- Cross-match of blood (if the bleeding is severe) or a blood group with serum held for cross-match if necessary
- Clotting screen

FIGURE 11.1 Placenta praevia and placental abruption (a) Placenta praevia: in practice, vaginal delivery is usually only possible in an anteriorly situated type I placenta: the descending fetal head compresses the placenta against the pubic symphysis and the bleeding is controlled. (b) Placental abruption occurs when a part of a normally situated placenta (in the upper uterine segment) becomes detached from the uterine wall, resulting in pain and bleeding. A small retroplacental bleed (concealed) can cause pain with abdominal tenderness if the placenta is on the anterior uterine wall, or backache if on the posterior wall. A bleed at the edge of the placenta will cause bleeding per vagina.

(a) Placenta praevia

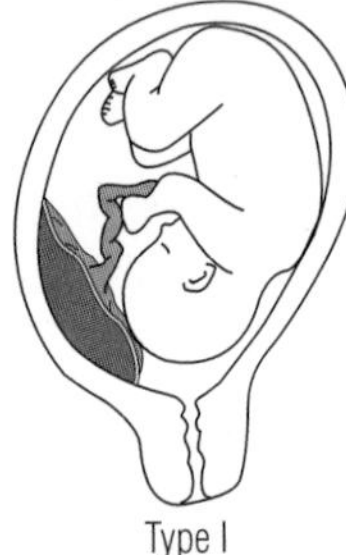

Type I

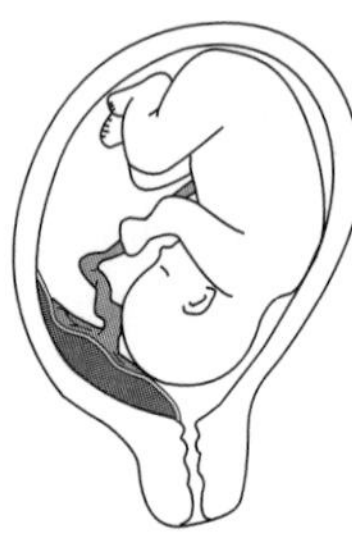

Type II

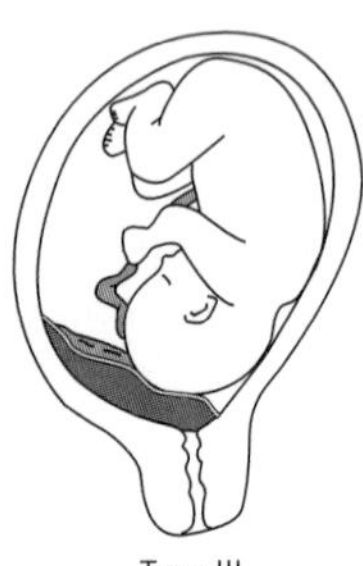

Type III

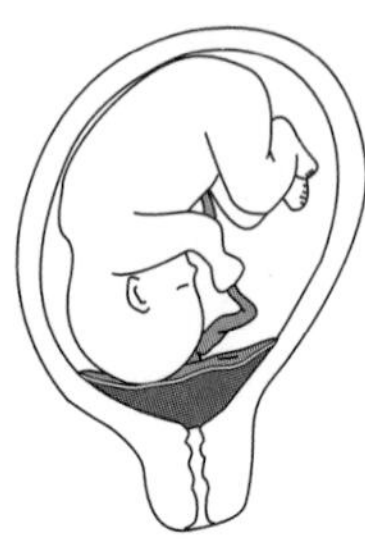

Type IV

Classifications:

	Classical	Ultrasound
Type I	Placenta encroaches on lower segment	Minor
Type II	Placenta reaches internal os	
Type III	Placenta covers internal os but not when dilatated	Major
Type IV	Placenta completely covers internal os even when dilatated	

(b) Placental abruption

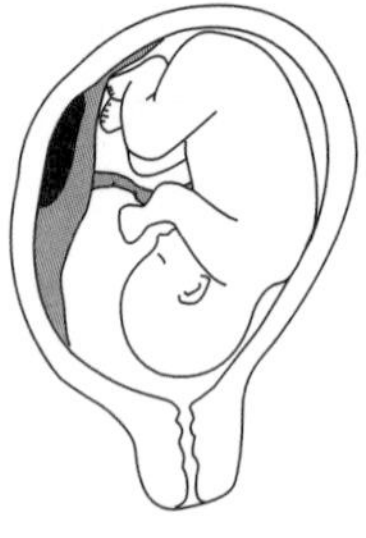

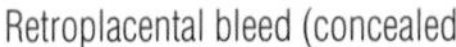

Retroplacental bleed (concealed)

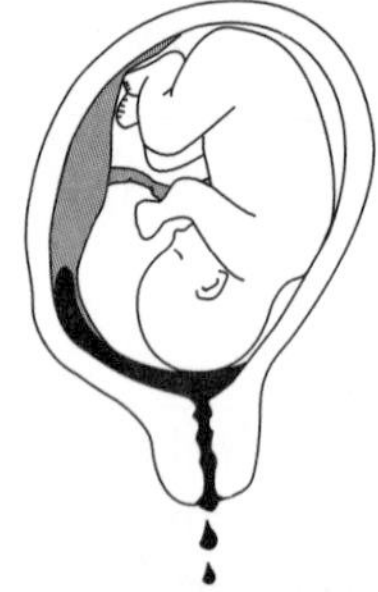

Placental edge bleed (revealed)

- A cardiotocograph should be started to check fetal well-being.
- An ultrasound scan will determine the position of the placenta but cannot exclude a placental abruption. Once the placenta has been confirmed not to be low-lying, a speculum examination should be performed to exclude

local causes. Only then may a vaginal examination be performed to check for signs of labour.

Placenta praevia

Placenta praevia is when the placenta embeds on the lower segment of the uterus. This is the part of the uterus that does not contract in labour but is stretched in response to contractions. The stretching and thinning in the third trimester may shear off part of the placenta. Placenta praevia is described in four grades (Figure 11.1). Vaginal delivery is sometimes possible in a minor anterior placenta praevia where the descending head will compress the bleeding placental bed. All other variants will require the baby to be delivered by caesarean section. The condition is more common in multiparous women, possibly in twin pregnancy and when there has been a previous caesarean section.

The placenta is low in about 5 per cent of women when scanned at around 20 weeks. The scan is usually repeated at 32 weeks and only 0.5 per cent of women have placenta praevia at delivery. In asymptomatic women there is some debate about the need for hospitalisation but bleeding with placenta praevia usually leads to admission to hospital. If the bleeding settles then the mother may be allowed home if she lives close to hospital. The high rate of major bleeding at caesarean section for placenta praevia means an experienced surgeon is needed. As the placenta is embedded in the lower segment, which does not contract, this leads to a high rate of postpartum haemorrhage. Hysterectomy is occasionally needed, particularly if the placenta is anterior and there has been a previous caesarean section.

Placental abruption

This is the premature separation of a placenta normally sited in the upper uterine segment. It occurs in around 1 per cent of pregnancies. If this involves over one-third of the placenta it is usually classed as major and is accompanied by fetal death. Placental abruption accounts for 10–15 per cent of perinatal deaths. Precipitating factors include hypertension, poor placentation, trauma, sudden uterine decompression, cocaine use and multiple pregnancy. Placental abruption can be concealed with no visible bleeding and this must be remembered when a woman presents with continuous pain. Early delivery is usually required. However, where the infant is preterm and the symptoms have settled, delivery may be delayed. When the baby is alive, often caesarean section is used but vaginal delivery is possible with continuous fetal and maternal monitoring. When there is no fetal heart, vaginal delivery should be the aim.

Placental abruption can lead to the development of a couvelaire uterus, where there is blood between the uterine muscle fibres. This makes it more difficult for the uterus to contract after delivery, leading to postpartum haemorrhage. There is often an accompanying disseminated intravascular coagulopathy increasing the problems of bleeding. Treatment of the bleeding requires the transfusion of blood, platelets, fresh frozen plasma and cryoprecipitate. In addition the risk of renal failure is increased.

CLINICAL PRESENTATION: Postpartum haemorrhage

Postpartum haemorrhage (PPH) is the loss of 500 ml or more of blood from the genital tract after delivery of the baby. Postpartum haemorrhage within the first 24 hours is termed primary PPH and occurs in up to 5 per cent of deliveries in developed countries. Some women may be more at risk than others (Box 11.1). It is important to remember that not all blood loss is revealed and that blood may be retained in the uterine cavity as clot, in the uterine muscle with a couvelaire uterus, and in the broad ligament with uterine rupture or a broad ligament haematoma. It most commonly presents within four hours of delivery.

BOX 11.1 Risk factors for postpartum haemorrhage

- Previous history:
  - Previous PPH
- Maternal factors:
  - Increased maternal age
  - High parity
  - Coagulation disorders
  - Anaemia
- Present pregnancy:
  - Antepartum haemorrhage
  - Multiple pregnancy
  - Large baby
- Labour:
  - Long labour
  - Syntocinon in labour
  - Operative delivery/caesarean section

The examination of a woman with a PPH needs to take into account the four T's: tone, trauma, tissue, thrombin. This means that in addition to checking that the woman is stable (BP, PR and RR) and commencing appropriate resuscitation (position, oxygen and intravenous fluids) it is necessary to check whether the uterus is firm and contracted, perform an examination probably under anaesthetic, and send blood to exclude coagulation defect, check the haemoglobin and arrange for cross-match (Box 11.2).

BOX 11.2 Management of postpartum haemorrhage

1. Insert 16 gauge IVI.
2. Send blood for cross-match, FBC, clotting studies.
3. Oxygen by face mask.
4. Insert urinary catheter (measurement of urine output, emptying the bladder aids compression of the uterus).
5. Check uterine fundus for atony—if present 'rub up' a contraction and give oxytocic.
6. Bimanual compression of the uterus can be used while waiting for drugs to take effect.
7. Check whether placenta is complete.
8. Arrange examination under anaesthesia in theatre to exclude genital tract causes.
9. If atony persists other drugs may be required (syntocinon IVI, haemabate, which is a prostaglandin, can be given intramuscularly or intramyometrial, misoprostol 800 μg rectally).
10. If haemorrhage persists, ultimately surgery may be needed. Conservative surgery to reduce blood supply to the uterus can be attempted but often hysterectomy is needed.

The best method of avoiding a PPH is prevention (Section 7). If a PPH occurs, the sequence of management is to give repeated doses of oxytocic while resuscitating the woman, excluding coagulopathy, and preparing for examination to exclude trauma and retained tissue (Box 11.3). If the placenta is retained, the management depends on the degree of associated haemorrhage. Where rapid bleeding occurs, a prompt response is needed, with manual removal of the placenta under general anaesthesia (Figure 11.2). If there is no PPH an infusion of syntocinon into the umbilical cord has been shown to reduce the need for manual removal. Beware of abnormally adherent placentae. With placenta accreta the villi penetrate into the myometrium; with placenta percreta they penetrate through to the peritoneum. Either of these conditions will need a hysterectomy.

BOX 11.3 Differential diagnosis of postpartum haemorrhage

- Atony of the uterus—the most common cause
- Lacerations of the vulva, vagina and cervix
- Retained placental tissue in the uterus
- Vulval or paravaginal haematoma (often 'concealed')
- Dehiscence of a previous uterine scar
- Uterine inversion
- Diffuse intravascular coagulation
- Amniotic fluid embolism

FIGURE 11.2 Manual removal of the retained placenta under general anaesthesia

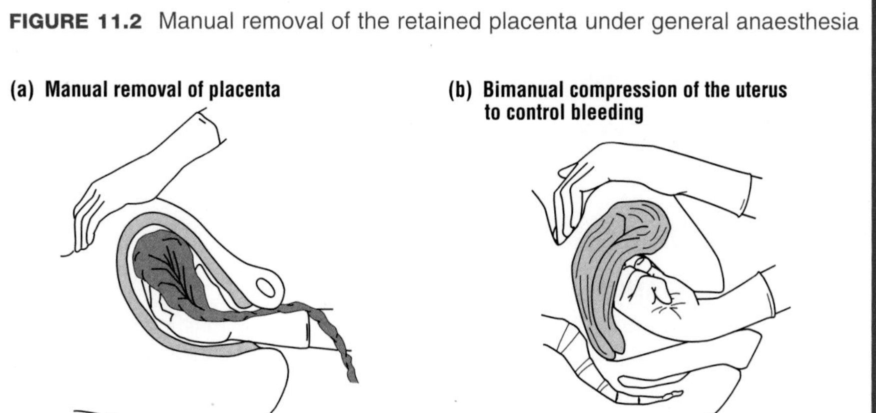

Prolapsed cord

CLINICAL PRESENTATION

Prolapsed cord occurs in about 1 in 300 deliveries. It is variously described, depending on the position and whether the membranes are ruptured (Figure 11.3). It occurs where there is room between the presenting part and the maternal tissues for it to slide down, resulting in fetal malpresentation, preterm birth, hydramnios. Once diagnosed, delivery needs to be effected if the fetus is alive. This will be by caesarean section in most cases, except where the cervix is fully dilated. While awaiting delivery, the woman should be placed in a knee–chest position to take the pressure off the cord.

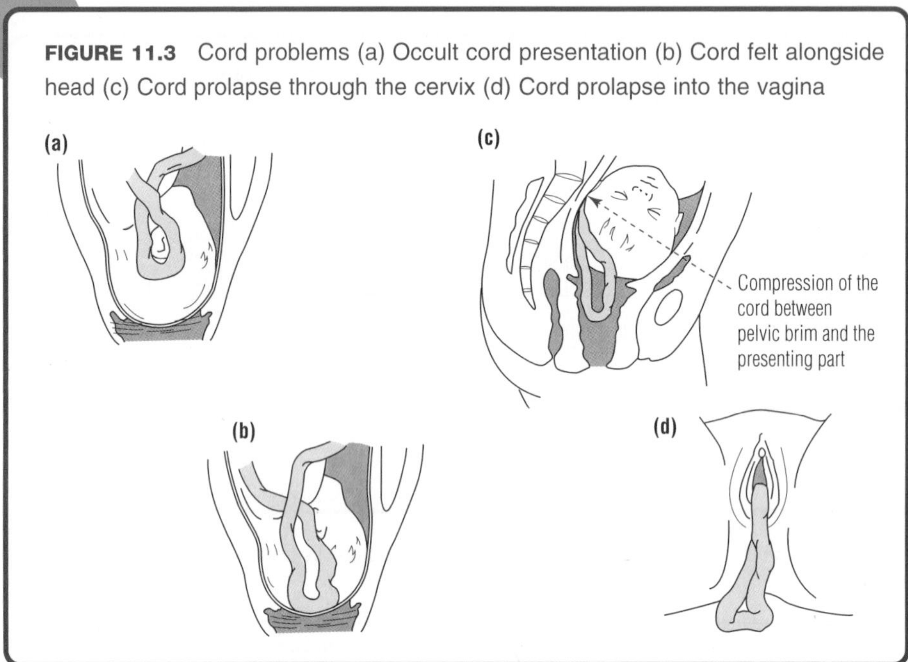

FIGURE 11.3 Cord problems (a) Occult cord presentation (b) Cord felt alongside head (c) Cord prolapse through the cervix (d) Cord prolapse into the vagina

Maternal collapse around delivery

CLINICAL PRESENTATION

Maternal collapse around delivery is an uncommon but serious event in maternity care. Prompt assessment, resuscitation, accurate diagnosis and nursing in an intensive care unit are vital to a good outcome. The initial assessment should be along the lines of the basic ABC of life support: airway, breathing and circulation. A team of people including obstetricians, anaesthetists, midwives and runners are needed to manage the situation. The first steps therefore are to call for help, ensure the airway and breathing, check pulse, blood pressure and oxygen saturation by pulse oximetry. Tilt the woman to avoid aortocaval compression if undelivered. Then establish an ECG and begin to consider the differential diagnosis (Box 11.4). If the mother has had a cardiac arrest and resuscitation does not lead to a pulse within five minutes then it is essential to effect delivery. This allows increased venous return by reducing aortocaval compression and facilitates effective resuscitation.

With maternal collapse the history should be taken from those attending the events. Particular attention is needed for complaints the woman had before collapse of bleeding, abdominal pain, headache, shortness of breath. The events just prior to collapse should be considered, particularly any drugs given or procedures performed. Signs such as vaginal bleeding, restlessness, cyanosis, respiratory distress, tachycardia and whether there was a seizure may suggest a specific diagnosis.

BOX 11.4 Differential diagnosis of collapse around delivery

Obstetric

- Most likely:
  - Haemorrhage (uterine atony)
  - Placental abruption
  - Pre-eclampsia/eclampsia
  - Embolus (amniotic fluid embolism)
  - Air embolus
  - Pulmonary embolus
- Less common:
  - Uterine inversion
  - Uterine rupture

Medical

- Epilepsy
- Asthma

Septic shock

- Cardiac event
- Cerebrovascular accident
- Peripartum cardiomyopathy
- Intracranial bleed or thrombosis
- Anaphylaxis
- Transfusion reactions
- Complication of regional anaesthesia

Uterine inversion

This is a rare complication when oxytocics are used for the third stage and the placenta delivered correctly. It can occur if excessive traction is put on the cord without supporting the body of the uterus during delivery of the placenta. It is more likely if the placenta is attached at the fundus. The fundus of the uterus dimples and descends through the cervix, often with the placenta attached (Figure 11.4). It presents with haemorrhage and/or immediate collapse. Once recognised the treatment is to replace the uterus quickly before it distends. If this fails, then an IV line is inserted, blood cross-matched and the hydrostatic method used: the forearm occludes the introitus and sterile saline is run into the vagina until the hydrostatic pressure builds up and turns the uterus back from inside out. Several litres of fluid are often required. If this fails then abdominal surgery is required.

FIGURE 11.4 Traction on the cord to the placenta that is fully or partially attached to the uterus causes partial or complete inversion of the uterus.

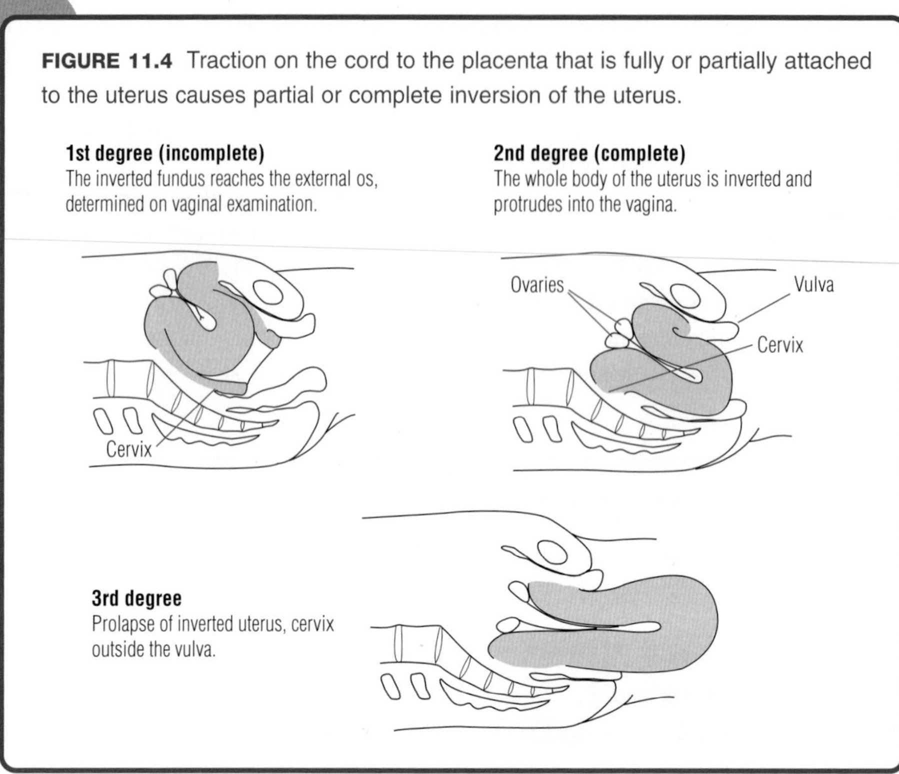

Uterine rupture

This is more likely in a woman with a previous caesarean section but can occur in women with an intact uterus, particularly in multigravida women treated with Syntocinon. Dehiscence of a uterine scar (without complete rupture) can occur with similar symptoms and rapid laparotomy may prevent fetal loss. The clinical signs are continuous low abdominal pain, vaginal bleeding, maternal tachycardia and fetal heart rate abnormalities. Laparotomy with repair of the uterus is required.

Pulmonary embolus

Pregnancy predisposes to venous thromboembolism (Section 9). Usually there will have been a period of immobility, the woman will be overweight or may have a personal or family history of thromboembolism. The first symptoms may be cough, shortness of breath and haemoptysis. Signs may include a tender, swollen leg, tachycardia, a pleural rub. Investigations may reveal ECG changes and lowered oxygen levels on blood gases. The diagnosis is made by either a ventilation perfusion scan or spiral computerised tomography. The treatment is anticoagulation with heparin or low molecular weight heparin followed by warfarin. In the most severe cases open thromboembolectomy may be considered.

Amniotic fluid embolus

This condition, while rare, accounts for up to 10 per cent of maternal deaths in developed countries. It is uncommon in women under 25 years of age. Mortality has previously been as high as 85 per cent but population studies now suggest approximately 30 per cent. It is characterised by hypotension, breathlessness, cyanosis and then haemorrhage associated with disseminated intravascular coagulation. This is followed rapidly by cardiorespiratory arrest and/or seizures. The woman should be given cardiopulmonary resuscitation and intermittent positive pressure ventilation. A transfusion of haemocel is started, and then blood when available. Most women who die do so in the first six hours after collapse.

Pre-eclampsia/eclampsia (Section 9)

Pre-eclampsia is a multisystem disorder. Collapse can be due to an eclamptic seizure, brain haemorrhage or thrombosis, pulmonary oedema or intrahepatic haemorrhage. Usually the woman will be known to be hypertensive. The treatment of eclamptic seizures is similar to severe eclampsia.

Septic shock

Endotoxic shock with chorioamnionitis or postpartum infection is usually associated with Gram-negative bacteria. The classic features of infection are fever, vasodilatation, hypotension, tachycardia and tachypnoea. However, the woman may also exhibit cyanosis, hypothermia, pallor and jaundice. Coagulation failure (DIC) can occur. Aggressive treatment with antibiotics, fluid resuscitation and intensive care are appropriate.

Complication of regional anaesthesia

Regional anaesthesia can be associated with allergic reactions to either the local anaesthetic or the opiate mixed with it. Epidural analgesia can be associated with an inadvertent spinal technique when a dural puncture has occurred and the anaesthetist is not aware of this. This then leads to a high block, which can cause respiratory embarrassment. Occasionally intubation is needed with ventilatory support until spontaneous respiration restarts.

Conclusion

Any bleeding or collapse of a woman during pregnancy, labour or post partum requires rapid assessment, resuscitation and specific management to avoid a maternal mortality or morbidity.

3 Obstetrics

A Listening to the fetal heart using a Pinnard's stethoscope

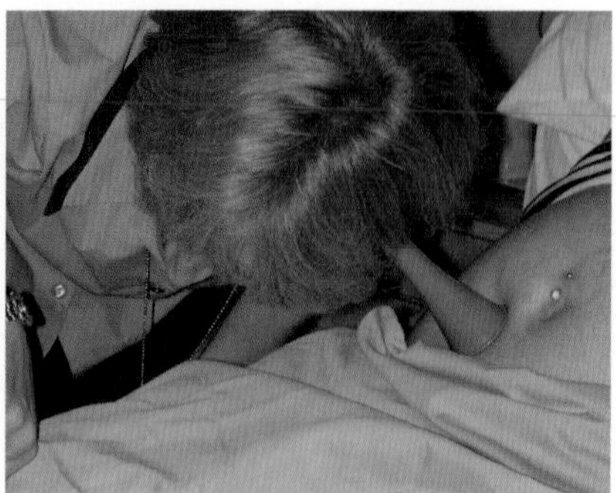

B Listening and recording the fetal heart using a cardiotocograph. Abdominal bands are recording the fetal heart rate and uterine contractions (seen on monitor printout).

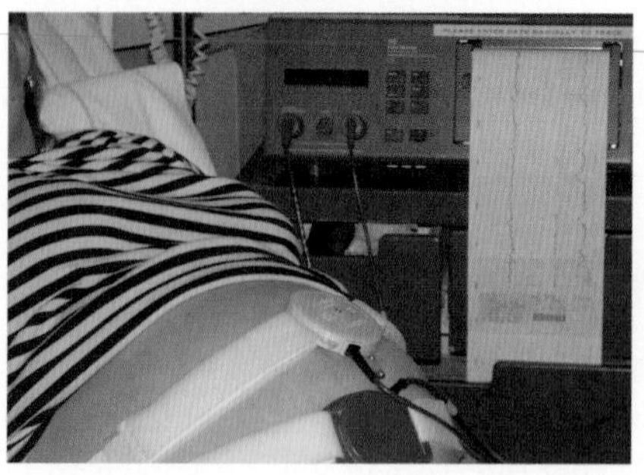

C Third stage of labour: delivery of the placenta. Gentle, firm traction in a downward direction is exerted on the cord while supporting the body of the uterus with the other hand on the abdomen.

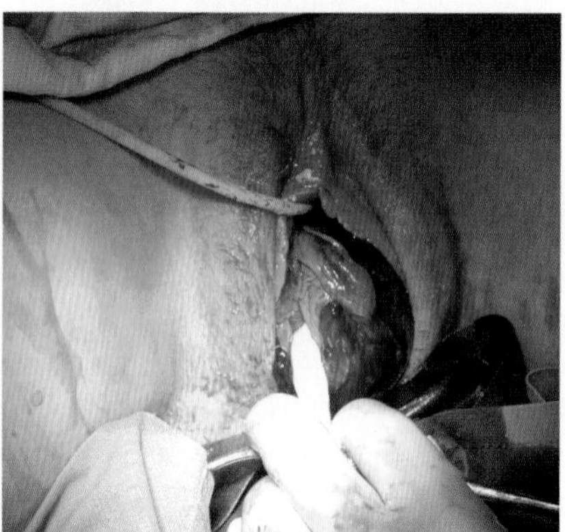

D Third stage of labour: control of bleeding. After the placenta is delivered, the uterine fundus is massaged to ensure that it is well contracted.

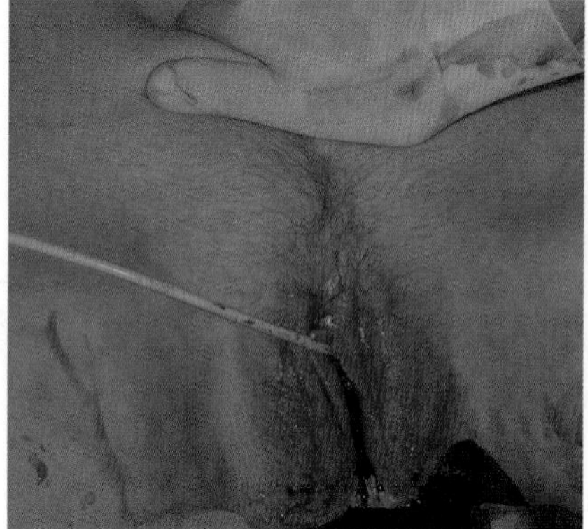

E Normal placenta—fetal side. Smooth surface with numerous blood vessels converging to meet in the umbilical cord. The fetus lies in the sac of membranes attached by the umbilical cord.

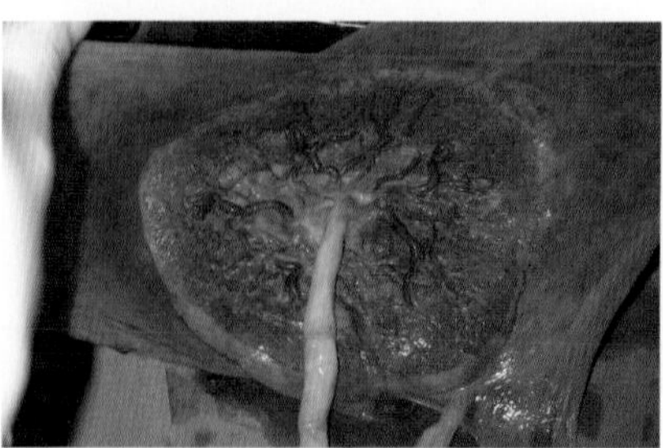

F Normal placenta—maternal side. Cotelydons of varying sizes can be seen. Checking that these are all present and not retained in the uterus is part of the examination of the placenta after delivery.

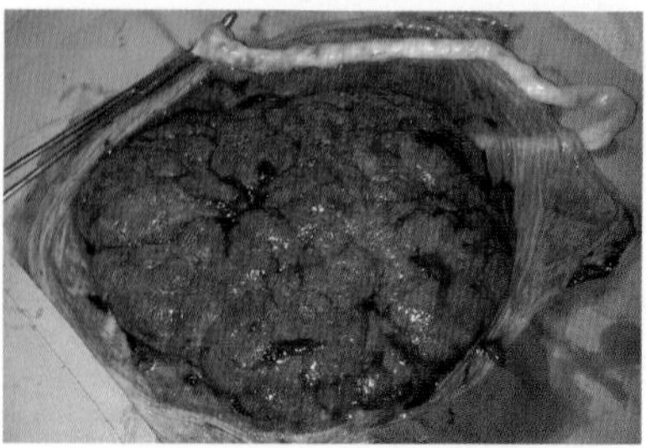

A Cephalohaematoma: bleeding has occurred beneath the scalp following a forceps delivery. Sometimes this can be marked and lead to a significant anaemia for the baby.

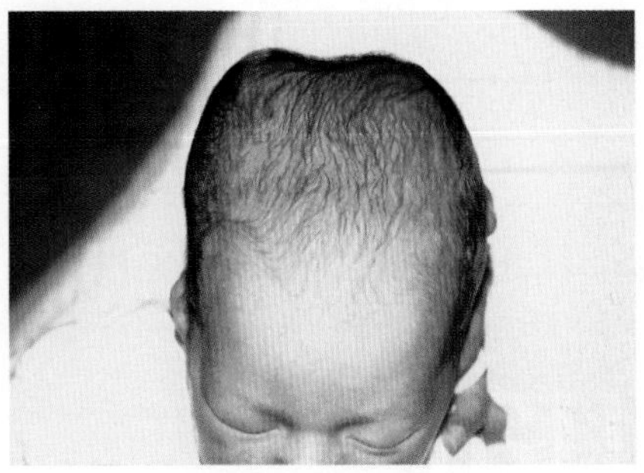

B Face presentation: a normal vaginal delivery but the soft presenting face has extensive bruising. This settled over a few weeks with no residual effects.

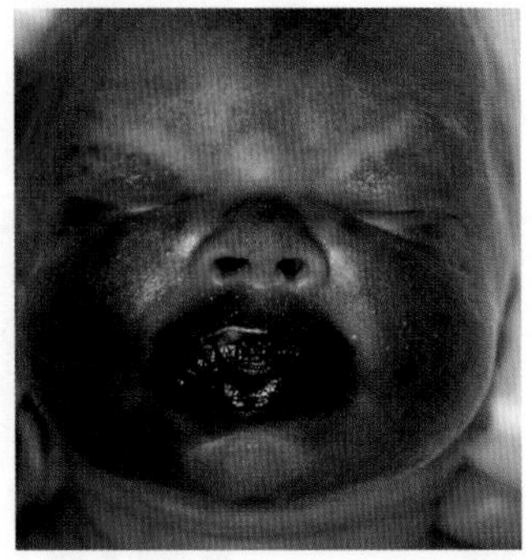

C A difficult delivery has resulted in a depressed skull fracture, suspected on palpation. This is confirmed on X-ray (see D).

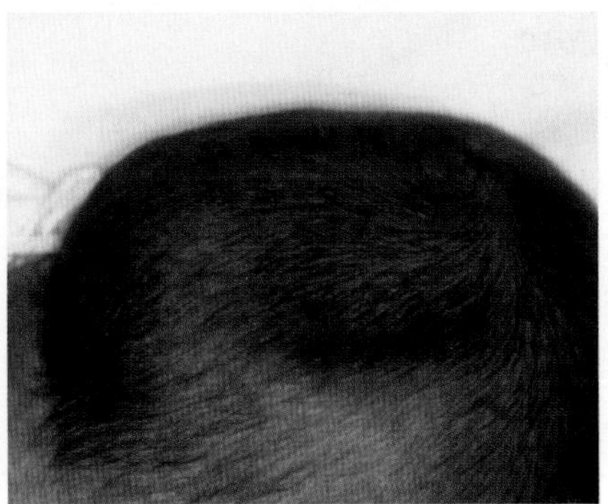

D Depressed skull fracture on X-ray.

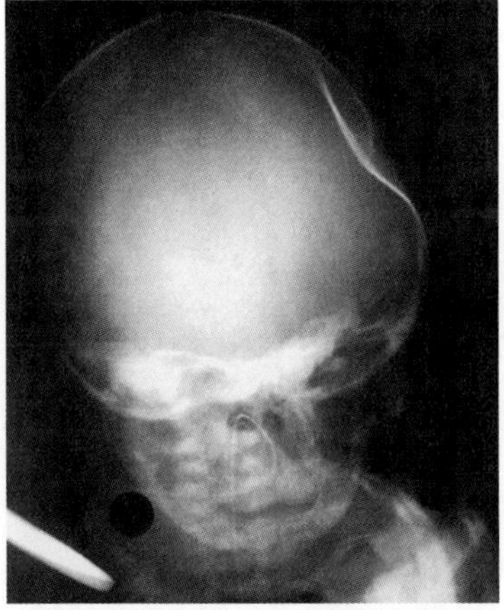

E Left Erb's palsy: compression of fibres of C5 and C6 of the brachial plexus resulting from a difficult shoulder delivery (dystocia or breech delivery). Occurs in fewer than 1 in 2000 births. Most cases resolve.

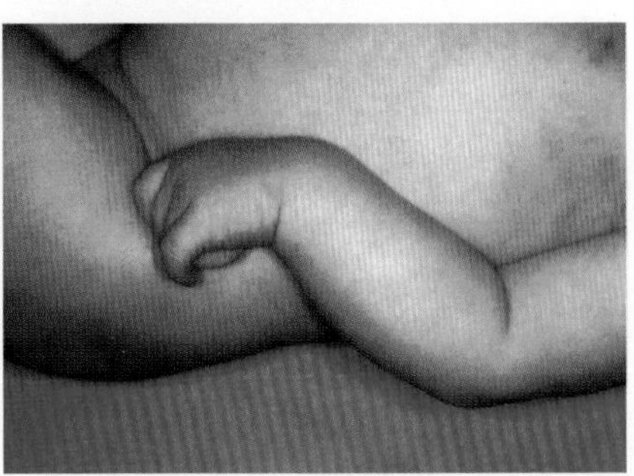

F Facial palsy: occasionally the facial nerve can be injured during a forceps delivery. Most cases resolve in 2–3 weeks.

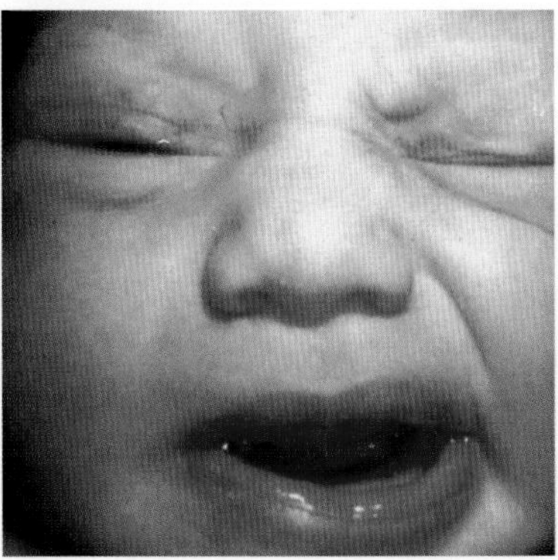

SECTION

12 Sexual health

Contraception

Choices through the reproductive years

Choice of a contraceptive method is influenced by a number of factors including age, medical history, relationship status, lifestyle, desire for a pregnancy in the future or family complete, likely exposure to sexually transmitted infections and the individual preferences of both the user and their partner. As circumstances change so too will contraceptive needs and choices.

CLINICAL PRESENTATION: Nulliparous women

If pregnancy is not desired within the next two to three years and oestrogens are not contraindicated, any hormonal method other than an intrauterine contraceptive device (IUCD) can be recommended. Condoms should be used in a new relationship or with multiple partners, either alone or in conjunction with hormonal methods.

In women with a contraindication to oestrogen any of the progestogen-only methods are suitable. An IUCD can be used by nulliparous women in mutually monogamous relationships where other methods are unsuitable or unacceptable side effects occur.

CLINICAL PRESENTATION: Women delaying pregnancy

If no contraindications exist, women who wish to become pregnant in one to two years should be advised to use an oral contraceptive or a barrier method. Depot medroxyprogesterone acetate (DMPA) is unsuitable because of the variable delay in the return of fertility. An IUCD or a long-acting progesterone subdermal implant can be used but the cost effectiveness of early removal needs to be kept in mind. There is no delay in return of fertility with these latter methods.

CLINICAL PRESENTATION: Women over 35 years

Women over the age of 35 years who are non-smokers can be prescribed low-dose combined oral contraceptives (COC) until the menopause. Recent studies have indicated that the mechanism of myocardial infarction in patients receiving COC is thrombotic or due to coronary arterial spasm rather than atherosclerotic.[1] Continuing oral contraceptive use until the menopause may have considerable benefit, as women in their forties often develop bleeding problems due to fibroids, adenomyosis or dysfunctional uterine bleeding. Combined oral contraceptives offer the best method for controlling such bleeding problems until the menopause.[2] The 50 per cent protection against ovarian and endometrial cancer, which continues for 10 to 15 years after ceasing oral contraceptive use, is also of particular benefit to older women. Combined oral contraceptives are also the best way for controlling hot flushes and other symptoms of the perimenopause since it is often difficult to tailor hormone replacement therapy (HRT) to a woman's naturally occurring cycle.

When to stop the pill in a perimenopausal woman is often difficult to determine. Many practitioners stop the pill at the age of 50, wait several weeks and then determine serum follicle-stimulating hormone (FSH) levels. If these are raised, the woman is certainly perimenopausal and may even be postmenopausal. It would be reasonably safe for her to stop contraception at this point and, if she so desired, change to hormone replacement therapy. If FSH levels are within the normal range then the pill should be continued for another year and the procedure repeated.

The levonorgestrel intrauterine system (Mirena IUS) offers considerable benefits to women in their forties without contraindications to IUCD use, especially if they suffer from dysfunctional uterine bleeding, common in this age group. Apart from its high contraceptive efficacy it considerably reduces menstrual blood loss. If perimenopausal symptoms such as hot flushes occur the woman can be prescribed oestrogens while having endometrial protection from the IUS and good contraceptive cover. Hormone replacement therapy alone does not provide effective contraception.

As women in their forties have reduced fertility, less effective methods such as progestogen-only pills and diaphragms have been shown to have lower failure rates than those seen in younger age groups. Older women are also likely to be more consistent in their use of these methods.

CLINICAL PRESENTATION: Women who have completed their families

For women who have completed their families or definitely do not want a child, highly effective methods such as subdermal implants, DMPA or Mirena will provide very effective contraception. Alternatively, vasectomy or female sterilisation can provide permanent contraception but couples need to be carefully counselled to consider life events such as loss of a partner or existing child, or breakup of the present relationship. Although these procedures may be reversible this cannot be guaranteed.

Hormonal methods

Since the introduction of the combined oral contraceptive pill in 1960 a variety of hormonal methods have been developed, providing greater choice and more effective contraception for women. The COCs available today contain a fifth or lesser dose of oestrogen and a tenth or lower dose of progestogen than the original pill, with a consequent reduction in side effects. Ethinyl oestradiol, a potent synthetic oestrogen in daily doses ranging from 20–50 μg, is combined with a variety of progestogens: norethisterone, levonorgestrel, desorgestrel, gestodene and norgestimate, to provide a variety of brands. It is not possible to compare progestogens by dose as the potency of progestogens varies. For example, levonorgestrel is ten times more potent than norethisterone weight for weight.

There are also different regimens.

- *Monophasic formulations*—the dose of oestrogen and progestogen does not vary during 21 days of active pill taking followed by seven pill-free days.
- *Biphasic formulations*—the dose of oestrogen remains the same in the 21 active tablets but the dose of progestogen is increased in the last 11 active tablets of the cycle.
- *Triphasic formulations*—the dose of oestrogen is increased in the middle of the cycle to lower the rate of breakthrough bleeding, while the progestogen dose is low initially but increases stepwise as the cycle progresses.

- *Progestogen-only formulations*—low-dose progestogen is taken continuously without a break.

Mode of action and efficacy of COC

Combined oral contraceptives are highly effective (theoretical pregnancy rate 0.5%)[3] due to their multiple effects on the reproductive system (Box 12.1). There are absolute and relative contraindications for COC use (Box 12.2), and there are a number of benefits (Box 12.3).

There are major adverse events associated with COC use. However, the thromboembolic risks need to be balanced against the same risks during a pregnancy (Box 12.4). Risk factors for arterial thrombosis include age, hypertension, smoking, obesity and strong family history of premature coronary artery disease. Use of COCs increases the risk of developing breast cancer (RR 1.24) during use, producing an excess of 11/100 000 in COC takers aged 40–44 and 17/100 000 in those aged 45 to 54 years. The risk returns to normal by 10 years post use.[4] Tumours developing in women while using COCs are usually localised, with a better prognosis. Many of the oral contraceptives taken by women in these studies were those used before the current low-dose formulations—the latter show less stimulation of the breast.[5]

BOX 12.1 Effects of the combined oral contraceptive pill

- Hypothalamic pituitary axis is suppressed by a synergistic action of oestrogen with progestogen, resulting in suppression of ovulation.
- Sperm penetration is inhibited by increase in the viscosity of cervical mucus by progestogen.
- Endometrial growth is suppressed by progestogen, making it unsuitable for implantation.
- Changes in tubal function.
- In typical use COCs have failure rates as high as 8%.

BOX 12.2 Contraindications to combined oral contraceptive use

- Existing or history of cardiovascular or cerebrovascular disease
- Diabetes with circulatory problems
- Complicated valvular heart disease
- History of thromboembolism
- Severe liver disease
- Breast cancer
- Uncontrolled hypertension
- Focal migraine
- Women > 35 years smoking > 15 cigarettes/day
- Prolonged immobilisation
- Malabsorption syndrome

BOX 12.3 Benefits of combined oral contraceptives

- Reduction in menstrual blood loss
- Decrease in anaemia
- Reduction in dysmenorrhoea
- Ability to manipulate menses
- Reduction of PMS in some women
- 50% reduction in endometrial cancer—protection lasts 10–15 years after cessation
- 40% reduction in ovarian cancer—protection lasts 10–15 years after cessation
- Reduction in benign breast lumps
- Reduction in functional ovarian cysts
- Some protection against pelvic inflammatory disease
- Helpful in management of endometriosis
- Fewer symptomatic fibroids
- Reduced benign breast disease
- Safe for long-term use in women without risk factors up to menopause except for smokers > 35 years

BOX 12.4 Major adverse events associated with COC

- Thromboembolic disease—risk of DVT in:
  - Non-users: 5–6/100 000
  - 2nd generation Pill users: 15/100 000
  - 3rd generation Pill users: 30/100 000
  - Pregnancy: 60/10 000
- Arterial thrombosis:
  - Thrombotic stroke
  - Haemorrhagic stroke
- Breast cancer

Side effects reported by women using COC

Although the reported side effects are not life-threatening they are the major reasons for discontinuation. They include breakthrough bleeding and spotting, increased irritability, decreased libido, increased hirsutism and acne, vaginal dryness, breast tenderness, nausea, bloating, chloasma, headaches and increased vaginal discharge. These can mostly be settled with an adjustment to the regimen (Table 12.1).

Weight change is variable, with some women reporting weight loss and some reporting weight gain, while the majority have no change.

Choice of COC

Oral contraceptives can provide a very effective and safe method of contraception provided a careful medical history is taken. The choice of formulation for the

TABLE 12.1 Common pill problems and their management

Problem	Management	Example
Nausea	a Reduce oestrogen dose b Change to progestogen-only method	30 to 20 mcg
Breast tenderness	a Reduce oestrogen dose b Increase progestogen dose	30 to 20 mcg Triphasic to monophasic
Breakthrough bleeding	a Change progestogen b Increase oestrogen	LNG to GSD Monophasic to triphasic
Dysmenorrhoea	a Decrease oestrogen b Increase progestogen dose	30 to 20 mcg Triphasic to monophasic
Menstrual migraine	a Reduce oestrogen dose b Oestradiol 100 mcg patch for pill-free week c Tri-monthly or continuous pill-taking regimen	30 to 20 mcg

individual woman depends on her medical history, with use of the lowest dose which is consistent with good cycle control and fewest metabolic changes recommended.[6] Women who are on enzyme-inducing drugs such as older anti-epileptics, rifampicin or griseofulvin should be provided with a higher oestrogen dose if prescribed a COC.

The general view is that levonorgestrel or norethisterone preparations, which are also cheaper, should be prescribed initially. Women with specific problems such as acne or who develop side effects need to be prescribed one of the newer COCs (containing desorgestrel, gestodene or cyproterone acetate), which appear to be more effective in reducing the severity of acne. Careful counselling is required when women start oral contraceptives, with instructions on how to take the pill and what to do if a pill is missed.

Progestogen-only pill (minipill)

For women who either cannot tolerate or do not want to take a COC the progestogen-only pill (minipill or POP) is a good alternative. The POP acts mainly by increasing the viscosity of cervical mucus with variable effects on ovarian function. In 40 per cent of cycles there is normal ovulation. There are relatively few contraindications to the POP and these include malabsorption syndromes, undiagnosed vaginal bleeding, previous ectopic pregnancy (because if pregnancy does occur with a POP there may be a greater incidence of tubal pregnancy), severe liver disease and taking enzyme-inducing drugs. The POP is taken continuously,

Adverse effects

The major adverse effect is unpredictable bleeding patterns. Women may have normal cycles, erratic short to long cycles or nuisance spotting. A small percentage will develop amenorrhoea. Other than bleeding irregularities, adverse effects of the POP are rare. However, some women may have follicular development without ovulation, resulting in follicular cysts. Women who elect to take the POP need to be meticulous pill takers.

Timing of pill taking

The efficacy of the POP depends largely on the effect on cervical mucus, which is maximal three hours after ingestion and starts to reduce 21 hours after ingestion. Consequently the pill should be taken at the same time each day and preferably some hours prior to the usual time that intercourse occurs. For instance, if intercourse usually occurs at night the POP should be taken each morning

Post-coital contraception

There are several regimens of emergency contraception using either high-dose COCs, known as the Yuzpe method, or levonorgestrel alone. Both methods are more effective the sooner after unprotected intercourse they are started. Women should be encouraged to return for a pregnancy test if their period is more than one week late. The mode of action of these methods is unclear but the major effect appears to be delay of ovulation and changes in the uterine environment making fertilisation unlikely. No evidence of histological changes in the endometrium has been demonstrated.

Yuzpe method

Seventy-five per cent of pregnancies resulting from unprotected mid-cycle intercourse can be prevented by prescribing two tablets each containing ethinyl oestradiol 50 mcg + levonorgestrel 250 mcg or four tablets each containing ethinyl oestradiol 30 mcg + levonorgestrel 150 mcg within 72 hours of unprotected intercourse and repeated 12 hours later. Approximately 60 per cent of women will experience nausea so an anti-emetic should also be prescribed. The next period may occur early in about 20 per cent of women. In 50 per cent of women it occurs at the expected time, but in 30 per cent of women it may be delayed as long as 3–4 weeks.

Levonorgestrel

A preferable regimen, since it has been shown to be more effective than the Yuzpe method, is levonorgestrel 750 μg given within 72 hours of unprotected intercourse and repeated 12 hours later. An emergency contraceptive pack consisting of two pills, each containing 750 μg levonorgestrel, is available.

Emergency contraception will not dislodge an implanted pregnancy, nor is there any risk of teratogenesis if unprotected intercourse has occurred earlier in the cycle, resulting in pregnancy. Because this formulation can avert a large number of possible pregnancies, it should be more widely available, particularly as a backup for women using barrier methods of contraception. In the UK the emergency contraceptive levonorgestrel (Levonelle) is sold by pharmacists without prescription.

Copper-bearing IUD

A copper-bearing IUD can be inserted up to five days after unprotected intercourse, with a failure to prevent pregnancy in 1 per cent of cases. It has the advantage of providing ongoing contraception for suitable women.

Long-acting methods

Advantages

Long-acting methods were developed to reduce user failure rates, since once initiated they require little or no further action on the part of the user. The newer methods use steady-state release mechanisms, giving more stable blood levels and enabling reduction of daily steroid dose. The majority are progestogen-only devices. There are contraindications to the use of progestogen-only methods (Box 12.5). The new long-acting methods are readily reversible, unlike depot medroxyprogesterone acetate (DMPA), which often requires 10–18 months after the last injection for the return of fertility.

BOX 12.5 Contraindications to use of progestogen-only methods

- Pregnancy: known or suspected
- Abnormal vaginal bleeding: undiagnosed
- Irregular bleeding or amenorrhoea unacceptable, especially for cultural reasons
- Hypersensitivity to any component
- Hepatic enzyme-inducing drugs (apart from women using DMPA)

Women with the following conditions require careful consideration because the potential risks of using a progestogen-only method may outweigh the benefits:

- Breast cancer: the influence of progestogens on progression is unclear
- Diabetes with vascular disease: progestogens may lower HDL-C and elevate LDL-C thus exacerbating the risk of arteriosclerosis
- Severe hypertension (> 180/110 mmHg) or hypertension with vascular disease
- Any severe liver disease: acute, chronic, benign or malignant tumours, as progestogens are metabolised by the liver.

Disadvantages

Long-acting methods require medical intervention for insertion and removal (for most), and they are more expensive, requiring initial higher outlay of costs, although given the longer lifespan of these devices they are cheaper over time than the COC. Most of the new long-acting methods contain only progestogen, resulting in altered bleeding patterns and therefore careful counselling is required prior to use.

Depot medroxyprogesterone acetate

Depot medroxyprogesterone acetate (DMPA) is administered by deep intramuscular injection into the gluteal or deltoid muscle in a dose of 150 mg every 12 weeks ± 14 days The initial dose should preferably be given in the first seven days of the cycle when no additional contraceptive protection is required. It may be given at other times in the cycle provided pregnancy is excluded. DMPA can be given immediately following abortion or post partum if not breastfeeding, or at six weeks post partum if breastfeeding.

Mode of action

The mode of action includes the following:

- The hypothalamic pituitary axis is suppressed, resulting in suppression of ovulation.
- Sperm penetration is inhibited by increase in the viscosity of cervical mucus by progestogen.
- Endometrial growth is suppressed by progestogen, making it unsuitable for implantation.

Bleeding patterns

Bleeding patterns are unpredictable, with 50 per cent of women developing amenorrhoea after 12 months of use and 70 per cent by two years of use. Frequent, prolonged or nuisance spotting may occur but this is less common than amenorrhoea and tends to revert to amenorrhoea over time.

Return of fertility

There is a delay in the return of fertility on cessation of use but with no permanent effect on fertility. The median conception time is 8–10 months after the last injection is given—that is, 5–7 months after the drug could have been expected to wear off. Seventy-five per cent of women conceive within 15 months of their last injection and 95 per cent within two years. Persistent anovulation, due to very slow metabolism and hence persistence of the drug, produces the delay in return of fertility. This is reversed as soon as the drug is cleared from the system. Prolonged duration of use does not increase the delay in return of fertility. Some women experience erratic and prolonged bleeding as DMPA wears off after the last injection, and some may develop follicular cysts as ovarian function returns. These require no treatment other than explanation and reassurance. If a woman does want to maintain regular cycles during DMPA withdrawal she can be prescribed a COC provided she is not desiring a pregnancy.

Bone density

Controversy exists about the effect of long-term DMPA use on bone mineral density (BMD).[7] Studies indicate that the majority of amenorrhoeic long-term DMPA users had slightly lower BMDs of lumbar spine and hip (96%) compared to age- and weight-matched controls, with 83 per cent of amenorrhoeic women having serum oestradiol levels below 100–150 pmol/l.[8] No correlation exists between duration of DMPA use, period of amenorrhoea or oestradiol levels and BMD. Nor do women on DMPA with low oestradiol levels exhibit symptoms of oestrogen deficiency such as hot flushes or dry vagina. Postmenopausal women who have formerly used DMPA have no significant difference in BMD compared to non-users.[9]

Concerns about hypo-oestrogenicity during long-term DMPA use and its possible effect on BMD have raised fears that its use in young women under 16 years may affect the post-menarche increase of BMD. These concerns need to be balanced with the obvious benefits of use of a long-acting method when counselling adolescents. Most problems can be easily managed (Table 12.2).

Other side effects reported by women using DMPA are weight gain, nervousness and depression.

TABLE 12.2 Managing problems associated with DMPA

Problem	Management
Bleeding disturbance	Oestrogens if not contraindicated
	Premarin 1.25 mg daily for 2 to 3 weeks
Cycle of COC	NSAID if oestrogen contraindicated
Delay in next injection	Exclude pregnancy
	Condoms for 14 days after last unprotected sexual intercourse
	Pregnancy test
Functional follicular cyst	Reassurance, as spontaneously regress

Etonogestrel implant

Etonogestrel implant (Implanon) consists of a single silastic rod 4 cm long and 2 mm in diameter, approximately the size of a match stick. The rod is contained in a sterile disposable inserter and has a sustained release of etonogestrel of 60–70 μg per day initially, gradually reducing to a release rate of 20–30 μg by the end of the third year. Women with low body weight tend to develop higher serum levels. It is a highly effective contraceptive that provides immediate cover if inserted on cycle days 1 to 5. It has a lifespan of three years and a pregnancy rate of 0–0.09 per 100 women years. With removal of the device there is rapid return of fertility, with undetectable levels of serum etonogestrel five days after removal.

The mode of action is somewhat different to that of progestogen-only pills. There is follicular development without ovulation as the progestogen suppresses the LH surge. Therefore, most women have early follicular-phase oestradiol production without ovulation until the third year, when ovulation may occur in approximately 4 per cent of women. There is an increase in cervical mucus viscosity within 24 to 48 hours of insertion, which is accompanied by a thin, proliferative but not atrophic endometrium. No significant metabolic changes have been reported to date.

Insertion

Insertion is simple once training has taken place. The device can be inserted in a doctor's surgery under local anaesthetic (Box 12.6). It is also readily removable if the woman requests this or if the device has come to the end of its three-year lifespan. Removal requires a small incision about 3 mm in length and is simple provided the device has been correctly placed. Occasionally a scar may develop at the insertion site.

BOX 12.6 Timing of etonogestrel implant insertion

- Day 1 to 5 of the menstrual cycle
- Changing from a COC during the pill-free week
- Changing from DMPA when the next injection is due
- Immediately after removal if the woman wants to continue its use
- Immediately following first trimester abortion
- Day 21 to 28 following delivery or second trimester abortion

Side effects

All users will have unpredictable bleeding patterns. Amenorrhoea and infrequent bleeding are the most common; frequent or prolonged bleeding episodes occur in 20 per cent of women. There is no effective treatment for frequent or prolonged bleeding. Bleeding patterns may improve over the first three months of use. If women find the bleeding unacceptable the device should be removed.

Other side effects are similar to those experienced with other steroid contraceptive methods. To date there has been no evidence of an increase in stroke, myocardial infarction or thromboembolism in women who have been using the etonogestrel implant.

Intrauterine devices

Modern IUDs are a safe, highly effective method, with failure rates of 1/hundred women years (HWY) for copper devices and 0.16/HWY for the LNG-releasing device (Mirena), providing long-acting, low-maintenance, low-cost contraception. There are two copper-bearing devices: the Copper T380A and the Multiload 375, with a lifespan of ten years and five years respectively. Mirena contains a column of levonorgestrel within a rate-limiting membrane, which is released at a rate of 20 μg over 24 hours, reducing to 11 μg over 24 hours after five years. The device has a lifespan of five years but in Swedish studies appeared to be effective for as long as seven years.

Mode of action

The exact mechanism is not understood but copper devices affect sperm motility, sperm and ovum transport and fertilisation as well as endometrial changes due to a foreign body response. Mirena also thickens the cervical mucus, impeding sperm migration through the cervix, uterus and fallopian tubes, endometrial atrophy and variable inhibition of ovulation in the first year of use in 5–15 per cent of cycles. All IUDs have contraindications to their use (Box 12.7).

Insertion

Intrauterine devices can be inserted in the first 17 days of a 28-day or longer cycle, immediately post abortion and 6–8 weeks post partum. Insertion is an office procedure which should only be carried out by practitioners trained in IUD insertion.

BOX 12.7 Contraindications to the use of IUDs

- Pelvic inflammatory disease: current or recurrent
- Pregnancy: known or suspected
- Infection of the lower genital tract until eradicated
- Postpartum endometritis
- Post-abortion infection during past 3 months
- Undiagnosed vaginal bleeding
- Women likely to be exposed to sexually transmissible infections
- Congenital malformations or distortion of uterine cavity, eg submucous fibroid
- Uterine or cervical malignancy
- Hypersensitivity to any of its components
- Inability or unwillingness to accept erratic bleeding pattern with Mirena
- Not first method of choice in nulliparous women but may be used if unlikely to be exposed to sexually transmissible infections.
- Antibiotic prophylaxis is required prior to insertion by women with congenital or valvular heart disease.

Bleeding patterns

Copper-bearing devices increase blood loss by 40–50 per cent. This can be treated with antifibrinolytic agents. Mirena reduces blood loss markedly over the first six months but produces erratic bleeding/spotting during the first months. Fifty per cent of women have infrequent bleeding by nine months and 10–15 per cent have amenorrhoea.

Pelvic inflammatory disease

Pelvic inflammatory disease (PID) directly related to IUD use is extremely low and confined to the first three weeks post insertion due to contamination of the uterus during insertion of the device. Other episodes of PID are related to STIs, not IUD use. Women need to be advised to use condoms in at-risk situations. The incidence of PID is lower with Mirena.

Other side effects

Pelvic pain in the initial period of use occurs in 1–2 per cent of women. Expulsion occurs in 2–10 per cent. Symptoms of partial expulsion include pain and bleeding. Expulsion can occur without the woman being aware. An increase in menstrual blood flow after some time of LNG-releasing IUD use may be an indication of expulsion. Functional follicular ovarian cysts may occur with Mirena but usually regress spontaneously.

Side effects reported with Mirena are similar to those of all hormonal methods, including an increase in acne, breast tenderness, weight gain, headache, nausea and mood changes. The ectopic pregnancy rate at 3–9 per cent of IUD pregnancies is lower than in non-contraceptors because of the low pregnancy rate of IUDs (1/HWY for copper devices and 0.1/HWY for Mirena).

Follow-up

Women should be reviewed four to six weeks after insertion to exclude post-insertion PID (rare) and to ensure that the strings have not lengthened, suggesting partial expulsion. They should then be seen annually and should be instructed to return immediately if they develop pelvic pain, deep dyspareunia or a dramatic change in bleeding patterns after the initial changes. If the strings of the device are not visible at follow-up and it is suspected that the device has been expelled or has perforated out of the uterus, pelvic ultrasound can usually determine the position or absence of the device.

Barrier methods

Condoms

Condoms are an effective method of contraception if used consistently. They are the only contraceptive method which also protects against sexually transmitted infections. Condom users need to be instructed in correct use and disposal.

Male condoms are traditionally made of latex but a polyurethane condom has become available. This has the advantage of being looser, the so-called 'baggy condom', conducting heat better than the latex condom, and providing an alternative for people with a latex allergy. However, it is more likely to slip off or split than the latex variety, resulting in a slightly higher failure rate. Condoms come in a variety of colours, some are impregnated with spermicide, and some are ribbed to provide extra stimulation for the female partner. In some countries different-flavoured condoms are available. Different brands are of varying sizes.

The female condom consists of a lubricated polyurethane bag which has a ring around its outer rim and a second unattached ring inside which is used to insert the condom into the vagina and help in anchoring it. The outer edge of the condom covers the labia majora, providing extra protection against herpes and genital warts compared to male condoms. It is considerably more expensive than the male condom but is the only method available for women to protect themselves against STIs.

Diaphragm

The diaphragm is a rubber dome with an outer ring that keeps it in situ. The theoretical failure rate is 4 per cent but user failure rates can be between 10 and 25 per cent. There are two types, one with a coiled spring and the other with a firmer double-coiled spring (the All-flex diaphragm). Diaphragms come in sizes ranging from 50 mm to 100 mm. The size required depends on the distance from the posterior fornix to the internal aspect of the symphysis pubis. The individual woman requires a fitting and needs to be shown how to insert the diaphragm and check that it is covering the cervix.

Diaphragms are unsuitable for women who have a latex allergy, large cystoceles or uterine prolapse, or are uncomfortable inserting their fingers into the vagina.

Side effects are rare. An increased incidence of urinary tract infections has been reported in users and if the diaphragm prescribed is too large the woman can experience discomfort during use.

The diaphragm can be inserted any time prior to intercourse but should not be removed in under six hours after the last ejaculation. There are no good data relating to the need for additional spermicide, so this is optional.

Periodic abstinence

Periodic abstinence refers to any method which avoids intercourse during the fertile period. This can be estimated by the calendar method, which is based on the length of the last six menstrual cycles, the taking of daily basal body temperature or detecting cervical mucus changes (Billings method). It is most reliable if all three methods are combined (sympto-thermal method).

Sterilisation

Male sterilisation (vasectomy) is a simple operation which can be performed under local anaesthetic as an outpatient procedure or general anaesthetic as a day-only procedure. The vasa differentia are occluded and cut through a central incision. Failure rates are 1 per 300 procedures. Side effects include haematoma and infection following the procedure and long-term granuloma formation and scrotal pain. Infertility is not immediate and generally a sperm count is done two months post surgery. If this is negative the couple can stop using alternative contraception. Reversal is possible, but only 50 per cent achieve a pregnancy following vasostomy.

Laparoscopic sterilisation is the most common form of female sterilisation, with the tubes being occluded by the Filshie clip. This produces immediate infertility. Recently the Essure device has become available. This is inserted into the ostia of both fallopian tubes by means of a hysteroscope under either local anaesthetic or a short-acting tranquilliser. Within three months of insertion both tubes are generally occluded. Immediate failure rates for female sterilisation are 1/1000.[10]

Women's choice

A woman needs to be fully informed about the contraceptive methods available to her, including the advantages, disadvantages and failure rate (Table 12.3). Individual preferences and medical history should be explored during the decision-making process.

TABLE 12.3 Summary of methods of contraception: comparative failure rates, advantages and disadvantages

Method failure rate: number of pregnancies that will occur if a method is used by 100 women for one year (HWY); is the failure rate inherent in the method of contraception used and is the lowest failure rate for that method. It occurs if the user receives correct instructions and follows these instructions conscientiously.

User failure rate: failure rate in actual use; varies according to user receiving and carrying out correct instructions.

Pearl Index: a method of comparing contraceptive methods; is calculated from formula:

Failure rate = (total accidental pregnancies X 1200)/total months of exposure.

(continued overleaf)

TABLE 12.3 continued

Method	Pearl index	Failure rate	Advantages	Disadvantages
Coitus interruptus	18	Not very effective	No health risks. Always available.	High failure rate. Requires good control of ejaculation. Not satisfying for many couples. May cause anxiety.
Natural family planning, sympto-thermal method	2–3	Although theoretical calculations may suggest these techniques can be relatively effective, in practice the failure rates are high.	No health risk. No financial costs. Acceptable to some religious groups. Increased self-knowledge and awareness. May be used to plan timing of conception	Failure rate higher. Takes time and training to learn method. May reduce spontaneity. Requires cooperation of both partners.
Male condom	3	If used properly and consistently, the failure rate can be as low as 2%. If used incorrectly, the failure rate can be as high as 20%. If used with spermicides, effectiveness is increased.	Readily available without prescription. No health risks. Protects against STIs. Can be used with spermicide.	May reduce spontaneity and sensitivity. Careful attention to instructions necessary to prevent breaking or slipping off. Requires continual motivation. Rare allergies to rubber may occur.
Female condom	5	Pregnancy rates similar to male condom if used consistently.	Only female method which protects against STIs. Can be inserted long before intercourse. Provides more extensive protection of genitals than male condom.	Expensive. Can slip into vagina or penis slip above the condom during intercourse.
Diaphragm (with spermicide)	6	Failure rate varies from 4 to 6%. Failure rates in general use 10–25%. Effectiveness depends on the motivation of the couple to use it correctly and at each act of sexual intercourse.	No health risks. Need not interfere with lovemaking. Good for infrequent sexual relationships.	Requires initial consultation for fitting. Occasional allergies to rubber or to spermicides. Requires continual motivation. Requires refitting weight gain or loss over 5 kg, and following pregnancy.

TABLE 12.3 continued

Method	Pearl index	Failure rate	Advantages	Disadvantages
Cervical cap	9	As for diaphragm	As for diaphragm	More difficult to insert than diaphragm. Sometimes knocked off cervix during intercourse. Not readily available in Australia.
IUD (intrauterine device)	0.1–1	Failure rate 1%	Effective. Requires no action at time of sexual intercourse. Provides continuous cover for 5–10 years depending on the device. Woman immediately fertile when device is removed. Suitable if continuous motivation is absent.	Periods may be longer, more painful and heavier. Risk of pelvic inflammatory disease. Insertion requires doctor's consultation and surgical procedure. Requires woman to check string monthly to confirm that IUD is correctly in place. Does not prevent ectopic pregnancy.
COC (combined oral contraceptive)	0.1	Highly effective with a failure rate of about 1% if taken according to instructions. Failure rate 2–6% in general use.	Convenient. Effective. Reduces pain and menstrual loss. Regular menstrual periods. Does not interfere with lovemaking. May improve acne.	Requires daily pill taking. Long-term health risks such as blood clots are related to thrombophilias, age and smoking. These are not common. Side effects may occur, eg breast tenderness, nausea, headaches, but usually pass in a few months. Effectiveness diminished by vomiting, severe diarrhoea, and some medications. Requires doctor's prescription. Requires continual motivation.
POP (progestogen-only pill)	0.5	Highly effective, with failure rate of 2%. Efficiency slightly lower than COC, especially in younger women. Efficiency is similar to COCs in women 35–40 years of age.	Convenient. Effective. Can be used during lactation. May be suitable for use in older women. Fewer side effects than COC.	Less effective than COC. Irregular bleeding patterns. Must be taken at same time each day. Requires doctor's prescription. Requires continual motivation.

(continued overleaf)

TABLE 12.3 continued

Method	Pearl index	Failure rate	Advantages	Disadvantages
Depo-Provera (progestogen-only injectable contraception)	0.3	Highly effective, with failure rate similar to Pearl index	Needs only be given every 3 months. Minimal motivation required. Does not interfere with lovemaking. Effective. May eliminate menstruation after 6–12 months.	Requires prescription and injection. Can result in irregular bleeding. Absence of periods may result in anxiety. Side effects, eg weight gain, nausea, breast tenderness. Not immediately reversible. Return of fertility may be delayed.
Mirena IUS	0.1	Highly effective. Cumulative pregnancy rate at end of 5-year lifespan 1.2%.	Long-acting, 5-year lifespan. Does not interfere with lovemaking. Reduces menstrual blood loss. Useful to manage dysfunctional uterine bleeding and pelvic pain.	Requires an experienced medical practitioner to insert and requires removal by a clinician. Some women experience progestogenic side effects, eg acne. May produce erratic bleeding, spotting or amenorrhoea.
Implanon	0.09	Most highly effective method available provided it is inserted at correct time in cycle. Provides contraception for 3 years.	Progestogen-only method. No action required on part of user following insertion. Rapid return of fertility.	Requires well trained clinician to insert and remove. All women have disruption of menstrual cycle. 20–30% of women have frequent or prolonged bleeding.
Tubal ligation	0.4	Highly effective, with failure rate less than 1%.	Immediately effective. Permanent.	Requires hospitalisation, risks associated with anaesthesia and surgical procedure. Generally irreversible.
Essure	N/A	Highly effective but requires 3 months after insertion to provide full tubal occlusion.	Irreversible. No anaesthetic or surgical procedure required for this method of tubal occlusion.	Requires highly skilled hysteroscopist to insert. Placement of device not always possible due to tubal spasm.
Vasectomy	0.1	Highly effective, with failure rate 0.1–0.5%.	Effective. Permanent.	Minor surgical procedure under local anaesthetic, therefore risks associated with surgery, eg infections, haematoma.

TABLE 12.3		continued		
Method	**Pearl index**	**Failure rate**	**Advantages**	**Disadvantages**
Vasectomy *(cont'd)*				Not immediately effective. Generally irreversible.
Post-coital contraception (emergency contraception)		Highly effective. Most effective if given in first 24 hours after unprotected intercourse, but still at least 58% effective at 72 hours. Yuzpe prevents 75%, levonorgestrel 83% of expected pregnancies following unprotected intercourse.	Effective. May reduce anxiety. Useful in incidents of unplanned sex, rape, broken condom, missed pill etc.	Requires prescription. Does not offer ongoing contraceptive cover. Yuzpe may cause nausea and vomiting, breast tenderness. Requires anti-emetic. Much lower incidence with levonorgestrel ECP. Pregnancy test is required if usual period or withdrawal bleeding does not occur.

Unplanned pregnancy

CLINICAL PRESENTATION

Control of reproduction is recognised as a woman's human right. Termination of pregnancy has legal, moral, ethical, social, political and medical aspects and is the subject of strong opinion. Termination of pregnancy is the outcome of approximately 20 per cent of pregnancies worldwide. The number varies within countries and is restricted by law in some and, where women have a legal right to abortion, there is often political and social controversy. Where women do not have a legal right to abortion, illegal abortion is the cause of considerable mortality and morbidity. The mortality rate from abortion, where this is legal and performed by accredited practitioners, is considerably lower than that of childbirth.

In the UK the Abortion Act was passed in 1967. A woman may have a termination of pregnancy if two practitioners are willing to certify that:

- the continuation of the pregnancy would involve a greater risk to the woman's life than termination
- a termination would prevent grave permanent injury to the physical or mental health for the woman or any existing child(ren) of the family of the pregnant woman
- the pregnancy has not exceeded 24 weeks gestation
- there is a substantial risk that if the child were born it would suffer from such physical or mental abnormalities as to be severely handicapped.

Since the introduction of this act, illegal abortion in the UK has virtually disappeared. In Australia, the legality of pregnancy termination varies by state and the data is incomplete (Section 5).

Psychological response to having an abortion

A woman's response to having an abortion will be influenced by the social context, the experience, the perceived degree of support for her decision, and the positive and negative aspects that the abortion has for her.[11]

The reasons for having an abortion vary with the woman's age, educational aspirations, socio-economic status, and whether or not she already has a family. It is influenced by:

- Personal situation—not ready, too young, health problems
- Circumstantial situation—relationship, financial, educational.

Counselling

Any women seeking a termination of pregnancy should receive counselling by a sensitive, sympathetic health professional. This should involve:

- An opportunity for the woman to discuss the reasons for the request and her concerns and fears
- Providing non-judgemental information about both termination of pregnancy and alternative courses of action (continuing the pregnancy and keeping the baby or considering adoption)
- A medical check to:
  - confirm the pregnancy and the gestation
  - screen for infection (*Chlamydia trachomatis* and other STIs)
  - take a Pap test
  - check the haemoglobin and blood group (give anti-D at the time of termination if the woman is Rhesus-negative)
  - check for a history of allergies, blood dyscrasias, or other relevant medical condition
- Support—discuss the relationship with her partner, family or friends who can offer her support
- Explain the procedure
- Arrange follow-up.

Methods of pregnancy termination

This depends on the gestation. The earlier the termination is undertaken, the less risk to the woman. However, this should not preclude adequate counselling. A curettage < 7 weeks gestation is three times more likely to fail than those between 7 and 12 weeks.[12] Ideally, women should be offered a choice of methods suitable to the gestation based on the evidence to support particular recommendations[13] (Figure 12.1).

Surgical

Suction curettage is performed on pregnancies < 14 weeks. A curettage < 6 weeks gestation may be less successful at complete removal of the products of conception (POC). The larger the uterus, the more dilatation is required to open the cervix and remove the POC. Where the cervix is firm and closed, vaginal prostaglandin may be

FIGURE 12.1 Methods of termination of pregnancy at different gestations

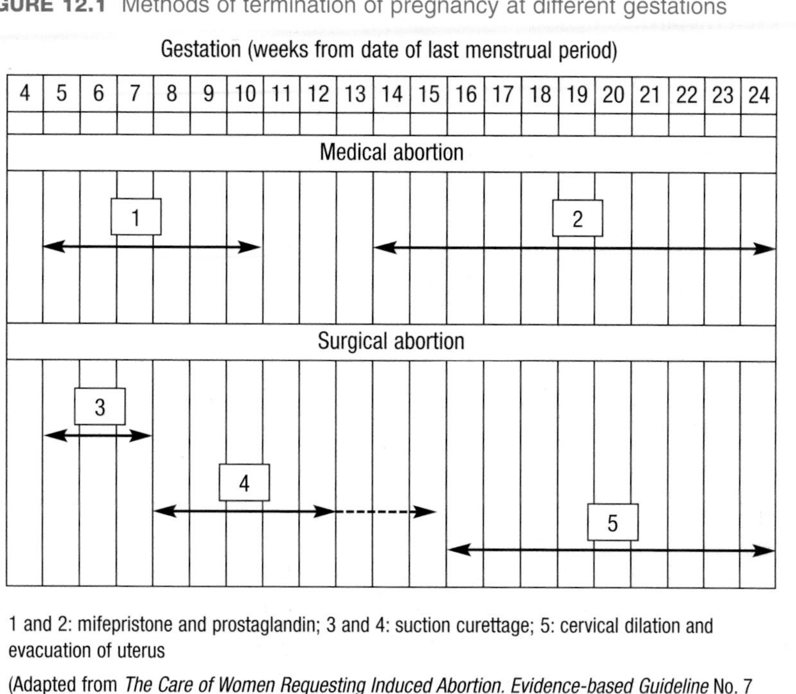

1 and 2: mifepristone and prostaglandin; 3 and 4: suction curettage; 5: cervical dilation and evacuation of uterus

(Adapted from *The Care of Women Requesting Induced Abortion. Evidence-based Guideline* No. 7 Due for Review 2003. Royal College of Obstetricians and Gynaecologists. Clinical Effectiveness Support Unit.)

given to soften the cervix and reduce the risk of trauma. Most women choose a general anaesthetic for this procedure.

Medical

A combination of RU486 (mifepristone) and prostaglandin can be used. The RU486 is an antiprogestogenic agent and the prostaglandin (PGE1—gemeprost, Cervigem) is used a few hours prior to the RU486 to soften the cervix. This regimen is effective in > 95 per cent cases, efficient (most abortions taking 6–8 hours), and therefore safer and more acceptable for women. However, it is not readily available in all parts of the UK, has not been approved for use in Australia, and is unavailable in many countries where unsafe abortion is practised.[14]

Complications

- Haemorrhage
- Incomplete abortion—may require an evacuation of the uterus
- Ectopic pregnancy—consider where minimal POC are obtained
- Failed abortion—continuing pregnancy
- Perforation of the uterus
- Infection—more associated with retained POC, or if an infection already present. Note: screen or give antibiotic cover for chlamydia and/or gonorrhoea

- Infertility – pelvic inflammatory disease can result from intrauterine infection
- Preterm birth – unlikely unless a late termination with marked dilatation of the cervix is performed.

Follow-up

- To check her medical and psychological health
- Plan for contraceptive and sexual health advice after the termination.

Sexually transmitted infections

CLINICAL PRESENTATIONS

The fact that sexual activity is involved in this wide group of diseases has implications other than for health. These are social, cultural, psychological and political as many become major public health issues. This group of infections is not constant over time or between cultures. While many are acquired through direct sexual contact, others may have significant non-sexual transmission. The clinical presentation of STIs varies, depending on which organisms and disease mechanisms are involved. Some may be asymptomatic. These are particularly important as complications can occur that may not be apparent until a later date. In fact, the most common scenario for women with STIs is that they are asymptomatic (chlamydia 70–90%, gonorrhoea 80%, trichomonas 90%). However, STIs can also present acutely, with less acute symptoms of a disease or as a chronic consequence of a disease (Box 12.8).

BOX 12.8 Clinical presentations of sexually transmitted infections

1. Detected from screening
2. Concern re STI contact
3. Vaginal discharge
4. External genital symptoms:
   - Pruritus
   - Dyspareunia
   - Dysuria
   - Pain/discomfort
   - Skin colour changes
   - Lump/swelling
   - Ulceration
5. HIV infection
6. Pelvic pain
   - Acute: ectopic pregnancy/PID
   - Chronic: PID
7. Dyspareunia
8. Sexual assault
9. Infertility
10. AIDS

General points

Sexual activity

- Current sexual activity is a more accurate measure of current exposure to the risk of STIs.
- Risk of exposure to an STI is directly associated not only with the number of infected sex partners, but also with the prevalence of STIs within one's pool of potential sex partners.

- The number of sex partners within a specific time period, often one to three months, has been shown to be a risk factor for having gonorrhoea, chlamydia, genital herpes and human papillomavirus infection.
- Some women are at risk of acquiring STIs because of their own risky sexual behaviour; others are at risk solely because of the sexual behaviour of their partners.
- Lifetime number of sex partners is associated with an increased risk of cervical and other genital tract cancers.
- The nature of sexual activity (vaginal, oral, anal sex) will affect the chance of acquiring specific infections.

Genital tract environment

- The normal vaginal flora has the acid-producing Gram-positive rods called *Lactobacillus* that produce lactic acid from glucose, keeping the vagina at an acid pH, which offers some protection against infection.
- Douching may adversely alter a woman's susceptibility to infection. Routine douching for hygiene has been shown to double the risk of acquiring bacterial vaginosis.[15]
- Cervical ectopy increases susceptibility to chlamydia and other infections. Cervical ectopy decreases with increasing age and increases with hormonal contraceptive use.

Diagnosis of an STI

Diagnosis of an STI not only has a profound effect on the individual but also has societal ramifications and many issues need to be considered (Box 12.9).

BOX 12.9 Considerations for STIs

- Concurrent STIs
- Confidentiality
- Counselling
- Contraception
- Condoms
- Compliance (adherence)
- Complications
- Cost
- Contact tracing

CLINICAL PRESENTATION: STI detected from screening

Whether or not screening is applied to the general population or to specific groups at risk for a particular disease needs to be based on the many different criteria for screening (Section 1). A number of sexually transmitted diseases cause serious long-term problems for the woman and/or a fetus. Most antenatal clinics screen for syphilis, hepatitis and some for HIV. A US study suggested that, for *Chlamydia trachomatis* infection, the most cost-effective strategy was age-based screening of all women under 30 years.[16] Screening was cost effective at any prevalence of chlamydia in asymptomatic women of 1.1 per cent or above, and at a prevalence of 11 per cent or above universal screening became most cost-effective. The prevalence of chlamydial infection in women in the UK ranges from about 2 to 12 per cent, with a weighted mean average of 5.3 per cent.[17] Screening can be simplified and made more acceptable by testing from the Thin Prep Pap test (approved for *Chlamydia trachomatis* and *Neisseria gonorrhoeae* tests by the FDA in the USA), from a urine test or from a self-collected swab.[18,19]

CLINICAL PRESENTATION: Concern about STI contact (asymptomatic)

Increased awareness of STIs has led more women to ask for a sexual health check, often after unprotected sex or if a new partner is involved in the relationship but without there being any specific symptom. This is with good reason—asymptomatic disease occurs in most cases of chlamydia, gonorrhoea and *Trichomonas vaginalis*.

An accurate history is an essential prerequisite to direct the examination and appropriate investigations.

History for a woman with STI concerns

Why is she concerned?

1 Unprotected sex (no barrier method used)
2 Partner concerns:
  - Symptoms
  - History of STI
  - IV drug user
  - Bisexual
  - Other partners (woman or her current partner)
  - Change in partner
  - Prisoner
3 Pregnancy concern.

Does she have any symptoms on direct questioning?

- Vaginal discharge
- Abdominal pain
- Dyspareunia or other sexual problem
- Dysuria
- Menstrual irregularity
- Vulval: itch, rash, ulcer, lump
- Rectal discharge or bleeding.

Additional information

1 Last menstrual period
2 Current contraception
3 Previous STIs
4 Medications, allergies, past medical and social history
5 Sexual behaviour:
  - Regular sexual partner
  - Last contact with other partner(s). This will be useful in assessing likelihood of infection considering the different incubation periods (Table 12.4).

- Sex without consent
- Gender of sexual partner(s)
- Any partner history of male-to-male sex
- Use of condoms
- Sexual activity: oral, vaginal, anal
- Overseas contact: USA, Asia, Africa
- Possible exposure to blood: tattoos, body piercing, IV drug user, needlestick injury, blood transfusion (dates).

TABLE 12.4 Incubation periods for sexually transmitted diseases

Infection	Time before onset of symptoms	Usual early symptoms*
Trichomoniasis	5–28 days	Women: vaginal discharge Men: urethritis
Gonococcal infection	Within a few days of exposure	Women: cervicitis, endometritis, PID, urethritis Men: purulent urethral discharge
Chlamydial infection	1–3 weeks after exposure	Women: cervicitis, endometritis, PID, urethritis Men: mucoid, watery or mucopurulent urethral discharge
Herpes simplex virus	2–14 days. The primary infection may be asymptomatic.	Genital vesicles and ulceration. Initial infection: multiple, widespread, bilateral, at different stages of development and resolution, and at sites of direct mucosal infection. Associated fever and malaise.
Syphilis	10–90 days (average 28 days) Four–ten weeks after primary disease	Primary disease: anogenital ulceration. Often not seen in women because chancre on cervix or fourchette. Secondary disease: disseminated rash and glandular fever-like illness, resolving over a few weeks. In 25% of patients it recurs in the 2nd year.
Chancroid	Usually 4–7 days	Ulcer, often missed by women, and inguinal tenderness
Genital warts	4–6 weeks	Warty lesions on anogenital area
HIV	1–3 weeks	Acute mononucleosis-like illness: headache, myalgia, sore throat, lymphadenopathy, fever and erythematous rash
Hepatitis A	Average 4 weeks	Malaise, fever, anorexia, jaundice
Hepatitis B	3–6 weeks	Malaise, fever, anorexia, jaundice

*Many are asymptomatic.

Clinical examination

An STI examination can be embarrassing and uncomfortable for many women. It is essential that the health care professional minimises these problems and creates a relaxed environment where the woman feels comfortable, safe and in control. The correct approach will encourage cooperation with treatment and follow-up. Privacy, a good light and equipment readily at hand for appropriate investigations are essential.

General system examination

An STI may produce extra-genital signs. Therefore check:

- General nutritional status
- Signs of needle exposure ('track lines', tattoos, body piercing)
- Lymphadenopathy
- Skin
- Mouth
- Abdomen
- Other systems as indicated from the history.

Genital examination

See Section 1.

Investigations

These should only be performed with the woman's knowledge and consent, after adequate counselling. Samples taken can be tested for microscopy and culture but these are insensitive tests. The development of the polymerase chain reaction (PCR) test has increased the detection of STIs.

PCR test

The PCR test is based on the fact that each species has a unique genetic sequence of DNA/RNA. The DNA can be extracted, amplified and new DNA detected. The PCR test has excellent sensitivity and specificity, is easy to take (urine sample or self-inserted swab), and does not depend on living organisms. It enables specimens to be collected without the necessity for cold storage. Negative issues include false positive results and not obtaining a drug resistance profile.

Office tests

Office tests are being developed to provide immediate answers. The sites sampled will depend on the specific infections sought from the history.

1 Swabs

- *Vaginal swab for PCR.* If the woman has had a hysterectomy, a first pass urine sample should be taken.
  - PCR for chlamydia and gonorrhoea
  - Gram-stained smear and culture (for antibiotic sensitivity). This may be taken if the gonorrhoea test is positive, before treatment with any antibiotic.
  - Can be taken during menstruation for chlamydia and gonorrhoea.

- *Vaginal swab from posterior vaginal fornix* for microscopy and culture. This will diagnose group B streptococcus, candidiasis, trichomonas and bacterial vaginosis.
- *Wet preparation and a high vaginal swab* for candidiasis, trichomonas and bacterial vaginosis. The vaginal secretion is mixed with two drops of normal saline on a slide and examined under 400 × magnification.
  A vaginal swab can also be smeared onto a microscope slide, air dried, heat fixed and Gram-stained and examined under 1000 × oil immersion. This allows precise identification of candidiasis and bacterial vaginosis (clue cells) but not trichomoniasis.
- *Anorectal mucosal swab.* Blind anal swabbing (ie without the use of a proctoscope) has been shown to be as sensitive as testing using a proctoscope.
- A *swab from genital ulcers* for herpes culture and HSV antigen detection. PCR testing is available for herpes and has been shown to be a much more sensitive test. It will also determine the herpes simplex type. Lymphogranuloma venereum (LGV) can also be detected using a PCR test.
- A *urethral swab* for chlamydia where there are urinary symptoms.

2 Vaginal pH

Vaginal pH suggests:

< 4.5	Normal
< 4, 4.0–4.5	*Candida albicans*
5.0–6.0	Bacterial vaginosis/*T. vaginalis*
> 6.0	Atrophic vaginitis

3 Biopsy

Biopsy may be required for vulvar ulceration or an unusual appearance of the cervix (usually by a specialist under colposcopic direction—see Section 16).

4 Blood test

Serology for syphilis, lymphogranuloma venereum (LGV), the hepatitis viruses A, B, C or Delta, and HIV infection. Specific herpes antibody tests are available but their place is unclear. Serological tests for chlamydia and gonorrhoea are rarely useful.

5 Urine test

For PCR and LCR for chlamydia—this specimen should be a first-pass sample. This is useful if a speculum examination is not undertaken, or for follow-up to check clearance of infection. A mid-stream urine can be taken to exclude bladder infection.

6 Pap test

The Pap test can be taken during a speculum examination. Yeasts, clue cells and trichomonads can sometimes be seen but this has a low sensitivity for vaginal infections and should not be used as a substitute test. Thin prep Pap test can detect *Chlamydia trachomatis* and *Neisseria gonococcus*.

Management

Immediate

Any results that are immediately available should be given to the woman. Once the tests are taken, a decision should be made as to whether immediate treatment should be given in the absence of a specific diagnosis. If a partner has an infection diagnosed or has non-gonococcal urethritis, the woman should be treated for that infection or with tetracycline even in the absence of the organism in the partner.

Follow-up

1 Results

The woman should be told the specific diagnosis, given information about the course of the disease, treatment and long-term implications of untreated disease covering specific aspects as requested (fertility, recurrence, transmissibility).

2 Advice

The woman should be advised to avoid intercourse until the treatment is complete, the partner treated and, ideally, follow-up tests negative. General advice taking into account the woman's age, lifestyle, beliefs, culture, sexual practices and social situation should be given. This could include safe sex practices (Box 12.10), fertility control, risk minimisation (eg needle exchange programs for IV drug users, avoiding contact until checked if an STI is suspected).

BOX 12.10 Safe sex practices

- Condom use: water-based lubricant with vaginal or anal sex.
- Condoms should be used for oral sex.
- Do not share bodily fluids: vaginal fluids, blood, semen.
- Negligible risk for kissing and masturbation.
- Oral sex is high risk for transmission of herpes but low risk for other STIs.
- Genital herpes, warts, pubic lice, HPV and scabies are transmitted by close body contact and are not prevented by condoms.

3 Partner notification

The woman is in the best position to contact partners. This may be made easier by providing her with a contact tracing letter that explains the infection, testing and treatment. In difficult situations assistance can be obtained from local sexual health clinics, health department counsellors, or health workers with contacts in specific cultural groups. Factors affecting the ability of the woman to contact the trace should be considered. These include explaining the purpose of contact tracing to prevent the woman being reinfected, prevention of long-term complications and preventing the spread of infection. The confidential nature of contact tracing should be discussed, should the health care worker perform this function. The woman may fear the repercussions of contact tracing, which may include violence, rejection or gossip.

4 Follow-up

A repeat test after treatment is the ideal but may not always be achieved. Where possible, single-dose treatment may benefit the woman who may be less likely to adhere to a course of treatment.

5 Counselling

Women with an STI may find an additional visit useful for asking further questions. Many women find a diagnosis of an STI a cause of anxiety and depression. This may affect their relationships both at the time and in the future. Monogamy between sex partners is one of the best methods of preventing STIs, but this may not be achievable. Encouraging communication between sexual partners and regular sexual health checks can reduce asymptomatic disease.

Notifiable STIs

It is the duty of the health care professional to notify the health authorities of specific STIs (Box 12.11). This is a public health requirement to monitor the prevalence of infections, the pattern of antibiotic resistance, and groups in the community who may be at risk and require specific education.

BOX 12.11 Notifiable* STIs

(*This may vary with the local authority.)

- AIDS (acquired immune deficiency syndrome)
- Chancroid
- *Chlamydia trachomatis* infection (genital, lymphogranuloma venereum, non-genital)
- Donovanosis (granuloma inguinale)
- Gonococcal infection (genital and non-genital)
- Hepatitis (A, B—acute and chronic)
- HIV (human immunodeficiency virus) infection

CLINICAL PRESENTATION: Vaginal discharge

Always check current symptoms against the background of what is 'normal' for that woman. This will vary with the individual, the menstrual cycle, pregnancy and time of life.

History

- What is this woman's 'normal' discharge like?
- When did this change?
- Describe the discharge:
  - Colour (clear, milky, bloody, yellow, green etc)
  - Consistency (thick, runny)
  - Quantity (scanty, copious, stains underwear, needs to wear protection)
  - Odour (fishy, yeasty, unpleasant)
- Relationship to menstrual cycle and sexual activity

- Recent travel overseas or contact with person who has travelled overseas
- Symptoms suggesting a complication of an STI: abdominal pain, dyspareunia, altered menstruation, arthralgia, rash
- History of sexual contact—has the woman a suggested contact time when an STI may have been acquired? (See incubation time of STIs, Table 12.4.)

Examination and investigations

See asymptomatic STI check and Section 1.

While the 'classic' appearances are described and sometimes seen (see photo section 4), specific infection can only be diagnosed accurately after microbiological testing.

Differential diagnosis

1 Physiological discharge:
   - 'Normal' discharge may be scanty or quite copious
   - 'Normal' for the individual may change throughout the life cycle
   - Cyclical changes: scanty after the period, 'egg white' at ovulation, white/creamy in the luteal phase and increasing premenstrually
   - Increases with: hormones: OCP, HRT and pregnancy, cervical ectropion, sexual arousal

2 Infective causes of vaginal discharge:
   - Vaginal infections (Table 12.5)
     - Candida
     - *Trichomonas vaginalis*
     - Bacterial vaginosis (the most common cause of abnormal discharge in women of child-bearing age).
     - Anaerobic organisms
     - Beta haemolytic streptococci
   - Cervical infections (Table 12.6)
     - *Neisseria gonorrhoeae*
     - *Chlamydia trachomatis*
   - Cervical lesions
     - Herpes
     - Warts
     - Syphilitic chancre
   - Rare:
     - Adult—toxic shock syndrome (*Staphylococcus aureus*)
     - Child—consider presence of a foreign body, sexual abuse, worm infestation

3 Non-infective causes of vaginal discharge:
   - Cervical cancer, endometrial cancer—foul-smelling discharge as a result of necrotic tissue
   - Cervical polyps, especially if the surface becomes eroded
   - Foreign body (tampon, condom, sex toy)
   - Trauma

4 Other issues that must be considered within the differential diagnosis of a sexual or gynaecological problem include:
- Anxiety or depression
- Relationship problems
- Abusive situation past or present.

TABLE 12.5 Main infective causes of vaginal discharge

	Candidiasis	Trichomoniasis	Bacterial vaginosis
Organism	*Candida albicans*: most common vaginal infection. Both cells and hyphae can be seen on a Gram-stained smear.	*Trichomonas vaginalis* is a flagellated protozoan. It is an anaerobe which generates hydrogen to combine with oxygen to create an anaerobic environment.	Characterised by an overgrowth of mainly anaerobic bacteria in the vagina. The normally predominant lactobacilli are reduced and replaced.
Symptoms	Itch—vaginal and vulval. Introital dyspareunia.	Asymptomatic 90%. Vaginal/vulval soreness. Dysuria. Offensive odour.	Offensive smell. Copious discharge. (No itching or discomfort.)
Odour	Yeast	Fishy	Fishy malodour more noticeable at time of sex or menses.
Colour	White	Yellow/green	Grey/white, thin homogeneous.
Consistency	Many clinical variants including thick 'cottage cheese', scant, and may have no associated discharge.	Varies from thin and scanty to thick and profuse. Classic frothy appearance in 10–30%.	Watery/profuse
Signs	Inflammation of vulva and vagina. Removing adherent plaques from vaginal wall may cause bleeding.	Inflammation of vagina and vulva. Colpitis macularis ('strawberry cervix').	No inflammation. Non-adherent, uniform, white/grey coating of vaginal walls.
pH	4–4.5	5–6	5–6+
Microscopy	Neutrophils. Pseudohyphae and spores (fungus).	Neutrophils. *Trichomonas vaginalis* (flagellate protozoan).	No neutrophils. Clue cells (vaginal squames covered with small coccobacilli).
Culture	*Candida albicans* responsible for 80–90%. Other species rare. Check candida species if recurrent infection.	*Trichomonas vaginalis* found in the vagina, urethra and paraurethral glands.	*Bacteroides* *Gardnerella vaginalis* *Mobiluncus* species *Mycoplasma hominis*

(continued overleaf)

TABLE 12.5 continued

	Candidiasis	Trichomoniasis	Bacterial vaginosis
Test	Wet prep or Gram-stained vaginal smear.	Direct observation on a wet preparation. Specific culture.	At least three of the following criteria should be present for diagnosis: 1 Thin, white, homogeneous discharge. 2 Clue cells on microscopy. 3 pH of vaginal fluid > 4.5.
		'Whiff' test: release of a fishy odour on adding alkali (10% KOH) to the sample. Also positive in presence of spermatozoa.	
Notes	Not an STI. Commensal from the bowel. Symptoms when overgrowth of organisms. Recurrent infection: consider underlying condition: diabetes mellitus, antibiotic use, immune suppression, HIV infection. Possible link to orogenital sex.	Sexually transmitted. Can be asymptomatic. Not a strong risk factor for miscarriage before 16 weeks gestation, but may be associated with miscarriage in the second trimester.[20]	Not an STI. Endogenous, overgrowth of organisms. Associated with sexual activity; in pregnancy with preterm rupture of membranes and preterm labour. Not uncommon in lesbian couples.
Partner	Secondarily infected. Symptoms of irritation, soreness and redness after sexual contact.	Treat. Asymptomatic in 15–50%. Or: urethral discharge and/or dysuria. Urethral irritation and frequency.	No need to treat if not troublesome.
Treatment	Topical anti-fungal cream/pessary course. Oral treatment for resistant, recurrent, or by choice (expensive). *C. krusei* is resistant to fluconazole. Long-term suppressive therapy if refractory.	All partners in previous 3 months should be treated. Metronidazole 2 g orally once or tinidazole 2 g orally once.	Treat if symptomatic or before invasive procedures (avoid PID complication). Pregnancy: metronidazole (except 1st trimester) or clindamycin 2% cream for 5 days.

TABLE 12.6 Main infective causes of cervical discharge

Infection	Chlamydia	Gonococcus
Symptoms	Most asymptomatic: 70–90%. Post-coital or intermenstrual bleeding can occur but has a low positive predictive value (PPV 19%) in women 25 years and older.[21] Lower abdominal pain.	Asymptomatic in up to 80%. Increased/altered vaginal discharge. Pelvic pain if upper genital tract involvement. Dysuria. Rare cause of intermenstrual bleeding or menorrhagia.
Signs	Nil/mucopurulent discharge/cervicitis.	Nil. Mucopurulent endocervical discharge and contact bleeding. Pelvic/lower abdominal tenderness.
Associated conditions	10–15% PID. May occur concurrently with gonorrhoea.	Coexistent anorectal and pharyngeal infection (also may be asymptomatic). Rectal infection can occur from posterior spread of vaginal secretions. 10–15% with PID. Coinfection with *Chlamydia trachomatis* common.
Organism	Obligate intracellular parasites.	Gram-negative diplococci, *Neisseria gonorrhoeae.*
Diagnosis	Endocervical swab: insert into canal, leave 15 seconds, and rotate as withdrawn. 10–20% additional positives will be detected by assaying a urethral swab or urine sample.	Endocervical swab for Gram-staining sent in Aimes or charcoal containing Stuart's medium. Urethral swab. Urine sample. Rectal and oropharyngeal swabs when symptomatic at these sites. Microscopy and culture should detect 90% of cases.
Tests	Direct fluorescent antibody (DIF): high sensitivity but labour intensive. Enzyme immunoassays (EIA): high specificity when combined with a confirmation assay, a variable sensitivity. Automated, inexpensive test. Culture. Nucleic acid amplification techniques (NAAT): high specificity and high sensitivity. Expensive.	Cell culture and selective culture media 85% versus microscopy 50–70%. Antigen detection tests 77%. PCR.
Male partner	Urethral discharge. Dysuria. Asymptomatic in 50%.	Asymptomatic in 10%. Urethral discharge/dysuria. Rectal infection may cause anal discharge or discomfort.

(continued overleaf)

TABLE 12.6 continued

Infection	Chlamydia	Gonococcus
Notes	Test of cure. Most common STI in the UK and Australia.	Penicillinase-producing infection (PPNG) is increasing—varies with country and area. Coinfection with *Chlamydia trachomatis* occurs in up to 40% of women and 20% of men. Combining effective therapies is therefore appropriate.
Treatment	Azithromycin 1 g orally as single dose (category B1 in pregnancy), or doxycycline 100 mg twice a day for 10 days *or* erythromycin 800 mg twice a day for 10 days (in pregnancy). PID: azithromycin and metronidazole followed by doxycycline.	Ciprofloxacin 500 mg orally as single dose *or* ampicillin 2 g plus probenecid 1 g orally as single dose. Agents effective against PPNG. Ciprofloxacin resistance widely reported, especially in SE Asia. Must culture. If no follow-up, offer ceftriaxone as treatment. Followed by anti-chlamydial treatment.
Complications	Upper genital, peritoneal, joint and ocular manifestations can occur. Epididymitis in the male. Neonatal conjunctivitis in 30–50% and pneumonia in 10–20% of neonates born to a mother with chlamydia from passage through an infected birth canal. Gonorrhoea should also be suspected with a 'sticky eye' in the neonate. Ophthalmia neonatorum (conjunctivitis within 21 days of birth) is a notifiable disease.	

Management

- Treat the infection diagnosed.
- Assess for other STIs.
- Trace and treat partners.
- Reinforce health education: safe sex, contraception, regular checks if at risk.
- Assess treatment efficacy—a test of cure should be considered three weeks after the end of treatment.
- A postmenopausal woman with an abnormal discharge needs an ultrasound scan and endometrial biopsy to exclude a malignancy.

KEY POINT

Vaginal discharge does not always indicate an STI.

Specific infections

Herpes

Diagnosis

PCR of swab taken from lesion. Viral culture and antigen detection may also be used—these are less sensitive tests.

Management
See Table 12.7.

There is no cure and no effective vaccine currently exists.

TABLE 12.7 Vulval lesions

Common/important infection	Herpes	Warts	Syphilis
Organism	Herpes simplex virus type 2 (HSV-2) in 70% or type 1 (HSV-1).	Human papilloma virus 2, 6, 11 (see Section 13).	*Treponema pallidum*
Local symptoms	Tingling in the skin Blister formation Painful ulceration Dysuria Cervical/urethral discharge Gingivostomatitis Proctitis	Irritation of skin. Development of raised lesions. Spread by touch and contact with adjacent skin. Increased vaginal discharge.	Primary syphilis • 2–10 weeks post exposure: characterised by a single, painless, indurated ulcer in the anogenital region, and regional lymphadenopathy. • 6–12 weeks: body rash, fever, headaches. Very infectious. • Atypical presentations may occur including multiple, painful, purulent, or extragenital ulcers.
Other symptoms/ presentations, notes	• Systemic symptoms of fevers, myalgia, and occasionally autonomic neuropathy, resulting in urinary retention and meningitis. • The patient may be asymptomatic. • Can infect fetus and cause skin lesions and meningitis. More likely if primary infection occurs during the pregnancy.	HPV may also cause: • Asymptomatic carriage. • Cytological changes. • Lesions apparent on colposcopy but not macroscopically. • Mother-to-baby spread in childbirth.	Congenital Acquired Early (< 2 years): Primary Secondary Early latent Secondary (6–12 weeks): fever, body rash, headaches, mucosal lesions, lymphadenopathy, very infectious. Latent: characterised by positive serology for syphilis, however no clinical evidence of infection. Late (> 2 years): Latent or secondary or tertiary neurosyphilis, cardiovascular syphilis, and gummata.

(continued overleaf)

TABLE 12.7 continued

Common/important infection	Herpes	Warts	Syphilis
Signs	Single or multiple ulcers. Vulva and perianal Exquisitely tender. Recurrent in 20% women. Cervical lesions are painless. May cause profuse, muco-purulent discharge. More common with first episode.	Anogenital area, vagina and cervix.	Vulval ulcer. Clinical examination is necessary to assess for the clinical manifestations of late infection, or for signs of congenital syphilis. Confirmation or exclusion of neurological, cardiovascular, or ophthalmic involvement is with: • Lumbar puncture to assess CSF • Chest X-ray to assess for aortic aneurysm • Ophthalmic assessment • Histologic evidence of gummata.
Treatment	Initial infection: Acyclovir 400 mg qid 5–10 days or valaciclovir 500 mg BD 5–10 days Topical lignocaine jelly 2% locally for 1–2 days Ice packs and salt baths for relief. Recurrent infection: Suppressive therapy —one of following for 3–6 months: Acyclovir 400 mg 12 BD Valaciclovir 500 mg BD Famciclovir 250 mg BD	Genital warts: • Spontaneous resolution can occur. • Antiproliferative agents: podophyllin, 5-fluorouracil. • Ablative: cryotherapy, cautery, laser. • Immune response enhancement: imiquinod cream.	*Early:* Procaine penicillin 1 g IM OD for 10 days, or benzathine penicillin 1.8 g IM single dose, or doxycycline 100 mg BD for 14 days. *Late:* Procaine penicillin 1 g IM OD for 15 days, or benzathine penicillin 1.8 g IM weekly x 3. Other forms: consult specialist.

First episode

Antivirals can be used if presenting within the first five days of the start of the episode or while new lesions are still forming. Acyclovir and valaciclovir for five days are effective in reducing the severity and duration of episodes. Topical agents show no benefit in reducing duration of lesions. The latter are more expensive. Supportive measures include saline bathing and analgesia. Hospitalisation may be required for urinary retention, meningism or systemic symptoms.

Recurrent genital herpes

Recurrences are self-limiting and generally cause minor symptoms. Asymptomatic viral shedding from the cervix can occur without the woman being aware of this. Management strategies include supportive therapy only, episodic antiviral treatments, and suppressive antiviral therapy if there are more than six attacks a year: this may include a topical or oral agent (monitor liver function tests for hepatotoxicity).

Pregnancy and herpes

See Section 9.

Warts

Diagnosis

Exfoliative lesions are often diagnosed on visual appearance. However, histological confirmation is recommended to exclude malignant change.

Human papilloma virus can be detected from:

1 Koilocytosis (halo surrounding cell nucleus) on a Pap test or biopsy is suggestive of HPV in the cell
2 Detection of viral DNA (research)
3 Polymerase chain reaction (PCR) highly sensitive (research).

In clinical practice, identification of a specific strain does not assist management.

Treatment

See Table 12.7.

Syphilis

Syphilis will develop in about one-third of people exposed to early disease and less where the disease is latent.[22] After the primary and secondary phases (Table 12.7) there is a latent period with few or no symptoms. About one-third of infected patients will go on to develop tertiary disease.

Diagnosis

Primary disease: be aware that a window period exists for serology.

1 Fluid from the lesion examined by dark ground microscopy. Only test to specifically diagnose very early syphilis.
2 *Specific tests:* may remain positive for life whether the disease has been treated or not. Fluorescent treponemal antibody absorption test (FTA-abs) first test to become positive. Treponema pallidum particle agglutination test (TPPA or MHA-TP) measures antibody level to surface protein of TP and is 90 per cent positive in early infection. These are expensive and difficult to perform.
3 *Non-specific tests:* Venereal Diseases Research Laboratory test (VDRL), rapid plasma reagin tests (RPR). This measures antibody to cardiolipin (a normal component of mammalian cells, modified by the TP). This reflects the activity

of the disease in early syphilis that disappears with treatment. The tests are reactive in most people after 4–7 days following the appearance of the lesions. It is reactive in most people with secondary disease. The levels decline over time with or without treatment and 25 per cent are non-reactive in the late stages. These tests are easy, cheap, sensitive and quantitative and can be used to monitor treatment.

Interpretation of test results

Always repeat positive non-specific tests and confirm the results with a treponemal test, as biological false positive serological tests occur in:

- Pregnancy
- Other treponemal infections—yaws
- Autoimmune disease
- Other viral infections such as glandular fever, chickenpox, mumps.

In secondary syphilis: RPR > 1:32, MHA-TP is always positive.

Treatment

See Table 12.7.

Follow-up

Review patient following course completion. Further duration of follow-up depends on stage of syphilis. Partner notification and treatment is essential, as are tests for other STIs.

Syphilis in pregnancy

Infectivity for the fetus when the mother has untreated syphilis is 100 per cent. Syphilis is transmitted vertically from mother to fetus. The outcome of a pregnancy for a woman with untreated syphilis may be spontaneous abortion, a stillborn infant, a child with congenital syphilis, or an unaffected child. The infectivity and severity become less with time. Prenatal infection and congenital disease is classified into early, latent and late. The typical stigmata include facial deformities and scarring in the eyes; it is a serious condition that can be fatal or cause permanent disfigurement or impairment. Penicillin during pregnancy has a cure rate of nearly 100 per cent.

CLINICAL PRESENTATION: HIV infection/AIDS

1 STI check after unsafe sex
2 Symptoms:
- Initial flu-like illness within two weeks of infection
- Later with symptoms after some years once the immune system is affected.

HIV and syphilis are sexually transmitted infections that both have a wide range of clinical manifestations. The relationship between the two diseases is complex. The presence of either disease can potentiate the transmission of the other and affect the diagnosis, outcome and management of the patient. They should be considered if the woman herself or a sexual partner's behaviour has put them at risk.

HIV antibody test

HIV can be found in the blood, vaginal fluids or semen of infected people. The virus can be transmitted to others:

- During sex
- When sharing needles and syringes
- By blood transfusion
- During childbirth and breastfeeding.

Antibodies to HIV appear approximately three months after infection and remain lifelong. Women with HIV can stay healthy for years and the onset of acquired immunodeficiency syndrome (AIDS) is delayed. AIDS occurs when the virus overcomes the immune system and the woman develops illnesses and infections that she would normally be able to resist.

Stages of disease

1 Initial infection ± symptoms:
   - Flu-like illness within two weeks of infection
   - Similar to glandular fever: headaches, fever, swollen glands, body rash
   - Lasts 3–14 days

3 Dormant phase for a number of years: asymptomatic carrier state

4 Immune system affected: fatigue, fever, weight loss, diarrhoea, gland swelling

5 AIDS: immune system severely affected and the body is overwhelmed by infections and cancers. The most common of these are pneumonia, Kaposi's sarcoma (rare in women) and lymphoma.

Progression of HIV

Why some HIV infections progress and others do not is not clearly understood. Factors that may be involved and for which advice may be given are:

- Other STIs—safe sex practices may be beneficial to the infected patient and their partner/s.
- Healthy lifestyle to maintain general health—well-balanced diet, exercise/physical activity balanced with rest.
- Avoid recreational drugs that may be immunosuppressant
- Stress may have an immunosuppressant effect. Minimise this by activities designed to manage stress.
- Avoid live vaccines
- Regular health monitoring.

After the primary infection the viral load stabilises at a 'set point'. The higher the set point viral load, the poorer the prognosis without treatment. The disease is monitored with HIV/viral load and CD4/CD8 lymphocyte counts. Rising viral load and falling lymphocyte count indicates the need for anti-retroviral therapy.

Treatment

Anti-retroviral therapy is constantly changing. It is common to use a combination treatment with three drugs. Specialist assistance should be sought to investigate and plan management.

Post-exposure prophylaxis (PEP)

Persons exposed to a significant risk (either through an occupational accident such as a deep needlestick injury or through lifestyle) may benefit from anti-retroviral therapy for one month, provided the drugs are commenced within 72 hours of exposure. This area is currently being researched.

Women and HIV

Women represent 21 per cent of adult cases in the USA, 5 per cent in Australia and low levels in the UK.[23,24] The ratio of females to males infected with HIV is increasing. Sexual transmission predominates, but vertical transmission (mother to baby) is increasing. In the developed world there have been three phases in the epidemiology of HIV: men having sex with men (MSM), intravenous drug users (IDU) and heterosexual transmission.[25]

Clinically there are differences between men and women with HIV.[26] In women:

- AIDS wasting is more common
- Diet is poorer
- Anaemia is common
- GIT pathology is more common.

The prognosis for women is worse than for men:

- Progress is faster for women (with a lower viral load and at a higher CD4 than men)[27]
- Viral loads stabilise at lower levels in women[28]
- Viral variants profile is different.[29]

This may be due to diagnosis later in the disease process, and having higher viral loads and lower CD4 at diagnosis.

Specific issues for women with HIV include:

1. *Cervical cancer:*
   - 50 per cent of HIV-positive women have high risk of HPV[30]
   - CIN development is related to the degree of immunosuppression[30]
   - Recurrence rates of CIN 2 and 3 are high[30]
   - 15–40 per cent of HIV-positive women have dysplasia on the Pap test, eleven times higher than HIV-negative women[31]
   - HPV in these women has higher prevalence, more persistent virus, more oncogenic subtypes.[32,33]
2. *Sexually transmitted infection:*
   - Increased prevalence of all other STIs
   - Increased susceptibility to HIV in the presence of genital ulcer disease.
   - PID is less responsive to treatment and tubo-ovarian abscess is more common.[33]
   - Unprotected ano-rectal sex is a risk factor for acquiring HIV and hepatitis B virus infection.
   - During vaginal intercourse, women seem to be at somewhat higher risk than men of acquiring HIV infection and several other STDs, probably including HSV-2 infection, gonorrhoea, chlamydia and others.

- Sex during menstruation may increase a woman's risk of acquiring HIV infection.

3 *Reproductive issues:* the diagnosis of HIV will affect the pregnancy outcome depending on whether this is made before or during pregnancy. More women choose to terminate the pregnancy when the diagnosis is first made after a pregnancy is under way.[34] Issues to be considered are the effects of pregnancy on the disease and the disease on the pregnancy, breastfeeding and subsequent contraception.

Counselling and testing for HIV

It is essential to discuss issues before the test and obtain informed consent from the woman. Advice about the rationale for testing reduces the risk of transmission to others and can improve long-term prognosis. Explain that there is a three-month 'window' from exposure to antibody development and therefore a repeat test will be necessary before it can be ascertained for certain that the test is negative. Confidentiality issues are important. A positive result may have implications for life insurance and immigration in addition to the serious social and psychological factors.

Sexually transmissible infections between women

Sexual activity between women carries a risk of transmission of infection. Women who identify as lesbian may have previously had male sexual partners. In one study of lesbians about one-third of women had had an STI,[35] and in another 17 per cent had had one or more STIs.[36] There are various methods of transmission including shared vaginal or cervical fluids through unprotected digital contact or the use of sex toys. This has the potential to transmit chlamydia, gonorrhoea, HPV, trichomonas, anaerobes of bacterial vaginosis and candida. Anal-to-genital contact, particularly sharing sex toys between the anus and vagina, can lead to transmission of anaerobes. Bacterial vaginosis (BV) is a very common condition among lesbians, with up to 35 per cent having had symptomatic BV.[37] It is found that 80 per cent of lesbian couples have the same BV status (either both negative or both positive).[38] This would strongly indicate that BV is sexually transmitted between women.

Genital-to-genital skin contact or oral-to-genital contact may transmit HSV, HPV or genital parasites. Cervical HPV infection has been reported in women who have never had sex with a man, notwithstanding the fact that many lesbians have had (or continue to have) sex with men. Therefore, advice regarding cervical screening is important for any sexually active woman. Vaginal penetration during menstruation or piercings as part of sex play can lead to transmission of blood-borne viruses including HBV and HIV.

The health care provider should be knowledgeable regarding lesbian safe sex practices.[39] There is little accessible information regarding safe sex, and this combined with a perceived immunity to STIs results in limited safer sex behaviours among lesbians. There are various forms of barriers available to prevent the sharing of genital fluids. A dam (or dental dam) is a rectangular piece of latex approximately 10 × 15 cm. This is placed over the genital area for protection during oral sex. Latex gloves can be used during digital penetration of vagina or anus, including regular change of gloves between events. Condoms can be used on sex toys and changed between partners to prevent transmission.

External genital symptoms

CLINICAL PRESENTATIONS

1 Pruritus

This is by far the most common symptom of vulvar disease but is quite non-specific. Thus, it can result from a multitude of causes and merges with other common descriptions such as discomfort, burning, stinging and soreness. It should go without saying that treatment should never be initiated on this symptom alone. *Candida albicans* is the most common cause of vulvitis and vaginitis. However, it is not the only cause of this symptom (Table 12.8).

TABLE 12.8 Vulvovaginal inflammatory conditions

More common infections	Non-infectious conditions
Fungal • Candidiasis • Tinea cruris or versicolor	Spongiotic disorders (characterised by intraepidermal oedema) • Irritant contact dermatitis • Allergic contact dermatitis • Atopic dermatitis (eczema)
Viral • Herpes simplex	Psoriasiform disorders • Psoriasis • Lichen simplex chronicus
Bacterial Gram-positive cocci • *Staphylococcus aureus* (folliculitis, furuncles, abscess) • Streptococci (erysipelas)	Lichenoid reactions (epidermal basal layer damage) • Lichen sclerosus • Erosive: lichen planus/vaginitis • Plasma cell vulvitis • Lupus erythematosus • Drug eruption
Gram-negative cocci • Gonococcal vulvovaginitis	Vesicobullous disorders • Including pemphigus, erythema multiforme, pemphigoid, herpes gestationalis and dermatitis herpetiformis
Gram-negative bacilli • Donovanosis • Chancroid	Granulomatous disorders • Including Crohn's disease and sarcoidosis
Spirochaetes • Syphilis	Vasculopathic disorders • Including Behcet's disease and urticaria
Mixed and non-specific • Bartholinitis	
Parasites • Trichomoniasis • Pediculosis pubis • Scabies	

Note: Bacterial vaginosis (*Gardnerella* infection) does not produce vaginitis. Streptococci and coliforms are not vaginal pathogens. Diabetes mellitus should be sought if appropriate.

2 Dyspareunia and discomfort at introitus (noticeable on tampon insertion)

Superficial dyspareunia is the most common symptom of vulvovaginal disease, after pruritus. It is often the most distressing. A substantial proportion of patients will have negative clinical and laboratory findings and the diagnosis may focus on a sexual problem.

The woman around menopause may present with atrophic vaginitis, and lactating women seldom suffer from candidiasis but may be sore from atrophic vaginitis and/or vulvar and perineal trauma.

3 Dysuria

Inflammation in the vestibular region may result in discomfort from contact with urine. This results in the symptom of vulvar dysuria and is one of the reasons why women should never be treated for urinary infection when dysuria is the only complaint, without at least performing a micro-urine.

4 Vulval pain and burning

The term 'vulvodynia' literally means 'pain of the vulva'. The International Society for the Study of Vulvar Disease (ISSVD) provides a more precise definition by describing vulvodynia as chronic vulvar discomfort that is characterised by burning, stinging, rawness or irritation. Vulval vestibulitis is a sub-type of vulvodynia and is characterised by pain when the vestibule is touched or pressured. These unpleasant symptoms, particularly burning, may occur in the absence of clinical and laboratory findings. In this case the likely diagnosis is genital dysaesthesia, a nervous system disorder for which no topical application is useful, but drugs such as the tricyclic antidepressants (eg amitriptyline) have a place. Imipramine is probably the most widely used.

'Splitting' usually equates with fissuring. Inflamed epithelium develops intraepithelial oedema (spongiosis), rendering it prone to tearing like wet tissue paper. These fissures can be exquisitely painful because they expose the nerve endings in the dermis. They occur most frequently in the interlabial sulci, fourchette and perineum. Candidiasis is by far the most common cause but it can be a non-specific clinical feature of any inflammatory disorder of the vulva.

5 Vulval change in colour

Changes in colour will occur in the presence of inflammation (redness), epithelial hyperplasia (whiteness) or as a result of disorders of pigmentation. The latter include melanocytic neoplasms (naevi, lentigo, melanosis or melanoma) or the patchy absence of melanin in vitiligo.

6 Vulval 'lump'

Vulvar lumps may be cystic or solid. The former may be congenital or acquired and vary from inconsequential skin appendage cysts to large cysts associated with obstruction of the duct of Bartholin's gland situated at the posterior end of the labium minus. The most common solid lumps are condylomata acuminata (warts) and the fibroepithelial polyp (skin tag). Malignancy must always be considered.

7 Vulval ulceration

See Table 12.9. Ulceration is one of the most serious manifestations of genital disease and must be diagnosed accurately, usually with laboratory confirmation. Self-inflicted excoriation is common in pruritic conditions and must be differentiated from bacterial (eg syphilis), viral infections (especially herpes), other infections, neoplastic disease and other pathology (lichenoid). If in doubt, take two biopsies of the lesion, one to be sent in formalin for histology, the other to be sent fresh in a sterile container for microbiology and immunofluorescence.

8 Discharge

Discharge is the most common symptom of vaginal and cervical disease. Unlike the highly pain-sensitive vulva, even extreme inflammatory disorders of the vagina and cervix may only be manifest by discharge because of the relative absence of pain fibres at this level. A large minority of patients complaining of discharge will be free of pathogens. The diagnosis can be made clinically with the addition of microscopy and culture (Box 12.12 and Table 12.10).

9 Odour

Odour is highly subjective and therefore may not always be helpful. It is the leading symptom of bacterial vaginosis. Also consider underlying anxiety or sexual problems that may be a cause or the result of the problem.

TABLE 12.9 Ulcerative conditions of the vulva

Condition	Notes
Excoriation secondary to irritation	Commonly seen. The history should seek the initiating factor to the problem although this may no longer be there.
Herpes simplex	Painful. Most common STI causing genital ulceration. See Table 12.4.
Syphilis	Painless, indurated lesions. Rare. Recent sexual contact in South East Asia or Africa. See Table 12.4.
Donovanosis *Klebsiella granulomatis*	More likely in Aboriginal women. Endemic in northern and central Australia. Diagnosis by demonstrating Donovan bodies with Wright's or Giemsa stain on a punch biopsy. Treat: azithromycin 1 g weekly 4–6 weeks.
Chancroid *Haemophylis ducreyi*	Multiple, tender, associated inguinal lymphadenitis. More likely if lesion acquired in Asia, India or Africa. These patients have an increased risk of HIV infection. Refer to sexual health clinic.
Lymphogranuloma venereum (LGV) *Chlamydia trachomatis* (different serotype to one causing cervicitis)	Transient ulcer 3–10 days after infection may not be noticed. May present weeks later with inguinal lymphadenopathy. Diagnose by demonstrating organism in fluid from gland or by serology. Treat: doxycycline 100 mg BD × 21 days.

TABLE 12.9 continued

Condition	Notes
Lichen sclerosis (LS) et atrophicus	Pale skin around the vulva and perianal areas. In later stages fusion of the clitoral hood and labia minora may occur.
Behcet's syndrome	Painful ulcers. Enquire about extra-genital symptoms, eg uveitis and arthralgia.
Drug eruption	Painful ulcers with a recent history of medication (remember over-the-counter and herbal preparations). Also toiletries, body sprays, antiseptics.
Trauma	Uncommon—see Section 3. May be evident from the history.
Pyogenic infection/folliculitis	Consider poor hygiene, underlying diabetes.
Scabies—secondarily infected	A common infestation with the mite *Sarcoptes scabiei.* Diagnosed clinically and confirmed with scrapings from the burrows. Check other sites for infestation, eg web spaces.
Squamous cell carcinoma	See Section 13. Also presents as a lump or with pruritus.

BOX 12.12 Preparation of a Wright-stained smear

1. The vaginal wall and/or introitus is wiped with a wooden spatula or cytology brush which is smeared on the slide.
2. Fix with the usual Pap smear fixative.
3. Apply 10–15 drops of Wright stain to the slide on a level surface. Leave for one minute.
4. Add an approximately double volume (20–30 drops) of water. Leave for three minutes.
5. Rinse with tap water for 10 seconds and dry (a hair dryer is ideal).
6. Examine with immersion oil or make the slide permanent by immersing in xylene and covering the smeared slide with mounting medium and applying a cover slip.

TABLE 12.10 Diagnostic categories from office cytology

Result	Observation	Presentation
Normal	Physiological vaginal contents: mostly mature vaginal squames. Polymorphs are few or absent and usually contained within strands of recognisable cervical mucus. Cervical mucus usually contains polymorphs after ovulation. Bacteria are mostly bacilli (rods).	Usually from patients complaining of discharge, pruritus or dyspareunia or with known vulvar dermatoses. These smears are complementary to routine microbiology. Culture of swabs may still grow pathogens such as *Candida albicans.*

(continued overleaf)

TABLE 12.10 continued

Result	Observation	Presentation
Atrophy	Without oestrogen, the vaginal epithelium does not mature (differentiate) so that cells from the deepest layer are found on the smears. These parabasal cells are easily recognised because they are relatively small, rounded and contain an open nucleus occupying about one half of the cell.	Dryness, dyspareunia, irritation may occur. Atrophy results from a lack of oestrogen and is associated with a very low incidence of candidal infection although trichomonads are in no way inhibited by oestrogen lack.
Infection	*Candida albicans*: basophilic filaments with a non-staining capsule and often budding. Trichomonads appear as well-demarcated round cells which stain as deeply as the surrounding epithelial cells. The flagellae will probably not be visible other than under oil immersion. Trichomonads are best identified in a wet mount because of their characteristic movement.	*Candida*: irritation, 'cottage cheese' discharge. *Trichomonas*: irritation, profuse vaginal discharge. (see STI section)
Epithelial erosion	It is possible to make a fairly confident diagnosis of erosive disorder (eg desquamative inflammatory vaginitis or lichen planus) on these smears. The characteristics are, in addition to inflammatory changes, the mixture of superficial cells (indicating premenopausal oestrogen levels) with parabasal cells from the depths of the epithelium. Regenerative atypia will be apparent in severe cases.	Pruritus, soreness, pain
Bacterial vaginosis	This condition can be confidently diagnosed on these smears so that culture confirmation may be unnecessary. A profusion of coccoid flora and a relative absence of polymorphs. The bacteria adhere to many of the epithelial cells so that their borders may appear ragged—the so-called 'clue cell'.	Vaginal discharge: fluid, profuse (see STI section). The absence of vaginitis is a feature of bacterial vaginosis.
Inflammation, no pathogens	1 A smear showing polymorphs in excess of differentiated epithelial cells but with no identifiable pathogen. 2 Polymorphs are mostly arranged in rows or clumps within the identifiable strands of mucus. Areas of epithelial cells unassociated with polymorphs are also present if cervical eversion is the only disorder.	1 Trauma or cervicitis can produce this picture. 2 A discharge from a cervical eversion (ectropion).

History

Specific points

- Duration of problem
- Degree of discomfort/pain
- Position of pain/discomfort (can the woman point to a specific area or is it more generalised)
- Relationship to sexual intercourse
- Lesions elsewhere
- Other associated symptoms
- Recent travel

General gynaecology

See generic notes. A general gynaecological and medical history is essential for good management. It is essential to assess psychosocial factors and take a sexual history.

Intercurrent disease: skin disease elsewhere

This may be relevant as there may be associated skin or mucosal disorders elsewhere. Thus, atopic eczema can affect the vulva and is associated with hay fever and asthma. Likewise, the clue to vulvar psoriasis may be the more characteristic extragenital lesions.

Medications

Vaginal and vulvar treatments

Contact dermatitis of the vulva is one of the most common diagnoses made in these patients so it is essential to know what prescribed and over-the-counter medications the patient has been applying. Getting the information can be difficult but has potential use in subsequent management. Anti-candidals can now be obtained without a prescription. These potentially irritating substances are also the most common cause of getting falsely negative swabs in recurrent candidiasis.

A history of any vulvar or vaginal surgery should be recorded and whether biopsy has been performed elsewhere. Diathermy, cryotherapy and laser can also have long-term sequelae in this area.

Systemic treatment

The older woman on HRT may still experience atrophic vaginitis from underdosage or poor absorption of oestrogen. *Candida albicans* is an oestrogen-dependent disorder. It therefore seldom occurs in healthy children, women who are breastfeeding or postmenopausal women unless they are on relatively high doses of oestrogen replacement therapy. The relationship between antibiotics and candidiasis is unarguable.

Clinical examination

A routine examination of the genital area is undertaken. Many conditions can be diagnosed on visual inspection with additional laboratory confirmation. If the patient is menstruating or there is much discharge it may be necessary to clean the area with wet cotton balls; otherwise erythema, fissures and small ulcers may be missed. Ask the woman to use the end of a cotton bud to indicate exactly the site of maximum discomfort. This may be the best way of selecting the site to take a biopsy and is useful diagnostically. The patient with 'vestibulitis syndrome' will place the swab stick in the region of the minor vestibular glands and the woman with vulvar dysaesthesia will indicate a wide, ill-defined area, often with a display of emotion.

Inspection

Inspection may reveal:

- General:
  - Eczema
  - Psoriasis
  - Lichen planus
- Genital:
  - Condylomata acuminata (exophytic warts)
  - Molluscum contagiosum (caused by the pox virus, transmitted by direct contact, and treated by direct ablation)
  - Sebaceous cysts
  - Bartholin's cyst
  - Naevi
  - Skin discoloration: white/red/brown
  - Vesicular lesions
  - Ulcerative lesions (Table 12.9).

Always consider neoplasia as a cause of any lesion.

Investigations

The importance of taking cervical and vaginal swabs and, if indicated, a vulvar biopsy before starting any treatment needs to be particularly emphasised to the patient. A two-hour postprandial blood sugar should be considered to exclude diabetes in women with pruritis vulvae and a haemoglobin A1c to check the control in an established diabetic woman.

Office pathology

Formal microbiology, cytology and histology will be required in most cases but the woman is likely to benefit greatly from the rapid narrowing of the differential diagnosis provided by the clinician using office microscopy, which takes five minutes. Examination of such smears has produced a useful list of diagnostic categories (Box 12.12 and Table 12.10).

Karyopyknotic index

When taking a cytological smear in ovulating women only cells from differentiated epithelium are obtained. These are called *intermediate* if some nuclear detail is visible, or *superficial* if the nucleus has become pyknotic. These cells are much larger than parabasal cells and the cytoplasmic border tends to be angulated. The ratio of parabasal to intermediate to superficial is known as the maturation or karyopyknotic index and is a fairly reliable indicator of oestrogen levels.

Specific tests

- Swab from ulcer
- Dark field examination for syphilis
- Direct fluorescent test for herpes
- PCR—consider as the first test as it is now very widely available
- Viral culture (± PCR for HSV 1 and 2)
- Microscopy and culture (for *Haemophylis ducreyi*)
- Cytology or histology from lesion (demonstrating Donovan bodies)
- Biopsy from ulcer or if appearance suggests malignancy.

Management

Management is covered under the description for each condition.

Candida vulvitis and vaginitis

Candida can reach the vagina via oral ingestion. It is not sexually transmitted. It is therefore unnecessary to recommend treatment of the male partner unless he has candidal balanitis or another form of cutaneous candidiasis in the genital area.

The infection almost always occurs within the insensitive vaginal lumen. The resultant 'burning' of the sensitive vulval epithelium is caused by the yeast's metabolites (seldom by infection of the vulvar skin). Treatment must be directed to the vaginal source of the infection. Applying antifungal preparations to the vulva will not only be ineffective but will also worsen the contact dermatitis which is a feature of the complaint.

Mixed pathology is common in the vulvar area. The most common combination is vulvar dermatitis exacerbated by bouts of candidiasis. Swabbing as often as necessary is the only means of selecting the appropriate treatment. The inappropriate use of antifungal applications can make the dermatitis worse as these products are relatively toxic to genital epithelium.

Candida species other than *albicans* are being diagnosed with increasing frequency. It is essential to identify the species in all cultures positive for recurrent or persisting *Candida*.

Treatment

- General care:
  - Avoid soaps, replace with normal saline, QV wash, sorbelene.
  - Do not use home remedies, over-the-counter preparations and non-prescribed medications.
  - In the sexually active, the avoidance of artificial lubricants should be discussed.
- Specific treatment:
  - A vaginal imidazole cream, inserted nightly for one week, is recommended as the standard treatment for candidal vulvovaginitis.

Recurrent candidiasis

There is no generally agreed definition of recurrent candidiasis. There are several strategies for the prevention of repeated infection. In the event of multiple recurrences, 14 days continuous use (including during menstruation) of a vaginal imidazole cream and a simultaneous course of ketoconazole 200 mg twice daily for five days are recommended.

Prophylaxis

The nightly insertion of 100 000 units of nystatin in a vaginal cream, tablet or pessary (including during menstruation) continued for six months can virtually be guaranteed to keep a woman free of candidiasis without producing any significant discharge during the day. It is the treatment of choice for pregnant women who have had more than one proven infection during the pregnancy.

Long-term oral therapy

There is evidence that fluconazole (150 mg twice weekly for prophylaxis) is the most effective and least toxic but it is expensive. This gives sustained levels in the vagina. Six months continuous treatment is recommended.

Dermatitis

Dermatitis is a common cause of chronic vulval symptoms. Treatment for dermatitis usually involves the use of a topical corticosteroid cream—initially a high-potency steroid cream for 2–3 weeks. Cool compresses and antihistamines may be used to bring relief from symptoms. If the dermatitis is thought to be due to an allergy or irritant, it is important that attempts are made to identify and avoid the substance.

Sexual feelings and behaviour

Most sexual behaviour is pleasurable and trouble free and does not come within the realms of clinical consultation. It is important to remember that sexual activity is enjoyed by people of any age, sexual orientation or ethnicity, by people living with chronic diseases and those with intellectual or physical impairments. A woman may choose to express her sexuality with different behaviours and in various social contexts: she may have multiple relationships, casual partners, or a monogamous relationship. Most women are heterosexual but approximately one in every thirty women appear to be exclusively homosexual in their desires and fantasies, while up to one in ten have some degree of sexual attraction and/or sexual fantasies involving women.[40,41] It is also important to appreciate that a substantial minority of women of all ages have no sexual partners at all, and for some this reflects a preference to be 'asexual'.

Although systematic research in this field is still in its infancy, it is clear that sexuality is as diverse as any other aspect of human personality. The most experienced clinicians in sexual health care have learned *not* to make broad generalisations about 'the typical sex life'. Successful consultations require trust and openness, and this is easier to attain if the clinician has an open mind and makes few explicit or implicit assumptions about what is usual or likely in the sexual lives of individual women.

The normal sexual response

It is important to feel comfortable discussing sex, to acquire a sound knowledge base, build good rapport, and employ active listening with appropriate empathy. Be willing to accept that the woman's or couple's knowledge and attitudes about sex may be different from your own. Most women will have gained information from numerous sources: their own sexual experiences, their partners, the media (including television, movies, the internet and magazines) and increasingly sophisticated books and advice manuals available from adult sex shops and conventional bookshops. Increasingly, Western societies are saturated with sexual imagery and personal stories. Women may have developed various expectations about what is normal or abnormal in terms of their sexual feelings and experiences. Mostly, this is not problematic. However, difficulties often arise where there is a wide discrepancy within a relationship as to what is viewed as normal.

Many clinicians find it useful to discuss with patients the underlying physiology of normal human sexual response. Figure 12.2 depicts the discrete phases in normal sexual response: desire, arousal, plateau, orgasm and resolution.

Desire waxes and wanes during the stages of the life cycle, and within each stage. Many factors can inhibit and enhance sexual desire for women. It may be inhibited by

- physical factors (eg tiredness, ill health, excess alcohol)
- psychological factors (eg low self-esteem, depressed mood, recent disagreement)
- situational factors (eg lack of privacy, shortage of time)
- emotional factors (eg lack of trust, loss of attraction).

It is also true that the opposite of these factors may enhance desire. In every situation it is therefore important to look at the woman's life in context: for example, loss of desire in a woman with a new baby who has colic in the daytime and

FIGURE 12.2 Sexual response cycle

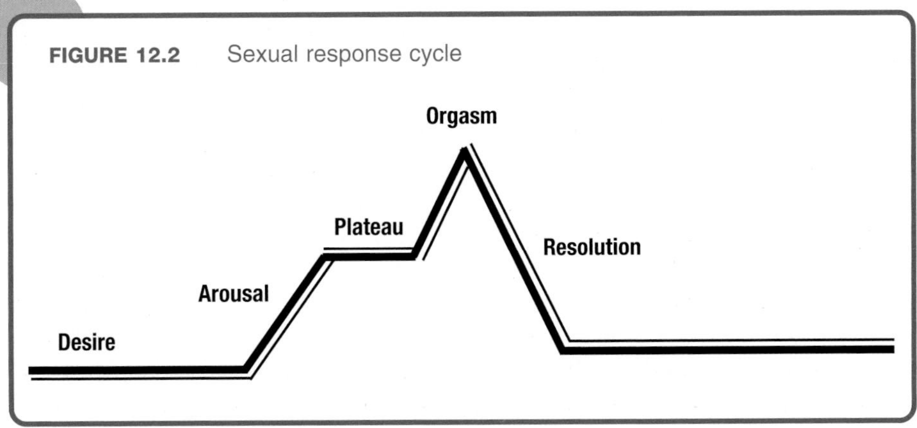

breastfeeds three times a night would be 'normal'. Discussion needs to centre on the practicalities of getting enough sleep and support.

The frequency and perceived 'quality' of sexual behaviour will vary with different women and also within the same individual woman at different times. This behaviour may be classified in the following ways:

- uninterested
- neutral
- available
- receptive
- initiatory.

Either partner in a relationship can be in a different zone to the other but the couple can still be sexually compatible. Most women are not initiatory in their behaviour and a woman's sex drive is more likely to be turned down by the stresses and strains of everyday life and love compared to a man's sex drive.

Sexual problems

People with acute or chronic disease often have sexual problems, and feel too embarrassed to talk about sex as they feel it is 'trivial' compared to their primary complaint. Often, clinicians avoid raising the issue altogether. However, studies have shown that, if given an opportunity to talk about sex and sexuality early on in their treatment, the psychosexual outcomes will be much better afterwards (see Sections 2 and 13).

Sexual problems vary widely and are caused by many factors. Some can be reported by patients more or less objectively, such as pain arising from sexually transmissible infections, vaginal discharges or erectile dysfunction. Others are more nebulous and subjective, such as loss of desire, excessive sexual fantasies or anxiety over sexual orientation. Some problems are debilitating, seriously impairing quality of life and relationships, while others may be relatively mild. Some will be discussed openly between doctors and patients, while others will remain hidden.

It is estimated that sexual problems affect between 10 and 20 per cent of the general population. A national survey of a representative sample of men and women between 18 and 59 years in Australia in 2000 included questions about common sexual problems.[42] These were compared to similar questions asked in a national sample in the United States.[43] The overall trends are very interesting and relevant to clinical consultations regarding sexuality. Both surveys showed that most people report at least one 'sexual problem' (53% of men and 60% of women). People with multiple problems are quite common and most problems remain untreated. For example, among Australian adults, 12 per cent of men and 20 per cent women reported three or more problems, and of these people, more than 60 per cent had not sought any clinical advice or treatment (see Table 12.11).

The surveys indicate the extent of the problems, and the low rates of treatment indicate that many people find it difficult to disclose problems of a sexual and intimate nature to their clinician. Very often these problems go undisclosed and undiagnosed and continue to trouble the couple for a very long time.

TABLE 12.11 Sexual dysfunction in the general adult population (aged 18–59 years) in Australia and the USA

During the past year has there been a period of several months or more where you …

Age group	Male Australian (%)	Male USA (%)	Female Australian (%)	Female USA (%)
Q: Lacked interest in sex				
18–29	19	14	27	32
30–39	17	13	40	32
40–49	14	15	35	30
50–59	16	17	34	27
Q: Unable to achieve orgasm				
18–29	7	7	23	26
30–39	6	7	17	28
40–49	5	9	17	22
50–59	9	9	26	23
Q: Climax too early				
18–29	30	30	7	–
30–39	44	32	9	–
40–49	39	28	13	–
50–59	43	31	9	–
Q: Physical pain during sex				
18–29	5	–	23	21
30–39	2	–	17	15
40–49	6	–	10	13
50–59	6	–	14	8
Q: Sex not pleasurable				
18–29	7	10	14	27
30–39	6	8	22	24
40–49	4	9	16	17
50–59	7	6	28	17
Q: Anxiety over performance				
18–29	14	19	14	16
30–39	13	17	15	11
40–49	12	19	7	11
50–59	9	14	18	6
Q: Females trouble lubricating				
18–29			18	19
30–39			17	18
40–49			23	21
50–59			33	27

The classic medical definitions of sexual dysfunction are listed in the DSM-IV 1994 and are divided into four categories:

1 Sexual desire disorders
2 Sexual arousal disorders
3 Orgasmic disorders
4 Sexual pain disorder.

These 'disorders' are then further subdivided into categories of:

- Lifelong or acquired
- Generalised or situational
- Psychological or medical.

These broad categories may be useful for evaluating a problem. In reality, a person or couple only has a sexual problem if they believe there is one. It is up to the health professional to whom that person divulges this information to elicit the nature of the problem and to put the behaviour into perspective for the couple.

In clinical practice, sexual problems can usefully be divided into two categories, problems of function and problems of desire. They are, however, frequently intertwined. If someone has a problem of sexual function they begin to lose desire, expecting failure and disappointment every time they try to have sex with their partner. Conversely, if the primary problem is lack of sexual desire, the patient often finds that even if they do try to have sex, they are either unable to do so or find it painful and difficult as they are physically withdrawn from their partner.

Women may present with either:

1 A *sexual problem*—a woman may feel comfortable in revealing a sexual problem as a specific complaint. The most common female problems that will be seen are vaginismus, loss of libido, anorgasmia and dyspareunia (pain on sexual intercourse).
2 A *gynaecological or other physical complaint* for which no organic cause is found. This could be, for example, vaginal discharge, a bleeding problem, pelvic pain or headaches. This is not to imply that whenever no organic disease is present, there must a psychological or 'psychosexual' explanation for the complaint. However, sensitive issues such as a sexual problem, abuse or anxiety should always be part of a differential diagnosis where the cause is not apparent—or even when it is! Sensitive issues are difficult to discuss and may require more time and good communication skills to elicit.

CLINICAL PRESENTATION: Vaginismus

The vagina has an anterior wall length of about 7 cm. It is a potential cavity with the walls being in apposition. The lining epithelium is in ridges (rugae) that permit distension for sexual intercourse and childbirth. The functional size is determined by the fibromuscular sheath that surrounds the lining epithelium and is under voluntary control in its lower third. Although there may be some individual variation, there is no anatomical problem (unless after surgery or injury) that prohibits normal sexual intercourse.

1 *Primary vaginismus:* vaginismus is involuntary spasm of the vaginal muscles, which is so strong that nothing is able to enter the vagina. If a woman has primary vaginismus the best key question to ask her is: 'Have you ever used a tampon?' In women with primary vaginismus the answer will always be no.
2 *Secondary vaginismus:* there has been previous vaginal entry, but she is now unable to have sexual intercourse. This may have an organic or psychogenic origin or some of each. For example, a vulvo-vaginal thrush infection may have caused irritation, soreness, dyspareunia and led to vaginismus. Even though the infection has been treated, the woman may have ongoing vaginismus.

Management

This consists of psychosexual counselling. It is important to exclude the physical condition of stenosis of the vagina. The latter may result from radiation treatment for gynaecological cancer or be part of vulval dystrophy; in these situations there may be benefit from the use of vaginal dilators and oestrogen cream.

CLINICAL PRESENTATION: Loss of libido

Loss of libido is loss of sexual interest and is related to many factors, including: socio-cultural, hormonal, past experiences and current relationship problems.

1 *Psychogenic:* Very often a woman with loss of libido is in a stable relationship. She will be unable to understand why, after a certain period of enjoying sex with her partner, she suddenly has no interest in any kind of sexual contact. The treatment for this in most cases is psychodynamic. Initially it is important to ascertain some background of the woman's life, her current relationship and past relationships. The treatment is to help the woman understand the origins of her problem as well as relationship counselling.
2 *Hormonal:* This area has been a topic of research only recently. There is some evidence for the use of hormonal treatment (oestrogen and testosterone) for loss of libido in some women who have undergone a natural or surgical menopause. It is well known that some women can describe loss of sexual interest when they are taking the combined oral contraceptive pill. This effect is not possible to predict for either the individual woman or for the preparation. Sometimes these women benefit from change of contraception so it is always worth offering them an alternative.

CLINICAL PRESENTATION: Dyspareunia

This is a condition of painful sexual intercourse and is often divided into two types to assist diagnosis.

1 *Superficial*—this refers to pain in the vagina on entry. It may be associated with vaginismus. The cause may be a local inflammatory condition or purely psychogenic.
2 *Deep*—this implies pain in the pelvic area and organic causes should be sought (See Section 13).

In the absence of physical findings the cause will almost certainly be psychosexual. The treatment again is to use psychodynamic or cognitive-behavioural therapy in order to help her understand and overcome her problem.

CLINICAL PRESENTATION: Anorgasmia

This is the lack of ability to achieve orgasm. It is often due to poor sexual technique. There are, however, some women who say they have never experienced orgasm. The first thing to do is have a discussion about the genitalia. Some women have never seen or touched their genitalia. Masturbation should then be discussed. The woman is far more likely to become orgasmic if she begins to understand the feelings of her own body. Most women feel sexual excitement through the clitoris; some women are able to have vaginal orgasms at the G spot, a small sensitive spot two-thirds up the vagina at the level of the urethral opening to the bladder. Sexual arousal is also dependent on cognitive input, and if the woman isn't 'turned on' by her partner or by fantasising, she would be unlikely to achieve orgasm.

It is important to explore the woman's belief's about sex. The woman may believe that once reproduction has finished, sexual activity should decrease or cease. It is important to give her 'permission' to feel sexual and indeed encourage her to have sexual thoughts; these can be stimulated by discussion, a book, a picture or a film if she wishes. Also discuss the health, feelings and attitude of her partner and the relationship between the couple. Never make any assumptions based on your own beliefs or jump to conclusions.

Case study

A 24-year-old woman has a male partner aged 36. They have been together for three years. She comes to the clinic and the doctor notices that she is due to have a cervical smear test. She declines. The doctor notices that she has been offered smear tests on a few previous occasions, but has made an excuse each time. When this is mentioned to the woman she suddenly becomes very upset. When the doctor proceeds a little further and asks if anything is wrong, she bursts into tears and discloses that she has never had sexual intercourse with this partner.

Scenario 1: *The doctor offers a vaginal examination. The woman is very hesitant and eventually agrees. She gets undressed behind the screens and then goes on to the couch and lies there in an almost fetal position with her knees drawn up. Despite reassurances from the doctor, she is obviously very anxious about the examination and even a one-finger insertion is not permitted. This woman has vaginismus.*

Scenario 2: *The woman is offered a vaginal examination. She agrees and is very relaxed. The genital examination is easy, there is no spasm of the vaginal muscles and everything is normal. The woman gets dressed, goes and sits back on her chair and bursts into tears. The doctor discovers eventually that the patient's partner has erectile dysfunction.*

Male sexual problems

It is important to have knowledge of male sexual problems, because this will affect any female partner that they might have.

CLINICAL PRESENTATION: Ejaculatory problems

The most common male sexual problem worldwide is premature ejaculation: the man ejaculates very quickly before either he or his partner has had satisfying sex. The mechanisms for this are poorly understood; however, counselling and psychodynamic therapy may help. A short course of an SSRI anti-depressant can be useful, utilising one of the known side effects of orgasmic delay.

Delayed ejaculation is sometimes a more difficult problem to overcome. As with all sexual problems it can be situational. It is useful to ask the man if he has a problem with ejaculation when he masturbates. Frequently he will only have the problem of inability to ejaculate when he is with his partner. The treatment is psychodynamic, helping him understand his problem. There is no 'quick fix' for this problem and the man will very often describe that he feels he 'cannot let go'.

CLINICAL PRESENTATION: Erectile dysfunction

Erectile dysfunction affects about 30 per cent of men aged between 40 and 70. It increases with age and with several clinical conditions. It can also be a side effect of various medications, such as antihypertensives and antidepressants. Some 60 per cent of erectile dysfunction is organic, 25 per cent of mixed psychogenic/organic origin and 15 per cent purely psychogenic. The treatment depends on cause, and is either mechanical, chemical or psychosexual or a combination of methods.

CLINICAL PRESENTATION: Male loss of libido

Loss of libido is a condition often suffered by men. The treatment is the same as with women. Individuals with loss of libido often suffer reduced self-esteem, which can be caused by some other major loss in their life. Situations such as bereavement, divorce or relationship break-up, and job redundancy can have a strong emotional impact on a man and lead to loss of interest in sex.

Fetishes

Some individuals, usually men, have unusual erotic triggers. It only becomes a problem when it is has a negative impact on a relationship. In order for sexual excitement to occur, the particular fetish object has to be present. Sadomasochism is a common form of sexual expression and is non-problematic between consenting adults. Under most legislation however, the infliction of grave physical punishment, even with consent, is not permitted.

Sexual counselling

A practitioner may choose to learn sexual counselling as part of their armamentarium or prefer to refer the woman or couple to a specific counsellor. For simple problems, being able to give permission to discuss the matter, provide information and assist the woman to make suggestions about management may be all that is required. Other more complex issues may need the time and the expertise of a sex therapist.

Conclusion

The key to treating sexual problems is heightened awareness of sexual issues by the clinician. A non-judgemental attitude will facilitate disclosure and acknowledgement of a problem in order to provide appropriate help.

Childhood sexual abuse: long-term effects

Sexual abuse in childhood has elicited a great deal of publicity, but there have been few population studies in this area. Australian studies reported by Fleming[44] and by Dunne and colleagues[45] suggest that the prevalence of unwanted sexual experience among Australian women is quite high, and comparable to rates in other Western nations. The extent of the problem in most developing nations and in many ethnic minorities remains largely unknown.

In the recent study by Dunne and colleagues,[45] the prevalence before the age of 16 years of any (self-reported) non-penetrative abuse was 15.9 per cent in males and 33.5 per cent in females; for penetrative abuse the prevalence was 4 per cent in males and 12 per cent in females. The survey, taken of a representative sample of the general population between the ages of 18 and 59 years, found that for males, the younger cohort were significantly less likely to report non-penetrative abuse, suggesting a decline in recent years. Although the pattern was less pronounced for females, there were several indications that, over time, girls are becoming somewhat less vulnerable. These findings complement data from the USA that showed the incidence of serious sexual assault of children to have declined across the 1990s.[46] Despite these positive signs, sexual assault of children remains common, and the broader moral and legal difficulties surrounding adult–child sex continue to cause serious problems across many levels of society, including health and welfare services.

Childhood sexual abuse is associated with a wide range of psychological and physical health problems. Numerous studies worldwide have compared the childhood sexual experiences of women with various mental and physical disorders with those of healthy women. The summary in Box 12.13 lists clinical disorders and emotional and social problems that have repeatedly been found in research to be more common in women sexually abused as children. This list is not comprehensive and there are other reviews.[47,48]

Does child sexual abuse cause these problems?

Given the sensitivity of child sexual abuse (CSA) to victims, families and in wider society, it is not easy to take a dispassionate stance on which health problems may or may not have been caused by these events. Clinically we can see clear links between sexual events and STI, pelvic pain, adolescent pregnancy and, among young children,

BOX 12.13 Possible long-term effects of childhood sexual abuse

- Emotional and social problems:
  - Anxiety disorders
  - Depression, low self-esteem
  - Suicidality
  - Dissociative disorders
  - Post-traumatic stress disorder
  - Excessive drug and alcohol use
  - Sexual dysfunction, including risky behaviours in adolescence
  - Early, unwanted pregnancy
  - Interpersonal relationships difficulties, including risk of divorce
  - Low academic achievement and unemployment
  - Risk of subsequent sexual abuse
- Physical health problems:
  - Sexually transmitted infections
  - Pain during intercourse as an adult
  - Chronic pain disorders
  - Pregnancy complications
  - Headache
  - Overweight/obesity
  - Anorexia nervosa
  - Gastrointestinal disorders

anxiety and social withdrawal. However, the number and range of women's health problems attributed by researchers and victims to CSA is so great that many people have become sceptical. There is a serious ongoing debate in medical research about whether many of the problems statistically associated with CSA are really best explained by other adverse life circumstances such as poverty, social disadvantage, physical abuse and emotional neglect (and associated risky behaviours like drug abuse and poor diet) that so often coincide with sexual exploitation of children and their later development.

A recent study of 3982 adult Australian twins (1991 twin pairs) has made progress in separating direct effects of CSA from the indirect effects of family environment.[49] The survey found an overall prevalence of CSA of 16.7 per cent for females and 5.4 per cent for males. In most twin-pairs neither twin was abused, although there were hundreds of pairs in which one twin self-reported CSA and the other twin did not. All twins had grown up in the same family environments. Detailed psychiatric history was assessed, on average, 19 years after the onset of sexual abuse. The most compelling finding was that, when one twin was abused and the other was not, psychological health was significantly worse for the abused twin on every measure (Box 12.14).

BOX 12.14 Significant differences between abused and non-abused twins[49]

- Suicide attempts
- Social anxiety
- Nicotine dependence
- Depression
- Alcohol dependence
- More likely to have been raped as an adult
- More likely to have been divorced

This twin study also replicated findings from other research showing that adverse family environment (eg parental alcohol abuse, parental fighting and parent–child physical abuse) predict poor mental health many years after childhood. In addition, though, there appears to be a direct, long-lasting effect of CSA on mental health, and risky behaviours such as smoking and alcohol dependence that pose serious risks for chronic disease.

Scientific studies of the causal chain linking child sexual exploitation and health of children and adults are important. However, many of the findings are complex and public arguments between researchers, lawyers, advocacy groups, politicians and social commentators can become vitriolic. From a clinical point of view, it is important to focus on the key elements: child sexual abuse is common, it affects a very broad diversity of women, for many victims it is traumatic and causes ongoing distress throughout life, and (regardless of whether it actually causes specific pathology) a history of CSA often diminishes personal resilience among women who are trying to cope with physical and mental disorders. Many women will reveal the problem to you, and for some it will be the first time they have disclosed to anyone. Be willing to discuss the woman's feelings and, if necessary, seek specialist advice.

SECTION 13 Common problems

Breast concerns

CLINICAL PRESENTATION: A lump found on self-examination or examination by a health professional (in women < 35 years)

Breast cancer is uncommon in these women, and while most young women have few breast problems those who do are far more likely to have a benign lesion (Section 15). While this is reassuring, breast cancer does occur even in women under age 20 and any significant clinical change must be regarded with suspicion and investigated seriously.

Benign conditions which occur more frequently in this age group:

- Fibroadenoma
- Cyclical hormonal changes (relating to menstrual cycles and the oral contraceptive pill)
- Simple breast cysts—uncommon in teens
- Inflammatory changes.

These are described in detail in Section 15.

Management

1. If doctor considers the palpable area or sign to be discrete or otherwise significant:
   - *Breast ultrasound* is the investigation of first choice[1] (mammography is often unhelpful due to breast tissue density but may be used in addition, especially in women 30–35 years).
   - *Needle sampling* (core biopsy or fine needle aspiration biopsy) is indicated if discrete solid lesion or if ultrasound appearances are even slightly atypical.
   - *Mammography* is contraindicated for women under 25 and undertaken in women > 25 only if diagnosis is considered uncertain following the above procedures or if malignancy has already been established, in order to assess disease extent and the contralateral breast.
   - *Early clinical review* (within one or two cycles) or second opinion if the above investigations do not clarify clinical concerns.
2. If doctor considers palpable area to be not significant:
   - Review by doctor in two to three months or seek a second opinion; document relationship of symptoms to cycles and if appropriate consider a change of oral contraceptive pill—low-dose monophasic pill is usually the best option. Reviewing the area early in the menstrual cycle is often helpful as breast tissue is less stimulated at this time by the hormonal milieu.

Subfertility

CLINICAL PRESENTATION

Infertility is defined as the failure to conceive after 12 months of exposure to the possibility of pregnancy. Some 90 per cent of couples should achieve conception in 12 months and 95 per cent within two years. These percentages depend on the normality of both male and female partner and most importantly on the age of the female partner.[2] Epidemiological evidence suggests an increasing incidence of infertility as women delay child-bearing.[3]

History

The history not only helps to identify potential infertility factors, but also educates patients who may be unaware of the wide variety of issues that can affect fertility. During the history many preconceived ideas about infertility may be discounted and the patient's views dealt with directly.

Menstrual history

Indications of ovulation:

- *Regularity.* A woman whose cycle is between 28 and 32 days on a regular basis is highly likely to be ovulatory. Irregular menses with uterine bleeding occurring more frequently than every 21 days, or less frequently than 35 days, is associated with irregular or absent ovulation.
- *Ovulation pain.* Mid-cycle unilateral abdominal pain, termed *mittelschmertz*, is related to the rupture of the follicle at ovulation.
- *Vaginal secretions.* Pre-ovulatory rise in oestradiol stimulates the mucus to be thinner, more alkaline and more copious. These changes promote the survival and transport of spermatozoa. Progesterone, secreted following ovulation, results in the thickening of the mucus, which becomes tenacious and cellular.
- *Premenstrual symptoms* including bloating, breast tenderness and irritability. This is also indicative that ovulation has occurred in that cycle.
- *Painful periods (dysmenorrhoea)* starting on or just prior to the commencement of bleeding and worse in the first 24 hours but then resolving, is a further hint that ovulation has occurred. This is called primary spasmodic dysmenorrhoea.

Age of the partners

The age of the woman is a vital factor in predicting the likely chances of conceiving, whatever the treatment modality required. More recently the age of the male has been suggested as a factor, perhaps as a result of increasing sperm chromosome defects with age. Delay in seeking assistance is also associated with reduced chances of success.

Previous pregnancies

- Recurrent abortions: after three consecutive first trimester losses, there is a need to further evaluate potential causes for this in addition to looking at the reason for infertility.
- Mid-trimester abortion also warrants more detailed investigation to check for cervical incompetence.

Frequency of intercourse and technique

- Normal rates of fertility occur with coitus every other day around mid-cycle when ovulation should be occurring. Normal sperm are capable of fertilising the oocyte for 48 to 72 hours after ejaculation, and the oocyte is fertilisable between 12 and 24 hours after ovulation. More frequent ejaculation may result in reduced sperm counts—this is only an issue if the sperm quality is suboptimal.

- It is normal for a large part of the ejaculate to escape from the vagina. Positioning of the female subsequent to intercourse in an attempt to improve her chances of pregnancy is a myth.
- There is a need to establish that penetration and ejaculation occur. There may be underlying psychosexual problems which can be exaggerated by the stress of failing to conceive and the need to perform at a given time in the menstrual cycle.

Timing

It is important to establish the patients' level of knowledge. Patients should be educated to the fact that ovulation occurs around 14 days prior to menstruation.

Contraceptive history

- Hormonal birth control methods have not been implicated as a cause of subsequent infertility, despite a generally held contrary view in the community.
- PID and intrauterine devices. This association may be related to the presence of symptomless infection at the time of insertion. A systematic review suggests that pelvic inflammatory disease may be overdiagnosed, and studies have not used an appropriate comparison group or taken the confounding effects of sexual behaviour into account.[4]

Medications

The major rationale for checking on medications taken by women is to identify those drugs that may be harmful in early pregnancy. There are very few drugs that actually impair fertility.

- Chemotherapy for childhood cancers can lead to premature ovarian failure.
- Medications that cause elevation in serum prolactin levels may cause anovulation in some women. These drugs include the phenothiazines.

Drug abuse

Drug abuse, and alcohol, marijuana and cigarette use, are associated with not only impaired semen quality but also reduced female fertility.[5–7]

Past medical history

- Previous surgery in the lower abdomen and pelvis, particularly with postoperative infection, can result in adhesion formation and therefore impairment of tubal patency and function.[8]
- Pelvic or abdominal infection such as a ruptured appendix, Crohn's disease, or a history of sexually transmitted diseases, including gonorrhoea and chlamydia, are all risk factors for scarring and damage to the fallopian tubes.

- A history of pelvic pain may be consistent with endometriosis or chronic pelvic inflammatory disease.
- Medical diseases such as liver disease, renal disease, heart disease and hypothyroidism can be associated with infertility.
- Polycystic ovarian disease (PCO) is suggested by irregular menses, obesity, acne and hirsutism, and results in anovulation. It is present in 90 per cent of women with oligomenorrhoea and 30 per cent of women with amenorrhoea.

Family history

A family history may point to genetic causes of female infertility such as premature menopause due to the fragile X,[9] or polycystic ovarian syndrome.

Examination

General examination

- Hair distribution: excessive hair growth in the male pattern (PCO suggested)
- Breasts: galactorrhoea
- Adipose tissue: adrenal hyperplasia (Cushing's syndrome), PCO, diabetes
- Thyroid: enlargement suggesting disease

Genital examination

- Vagina:
  - Structural abnormalities of the vagina or the cervix
  - Muscle spasm
- Pelvic organs:
  - Fibroids, which can inhibit implantation and cause early miscarriage
  - Ovarian cysts
  - Endometriosis: tenderness, nodular areas of scarring posterior to the uterus
  - Tenderness: suggestive of pelvic inflammatory disease or endometriosis.

Investigations

See Table 13.1.

TABLE 13.1 Investigations for subfertility

Investigation/purpose	Event	Outcomes/notes
Ovulation		
Progesterone	7 days before menses	> 30 nmol/l
Temperature chart	½°C rise in luteal phase	No evidence that use improves outcome.[10]
Cervical mucus	Midcycle mucus becomes thin to allow penetration by sperm.	Postcoital test not recommended as routine investigation.[10]

(continued overleaf)

TABLE 13.1 continued

Investigation/purpose	Event	Outcomes/notes
LH monitoring	Monoclonal antibody urine test Ferning in the saliva	Over the counter (OTC) kits: no evidence that use improves outcomes.[10]
LH	Day 2–5 of menstrual cycle	Raised LH, normal FSH, raised testosterone, low SHBG = PCOS
FSH	Day 2–5 of menstrual cycle Checks ovarian reserve	> 10 IU/l refer to specialist. May respond to IVF
Prolactin	Raised with amenorrhoea Slight raise with regular cycle	? Prolactinoma ? PCOS
Follicle tracking	Transvaginal ultrasound in fertility clinics	Follicle ruptures at 20–25 mm diameter, collapsed follicle after ovulation
Laparoscopy: ovulation	View corpus luteum	GA required
Tubal damage		
Laparoscopy	Check uterine tubes Check for adhesions and endometriosis	Methylene blue dye through tubes Divide adhesions, treat endometriosis
Hysterosalpingogram	Assess tubal patency, uterine cavity	Discomfort/pain for woman Used for women at low risk
Sonohysteroscopy	Injection of microspheres which reflect sound waves	Observe tubal patency on ultrasound
Chlamydial serology	For infective damage Normal < 1:128	Titre > 1:256 treat both partners Screen or cover with antibodies before uterine instrumentation
Sperm		
Postcoital test	Checks sperm function, cervical mucus and coitus	Normal: > 1 motile progressing sperm per HPF 8–18 hours post coitus
Seminal analysis: 3 days abstinence, masturbated sample, sterile container, keep at body temperature, reach laboratory within one hour	Normal: • Sperm count > 20 million/ml+ • Motile, forward progression > 50% • Morphology normal > 15%	Abnormal result: repeat after 3 months. *Karyotype:* Oligospermia < 10 million: eg XXY Klinefelter syndrome *Azoospermia:* micro-deletions on Y chromosome, cystic fibrosis (also absent vas deferens). Antisperm antibody test not recommended as a routine investigation.[10]

Management

1 Ovulatory defects

Polycystic ovarian syndrome

The most common ovulatory defect is treated with clomiphene citrate tablets or, in resistant cases, FSH injections to induce ovulation. Clomiphene is given for five days in the early proliferative phase. It acts as an anti-oestrogen at the pituitary, resulting in increased FSH secretion and thereby stimulating follicular growth and ovulation. Once ovulation is established, pregnancy rates consistent with normal fecundity should result (ie 70–80% in 12 cycles). Some 10–15 per cent experience side effects including hot flushes, nausea and headaches while taking the tablets, mid-cycle pain due to ovulation, exaggeration of premenstrual symptoms and, should pregnancy occur, multiple gestation (3–5 per cent compared with 1 per cent in natural conception).

Hyperprolactinaemia and hypothalamic amenorrhoea

See Amenorrhoea, page 466.

2 Mucus hostility

To stimulate cervical mucus production and augment oestrogenic changes, daily ethinyl oestradiol (10 µg tablet) has been used in the few days leading up to ovulation. There is no evidence to support its use except when clomiphene has been used in that cycle, as clomiphene exerts an anti-oestrogenic effect on cervical mucus. Intrauterine insemination is used for cervical factor problems.

3 Tubal problems

Tubal surgery

Microsurgical techniques: even in the best units with selection of the least damaged cases, results never exceed 40 per cent long-term pregnancy rates[11,12] and carry an increased risk of ectopic pregnancy (10%). The only cases where operative intervention is indicated are:

- Reversal of clip sterilisation where long-term pregnancy rates range from 60 to 80 per cent
- Laparoscopic division of adhesions to open the fimbrial end of the tubes
- Women with blocked tubes at a single site who cannot afford IVF or have religious or moral objections to its use.

The main reason for the poor results with surgery is that the inflammatory process that has caused the blockage has also caused permanent damage to the mucosal microstructures of the tubes. These provide vital nutrient functions to the oocyte and subsequently the early embryo. In addition, recurrence of adhesions is common.

In vitro fertilisation

In vitro fertilisation (IVF) is now used in the management of almost all causes of infertility.

In IVF, the woman is treated with FSH by daily injection, which stimulates the development of a cohort of multiple oocytes within the ovaries (termed *superovulation*). This stimulation requires careful monitoring with ultrasound and/or serum oestradiol levels to avoid overstimulation. In modern treatment the use of gonadotrophin-releasing hormone analogues (GnRHa) in conjunction with FSH have allowed controlled programming of cycles. GnRHa suppresses the normal LH surge that precedes ovulation. Thus the oocytes can be brought to maturity at a time convenient for the clinician and laboratory. The final maturation, which involves exposure to LH, can be timed precisely. The oocytes are collected by transvaginal ultrasound-guided aspiration of each follicle. Each retrieved oocyte is inseminated with sperm. Fertilisation is confirmed after 24 hours with the development of a normal pro-nuclear phase. By 48 hours the embryos should have cleaved to produce a four-cell embryo. One, two or at most three embryos are replaced into the uterus via the cervical canal. This transfer is conducted as an office procedure. Excess good-quality embryos can be cryopreserved for future use. Current clinical pregnancy rates for IVF vary from 20–40 per cent per cycle depending on the clinic and the patient population.

Complications of IVF

1 *Ovarian hyperstimulation syndrome (OHSS)* is the most serious complication of IVF. This condition is associated with excessive levels of oestrogen, which occur when large numbers of follicles are stimulated by FSH. This is particularly a problem in women with polycystic ovarian disease whose ovaries are particularly sensitive to supraphysiological levels of FSH.
   - *Mild OHSS:* bloating and abdominal discomfort with minimal ascites. Some 5 to 10 per cent of women undergoing IVF experience these symptoms.
   - *Moderate OHSS* includes presenting symptoms of abdominal distension, nausea and vomiting, and mild ascites, and is associated with changes in haematology and blood chemistry.
   - *Severe OHSS:* these symptoms are further exaggerated with substantial ascites leading to pain that requires hospitalisation, pleural effusions, pre-renal kidney failure with oliguria or, at worst, anuria. OHSS can be a life-threatening situation requiring expert medical management.

   The pathophysiology of OHSS is not clearly understood. High oestrogen levels plus the presence of high LH/HCG levels predispose to the condition. The condition is self-limiting if pregnancy does not occur. As oestrogen levels fall, the situation reverses itself spontaneously. Pregnancy can cause persistence of the problem for several weeks.

   Prevention of OHSS is a primary goal. The optimum strategy is yet to be determined.

2 *Multiple pregnancy*. A balance between maximising the chances of conceiving and the incidence of multiple pregnancy has always been difficult to achieve. Now even with a two-embryo transfer, the chances of a twin pregnancy are in the order of 20–30 per cent. The perinatal outcome is poor, with the risk of perinatal death up to four times that of a singleton pregnancy. For triplets there is a 10-fold increase in risk of perinatal mortality. Not surprisingly, there is an

increasing move for single-embryo transfer to avoid the risk of multiple pregnancy.

3 *Perinatal mortality and morbidity.* Even in a single pregnancy IVF appears to be associated with growth retardation and a higher perinatal mortality rate than normally conceived singletons.[13,14] This has not been explained. The perinatal outcome overall from IVF because of the multiple pregnancy rates appears to be compromised with higher rates of cerebral palsy. Most studies suggest that this effect is a reflection of prematurity, but there has been at least one recent study suggesting that this is an overall problem with IVF and intracytoplasmic sperm injection (ICSI)—the issue remains controversial.[15]
4 *Long-term effects for the woman.* Concerns about exposure of women to supraphysiological levels of gonadotrophins and oestrogens have been raised. An Australian study prospectively following up 16 000 infertile women has as yet shown no increase in risk.[16]

Unexplained infertility

Women in whom there is no obvious cause account for some 10–20 per cent of infertile couples. A couple has an 80–90 per cent chance of conceiving in the first year. With no obvious cause for failure to conceive after 12 months of trying, a couple has a 40–50 per cent chance of conceiving spontaneously in the subsequent 12 months. Various interventions to improve this rate have been suggested.[17] Clomiphene has been shown to slightly enhance the monthly success rate.

Intrauterine insemination

This treatment is used primarily for the treatment of unexplained infertility but it can also be employed when there is a mild male factor problem. The aim of intrauterine insemination is to maximise all the elements that contribute to a natural conception. The cycle is monitored initially with ultrasound and later by LH assessment to establish the time of the LH surge and so ovulation. This timing allows the insemination to occur when an oocyte should be in the process of transport down the fallopian tube. The sperm are injected via a catheter through the cervix into the uterine cavity. This procedure is done in an office setting. With this technique, pregnancy rates of 15–20 per cent per cycle are regularly reported.

Psychology of infertile couples

Infertility produces significant stress in virtually all couples who are trying to conceive, albeit greater for the female than her partner. The process of treatment and failure can be an emotional roller coaster. In IVF, once the embryos have been replaced, women commence two weeks of unparalleled uncertainty. This period is acknowledged as the hardest part of the treatment. Joy will follow if pregnancy is achieved; frustration and the anger of failure are precipitated by the onset of menses. A quality infertility unit will provide the couple with access to emotional support and counselling before, during and after treatment. Dealing with recurrent failure in a treatment program is a demanding facet of care. Couples need support in carrying on with further treatment, together with realistic advice as to future options, which may include acceptance of childlessness or exploration of the possibilities of adoption.

Age as a factor in infertility

In relation to fertility, cumulative pregnancy rates clearly show the effect of increasing age (Table 13.2). An interesting study of the factors involved in reduced fertility with age is the use of egg donation using younger women's oocytes in this older age group. This study clearly shows that oocyte quality is the major factor.

The same negative effects of age in the artificial reproductive technology (ART) situation are present, as they are in women attempting a natural conception. In counselling women in an ART program in later years, a realistic view of their chances of success must be imparted. However, no matter how negatively one puts the situation, in many cases the woman's desire to attempt to have a child is so great that even the very low odds that exist will not deter her from at least attempting one IVF cycle. It certainly is a necessary step for most women to have tried all possibilities before finally accepting childlessness.

There is an increased incidence of chromosomal abnormalities with age. These are primarily related to chromosomal defects, predominantly trisomies and monosomies.

Obstetric problems: the woman may have developed hypertension, diabetes and thyroid disease. The fetus is at higher risk of having growth retardation due to poor placentation and carries an increased perinatal mortality rate, with a greater incidence of stillbirths and early neonatal deaths.

There is certainly a significant need for education of those women whose long-term plans include being mothers. From the fertility doctor's perspective, when a woman is in the later reproductive age, it is vital to move rapidly to establish the normality of the factors that may inhibit conception, and commence early treatment.

TABLE 13.2 Effects of age on fertility

Age (years)	Chance of fertility in 12 months (%)	Chance of miscarriage	FSH in first 3 days of menstrual cycle
25	90		1 Normal: conception
35	75	30 years: 1 in 6	5–10% per cycle
40	50	40 years: 1 in 4	2 > 15 IU/l conception
45	10	45 years: 1 in 2	< 1–2% per cycle

Male infertility

Male infertility accounts for some 40 per cent of the causes of infertility. A semen analysis will define the problem in 99 per cent of cases.

History

- Past medical history: operations for undescended testes or hernias that may have compromised testicular blood supply, trauma to the testes, testicular tumours, infections such as epididymo-orchitis associated with mumps, STIs (in particular gonococcal infection).
- Current medical illnesses such as diabetes may affect the sperm quality as well as erectile problems.
- Drugs also can impair spermatogenesis; for example, salazopyrin used in ulcerative colitis, beta blockers can reduce motility and anabolic steroids can suppress spermatogenesis.
- Recreational drugs including nicotine, marijuana and alcohol are associated with reduced sperm quality.
- A family history may indicate other men in the family with poor sperm quality, suggesting a genetic link.
- Environment: workplaces may be associated with reduced spermatogenesis; this is thought in part to be related to temperature.[18] Thus men who work in or near furnaces, such as steel workers or bakers, or where they are sitting down for long periods of time, such as long-haul lorry drivers, have been reported to have reduced sperm quality. Exposure to chemicals has also been implicated in agricultural workers.
- Stress: there is good evidence that significant stress can result in reduced sperm quality.
- Sexual dysfunction: premature ejaculation or erectile impotence is rare as a cause of infertility.

Physical examination

A general approach to male infertility is to undertake a semen analysis and, if this is normal, to not proceed to a physical examination. When a sperm count is reported as suboptimal, examination is embarked upon.

Semen analysis

See Box 13.1. If the first test falls below these levels, a repeat test is worthwhile to confirm the problem since semen quality varies on a daily basis. Once a semen analysis has shown a poor result then further investigations are warranted not only to help define the cause but also to predict future prognosis and potential treatment modalities.

Endocrine assessment

Follicle-stimulating hormone plays a vital role in spermatogenesis. Elevation of FSH in the serum correlates with spermatogenic failure similar to the elevation

BOX 13.1 Semen analysis[19]

- Checks sperm production.
- Normal values:
  - volume > 2.5 ml
  - sperm count > 20 million/ml
  - motility > 50%
  - morphology > 15%
- Calculate result as motile normal sperm concentration (count × (% motile) × (% normal ml): normal value > 1 million/ml)
  - *Low volume:* check sample complete or possible retrograde ejaculation
  - *Azoospermia:* repeat sample; testicular examination for reduced size, consistency and presence of vas deferens; check FSH and karyotype and (if possible absence of vas) test for cystic fibrosis
  - *Oligospermia* (< 10 million/ml): check karyotype; early specialist referral if repeat sample abnormal

of FSH seen in menopausal women with ovarian failure. A high FSH carries a poor prognosis.

Genetic investigations

A rapidly expanding area of knowledge is the genetic cause of male infertility.

- Micro deletions on the Y chromosome have become much more specific. In men with counts of less than 5 million per ml, some 15 per cent have been shown to have micro-deletions. This rises further in the azoospermia group.
- Karyotyping should be done in all men with azoospermia and perhaps even those with severe oligospermia (ie less than 2 million per ml): Klinefelter syndrome (XXY) can be detected.
- Cystic fibrosis (CF): when there is absence of the vas deferens. Clearly this has implications for treatment with the man's sperm if the female partner is also a carrier of CF genes.

Ultrasound can be used to visualise the seminal vesicles, prostate and ejaculatory ducts. It also is useful where a swelling of the testes has been detected.

Treatment

Idiopathic

The majority of sperm problems still remain without a specific cause and are defined as idiopathic. No randomised controlled studies of any drug therapy have shown a significant effect. The other problem is that even with very low counts, pregnancies can still occur, albeit at a reduced rate.

Intracytoplasmic sperm injection

Intracytoplasmic sperm injection (ICSI) has revolutionised pregnancy achievement with severe male infertility. The technique involves the selection of an individual sperm by the embryologist, its immobilisation and injection into the ooplasm of oocytes with extremely fine micro pipettes. Fertilisation occurs in some 60 per cent of injected oocytes. Indications for this now include:

- Male factor infertility where the count is so low as to be unlikely to produce normal fertilisation
- When sperm are retrieved directly from the testes or epididymis post vasectomy or blockage due to infection[20]
- Where there has been failed fertilisation despite apparently good semen parameters in an IVF cycle and where there are high levels of anti-sperm antibodies.

Summary

Infertility is a common problem, particularly as women delay child-bearing. To fail to conceive is stressful for both partners, and appropriate and timely investigation is paramount. Application of modern technologies in assisted reproductive therapies now offers couples better than ever opportunities to achieve their desired child.

Lesbians and fertility/parenting

The past 20 years has seen a societal shift towards acceptance of lesbian relationships, with women forming long-term lesbian relationships earlier, and desiring children within these relationships. Some couples and single lesbians foster children, and some would choose adoption, but this is currently not legal in Australia or the UK for lesbian couples. Some states in the USA have legalised adoption by gay and lesbian couples. Most lesbians desiring children choose pregnancy.

Choosing a known sperm donor and self-inseminating is a common practice. This method is chosen for a number of reasons including a desire for the child to know his or her biological father, a need for privacy and control over the process, and lack of access to donor insemination clinics. This may be due to specific legislation that actively excludes lesbians and single women from these programs or because they cannot afford the expense of clinic-based donor insemination. Self-insemination with a known donor usually involves detailed negotiation with the potential sperm donor as to his degree of involvement in the family and his rights and responsibilities.

The health care practitioner fulfils a number of roles for these families. Referral to donor insemination clinics, particularly those that are lesbian-sensitive, is straightforward. Other advice about safe insemination is invaluable:

- Pre-pregnancy advice and screening for the biological mother
- Safe self-insemination procedures
- Screening of the sperm donor for sexually transmissible infections
- Safe sex practices for the donor throughout the insemination period
- Information about insemination technique
- Recognition of ovulation to ensure optimal timing for insemination, which may include the use of urine LH testing
- The need to ensure as short a time as practicable between ejaculation and insemination

- Method of insemination, using a 5 ml syringe
- Orgasm immediately prior to insemination may assist sperm movement through the cervix.

The practitioner can also assist with providing psychosocial support for prospective and current lesbian families.

Menstrual disturbance

CLINICAL PRESENTATION: Infrequent periods (oligomenorrhoea) or absent periods (amenorrhoea)

Amenorrhoea is defined as the absence of menses and is arbitrarily set at six months. The 'normal' length of the menstrual cycle is 21–36 days; the woman is said to have oligomenorrhoea when the menstrual cycle occurs every 36–180 days. Some women with regular cycles may present for evaluation before 180 days of amenorrhoea and are worthy of evaluation to exclude, at least in the first instance, physiological causes. Primary amenorrhoea is the absence of menses by the age of 16 or within two years of the onset of breast development. Primary amenorrhoea is rare, secondary amenorrhoea is common. Secondary amenorrhoea is the absence of menses for six months or greater where the woman has previously menstruated spontaneously.

Causes of secondary amenorrhoea and oligomenorrhoea may be physiological, iatrogenic or pathological (Box 13.2). The evaluation should involve the relevant history, examination and investigations.

BOX 13.2 Causes of secondary amenorrhoea

- Physiological:
  - Pregnancy
  - Lactation
  - Menopause
- Iatrogenic:
  - Contraception (Depo-Provera, Implanon, Mirena)
  - After ceasing contraception
  - Asherman's syndrome
- Pathological:
  - Hyperprolactinaemia
  - PCOS
  - Cushing's syndrome
  - Hypothalamic (weight change, exercise, stress)
  - Premature ovarian failure
  - Other endocrine disorders

History

- Age of menarche
- Pre-existing menstrual function
- Use of hormonal contraception
- Risk of pregnancy
- Galactorrhoea
- Hirsutism
- Headaches
- Hot flushes
- Weight loss and gain
- Exercise.

Essential investigations

- Beta HCG
- Prolactin
- Thyroid function tests
- LH, FSH and oestradiol
- If clinically indicated:
  - DHEAS or free androgen index (total testosterone and sex hormone binding globulin)
  - Chromosomal analysis
  - Pelvic ultrasound scan (transvaginal if sexually active).

Examination

- Calculation of body mass index
- Inspection for features of anorexia nervosa and bulimia (lanugo, dental caries, parotidomegaly, bradycardia) and hyperandrogenism (hirsutism, clitoromegaly)
- Gynaecological examination: clitoromegaly, acanthosis nigricans and evidence of vaginal atrophy
- Breast examination for hirsutism and the presence of expressible galactorrhoea.

Physiological amenorrhoea

1. *Pregnancy* is the most common cause, and is essential to exclude initially and indeed throughout the evaluation (sometimes oligo-ovulatory women conceive during the evaluation of the menstrual disturbance!).
2. *Lactation* is frequently associated with amenorrhoea although ovulation rapidly resumes in women consuming a Western diet when solid foods are introduced to the baby. Bone density may decrease during this time but seems to recover following the cessation of lactation. Contraceptive advice may be appropriate as ovulation can resume at any time.
3. *Menopause:* the natural age is from the mid-40s to the mid-50s and amenorrhoea retrospectively defines the menopause.

Iatrogenic amenorrhoea

1 *Using hormone contraception.* Women need to be reassured in these circumstances and decide whether the side effect of amenorrhoea is acceptable to them. Sometimes women on the COCP present with amenorrhoea—often they have a history of menses that have become progressively lighter and shorter as the duration of use of the COCP has increased. Once pregnancy has been excluded these women can be reassured that medically there is no requirement for a withdrawal bleed during the pill-free interval. The mechanism of amenorrhoea is usually endometrial atrophy.
2 *Ceasing hormonal contraceptives.* Older textbooks will describe 'post-pill amenorrhoea'—this is a misnomer and investigation of the amenorrhoea is required after cessation of hormonal contraception as it is at any time of a woman's life. These women frequently have a history of pre-existing menstrual disturbance which had been subsequently masked by hormonal contraception. Women should be advised of this prior to usage. Implanon and oral progestin-only contraception are not associated with delay in the return of ovulation.
3 *Asherman's syndrome* is a rare cause. This is complete or partial loss of the endometrium due to excessive curettage. It should be considered in women with a history of uterine manipulation (repeated curettage post partum, termination of pregnancy, particularly those associated with uterine infection). Careful vaginal ultrasound may be helpful in identifying islands of endometrium. The diagnosis requires hysteroscopy and/or hysterosalpingography.

Pathological amenorrhoea

1 Hyperprolactinaemia

This is a common cause of secondary amenorrhoea that must not be missed. As prolactin rises, the degree of menstrual abnormality rises, progressing through oligomenorrhoea due to luteal insufficiency, oligoovulation to anovulation and finally amenorrhoea.

History

- Galactorrhoea is present in the minority of women, particularly in the nullipara and in those with oestrogen deficiency.
- Sometimes headaches are present.
- Pre-existing menstrual function is often normal, although the condition may have been present and unrecognised for many years.
- Drug history (Box 13.3)
- Rarely: unrecognised hypothyroidism should not be missed.

Investigations

- Mild elevation of prolactin (less than twice the laboratory upper limit of reference range) is common and is often due to stress. Repeat measurement on two or three occasions separated by a few weeks will usually establish this minor elevation.

- If a pathologically elevated prolactin, check a drug history.
- Imaging of pituitary by either MRI or CT scanning, for micro- or macro-adenoma, is appropriate where pathological hyperprolactinaemia exists.

Treatment

- If a microadenoma or macroadenoma is diagnosed, use of dopamine agonists such as bromocriptine or cabergoline is associated with reduction in the tumour secretion of prolactin and often tumour shrinkage also.
- The patient needs to be counselled about side effects of the drug therapy. The dose should be increased gradually and the patient warned that ovulation frequently resumes promptly with its attendant risk of pregnancy. These women may be at long-term risk of osteoporosis, depending on the degree of hypo-oestrogenism, and measurement of bone mineral density may be appropriate.
- Surgery is rarely required for pituitary adenomas, which are composed of prolactin-secreting cells.

BOX 13.3 Drugs that may cause hyperprolactinaemia

- Phenothiazines
- Butyrophenones
- Atypical antipsychotics (eg risperidone >> olanzapine)
- Tricyclic antidepressants
- Oestrogens
- Verapamil
- Methyldopa
- Metoclopramide
- Opiates (eg heroin abuse)

2 Polycystic ovarian syndrome

Polycystic ovarian syndrome (PCOS) is a common cause of oligomenorrhoea and amenorrhoea. Approximately 6–9 per cent of women have PCOS. The diagnostic criteria for the disease are disputed but confirming a state of chronic anovulation with hyperandrogenaemia where other causes (such as hyperprolactinaemia and Cushing's syndrome) have been excluded is a useful working definition adopted by NIH consensus in 1990. The place of ultrasound in the diagnosis is debated, as the sonographic features are non-specific and can be present without hyperandrogenaemia or present in other conditions such as Cushing's syndrome.

History

There is frequently a history of increasing weight gain with the worsening of the menstrual disturbance. These women are at particular risk of endometrial hyperplasia that probably parallels the duration of the amenorrhoea.

Differential diagnosis

Approximately 60 per cent of women with Cushing's syndrome present with menstrual disturbance, and although Cushing's syndrome is a rare condition its diagnosis should be considered. Ultrasound evidence of polycystic ovaries is seen in Cushing's syndrome but tests suggestive of Cushing's syndrome include elevation of 24-hour urinary free cortisol or failure of early-morning cortisol to suppress after administration of 1 mg of dexamethasone at 11 pm the preceding night. Random cortisol measurements are not particularly useful.

Long-term implications of the diagnosis of PCOS:

- Increased risk of developing diabetes mellitus, particularly with increasing obesity, should be discussed with the woman.
- Women with PCOS and oligomenorrhoea should be advised to seek medical advice with the subsequent development of amenorrhoea because of the risk of endometrial hyperplasia.

Investigations

- *Endometrial sampling.* If there is a history of amenorrhoea followed by the development of heavy and prolonged irregular bleeding it is appropriate to refer the patient for endometrial sampling. Outpatient sampling of the endometrium may miss endometrial hyperplasia with atypia.
- *Ultrasound.* The place of measurement of endometrial thickness with transvaginal ultrasound is not well evaluated in this group of women.

Treatment

- It is important to arrange some form of endometrial protection such as the COC or cyclical progestin to induce secretory change and withdrawal bleeding. Suitable currently available progestins are dydrogesterone 10 mg, medroxyprogesterone acetate 5–10 mg, and norethisterone 1.25 mg daily for two out of four weeks.
- Irregular bleeding may indicate spontaneous ovulation, pregnancy or development of endometrial hyperplasia. Women need to be reminded that cyclic progestin is not contraceptive.
- In PCOS, obesity is common and weight reduction is frequently associated with resumption of ovulation.
- Screening for diabetes mellitus, hypertension and hyperlipidaemia is appropriate. Annual measurement of fasting blood sugar level in obese women with PCOS (although the most efficient screening tool is not yet confirmed).
- Counselling on lifestyle modification to have a healthy low-fat diet and regular exercise is important. There is some evidence that supportive medical relationships assist patients in this very difficult endeavour.

3 Hypothalamic amenorrhoea

- Weight reduction following intense dietary restriction or excessive exercise is often associated and probably contributes to the aetiology.

- Psychosocial stress may also contribute.
- Consideration of the diagnosis of an eating disorder is important.

Investigations

- Low or very low gonadotrophins with low oestradiol.
- Imaging of the brain to exclude brain lesions is mandatory, (although positive findings are uncommon in this group), before a gentle but honest discussion with the patient.
- This group is at particular risk of reduced bone density and therefore bone density should be measured, often serially.
- Rarely anosmia may be associated; the condition is a genetic cause of primary amenorrhoea.

Treatment

Some women are resistant to lifestyle modification resulting in weight gain, and therefore calcium and oestrogen supplementation should be encouraged.

4 Premature ovarian failure

A minority of women with secondary amenorrhoea will have premature ovarian failure (POF)—approximately one per cent of women aged less than 40 years.

Investigation

- Very high levels of serum FSH and low serum oestradiol.
- There is sometimes a family history of POF and chromosomal study is relevant to detect deletions of all or part of the X chromosome. If a karyotypic abnormality is found, family studies and genetic counselling of female relatives may be required. If the diagnosis of XO dysgenesis (Turner's syndrome) is made, evaluation of the associated consequences including aortic root dilatation and associated renal, thyroid and other endocrine disorders is appropriate.

Prognosis

- Spontaneous fertility after the diagnosis of premature ovarian failure is very uncommon. Some women achieve pregnancy though use of donated oocytes.
- Women with POF without replacement of oestrogen are at long-term risk of osteoporosis and premature atherosclerosis.

5 Other endocrinopathies

Other causes to consider:

- Addison's syndrome (suggested by fatigue, nausea, vomiting, diarrhoea, weight loss, increasing pigmentation, lymphocytosis and electrolyte disturbance)
- Thyrotoxicosis and centrally based hypogonadism from perhaps a non-functioning pituitary tumour
- Hypothyroidism can be associated with oligomenorrhoea and anovulation but rarely amenorrhoea.

Hirsutism

CLINICAL PRESENTATION

Hirsutism is an excess of body hair in the androgen-dependent areas of the female body.

A woman's perception of increased body hair is affected by cultural and social expectations. There is wide variability in amount and quality of hair in the androgen-dependent areas according to ethnic extraction, with women of Mediterranean descent having more hair in androgen-dependent areas and Asian women having less. It can be defined in a semi-objective manner by use of charts such as that proposed by Ferriman and Gallwey (Figure 13.1).[21] Drug therapy (Box 13.4) and hormonal status are significant aetiological influences.

BOX 13.4 Drugs associated with hirsutism

- Androgens and derivatives such as danazol
- Corticosteroids
- Cyclosporin and derivatives
- Phenytoin
- Minoxidil

The body hair cycle has three phases:

- *Anagen*, the growth phase, which lasts months to years
- *Catagen*, which lasts two weeks when the hair follicle undergoes apoptosis and the hair stops growing
- *Telogen*, the resting phase, which lasts up to three months while the hair follicle is attached to the follicle and then sheds. Anagen of the hair follicle then ensues.

With such a long normal cycle the development and response to treatment of hirsutism is slow. Recruitment to the growth phase, coarsening and darkening of the hair shaft and and increased rate of growth of the hair shaft are stimulated by androgens.

The amount of active androgen present is determined by the amount of sex hormone binding globulin (SHBG) and other plasma proteins. Only free or bio-available androgens are active at the hair follicle. Influences on SHBG are therefore significant influences on the level of free androgen (Section 4). The effect of change of free androgen status on the hair follicles is slow and may not be seen for 3–6 months as changes in body hair quality, amount and distribution.

Clinical assessment

- Hirsutism is frequently a most distressing symptom for women and presentation is at any age. The woman may have noted increased facial, abdominal and chest hair over a period of time. Appropriate clinical evaluation includes

FIGURE 13.1 Scoring systems can assess the severity of hirsutism.[21,22] The Ferriman-Gallwey model quantitates the extent of hair growth in nine key anatomic sites (seven of them are shown). Hair growth is graded using a scale from 0 (no terminal hair) to 4 (maximal growth), for a maximum score of 36. A score of eight or more indicates the presence of androgen excess.

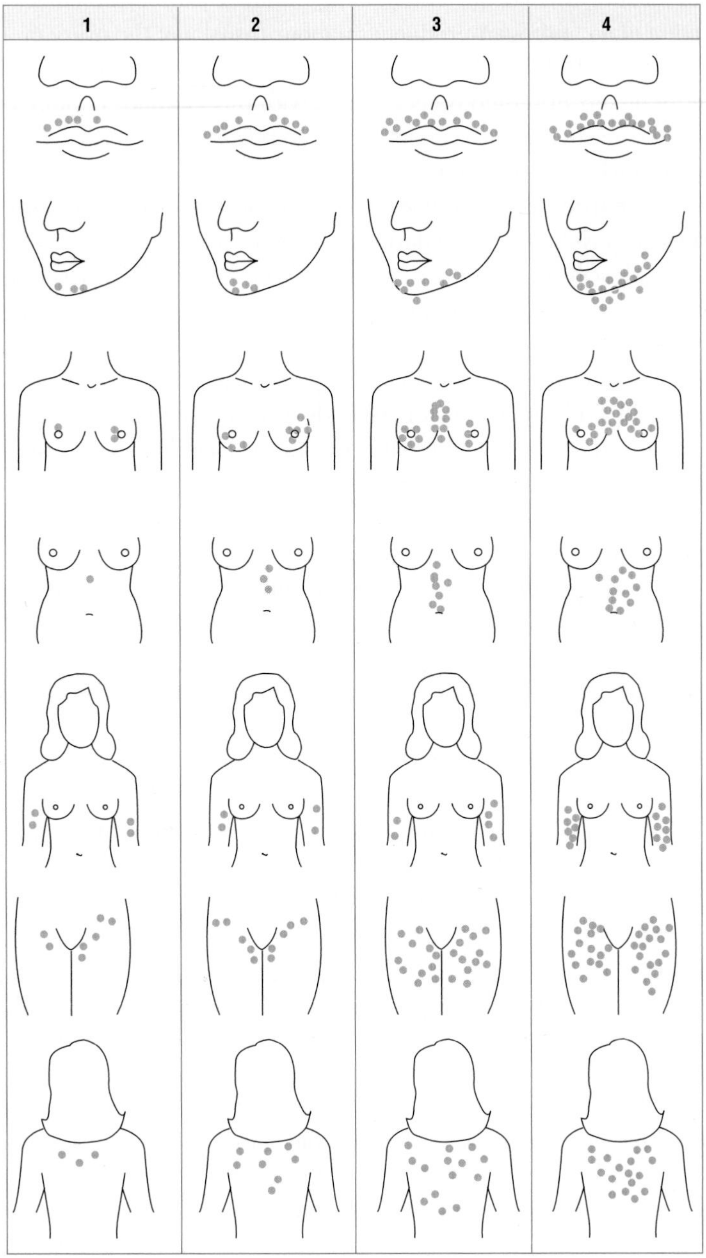

1	2	3	4

noting the age at which hirsutism was first noted, at what age local treatments were first used (waxing, shaving, bleaching, depilatory creams, electrolysis) and how frequently these were used initially and how frequently they are used now. In such a way the clinician can determine whether the degree of hirsutism is rapidly or gradually worsening, or is relatively constant.
- While hirsutism is not life-threatening, rarely it can be the clinical manifestation of an androgen-producing tumour (usually of the ovary or adrenal gland), which itself may be life-threatening. Therefore evaluation and treatment of hirsutism should be performed with this in mind. Rapidly worsening or new-onset hirsutism is more likely to reflect a tumour than long-term, mild or slowly worsening hirsutism.
- Severe hirsutism associated with deepening of the voice and clitoromegaly (termed *virilisation*), particularly if rapid in onset, is likely to reflect a tumour. Most hirsutism is associated with menstrual disturbance and this should be specifically sought in history taking and appropriate management instituted.
- Gradually worsening hirsutism is frequently associated with progressive weight gain, and so a life history of body weight should be obtained. Other endocrinopathies associated with hirsutism include acromegaly, hypothyroidism and premature ovarian failure.

Examination findings

- General: measurement of body mass index, use of a semi-objective measurement tool of hirsutism, and examination of the body habitus for stigmata of Cushing's syndrome.
- Androgenic alopecia should be sought and parallels more severe hyperandrogenism.
- Acanthosis nigricans is a marker of insulin resistance, which may suggest polycystic ovarian syndrome as a possible cause.
- Abdominal examination for abdominal masses is prudent but is frequently normal.
- Genital examination for evidence of clitoromegaly.

Investigations

There is considerable variability between countries in terms of assay availability and so it is hard to be prescriptive about what tests should or should not be performed.

1. Cushing's syndrome if clinically considered should be screened for by measurement of 24-hour urinary free cortisol, measurement of cortisol creatinine ratio in the urine or response of early morning serum cortisol to administration of 1 mg of oral dexamethasone at 11 pm the preceding night.
2. Confirmation of hyperandrogenaemia may be useful and is available in Western societies but androgen assays are expensive and of limited usefulness in clinical practice.

3 Very high or rising androgen levels may prompt the clinician to consider adrenal or ovarian tumours. Normal androgen levels may reflect genetic predisposition to hair growth as seen in certain racial groups (a condition termed *idiopathic hirsutism*).
4 Some measure of bio-available testosterone (the most potent androgen in serum) can be used, such as free androgen index (FAI), which is a value calculated from measurement of total testosterone and SHBG, and DHEAS (which is almost all adrenal in origin). Free testosterone assays if reliable can be used instead of FAI (Section 4).

Management

Local treatments although often inconvenient and uncomfortable and do not have systemic side effects, and this should be explained to the patient. Even where drug therapy is entertained, women should be encouraged to continue with local treatments. There is no objective evidence that local treatments worsen the hirsutism, although women will often associate their increasing use of local treatments with worsening hirsutism. It is likely that the converse is true—the hirsutism worsened and local treatments were increased. In general, medical treatment with its attendant side effects is not recommended for hirsutism alone when the Ferriman and Gallwey score is less than 8. Women with moderately severe hirsutism (F&G score > 15) frequently require long-term treatments.

It is essential that at the initiation of drug treatment for hirsutism it is clearly explained to the woman that the onset of treatment effect is slow (six months) and that hirsutism is likely to recur within six months after cessation of the drug treatment unless the predisposing cause has been treated (eg there has been significant weight loss in a woman with PCOS). Where drugs are implicated, change in drug therapy may be appropriate if possible, and clearly Cushing's syndrome and other tumours should be treated.

- Combined oral contraceptive pill. This works by at least two mechanisms: induction of SHBG by the liver, which reduces the free androgen levels, and also by suppression of ovarian production of androgens. Sometimes the progestogen component of the COCP is an anti-androgen such as cyproterone acetate which acts further at the level of the hair follicle to competitively inhibit the action of any free androgen. Randomised controlled trials (RCTs) suggest that most of the effect is due to the first two mechanisms and therefore if cost is a major constraint, addition of cyproterone may be undesirable. Severe hirsutism sometimes requires the addition of higher doses of cyproterone acetate. Traditionally this has been done in what is called 'the reverse cyproterone regimen' when cyproterone 25–50 mg per day is given from days 1 to 10 of the COC cycle. This relates to the long duration of action of cyproterone.
- Other anti-androgens such as flutamide have been studied in clinical trials with promising effect but are not yet available for such use in Australia and New Zealand.

- Spironolactone has been used as an anti-androgen but meta-analysis of RCTs reported in the Cochrane Collaboration suggests that the benefit of spironolactone over the COC is uncertain until further trials have been performed. Spironolactone may have a place in the management of a woman who does not wish to take the COC or cannot take the COC (eg exacerbation of migraine headaches or smoker aged > 35 years). Where anti-androgens are taken without the COC, adequate contraception must be used because of the teratogenic risk to the male fetus.
- Postmenopausal women who decline HRT may notice increasing hirsutism related to the relative excess of free androgens as oestrogen and SHBG levels fall. This is a major concern if the woman desires androgen replacement for reduced libido in the absence of HRT. Introduction of oestrogen replacement with use of a progestogen with few androgenic side effects such as dydrogesterone may be helpful in postmenopausal women complaining of hirsutism.
- Women with PCOS may benefit from weight loss (RCTs pending) and currently there is no evidence that use of insulin sensitisers such as metformin have a role in the improvement of hirsutism.

Pelvic pain

CLINICAL PRESENTATION: Acute pelvic pain

Acute pelvic pain is a common indication for emergency referral. Because of the diversity of problems which may present in this way (Table 13.3, page 478), it can provide a considerable diagnostic challenge. The need for emotional support as well as professional clinical care and a holistic approach cannot be overemphasised.

Rapid clinical assessment

Quick assessment is made of the degree of distress of the patient and her general clinical state. Observations should include:

- Level of consciousness
- Routine: pulse, blood pressure and temperature
- Vaginal bleeding should be noted if present, and an estimate made of the degree of blood loss
- Signs of intraperitoneal haemorrhage or perforation (abdominal wall rigidity/rebound tenderness).

If there are signs of shock, resuscitation should be commenced with IV access and blood sent urgently for a full blood count and cross matching. Intraperitoneal haemorrhage requires surgical intervention as a matter of urgency. However, most women presenting with pelvic pain are clinically stable, enabling a more relaxed approach to assessment.

Relevant history

This must include:

- Pain: a description of the onset, site, nature, intensity, duration, radiation and any associated factors
- Menses: LMP and any change in normal pattern
- Contraception
- Pregnancy symptoms (see early pregnancy, Section 6)
- Other relevant symptoms: vaginal discharge, dyspareunia, urinary or gastro-intestinal symptoms will help in clarifying the source of the pain.

A gynaecological, obstetric, medical and social history should be taken.

Relevant clinical examination

- Routine observations of the rapid clinical assessment
- Abdominal examination is performed to confirm the site and radiation of the pain, tenderness, signs of peritonism and palpable masses
- Speculum and vaginal examination. If the woman has a history suggestive of miscarriage, vaginal examination should be performed to assess the size of the uterus and the state of the cervix.

The history and examination will direct investigations. Pregnancy must always be suspected in a woman of reproductive years, and ectopic pregnancy excluded.

Relevant investigations

- Urinalysis should be performed prior to clinical examination, together with a rapid urinary HCG test
- Mid-stream urine for culture if a urinary tract infection is suspected (symptoms of urinary frequency and dysuria)
- Blood should be taken for a full blood count, group and save (or cross match if there is a concern about blood loss)
- Quantitative serum HCG assay if ectopic pregnancy is suspected
- Endocervical swabs should be taken to detect infection (including chlamydial polymerase chain reaction test)
- Ultrasound scanning will enable a definite diagnosis of intrauterine pregnancy and its viability to be assessed. It can also identify the presence and nature of a pelvic and adnexal mass (see Pelvic mass) and the presence of fluid in the pouch of Douglas may be suggestive of a ruptured cyst, bleeding from an ovarian cyst or ectopic pregnancy.
- A diagnostic laparoscopy may need to be performed to make a diagnosis or exclude a gynaecological cause.

Differential diagnosis

See Table 13.3. There are many causes of acute pelvic pain and the individual conditions are discussed in detail elsewhere. Although the diagnosis may be very clear from the clinical features, backed up if necessary by ultrasound and biochemical tests, in many cases the clinical picture is vague and non-specific and is eventually classified as 'non-specific abdominal pain'.

TABLE 13.3 Differential diagnosis of acute pelvic pain

Category	Diagnosis
Gynaecological	
1 Pregnancy-related (Section 9)	Ectopic
	Miscarriage (eg inevitable, incomplete, septic)
	Fibroid degeneration—rare
2 Ovarian	Mittelschmerz (ovulation pain)
	Accident to a cyst (torsion, rupture, haemorrhage)
	Ovarian hyperstimulation syndrome
3 Tubal	Pelvic inflammatory disease
4 Uterine	Dysmenorrhoea
5 Pelvic	Endometriosis
Non-gynaecological	
1 GIT	Appendicitis
	Inflammatory bowel disease
	Irritable bowel syndrome
	Diverticulitis
	Constipation
	Adhesions
	Hernia—strangulated
2 Urinary tract	Infection
	Calculus
	Retention

CLINICAL PRESENTATION: Chronic pelvic pain

Chronic pelvic pain has many possible causes, both gynaecological and non-gynaecological, the list of non-gynaecological causes outnumbering those which are gynaecological in origin (Table 13.4). In many cases the distinction may be obvious but assessment and management of women with chronic pelvic pain can be challenging, sometimes involving referral to a multidisciplinary team which can offer a holistic approach. The prevalence of chronic pelvic pain among women of reproductive age is reported to be around 15 per cent.

Clinical assessment

The history must include:

- *Pain:* a detailed description of the nature, site and radiation of the pain, its frequency and duration, relationship to the menstrual cycle, to sexual intercourse and any other aggravating or relieving factors. It is necessary to assess the severity of the pain (some health professionals ask the woman to assess this on a scale of one to ten, with ten being the worst she has ever experienced or could imagine). It is valuable to assess the impact it is having on lifestyle, for example on social function or on sexual relationships.

TABLE 13.4 Differential diagnosis of chronic pelvic pain[23]

Category	Diagnosis
Gynaecological	
1 Physiological/functional	Dysmenorrhoea Mittelschmerz Pelvic congestion syndrome Inflammation
2 Pelvic inflammatory disease	Endometriosis (chocolate cysts, minimal disease)
3 Tumour	Benign (ovarian cysts, fibroids) Malignant Non-gynaecological
4 GIT	Irritable bowel syndrome Inflammatory bowel disease Diverticulitis Constipation Adhesions
2 Urinary tract	Infection Retention
3 Psychosocial	Somatisation Depression/anxiety Childhood sexual abuse Domestic violence Psychosomatic Munchausen's syndrome
4 Orthopaedic	Back or hip disease

- A detailed menstrual, gynaecological and sexual history is important, together with obstetric, medical and social history and details of previous therapies and their effectiveness.

Relevant clinical examination

During the consultation a general impression of the patient's attitude and demeanour is relevant. A general and gynaecological examination is undertaken (Section 1). Young women who have never been sexually active should not be subjected to vaginal examination.

Relevant investigations

Further investigation will depend on the differential diagnosis made from the history and examination. An ultrasound scan and diagnostic laparoscopy may be considered.

Aetiology

- A gynaecological cause is more likely if the pain is related to specific phases of the menstrual cycle and to sexual intercourse.

- In women with chronic pain unrelated or only partially related to the menstrual cycle, urinary, gastrointestinal and musculoskeletal symptoms should be elicited.
- Psychosocial factors may need to be explored in detail but not necessarily at the initial visit. Sensitive enquiry into a possible abusive relationship, either current or in the past.
- Many women are simply seeking reassurance that there is no serious underlying cause; others may be anxious about possible impact on fertility; in others the situation may be complex.
- Endometriosis is the most common gynaecological cause of chronic pelvic pain, occurring in around one-third of laparoscopies carried out for this indication (Box 13.5).
- One-third of laparoscopies carried out for the investigation of pelvic pain are negative, implying non-gynaecological causes.
- Irritable bowel syndrome is more common in women than men and is often confused clinically with endometriosis because there may be dyspareunia and premenstrual exacerbation of bowel symptoms.
- Psychosocial factors are also important. Factors such as personality traits, coping strategies and health beliefs may predispose an individual to the development of chronic pain.
- There is also a high prevalence in women with a history of physical or sexual abuse.
- Pelvic venous congestion is a condition described in multiparous women of reproductive age.[24] Chronic dull, aching pain is characteristically exacerbated perimenstrually by activity and by sexual intercourse, and relieved by lying down. It is attributed to the presence of dilated veins in the broad ligament and ovarian plexus. Typical appearances have been described at venography and reported with both ultrasound and MRI. However, there is no universal agreement about the existence of the condition as an entity distinct from unexplained chronic pelvic pain.

BOX 13.5 Laparoscopy for chronic pelvic pain[25]

- Results of 1524 laparoscopies for pelvic pain:
  - Normal findings (35%)
  - Endometriosis (33%)
  - Adhesions (24%)
  - Chronic PID (5%)
  - Ovarian cysts (3%)
  - Pelvic varicosities (1%)
  - Fibroids (1%)
  - Other (4%).

Endometriosis

Endometriosis is the condition in which endometrial glands and stroma are found in locations outside the uterine cavity. It is variable in both its surgical appearance and clinical manifestations, often with poor correlation between the two.

CLINICAL PRESENTATION

1 *Asymptomatic endometriosis.* Factors associated with a reduced risk of endometriosis are an irregular cycle, two or more births, and one or more induced abortions. A subgroup of asymptomatic women will present with an adnexal mass and require further investigation to prevent cyst complications and in the older woman to exclude malignancy.

2 *Pain.* There is often poor correlation between symptoms and extent of disease at laparoscopy which remains unexplained. The classic history is of progressively increasing dysmenorrhoea, dyspareunia and chronic pelvic pain. These are common symptoms and a causal relationship cannot be assumed. Some studies have attempted to correlate the depth of invasion of endometriosis with the degree of pain.

3 *Infertility*. Possible mechanisms include:
- Interference with ovum transport
- Mechanical disruption of the normal tubo-ovarian anatomical relationship
- Impaired oocyte quality
- Iatrogenic factors including suppressive hormone therapy and destructive surgery.

4 A *history of cyclic bleeding* in any organ system may be due to endometriosis.

Consumer groups have documented a wide range of symptoms in women diagnosed with endometriosis, such as painful bowel movements during menstruation.

Examination

This can range from a normal finding to a fixed retroversion of the uterus (uterus adherent to bowel and pelvic walls), tender nodularity of the uterosacral ligaments and the presence of ovarian endometriomas.

Investigations

Endometriosis can only be accurately diagnosed by direct visualisation by laparoscopy and could be confirmed by histology of a biopsy or after tissue sample. However, tertiary ultrasounds can detect small endometriomas within the ovary and some ultrasonologists can diagnosis the presence of pelvic adhesions by a lack of mobility of the bowel.

Incidence

As endometriosis can only be diagnosed by laparoscopy (visual appearance and histology), neither the incidence nor the prevalence is accurately known. The incidence does vary among different groups of women, depending on the occurrence of menstruation. Previously described variations among different ethnic groups can be explained in that endometriosis is less likely in amenorrhoeic women. There is also some variation in the reported incidence due to operator expertise and knowledge of the variable visual characteristics of the disease. It is important to remember that endometriosis has been described in a significant proportion of teenage women. Also the condition can (rarely) occur in postmenopausal women.

Sites

The most common sites affected by endometriosis are the surface of the ovaries and the uterosacral ligaments. This probably represents the link between endometriosis and retrograde menstruation. However, endometriosis has been described in every system of the body.

Pathogenesis

Retrograde menstruation

The implantation of refluxed endometrial tissue was first proposed by Sampson in the 1920s.[26] Retrograde menstruation is in fact quite common in women, having been described in up to 80 per cent of menstrual cycles.

Immunological theory

The interplay of enhancing and suppressing genes and environment is an attractive theory to explain why some women continue to have mild endometriosis, while in others the disease rapidly progresses to the severe form, and others with retrograde menstruation do not express endometriosis at all. A familial pattern has been described.

Abnormal proliferation

Angiogenesis, release of cytokines and inflammatory mediators appear to be part of the disease process and are associated with pain and tissue damage.[27]

Direct spread

Endometriosis can be distributed via surgical transplantation, via blood vessels and lymphatic vessels. This would explain the remote locations and also its not uncommon description in episiotomy wounds and abdominal wounds.

Metaplasia

This was an embryological theory: constant irritation by retrograde menstruation may cause metaplasia of similarly derived embryonic tissue such as the pelvic peritoneum.

Natural history

The definition made at laparoscopy has changed to encompass microscopic lesions, clear blister-like lesions, haemorrhagic and petechial areas, to the classic blue-brown and black spots. If the disease progresses it can involve blood-filled cysts within the ovarian tissue (endometriomas), dense adhesions throughout the pelvis, and infiltration of disease into the tissues. Oestradiol (in the normal menstrual cycle) is generally believed essential for the progression of the endometriotic lesions.

Classification

Mild disease is generally described as that in which neither fallopian tubes nor ovaries are compromised in their normal function. Severe disease is where extensive adhesive formation has occurred or an altered function of an affected organ is clearly demonstrated. The American Fertility Society has a complex scoring system that is a result of an expert committee attempting to correlate the extent of the disease with impairment of fertility. This does not include information about depth of infiltration.

Management

This will depend on the woman's age, the presence of symptoms, and past and future fertility plans.

1 *Asymptomatic endometriosis.* There is no current data suggesting that this should be treated.[28] The exceptions are an adnexal mass where complications from this are a concern and the exclusion of malignancy is necessary.
2 *Pain.* This may involve symptom relief, disease suppression or both. It is frequently stated that the extent of the disease does not correlate with the symptomatic presentation of the disease. The depth of infiltration of endometriosis has some correlation with pain.[29] Secondary dysmenorrhoea in young women may continue on from primary dysmenorrhoea with no clear distinction. Both medical and surgical treatments may be effective for pain relief.
3 *Infertility.* Medical treatment will not enhance fertility.[30] Laparoscopic surgery has benefits for infertility with a sustained effect over 36 months.[31] In vitro fertilisation does not have a good outcome for women with endometriosis.

Medical management

- The COCP can be particularly effective for women with dysmenorrhoea. The pill can be administered in a four-monthly cyclic regimen or continuous regimen achieving amenorrhoea.
- Progestogens (medroxyprogesterone acetate and danazol) can be used in high doses over six months to inhibit ovulation, thereby suppressing menstruation and resulting in constant low levels of oestrogen. This results in significant reduction in the size of the endometriotic deposits, and pain relief.[32]
- A second method of achieving reduction in the size of endometriotic deposits is administration of GnRH analogues, which results in a menopausal level of oestradiol. Because most of these drugs are used in high dosages there are significant side effects, including progestogenic, androgenetic and menopausal symptoms.

Surgery

Surgery is divided into conservative (preserving reproductive function) and radical.

- The current favoured treatment is to ablate (electrocautery, laser) visible endometriotic deposits and excise endometriomas. The division of adhesions to reconstruct the normal anatomy is certainly of benefit for patients presenting with infertility. However, the Cochrane Libraries Randomised Controlled Register would indicate that there is no proven benefit for division of adhesions for symptoms of pain.

- Women presenting with the symptoms of dysmenorrhoea and who have completed their families can discuss the benefits of a hysterectomy. Frequently a discussion of bilateral oophorectomy is needed, as cyclic symptoms will continue if the ovaries remain and thereby cyclically release increasing levels of oestradiol.
- The routine performance of complementary denervating procedures cannot be recommended on the evidence available.[33]
- Should a woman conceive and be successful, lactation is to be encouraged, because during lactation very low levels of oestradiol are present and therefore this is a treatment of endometriosis in itself.
- Complementary therapies are used by a significant proportion of women, with many reporting benefits. There is a lack of appropriate studies.
- There are significant opportunities for symptomatic treatment, including analgesia for pain and dysmenorrhoea.

Support

Support groups are available for women internationally and their charter is to encourage women to take charge of their own health. The groups assist this process by providing information, networking opportunities, crisis call helpers and information on an exhaustive range of treatment options.

Communication

The management of endometriosis is a complex issue involving many different forms of surgery and medical treatment options. A high level of communication skills is frequently necessary for dealing with women who have endometriosis, as the symptoms have been described as being present for up to nine years prior to diagnosis in a significant proportion. Not uncommonly such women have tried many different symptomatic treatment regimens with variable success and can be angry at the apparent delay in diagnosis of endometriosis.

However, it is unfortunately true that the medical and surgical approaches to endometriosis do not always resolve the symptoms. It is important to encourage the patient to take ownership of the problem and work with the medical team to resolve the symptoms. In this respect it is very useful to adopt an approach that includes healthy lifestyle factors.

Pelvic mass

CLINICAL PRESENTATION

1. *Pressure symptoms:* feeling of abdominal fullness, pressure on bladder (frequency of micturition), rarely bowel symptoms
2. *Incidental finding:* on routine examination (eg at the time of a Pap test)

Detection of a pelvic mass inevitably raises concerns about possible malignancy, although most masses of gynaecological origin are benign fibroids or benign ovarian cysts. The possibility of pregnancy must not be overlooked and although presentation with an advanced undiagnosed pregnancy is uncommon, this diagnosis may be unsuspected by older women who mistake the amenorrhoea for onset of the menopause. Pelvic masses in postmenopausal women are more likely to be associated with malignancy. Non-gynaecological causes of a pelvic mass are unusual.

Rapid clinical assessment

Most women who present with a pelvic mass are asymptomatic. When there is acute pain, rapid general assessment is needed as active intervention will be required. In the absence of pain or tenderness, the approach to management can be more relaxed, although it is important to elicit worrying features which may point to an underlying malignancy.

Relevant history

A full gynaecological, obstetric, medical and social history should be taken. In addition:

- The circumstances of discovery of the mass should be documented.
- Associated features such as amenorrhoea or menstrual abnormalities, pain, urinary or gastrointestinal disturbances, fever, systemic illness or weight loss.
- Pregnancy symptoms, contraception and sexual activity.

Relevant clinical examination

- General assessment of the physical state of the patient and her level of anxiety.
- Detailed inspection and palpation of the abdomen and pelvic examination. Note should be made of the size and consistency of the mass, whether it is fixed or mobile, presence of tenderness and whether it is separate from the uterus (Section 1).
- If features are suggestive of malignancy (signs of weight loss; ascites) a more detailed systemic examination is needed (Section 16).

Relevant investigations

- A rapid urinary HCG assay if pregnancy is suspected.
- Ultrasound. If the scan confirms a diagnosis of an ovarian cyst or tumour, even if there are no initial signs of malignancy, blood should be taken for tumour markers.
- In some cases where the diagnosis remains uncertain, more detailed imaging by MRI or CT scanning or direct visualisation by laparoscopy may be indicated.
- A suspected abscess or malignancy requires urgent attention.

Other initial investigations will depend on the history and clinical findings.

Differential diagnosis

See Table 13.5.

- Size: a pelvic mass may be confined to the pelvis, be palpable abdominally arising from the pelvis, or in some cases be so large that it fills the entire abdomen.
- A mass large enough to be palpable abdominally suggests: intrauterine pregnancy, ovarian cysts and tumours, uterine fibroids, sarcomas and some inflammatory masses.
- Gynaecological masses arising from the pelvis normally lie centrally, although uterine fibroids may be eccentric. An over-distended bladder will also be central but masses arising in the bowel or kidneys are usually more lateral.
- A tender mass confined to the pelvis is most likely to be a torted or haemorrhagic cyst or an inflammatory mass (abscess or pyosalpinx), which may present without obvious signs of infection.
- A palpable mass is unusual with ectopic pregnancy, but may be secondary to the presence of a haematoma that has beome 'walled off' from the rest of the pelvis by surrounding omentum.
- A rare condition presenting in young women is a haematometra (blood-filled uterus) secondary to obstruction of blood flow from the uterine cavity during menstruation. This may be due to an imperforate hymen, when there will be a history of cyclical pain and amenorrhoea; or, more rarely, there may be obstruction at the level of the cervix or a congenital uterine abnormality (Section 5).

Uterine fibroids (leiomyomata)

Uterine fibroids are common benign tumours of the uterus which are present in up to 25 per cent of women of reproductive age. They may be single or multiple and of varying sizes, in some cases producing very bizarre distortion and enlargement of the uterus.

CLINICAL PRESENTATION

The presentation and symptoms of fibroids vary according to their size and position.

- Asymptomatic even when large (an incidental finding during routine pelvic or ultrasound examination)
- Heavy menstrual bleeding: submucous fibroids that enlarge or distort the endometrial cavity
- Increasing girth with or without pressure symptoms (urinary frequency or backache), rarely urinary retention from retroverted impacted fibroid uterus)
- IMB and PCB from a submucous fibroid
- Complication of fibroids:
  - In pregnancy:
    - Acute abdominal pain due to red degeneration

TABLE 13.5 Differential diagnosis of a pelvic mass

	Category	Diagnosis
Gynaecological		
1 Ovarian	Physiological	Corpus luteum cyst
		Follicular cyst
	Inflammatory	Endometriotic cyst
	Benign	Epithelial
		Germ cell
		Sex-chord stromal
	Borderline	
	Malignant	Primary/secondary
2 Uterine tube	Pregnancy	Ectopic
	Inflammatory	Pelvic abscess
		Pyosalpinx/hydrosalpinx
	Malignant	Cancer—rare
3 Uterus	Benign	Pregnancy
		Fibroids
		Haematometra
	Malignant	Adenocarcinoma
		Sarcoma
Non-gynaecological		
1 GIT		Constipation
		Volvulus
	Inflammatory	Abscess (secondary to diverticular or Crohn's disease, appendicitis)
	Malignant	Carcinoma of bowel
2 Urinary tract		Retention of urine
		Pelvic kidney
	Malignant	Bladder tumour

  - If situated low in the uterus or in the cervix they may cause malpresentation or may be a cause of pre-term labour or miscarriage (double the risk for submucus fibroids compared to no fibroids).[34]
 - Acute abdomen: rare torsion of a subserosal fibroid or urinary retention from retroverted impacted fibroid uterus
 - Prolapse through the cervix of pedunculated submucosal fibroids causing prolonged bleeding, discharge and crampy pain. This may occur spontaneously or as a consequence of treatment with a GnRH analogue or following embolisation.
- Anaemia secondary to menorrhagia
- Prolonged infertility is associated with the development of fibroids.[35]

Aetiology, pathology, epidemiology

Fibroids are composed of smooth muscle and connective tissue and may be intramural, subserosal or submucosal (Figure 13.2). Subserosal and submucous fibroids can become pedunculated. Fibroids commonly outgrow their blood supply and undergo degeneration. This is particularly common after menopause when they may become calcified and visible as solid lumps on a plain abdominal X-ray.

The cause of fibroids is unknown. Risk factors tend to be associated with oestrogen (Box 13.6). They are hormone dependent for their growth, do not occur prior to puberty and shrink after the menopause. Fibroids tend to be larger and more numerous in nulliparous women. There is also a genetic predisposition as they are more common where there is a family history or in black women, in whom they occur at a younger age. Smoking and long term use of the COCP and Depo-Provera are associated with a reduced risk. Sarcomatous change is unusual (< 1%).

FIGURE 13.2 Fibroids
1 Pedunculated. 2 Subserosal.
3 Intramural. 4 Submucosal.

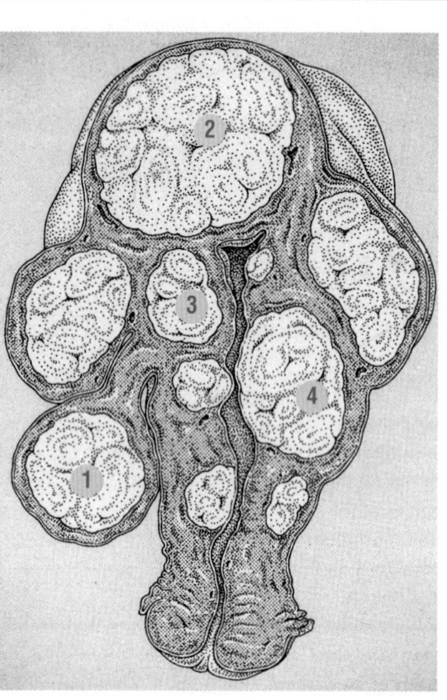

Clinical assessment

- Abdominal and pelvic examination: usually firm in consistency but can be soft (where there is hyaline or cystic degeneration) or hard (where there is calcification). Single or multiple with a regularly enlarged uterus (intramural and submucous), or an irregular uterus (subserosal or large intramural).
- Abdominal or transvaginal ultrasound examination confirms the diagnosis and delineates the numbers, sizes and positions of individual fibroids.
- Small submucosal fibroids may only be detected by transvaginal ultrasound, saline infusion sonography or at hysteroscopy.

BOX 13.6 Risk factors for uterine fibroids[36]

- Increased risk (increased oestrogen):
  - Age (until menopause)
  - Family history (× 3 in first-degree relatives)
  - Ethnicity (increased risk in Afro-Caribbean-American women)
  - Obesity (× 3 in women > 70 kg compared to those < 50 kg)
  - Menarche (younger age)
- Reduced risk:
  - Multiparity
  - Smoking (decreases circulating levels of oestrogen)
  - Menopause
- Uncertain risk:
  - Oral contraceptives
  - Low parity (inverse relationship between number of pregnancies and fibroids)
  - Infertility (× 2 risk of fibroids)

- If the fibroids are very large there could be obstruction or distortion of the ureters. Renal ultrasound and urea and electrolytes should be checked to assess renal function.

Clinical outcomes

The outcome of fibroids is influenced by:

- the woman's age
- symptoms
- fertility history and future plans
- attitude to the problem.

Fibroids are frequently asymptomatic and of no clinical significance.

Conservative and medical treatment

Symptomatic treatment of menorrhagia associated with fibroids includes the use of oral iron to treat anaemia, together with antifibrinolytics (Section 14) to reduce menstrual blood flow. Other options are available but less predictable (Table 13.6).

Asymptomatic fibroids can be managed conservatively regardless of their size.

Surgical treatment

1 *Hysterectomy* offers a permanent cure for women with fibroids who have completed child-bearing.
2 *Myomectomy* aims to remove the fibroids and preserve the uterus and can be performed via a laparotomy or a laparoscopy. After myomectomy fibroids may recur in up to 27 per cent of women over a 10-year period. The rate is lower in women with fewer fibroids at the time of surgery and for those who give birth after the myomectomy. Pregnancy outcomes after myomectomy are favourable,

TABLE 13.6 Hormone therapies, fibroids and heavy menstrual bleeding

Hormone	Effect on fibroids/HMB	Problems/role
OCP	Not effective in decreasing size May reduce HMB	
HRT	Not effective in decreasing size	
Progesterone	No benefit	
GnRH analogues	50% reduction in size (maximal at 12 weeks) HMB reduced	Heavier women require larger doses Size 'rebounds' on stopping HMB returns on ceasing therapy Hypo-oestrogenic effects: demineralisation of bone, hot flushes, vaginal dryness Therapy limited to 6 months
GnRH + 'add back'	Benefits as for GnRH analogues	Avoids side effects Reduces size preoperatively Easier surgery Reduces blood loss
HRT at 12 weeks	Possible use preop for fibroids >18 weeks, if anaemia present, or to avoid midline incision	
Danazol	Reduction in size (less than GnRH) ? Stops rebound growth	Androgenic side effects Use limited to 6 months
Gestrinone	Reduction in size and HMB	Androgenic side effects Effect lasts one year after stopping treatment
Mifepristone (RU486)	Reduction in size	Few studies Not available Australia and New Zealand
LNG-IUS	Users had decreased fibroid development and hysterectomy rates	Further studies required

HMB: heavy menstrual bleeding
Source: adapted from Farquar et al 2001.[37]

with scar rupture uncommon (0.5% of cases). Caesarean section is usually recommended if multiple fibroids have been removed or the uterine cavity entered, although there is no evidence to support this position.

Heavy blood loss is a potential problem at myomectomy and women need to be warned of the possible need for blood transfusion and, in extreme cases, emergency hysterectomy.

3 *Uterine artery embolisation* has recently been introduced as a line of treatment for uterine fibroids. Its use is new and needs more collaborative studies, particularly RCTs comparing it to other surgical procedures.[38]

Fibroids cause surprisingly few complications in pregnancy. The most common complication is red degeneration, which presents with acute pain and tenderness, usually in the mid trimester of pregnancy. Management is conservative with rest and analgesics.

Prevention

In common with other gynaecological disorders, fibroids are more common in nulliparous women and those with longest exposure to natural menstrual cycles. Thus women who delay child-bearing can, in theory, reduce the risk of developing fibroids by use of agents which suppress natural menstruation such as the combined pill, Depo-Provera and progestogen-releasing IUS. It is unclear whether these strategies would be effective in women with a strong genetic predisposition towards the development of fibroids.

Attitudes to the management of fibroids have changed greatly in recent years. Fibroids used to be regarded as an indication for surgery, usually hysterectomy, because of difficulty in diagnosis and concern about possible malignancy. It is now recognised that fibroids rarely, if ever, undergo malignant change and the widespread availability of imaging techniques such as ultrasound enable fibroids to be distinguished from other causes of a pelvic mass and managed more conservatively.

Benign ovarian cysts and tumours

Ovarian cysts are a common cause of gynaecological referral. It is important to make a distinction between simple physiological (functional) cysts and those with a more complex structure which are pathological (see Box 13.7). Although 90 per cent of ovarian tumours are benign it is important to be aware of the possibility of malignancy. Malignancy is very rare in women under 35 but rises with age: 45 per cent of ovarian tumours in postmenopausal women are malignant. One of the priorities of management is to exclude malignancy without compromising ovarian function and fertility in younger women.

CLINICAL PRESENTATIONS

1 Acute abdominal pain

This may be:

- *Rupture or leaking.* Physiological cysts may present with acute rupture followed by rapid resolution.
- *Torsion.* Suspicion of torsion is an indication for early surgical intervention because of the risk of infarction from occlusion of the blood supply. Intermittent abdominal pain, possibly associated with vomiting, may occur that becomes continuous once there is a complete torsion.
- *Infection.* This is usually accompanied by other systemic findings.
- *Haemorrhage* into a physiological luteal cyst.

BOX 13.7 Pathology of benign ovarian tumours

- Physiological cysts:
  - Follicular cysts
  - Luteal cysts
- Benign germ cell tumours:
  - Dermoid cyst
  - Mature teratoma
- Benign epithelial tumours:
  - Serous cystadenoma
  - Mucinous cystadenoma
  - Endometroid cystadenoma
  - Brenner tumour
- Benign sex cord stromal tumours
- Theca cell tumours:
  - Fibroma
  - Sertoli-Leydig cell tumour

2 Vaginal bleeding

This may be heavier bleeding after a short episode of amenorrhoea. This can occur from a follicular cyst if oestrogen and progesterone are produced from the granulosa cells. Alternatively, a corpus luteum cyst may continue to produce progesterone. The presentation may mimic an early miscarriage or an ectopic pregnancy.

3 Non-acute presentation

An incidental finding on:

- Abdominal or bimanual examination
- Ultrasound.[39]

Diagnosis and investigation

Tumour markers

Tumour markers are helpful in assessing the likelihood of malignancy. CA-125 (a serum antigen recognised by a murin monoclonal antibody produced by ovarian cancer cells) is especially useful post menopause.[40] In the younger woman it can be normal in up to 50 per cent of stage 1 malignancies. It is also raised in pregnancy, pelvic inflammatory disease, endometriosis, menstruation, pancreatitis and liver cirrhosis.

Imaging

Ultrasound will identify most physiological cysts and may detect features suggestive of malignancy: papillary growth, mixed solid and cystic areas, increased blood flow on Doppler ultrasound.[41] Predominantly solid tumours are more likely to be malignant than those which are largely cystic. Computerised tomography or MRI scanning may be helpful if the nature of the lesion remains unclear. In most cases an accurate diagnosis is not possible until after its removal and examination by the pathologist.

Management

- Asymptomatic physiological cysts < 5 cm in diameter usually resolve spontaneously, and repeat ultrasound should be performed after an interval of 2–3 months. If persistent, a physiological cyst can be aspirated (when there is a risk of recurrence) or removed by ovarian cystectomy, performed either by laparoscopy or by laparotomy depending on the size of the cyst and the preferences of the gynaecologist and the woman.
- Acute symptoms secondary to a haemorrhagic or ruptured cyst often resolve spontaneously and can be managed conservatively with analgesics.
- Severe symptoms, or marked tenderness combined with clinical signs of shock, is indicative of intraperitoneal bleeding secondary to a ruptured luteal cyst, necessitating emergency laparoscopy or laparotomy.

Surgical management should be as conservative as possible in young women, although following torsion with impairment of the blood supply to the ovary or with a very large tumour it may be impossible to conserve the ovary.

Pathological cysts should be removed, usually by laparotomy because of the risk of rupture and spill of cyst contents if laparoscopic techniques are used. If malignancy is suspected, a frozen section of the cyst can be examined in the operating theatre. The woman should be counselled beforehand and consideration given to more extensive surgery if malignancy is confirmed.

In the acute situation it may be difficult to counsel the patient adequately about her condition and the likely surgical procedure and for her to give fully informed consent, particularly if she is distressed by pain or sedated with analgesics. Involvement of a partner or close relative is important.

Classification of benign ovarian cysts and tumours

Physiological (functional) cysts

These are a common occurrence of the normal cyclical function of the ovary. They may be follicular, theca lutein or corpus luteum in origin. Prior to ovulation the ovarian follicle measures up to 3 cm in diameter; a functional cyst is by definition a unilocular cyst greater than 3 cm in diameter. Such cysts rarely become larger than 10 cm. They are usually single unless they occur following the use of drugs to stimulate ovulation or in the presence of trophoblastic disease, when multiple follicular or luteal cysts may occur (Section 9). Functional cysts are more common in users of progestogen-only contraceptives, around the time of menarche and perimenopause. The COCP suppresses follicular development. If uncomplicated, they resolve spontaneously within 8–12 weeks and active surgical management is rarely necessary.

Pathological (neoplastic) ovarian cysts and tumours

These are classified histologically according to their site of origin within the ovary (Section 16).

Benign epithelial tumours

These arise from the surface epithelium of the ovary and are most common in women over the age of 40. They are classified according to their tissue of origin and the nature of the cyst contents. Epithelial tumours are most commonly asymptomatic, and are less common in multiparous women and those with a late menarche and early menopause. The risk of malignancy rises with increasing age.

1 The serous cystadenoma is bilateral in 30–50 per cent of cases. It is unilocular and has papilliferous projections that may fill the whole cyst. It is usually benign but malignant change can occur.
2 The mucinous cystadenoma is multiloculated, unilateral in 90 per cent of cases, large but rarely forms adhesions. Papillary ingrowths are rare and may suggest malignant change to an adenocarcinoma, which occurs in 5–10 per cent of cases. Pseudomyxoma peritonei is a rare complication of these cysts. This occurs when the cyst leaks and cells from within the cyst implant on the peritoneum and continue to secrete mucus. Adhesions, reformation of the cysts after removal and eventually cachexia and death occur.

Benign germ cell tumours

Dermoid cysts may contain tissue that arises from all embryological layers: ectoderm, mesoderm and endoderm, and typically contain tissues such as skin, hair teeth, cartilage and even intestinal and thyroid tissue. They are a very rare cause of thyrotoxicosis. They occur in young women, are bilateral in 10 per cent of cases and rarely grow bigger than 12 cm. Most dermoid cysts are asymptomatic but because of the risk of torsion should be removed surgically.

Malignant germ cell tumours are very rare (less than 3 per cent of germ cell tumours) but occur most frequently in very young women under the age of 20.

Benign sex cord stromal tumours

These are extremely rare and may occur at all ages. Theca cell tumours may secrete oestrogen and Sertoli-Leydig cell tumours secrete androgens. Granulosa cell tumours are also oestrogen secreting but are classified as malignant. Benign fibromas form five per cent of ovarian neoplasms. In 20 per cent of cases they are associated with ascites. Meig's syndrome is the triad: ovarian fibroma, ascites and hydrothorax; it is cured by removal of the fibroma but causes concern initially as it resembles a malignancy in presentation.

Endometriomas

Endometriotic cysts fall into a different category from those described above, as they are retention cysts which develop as a consequence of active ovarian endometriosis. They may be confused with both physiological (luteal) and neoplastic cysts and even with ovarian cancer as CA-125 levels are commonly raised in endometriosis.

Prevention

Ovarian suppression by repeated pregnancies or long-term use of the COCP reduces the incidence of functional cysts and epithelial tumours. Use of the COCP may be of particular relevance to women deemed to be at additional risk by virtue of their past history or, in particular, a known genetic risk of epithelial carcinoma.

Pelvic inflammatory disease

Pelvic inflammatory disease (PID) is upper genital tract infection of the uterus, fallopian tubes and other pelvic organs. Pelvic inflammatory disease has a major impact on women's health, both globally and at a personal level. The number of cases of PID is increasing worldwide and it is a major cause of gynaecological morbidity. The most common pathogens causing PID are *Chlamydia trachomatis* and *Neisseria gonorrhoeae* (60–80 per cent in women aged < 25 years).[42] Polymicrobial PID (in the absence of chlamydia or gonorrhoea) is usually from the patient's own microflora. Tuberculous PID may occur in endemic areas.

Long-term sequelae of PID make detection and treatment of asymptomatic and early infection of vital importance. However, the diagnosis may be difficult.

CLINICAL PRESENTATION

- Asymptomatic detected on ultrasound. Where severe PID has resulted in tubal occlusion, the tube may become distended with clear sterile fluid, known as a hydrosalpinx.
- Pelvic pain: acute, subacute or chronic. In most cases the pain is bilateral, dull and aching and associated with deep dyspareunia.
- Dyspareunia or dysmenorrhoea
- Menorrhagia
- Ectopic pregnancy may result from the tubal damage.
- Infertility: during investigations for tubal patency occlusion due to previous PID may be diagnosed. The proportion of women with salpingitis who develop tubal occlusion rises from 10 per cent after one attack to 75 per cent with three or more.[43]

Clinical criteria for diagnosis of PID

These may be minimal (especially with a bacterial infection) and a high index of suspicion is necessary not to miss the diagnosis. By definition symptoms include:

- All of the following:
  - Lower abdominal pain
  - Cervical motion tenderness
  - Adnexal tenderness
- Plus one of the following:
  - Temperature > 38°C
  - White cell count > 10.5
  - Increased ESR or CRP
  - Pus from culdocentesis
  - Tender mass on bimanual examination
  - Isolation of *N. gonorrhoeae* or *Chlamydia*
  - Histological evidence of infection (eg plasma cells)

Examination

Signs may include:

- Fever
- Abdominal tenderness on deep abdominal palpation with rebound tenderness in more severe cases
- Adnexal tenderness (a sensitive marker of endometritis)[44]
- Adnexal mass (inflammatory or pyosalpinx)
- Cervical excitation
- Purulent cervical discharge.

Investigation

Investigation of suspected PID should include the following:

- STI screen, particularly chlamydia and gonorrhoea
- Blood cultures if there is systemic upset
- Ultrasound. This is useful where there is a fluid collection (eg tubo-ovarian abscess). The use of Doppler ultrasound to measure the blood flow in the tubes (increased in the presence of inflammation) is a good predictor of less severe disease but requires ultrasonic expertise.[45]
- Exclude other possible causes of pain (see above)
- Diagnostic laparoscopy is helpful in clarifying the diagnosis if there is no response to treatment.

Long-term problems

These include all the possible presentations in addition to psychological sequelae and financial costs to the individual and the health system.

Pathogenesis

Pelvic inflammatory disease primarily involves the fallopian tubes. There is acute inflammation of the mucosal lining, the tube appears red and swollen and there may be a purulent discharge from the fimbrial end. If treated at this stage, the changes may resolve completely but more prolonged or recurrent infection may result in the development of adhesions involving the tubal mucosa, the fimbriae and the adjacent ovary, leading to tubal block and peritubal adhesions. The occluded tube may be filled with fluid (hydrosalpinx) or in severe cases with pus (pyosalpinx). This advanced inflammatory process may involve the ovary (tubo-ovarian abscess) or a pelvic abscess may develop in which the uterine tube and ovary become walled off by omentum and adherent to bowel and adjacent structures. This may present as a pelvic mass—a 'cold abscess'.

Management

It is usual to commence antibiotic therapy prior to obtaining the results of culture as there is concern that delay may lead to greater risk of long-term sequelae.[46] In many cases the results of culture are negative. Sexual partners should also be treated, preferably after STI screening.

Many places have locally recommended protocols or guidelines.[47] Because the sensitivity of micro-organisms to antibiotics may vary, ongoing review of protocols is important.

The use of the NSAID diclofenac has been shown to down-regulate acute inflammation in the uterine tube and may provide some benefit.[48]

Hospitalisation and intravenous antibiotic therapy is necessary if there is a systemic illness; otherwise outpatient management is appropriate. Antibiotic treatment should effect a marked improvement within 48–72 hours. At that stage treatment should be reviewed, taking the microbiological results into account. If there is no clinical improvement, a laparoscopy is indicated. Adequate analgesia should be prescribed and the patient is advised to stay off work and refrain from intercourse until her symptoms have settled. Poor compliance with antibiotic therapy is a potential problem and follow-up no later than two weeks after presentation is important in order to assess whether there has been an adequate response.

Prevention

Prevention of PID centres around prevention of STI through health education backed up by screening for early asymptomatic infection.[49] Screening for asymptomatic infection prior to uterine instrumentation (termination of pregnancy, IUCD insertion, fertility investigations) is well established and young people should be encouraged to attend for STI testing if they have concerns about possible risk.[50]

Advice

- Safe sex
- Douching: this is predominantly done for hygiene or to prevent or self-treat infection. US data indicates that 37 per cent of US women of reproductive age (15 to 44 years) douche regularly, about half at least once a week. Pelvic inflammatory disease has an estimated cumulative incidence of 10 per cent up to 45 years of age. Women who douche have a 73 per cent increased risk of PID while those who douche at least once a week have a risk increased by about four-fold. Vaginal douching is unnecessary in routine feminine hygiene.[51]

Unresolved issues

Long-term sequelae are ectopic pregnancy, infertility and pelvic pain (Box 13.8). The major problem in the management of PID is the difficulty of diagnosis—the fact that many infections are asymptomatic and, even in symptomatic cases, microbiological culture may be negative.

BOX 13.8 Long-term complications of PID

- Long-term complications of PID include:
  - Infertility (20%)
  - Chronic pelvic pain (18%)
  - Ectopic pregnancy (9%)
  - Chronic infection
  - Fitz-Hugh-Curtis syndrome (peri-hepatic adhesions).

4 Gynaeocology

A Normal ovary with corpus luteum indicating that ovulation has occurred

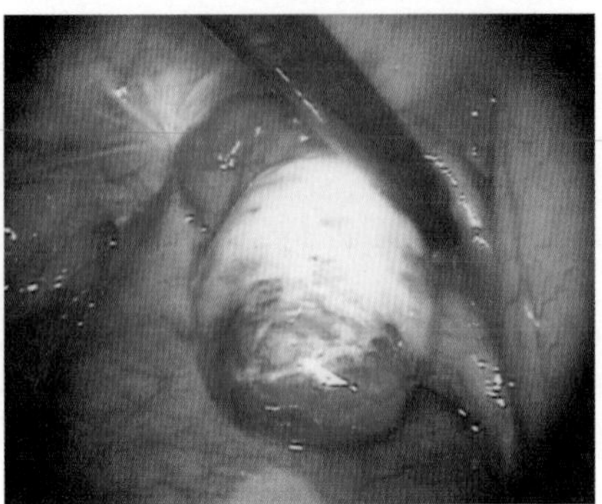

B Ovulatory mucus: 'egg-white' mucus at ovulation facilitates sperm transport.

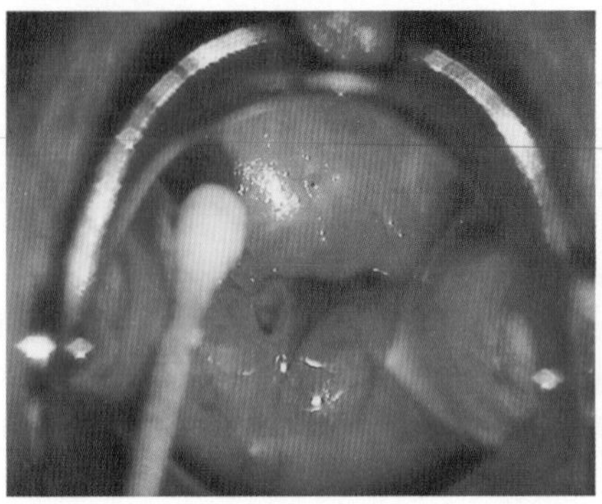

C Torsion of ovary

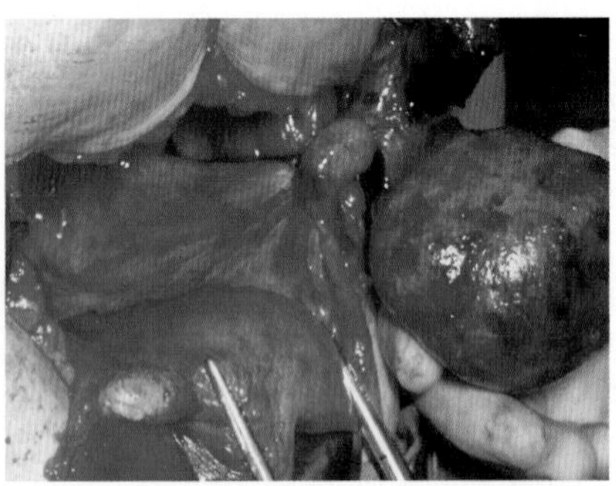

D Ectopic pregnancy: an opened uterine tube showing the presence of a fetus

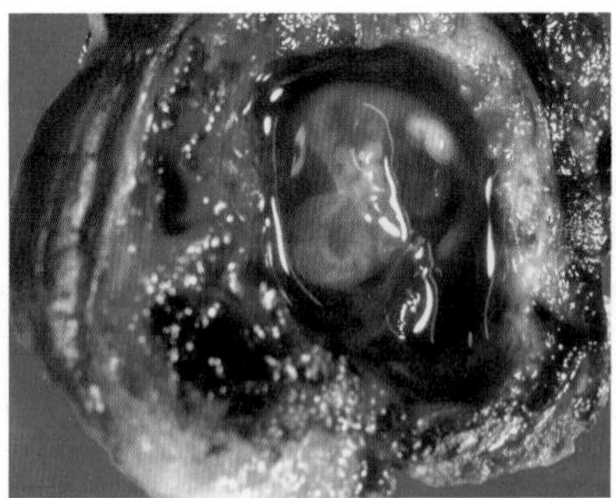

E Mastitis: an infection of the breast post partum, most often caused by *Staphylococcus*. The breast shows an inflamed segment that is firm and tender on examination.

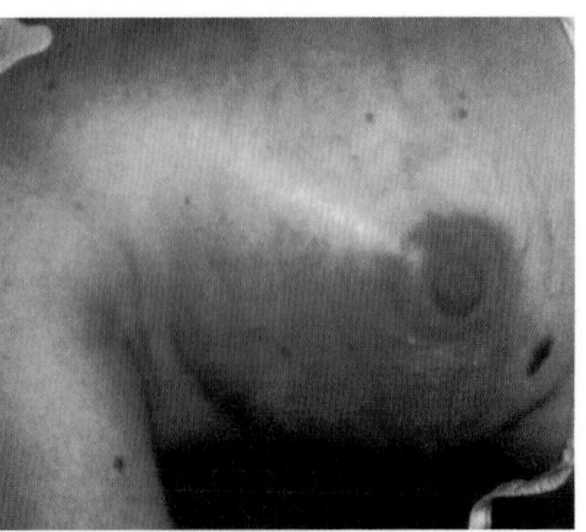

F Endometrial polyp at hysteroscopy. This can cause intermenstrual bleeding and vaginal discharge. It can be removed through the hysteroscope.

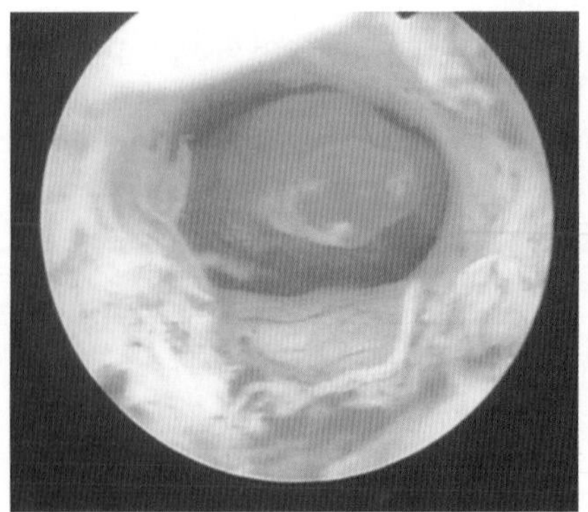

A Vaginal discharge due to bacterial vaginosis

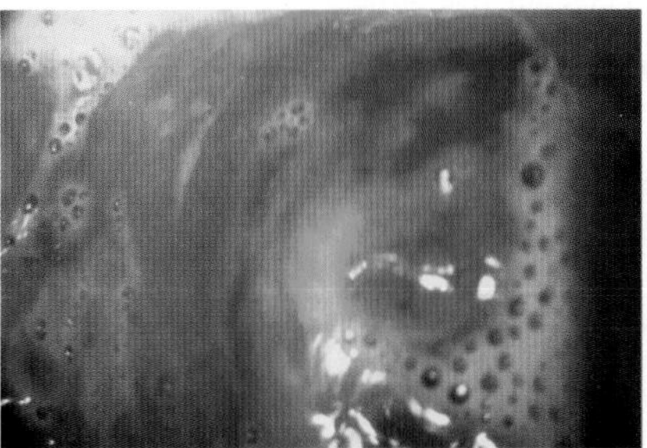

B Ulcer of primary syphilis in perianal area

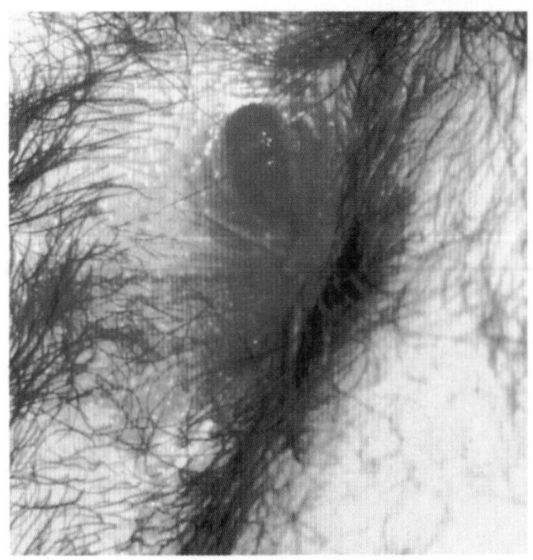

C Genital herpes: multiple ulcerated lesions on the vulva. The woman was unable to pass urine because of the vulvar pain and required catheterisation.

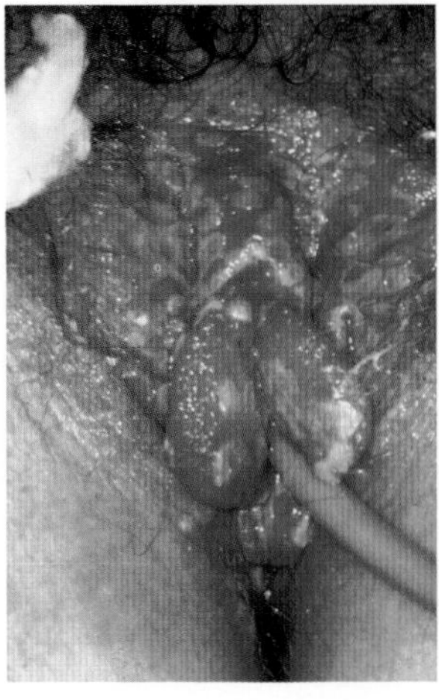

D Genital warts on the vulva

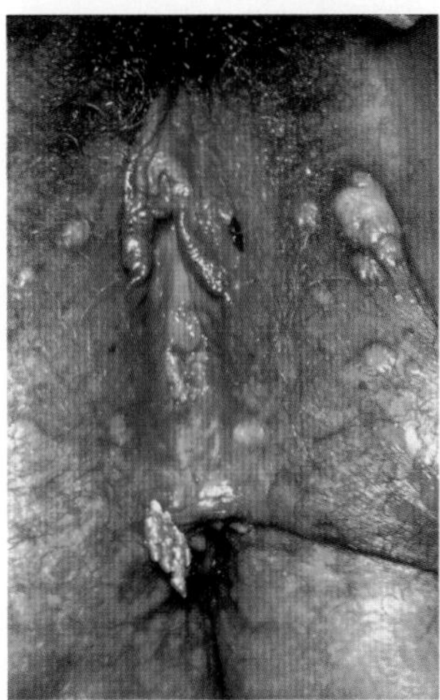

E Monilia of vagina: thick 'curd-like' discharge adherent to the vaginal wall

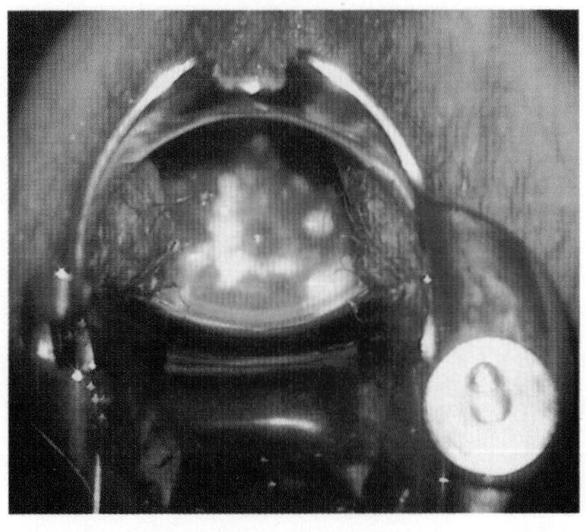

F Yeast infection showing erythema and characteristic satellite lesions

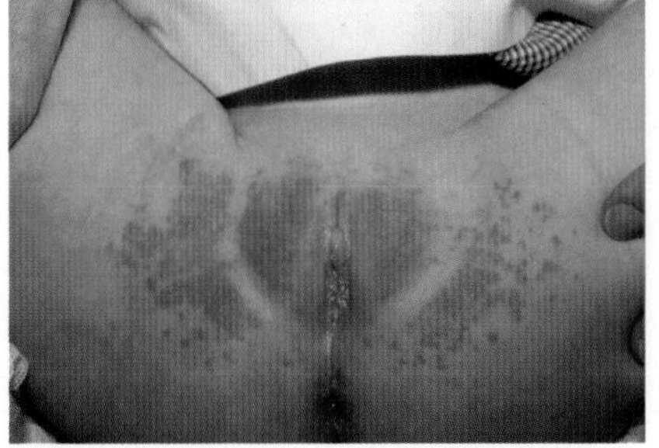

A Uterus lifted out from the abdominal cavity, showing one very large and several smaller subserosal fibroids

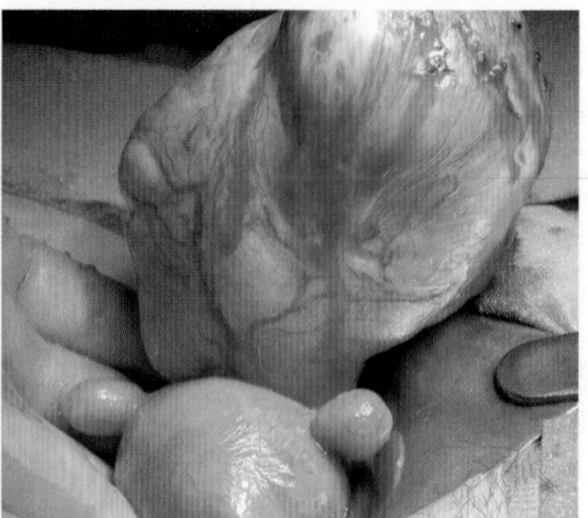

B Bisected uterus during vaginal hysterectomy, showing the presence of an intrauterine device

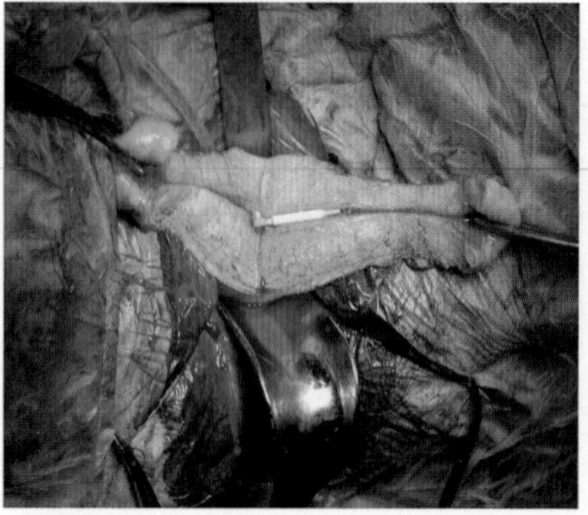

C Examination of abdominal mass

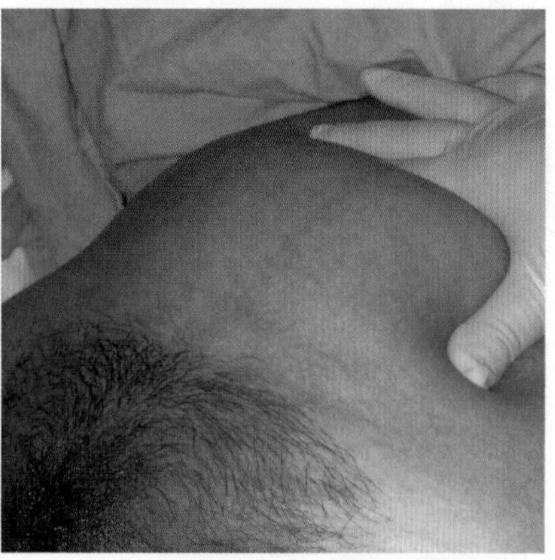

D Abdominal X-ray showing teeth in dermoid cyst. This appears on the X-ray to lie on the patient's left side.

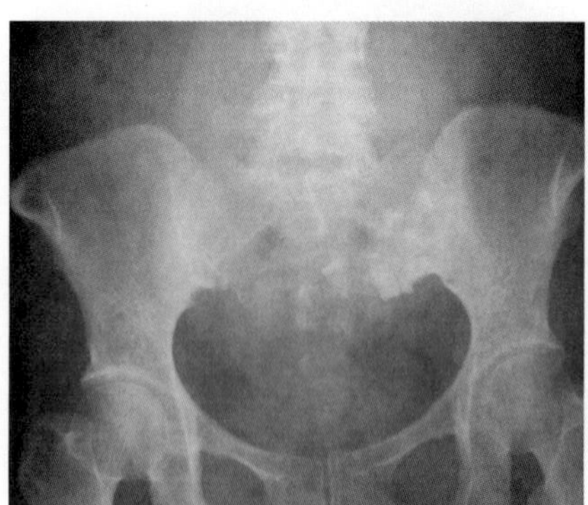

E Cyst arises from the right ovary at laparotomy (large size explains X-ray appearance in slide D). Note protrusion of bone and cartilage in cyst.

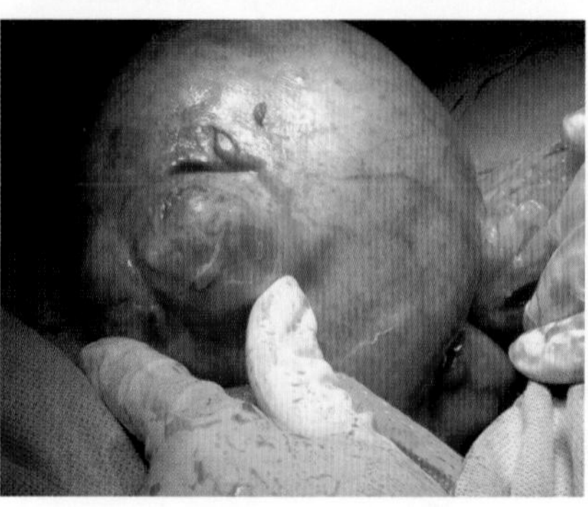

F Opened dermoid cyst demonstrating teeth, cartilage and bone

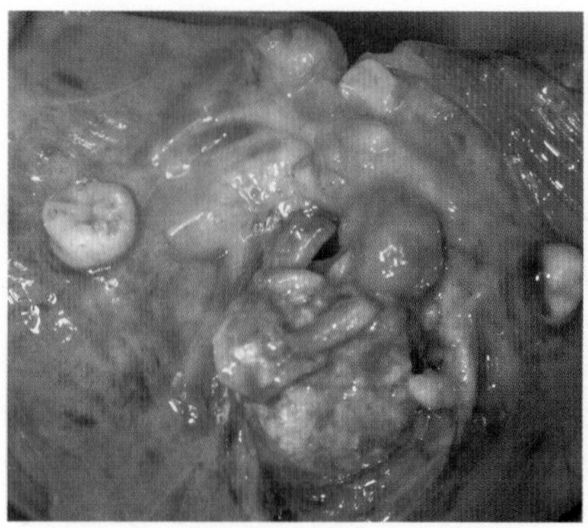

A Normal large vaginal squames with hyphae

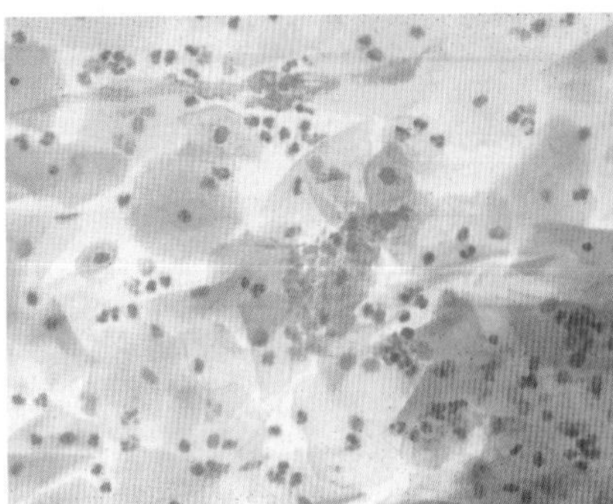

B Cytology: CIN I

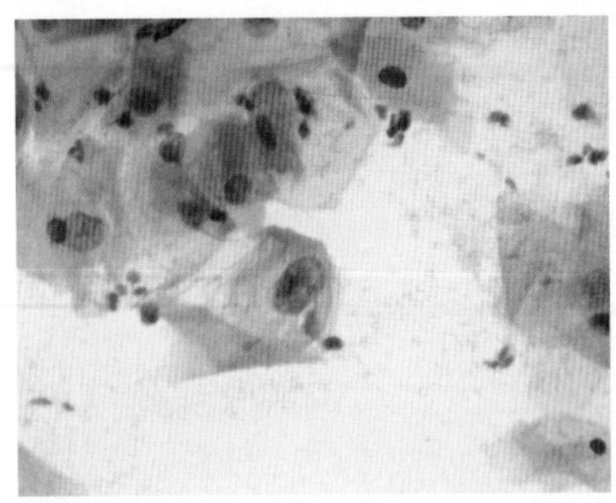

B to D Increasing density of the nucleus and changing cytolasmic : nuclear ratio as changes from CIN I to CIN III.

C Cytology: CIN II

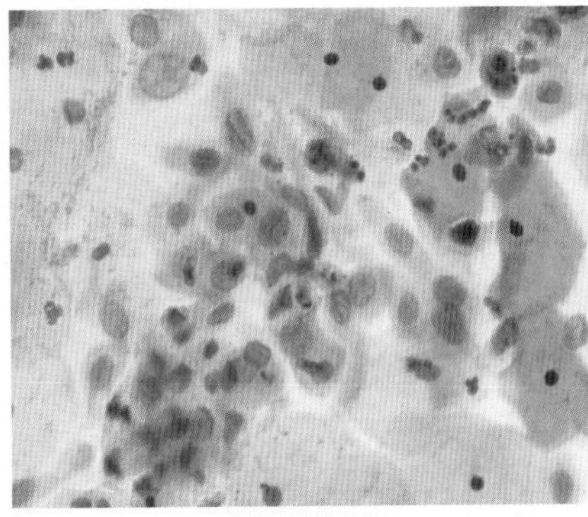

D Cytology: CIN III

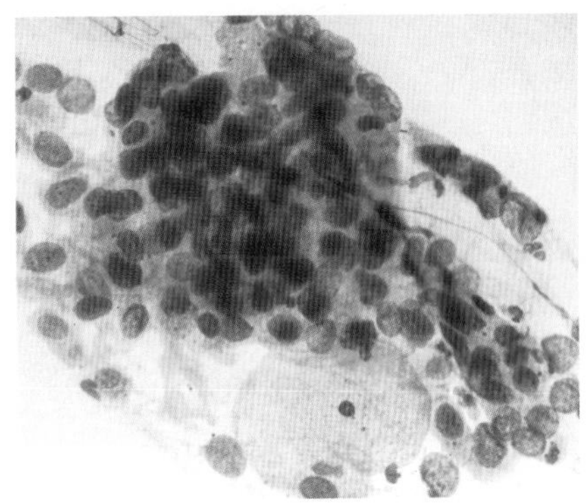

E Acetowhite showing CIN II

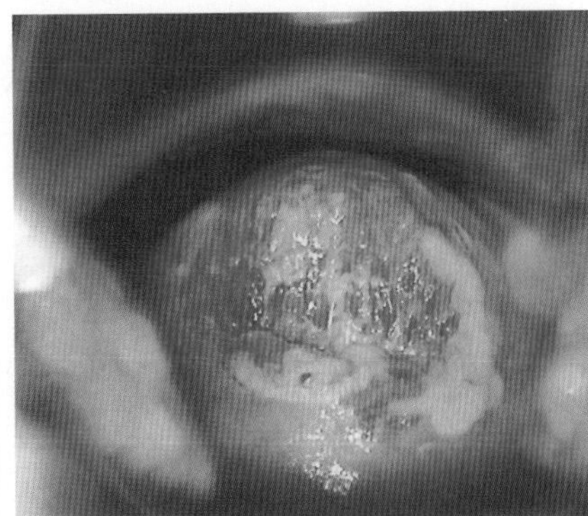

F Iodine negative CIN II

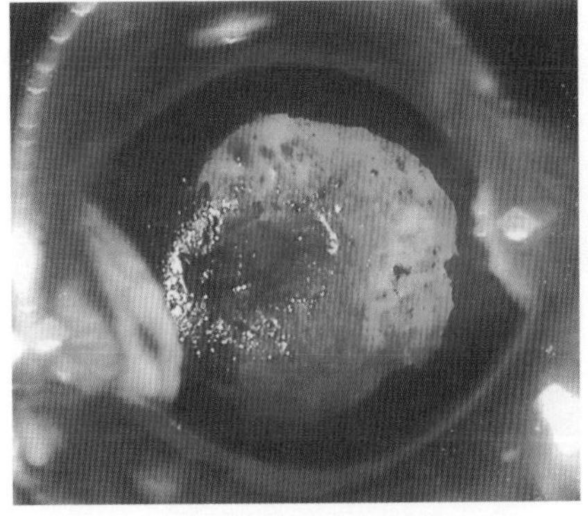

A Acetowhite showing VIN II

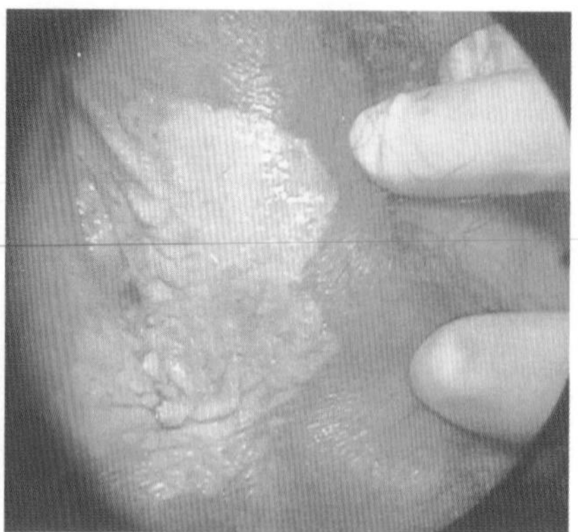

B Protuberant cancer of anterior vulva

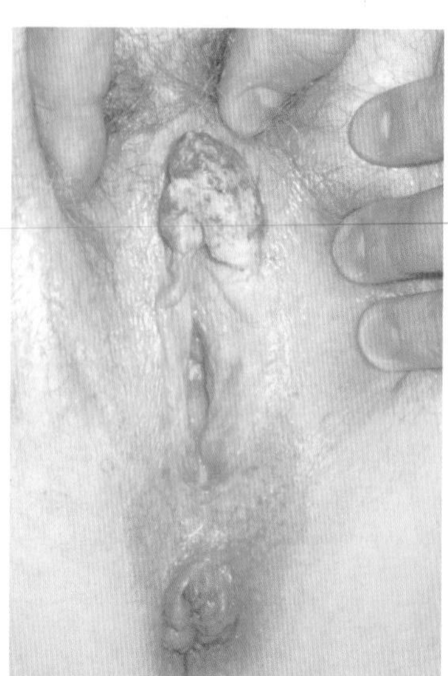

C Cancer inside cavity of uterus

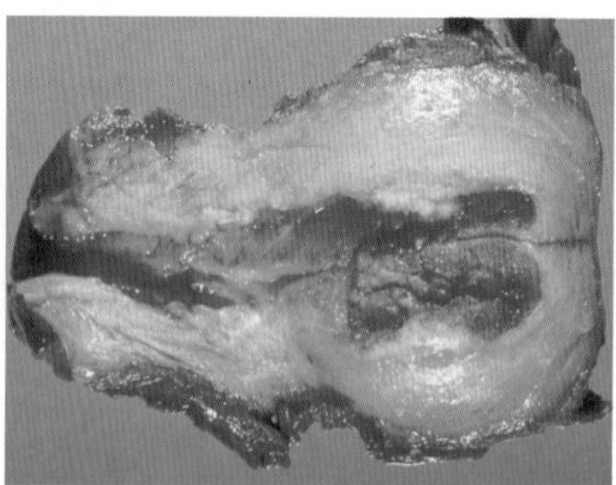

D Ovarian cancer—involvement of both ovaries at laparotomy.

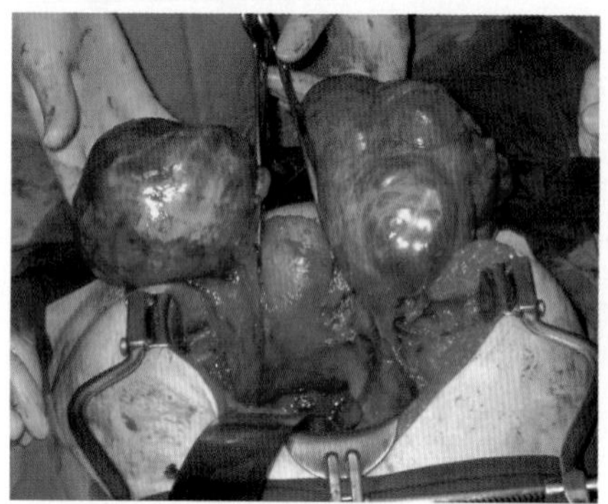

E Cancer of the cervix—operative specimen.

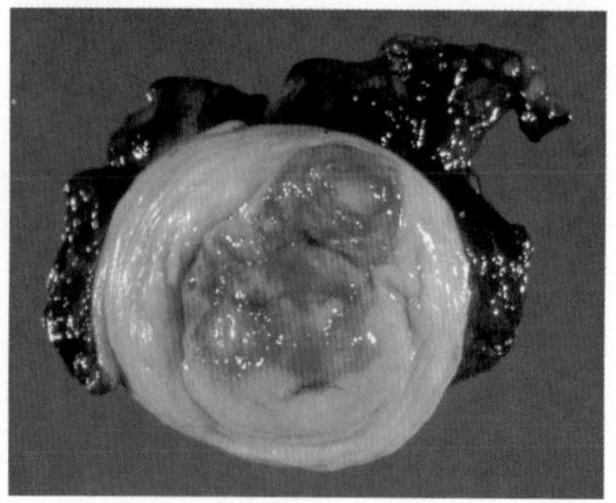

F Locally advanced breast cancer with Paget's disease of the nipple

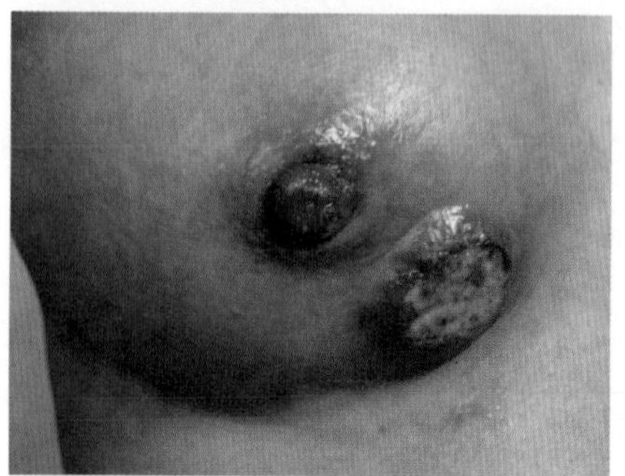

A Simple ovarian cyst with normal-sized ovary

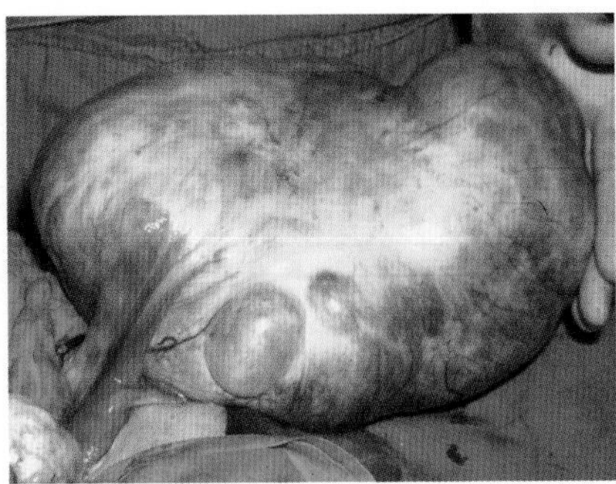

B Hydrosalpinx: fimbrial end of tube outlined by methylene blue dye which does not flow freely from the end of the tube

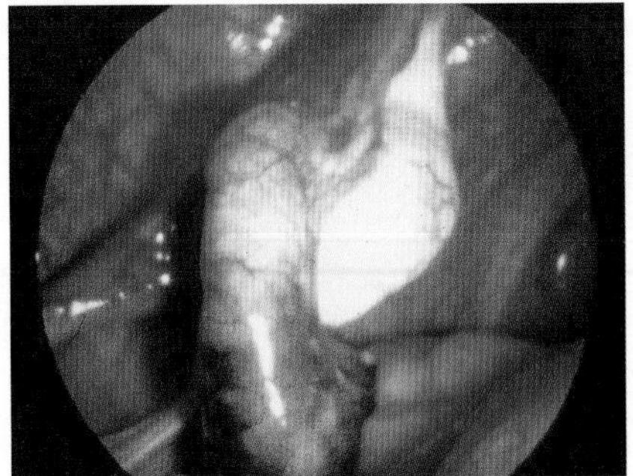

C Early endometriosis: clear 'vesicles' and areas of inflammation are seen

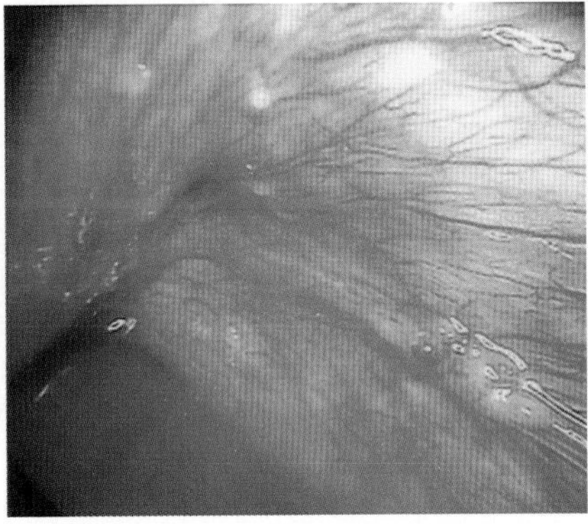

D Pelvic varicosities, a possible cause of pelvic discomfort

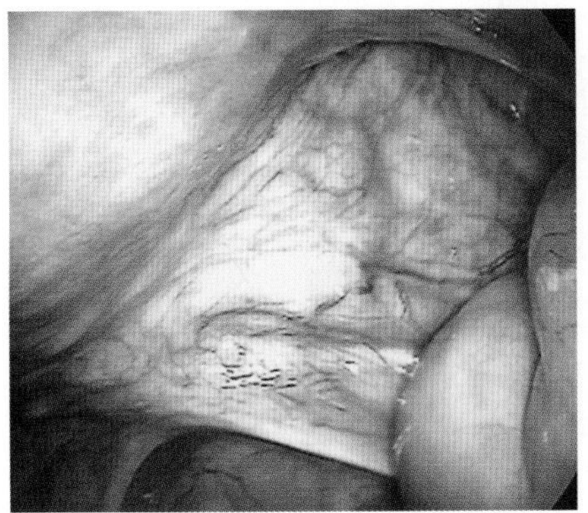

E Pelvic inflammatory disease: inflamed enlarged uterine tubes, exudate in the pouch of Douglas, and adherence between tissues

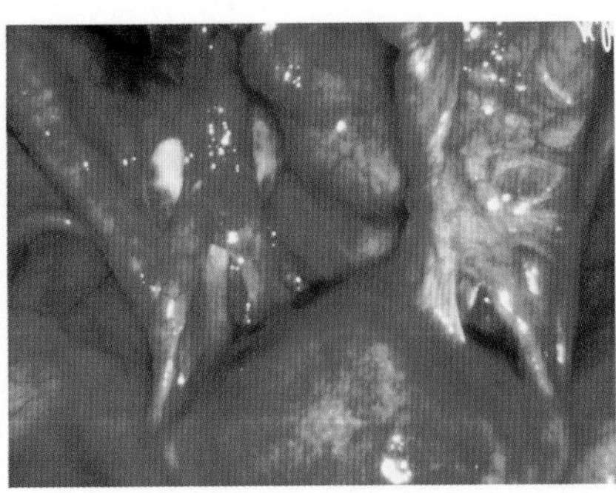

F Liver adhesions due to *Chlamydia* (Fitz-Hugh-Curtis syndrome)

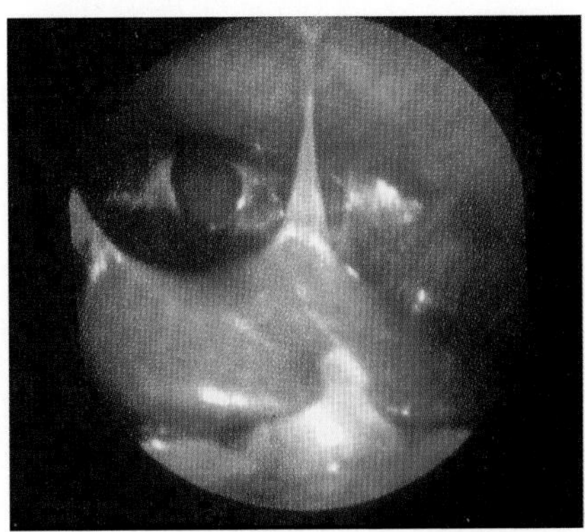

SECTION 14

Part 4
The middle years

Health maintenance and disease prevention

The well woman

Although the 'well woman' may request a health check (Pap test, blood pressure etc), she may wish to discuss other concerns (Box 14.1). These might be symptoms that she thinks are menopause-related. Many women might not be seeking treatment but simply information and discussion about health improvement and health maintenance as they reflect on this phase of life. An ideal opportunity exists for health promotion and disease prevention activities.

BOX 14.1 Middle years: checks and discussion points

- Current concerns: symptoms, lack of knowledge, sexual health, anxiety and stress, depression, abuse
- Current health status review: drug use (prescribed, self-medication), established medical conditions
- Family history: cardiovascular disease, cancer, osteoporosis, diabetes, hypertension
- Risk factors for disease: smoking, alcohol, overweight, diet, minimal activity
- Recommendations (individualised):
  - Tests—Pap test, mammogram, bone mineral density, lipid profile
  - Lifestyle changes
- Social situation: finances, work, relationships, family

Breast screening

The cumulative lifetime risk of a woman in Australia or the UK developing breast cancer by the age of 75 is approximately one in eleven and in the USA approximately one in nine. It is a common cause of cancer death for women. Over the past 10 years the incidence has increased, largely due to earlier detection through mammographic screening.[1] Mortality rates from breast cancer changed very little until 1994 when breast cancer deaths in Australia began falling. In the UK and USA, breast cancer mortality rates have been falling over the past decade. Although uncommon, breast cancer also occurs in men. Male breast cancer is responsible for less than 1 per cent of all breast cancers.

Studies of screening by breast self-examination have indicated that cancers can be detected at an earlier stage but these studies have not demonstrated any survival benefit.[2,3] However, screening by mammography has shown significant benefits in terms of earlier diagnosis and reduction in overall mortality ratios.[4,5]

Although there has been some debate recently about the evidence for benefit of mammographic screening, the criticisms relate more to technical (statistical) design of the randomised controlled trials. The fact is that technology is now available to detect very small cancers, and more than 90 per cent of these women are alive and free from metastatic disease 20 years later.[6]

Who should be screened?

To be cost effective, screening should be targeted at populations where the incidence of breast cancer is high. Apart from female gender, increasing age is the most powerful risk factor for breast cancer; therefore, in Australia, biannual mammographic screening is offered to women from 40 years of age. In the UK government-initiated screening for breast cancer program, a mammogram is undertaken three-yearly in the 50–64 year age group; the American Cancer Society Guidelines recommend annual screening for women over the age of 40.

Screening mammography in the 40–49 year age group is controversial and the benefits may be smaller than in the 50–69 year age group, as the breast cancer incidence is lower in this age group, while the incidence of benign breast disease is high. Nevertheless studies have demonstrated significant reduction in breast cancer mortality in this age group with regular mammographic screening.[6] Controversy also exists as to the value of mammographic screening in the woman aged > 75 years due to her shorter overall life expectancy at this age. A reasonable guide would be that if the life expectancy for a woman is 5–10 years, she should undergo mammographic and clinical breast screening.

Screening method

Clinical breast examination alone will detect 50 per cent of cancers, while screening mammography detects 90 per cent. Ten per cent of clinically detected cancers are missed by mammography and therefore breast examination by the clinician should be undertaken on an annual basis.

Screening mammography using two standard views of each breast (the craniocaudal and the medio-lateral oblique) has been adopted in over 20 countries worldwide since commencing in Sweden in 1985 (1991 in Australia). Ultrasound for screening is not routinely used as it is time consuming, highly operator-dependent and will not usually detect ductal carcinoma in situ.

Frequency of mammograms

Two years is an acceptable interval between examinations for women after the menopause; annual screening is recommended in younger women (40–50 years) and for women at higher risk (family history of breast cancer, previous history of breast cancer or atypical or proliferative hyperplasia) and possibly for women using hormone replacement therapy.

Benefits and risks

An important but complementary concept of harm minimisation must be understood and taken into account when screening and early detection methods are promoted to the community. This includes the anxiety generated from over-zealous promotion of diagnosis and screening and the anxiety and cost associated with working up asymptomatic lesions that later prove to be benign. Women need to understand the possibility of obtaining false-positive results when they have screening mammograms.

Around 10–15 per cent of all breast cancers are not detected on mammogram; therefore careful clinical breast examination should be undertaken annually. Information presented to women must be based on the best available evidence.

Women with prostheses

Women with prostheses require special consideration with regard to optimal diagnostic methods. Because the value of mammography in identifying breast cancer is reduced, greater dependency is placed on ultrasound and clinical examinations. The 'reliability' of mammography is reduced by varying degrees depending on the amount of 'free' soft breast tissue lying anterior to the implant, which determines how effectively implant exclusion 'push-back' mammographic views can be done.[7] This relates to the degree of capsule formation, and also to the relative size and position of the implants. However, even in difficult cases special localised mammographic views may be taken to provide further information about a specific area of concern identified by clinical or ultrasound examination. Magnetic resonance imaging may be of assistance with deep lesions lying close to the prosthesis. Needle sampling may be more difficult depending on the position of a focal lesion.

In many instances these women are extremely anxious about themselves and their breasts and also about their prostheses, and so special degrees of reassurance may be required.

Women with dense breasts/effect of HRT/size of breasts

Breast tissue is usually denser in the premenopausal woman; therefore there is reduced sensitivity for detecting cancers compared with older women who have predominantly fatty breasts. Breast density will increase in approximately 30 per cent of women taking HRT. In these instances and in the woman aged < 49 years, some advocate annual screening.

Mammography can be performed on breasts of all sizes, including small-breasted women and the male breast. For very large-breasted women, more views may be required to image the whole breast. This is often achieved by imaging the anterior and posterior sections of the breast in separate views.

Prevention

Few of the well-established risk factors for breast cancer are modifiable. Low rates of breast cancer occur in African and Asian women which, on migration, approximate over time to that of the host country. This has prompted the suggestion that lifestyle factors such as diet may be related and has led to lifestyle recommendations. However, whether other factors are involved or whether risk can be modified by short-term changes rather than lifelong adherence remains to be fully evaluated. Some of the findings so far include:

- *Exercise.* For premenstrual women exercising more than 4 hours per week the relative risk of breast cancer is 0.40.[8]
- *Diet.* Asian women eating a traditional diet have 20 per cent of the breast cancer risk compared to Western women. No specific correlations have been made between breast cancer and animal fat.[9,10]

- *Alcohol.* A positive association between alcohol consumption and breast cancer has been observed.[11]
- *Selective oestrogen receptor modulators (SERMs).* Tamoxifen used in the treatment of breast cancer has been shown to decrease the risk in women > 35 years who are at an increased risk of breast cancer.[12] Further studies are under way on both tamoxifen and raloxifene.
- *Bilateral mastectomy* has also been demonstrated to reduce the risk for hereditary breast cancer.[13]

Menstrual problems

CLINICAL PRESENTATION: Menorrhagia (heavy menstrual bleeding)

Women may complain of an increased amount of blood, passing clots, flooding or their periods lasting longer.

History

A careful detailed history has been shown to reliably indicate the presence of menorrhagia (Box 14.2). A targeted history can suggest the presence of specific organic pathology or indicate specific investigations (Box 14.3). For women reporting

BOX 14.2 History to establish presence of menorrhagia[14]

- Number of pads/tampons: 'super', double, incontinence
- Frequency of pad change: every half to two hours
- Clots/flooding: soaking the bed/clothes
- Duration: > 4 days heavy/ > 9 days total
- Frequency: more than once in 21 days
- Prolonged irregular or intermenstrual bleeding (IMB)

BOX 14.3 History for underlying causes of menorrhagia

- Bleeding tendencies (challenges: pregnancies, tooth extraction, easy bruising)
- Family history of bleeding tendencies
- Excess oestrogen (exogenous, endogenous: obesity, PCO)
- Indications of underlying pathology:
  - Pelvic pain (endometriosis, PID)
  - Pressure/mass (fibroids)
  - Infertility (endometriosis, PID)
  - Intermenstrual (IMB), postcoital (PCB) (polyps, STI, malignancy)
- Symptoms associated with thyroid disease
- Consequences of menorrhagia: anaemia—tiredness

menorrhagia but in whom the examination and blood tests are normal, a pictorial blood loss assessment chart (PBAC) can be used for one cycle (Figure 5.3). This has been shown to have good sensitivity and specificity for blood loss.[15]

Examination

Apart from a check for anaemia and systemic disease, an abdominal and pelvic examination will reveal most of the likely pathologies causing menorrhagia (Table 14.1). There is also the opportunity to take a Pap test, culture swabs for chlamydia and other infections, and an endometrial sample. Normal findings do not exclude the possibility of endometrial pre-cancer or cancer.

Referral for menorrhagia is associated with a 60 per cent probability of hysterectomy in the next five years, and therefore it is essential that women with menstrual-related complaints be carefully assessed and managed to avoid unnecessary surgery. Menorrhagia has been defined as blood loss > 80 ml per cycle. This upper limit may be higher in a well-fed population and a loss of 115 ml per cycle may be a more realistic estimate of menorrhagia or heavy menstrual bleeding (HMB).[16] The level reflects the 'upper tolerance level' of bleeding indicating no anaemia or iron depletion. Obviously in societies or groups within societies with depletion of iron stores, the 'upper tolerance level' that constitutes menorrhagia would need to be adjusted to reflect this.

TABLE 14.1 Examination of a woman with menorrhagia

Examination		Possible diagnoses
General		
Hands	Mucous membranes	Anaemia
Thyroid gland		Thyroid disease
Abdominal		
Observe:	Protrusion, varicosities	Fibroids, tumour
Palpate:	Tenderness	Inflammation
	Mass	Fibroids, tumour
	Ascites	Inflammation, malignancy
Speculum*		
Observe:	Discharge	Infection
	Bleeding	Cancer, pre-cancer, inflammation
Bimanual		
Uterus	Enlarged and smooth	Adenomyosis, small intramural fibroids
	Enlarged and irregular	Fibroids
	Tender	
	Retroverted and fixed	Endometriosis, PID
Adnexae	Tender	Hydrosalpinges, pyosalpinx
	Enlarged	Ovarian endometrioma

*Take a Pap test/endometrial sample/culture swabs from the cervical canal.

Underlying pathophysiology

Menorrhagia can result from a number of conditions (Box 14.4). Those most commonly cited are fibroids and endometriosis. Thyroid disease as a cause of menstrual problems is unlikely unless there are other indications of thyroid disease on the history and examination. Acquired and congenital bleeding disorders are causes of menorrhagia in adolescent girls but should also be considered in other age groups. Severe anaemia is a frequent complication of this cause of menorrhagia. A deficiency such as von Willebrand's disease might be amenable to treatment with desmopressin nasal spray.

BOX 14.4 Causes of confirmed menorrhagia

Organic causes: 60%

- Pelvic pathology:
  - Uterine leiomyoma
  - Adenomyosis
  - Endometriosis
  - Endometrial polyps
  - Pelvic inflammatory disease
  - Endometrial hyperplasia
  - Endometrial cancer
  - Cervical cancer
- Systemic disease:
  - Coagulation disorder
  - Systemic lupus erythematosus
  - Hypothyroidism

No cause found: 40% dysfunctional uterine bleeding

- Most ovulatory and chronic
- Anovulatory: < 20 and > 40 years, irregular cycle

In a woman aged under 40 years with menorrhagia the number needed to investigate (NNI) to detect one case of endometrial hyperplasia is 23 and for endometrial cancer 206. If women with menorrhagia are selected on risk factors for endometrial cancer (weight > 95 kg, infertility, age > 45 years, a family history of colonic cancer) the number needed to investigate (NNI) is 8–13 for a case of hyperplasia.[17]

For other women with menstrual problems, where no specific underlying pathology can be determined, the term *dysfunctional uterine bleeding* (DUB) is used. Dysfunctional uterine bleeding is cited less commonly in the USA than in the UK as a cause of hysterectomy (6–18% compared to 29–37%).

Investigations

- A haemoglobin estimation is best accompanied by a serum ferritin level to reflect the iron stores.

- Pelvic ultrasound may be particularly useful in specific situations (Box 14.5) and may provide information to support a specific diagnosis (Box 14.6). Ultrasound examination is less satisfactory at identifying areas of endometriosis or inflammation unless accompanied by anatomical distortion from complications. The expertise of the ultrasonographer is crucial—in expert hands most of the underlying pathological causes of menorrhagia can be identified.
- Sampling the endometrium in the surgery can be a useful procedure if a positive result is obtained. If it is negative (due to failure to enter the endometrial cavity or obtain an adequate tissue sample) then a further procedure is indicated. Endometrial sampling via the hysteroscope remains the gold standard to check for endometrial pathology.[18] A dilatation and curettage is a diagnostic and not a therapeutic test, and should be accompanied by a hysteroscopy and be considered in specific situations (Box 14.7).

BOX 14.5 Indications for transvaginal ultrasound examination[19]

- History: intermenstrual and postcoital bleeding
- Abnormal examination: masses, tenderness
- Normal pelvic examination + risk factors for endometrial pathology*
- Investigations: abnormal histology, severe anaemia
- Failed medical treatment in reproductive years

*Woman > 45 years/obesity > 90 kg/PCO/diabetes mellitus/PH infertility/FH colonic and/or endometrial cancer.

BOX 14.6 Transvaginal ultrasound diagnostic features

- Endometrium: thickness and symmetry—depends on stage of cycle (consider: hyperplasia, cancer, polyps, submucous fibroids)
- Myometrium: thickness/irregularities (consider: fibroids, adenomyosis)
- Ovaries and uterine tubes: cysts, cancer, results of inflammatory disease
- Mass: nature, structure, blood flow, integrity of surrounding organs

BOX 14.7 Indications for dilatation and curettage and hysteroscopy in women with menorrhagia

- Over 40 years of age
- Under 40 years with persistent IMB
- Under 40 years with failed medical treatment
- Abnormality suggested on transvaginal ultrasound
- Abnormal endometrial sample

Models of menorrhagia

Any woman presenting with menorrhagia could be found to have definite underlying pathology or DUB. However, approximately half of women complaining of menorrhagia do not have the complaint confirmed. The reasons that these women present with the complaint of menorrhagia include: lack of information about normal menstrual variations, concern about possible underlying pathology, and as an opening to discuss other matters.[20] A 'model' is suggested to consider which would be most appropriate for each woman (Box 14.8). Determining the model is not to 'label' women but to assist the woman and her health practitioner in the appropriate decision-making pathway and avoid unnecessary intervention. To this end it is important to determine her particular needs for management (Box 14.9).

Medical and surgical management options for menorrhagia

Women now have a range of options for the management of heavy menstrual bleeding (HMB) (Table 14.2). Women with DUB can consider a wide range of medical options as first choice. If these are unsatisfactory then consideration should be given to an ablative procedure to remove the endometrium. Hysterectomy now forms a second-line surgical treatment for many women. However, where there is significant pathology hysterectomy may be the ideal option. Hysterectomy is mostly undertaken to improve quality of life, and a marked improvement does occur following symptom relief.[21] The decision-making process will need to take into account the diagnosis, the woman's past medical and surgical history, aims of treatment and her health beliefs. The latter may be based on her knowledge, past experiences and current expectations, and the views of friends and relatives. The attitude and approach of the medical practitioner will also affect her decisions.

BOX 14.8 Models of menstrual loss[22]

- Disease model:
  - Underlying pathology
  - Medical effects: anaemia
  - Specific medical solution (eg hysterectomy for large fibroids)
- Illness model:[23]
  - No underlying pathology (DUB)
  - History suggests HMB
  - Investigations support HMB
  - Woman's perception of HMB
  - Medical and surgical options
- Experience model:
  - No underlying pathology
  - History does not support HMB
  - Investigations normal
  - Woman's perceptions of menstrual loss
  - Explanation, education, acceptance, solution

BOX 14.9 Aims and needs for the management of menorrhagia

1 End points:
- Stop or decrease HMB
- Stop or decrease pain (dysmenorrhoea, dyspareunia, pelvic pain)

2 Answer individual needs:
- Fertility issues
- Premenstrual syndrome
- Ovarian cysts
- Anaemia

3 Avoid short- and long-term problems of treatment

4 Minimise side effects of medications

5 Address any other psychosocial issues

6 Improve quality of life
- Relationship/sexual
- Professional/working
- Social/family
- Costs: time, financial, psychological

TABLE 14.2 Dysfunctional uterine bleeding: treatment options

Surgical	**Medical**	
	Non-hormonal	**Hormonal**
Endometrial ablation	Prostaglandin synthetase inhibitors (eg NSAIDs)	Synthetic progestogens Combined OCP
Hysterectomy	Inhibitors of fibrinolysis (eg tranexamic acid) Reducers of platelet fragility	Danazol GnRH inhibitors LNG-IUS (levonorgestrel-releasing intrauterine system)

Specific diagnoses

Fibroids

The relationship of HMB and fibroids is not clear. Some women with higher volumes of menstrual blood loss have an increased frequency of fibroids and submucous fibroids in particular. The diagnosis of fibroids is often also made on routine examination of the asymptomatic woman. The exact prevalence is unknown but stated to be between 20 and 40 per cent of women in the reproductive years (Section 13).

Dysfunctional uterine bleeding

This is the term given to HMB where no specific pathology has been found. It may be the cause most amenable to other treatment options that can avoid hysterectomy (Table 14.3). Surgical alternatives for DUB include a variety of endometrial ablative techniques. Medical options for DUB are currently under-utilised by medical practitioners and women. Many have considerable benefits for HMB and should be discussed as a first-line option.

TABLE 14.3 Medical options for dysfunctional uterine bleeding[24]

Drug	Mean reduction in blood loss (%)	Women benefiting* (%)
LNG-IUS	94	100
Progesterone (oral day 5–24)	87	86
Tranexamic acid	47	56
NSAIDs	29	51
OCP	43	50
Danazol	50	76

* Proportion with MBL < 80 ml.

Medical treatment options

1 Non-hormonal treatments

Many women prefer not to take hormone treatments. They are also attracted by treatment that is only required at period times as opposed to all the time. A number of options exist for these women.

Tranexamic acid

The action of this drug is to block the attachment of plasmin to fibrin and this prevents the 'secondary' bleed that occurs when the clots dissolve. The total amount of bleeding is reduced by 35–55 per cent. Side effects occur in 30 per cent of women and include dizziness, headache and leg cramps (dose-related), and gastrointestinal problems as in the NSAIDs. Tranexamic acid needs only to be taken when the bleeding occurs but is required for the entire course of bleeding. The action ceases when the drug is ceased. It does not cause clotting in non-bleeding vessels or elsewhere in the body.

Non-steroidal anti-inflammatory drugs

The NSAIDs inhibit prostaglandin synthase, reduce the production of vasoactive substances and have a direct effect on prostaglandin receptor sites. Menstrual loss is reduced by up to 20–50 per cent and there is benefit on pain and PMS. Side effects include headache and GIT symptoms with contraindication for use in women with gastric ulceration or asthma. As NSAIDs are OTC drugs it is particularly important to explain to women that they should not be used as a regular analgesic but taken regularly before the bleeding and pain occur.

2 Hormonal treatments

Levonorgestrel intrauterine system (LNG-IUS)

The LNG-IUS offers a therapeutic concept that combines a highly efficient contraceptive with a treatment that reduces menstrual blood loss in both normal women and those with menorrhagia. The main mechanism of action is at the level of the endometrium, where the high dose of local progestogen causes decidualisation, epithelial atrophy and direct vascular changes. This is reversible and the endometrium regenerates within 30 days after removal of the device. While some women experience systemic hormonal effects, circulating concentrations of levonorgestrel are low in comparison to the levonorgestrel progestogen-only pill. The LNG-IUS is ideal for dysfunctional uterine bleeding and has other advantages (Box 14.10). The main side-effect of the LNG-IUS is irregular breakthrough bleeding in the first 3–6 months after insertion. Detailed counselling is crucial to reduce unnecessary discontinuation of treatment. After six months' treatment with the LNG-IUS, 50 per cent of women become amenorrhoeic. Again, it is important to explain that this is an expected phenomenon, not a disorder, and that this 'bleed-free' status should be viewed as a positive feature in its own right.

BOX 14.10 Levonorgestrol intrauterine system (LNG-IUS)

- Action: LNG absorbed by endometrium
- Endometrium unresponsive to oestradiol
- Side effects: initial light bleeding, nausea, weight gain, breast tenderness
- Contraindications: undiagnosed abnormal bleeding, pregnancy, malignancy, infection, thromboembolic disease
- Uses: menorrhagia, contraception, oppose oestrogen in HRT, pelvic pain. Evaluation required for endometriosis, adenomyosis, fibroids, endometrial hyperplasia.
- No significant changes in blood pressure, lipids, coagulation factors, liver function tests or carbohydrate metabolism

Combined oral contraceptive pill

The COCP may prove ideal for many women with menorrhagia as it reduces the volume of endometrium and prostaglandin production. The 30 microgram pill decreases menstrual loss by 40 per cent. In addition, the COCP has other advantages for women (Box 14.11). In women without contraindications for its use the pill has been used until the age of 50 years, and the newer 20 microgram pill may be ideal for the woman with bleeding problems, cycle irregularity and menopausal symptoms (once underlying pathology has been excluded).

BOX 14.11 Benefits of the combined oral contraceptive pill

- Decreased menstrual loss
- Regular cycles
- Contraception
- Dysmenorrhoea control
- Relief of PMT and perimenopausal symptoms
- Prevention of ovarian cyst formation
- Reduction in ovarian cancer risk

Progestogens

These have not been shown to be of value in the treatment of menorrhagia when given in the luteal phase only. They may have a place for some women when used for longer (eg norethisterone acetate 5 mg bd/tds from day 5–25 cycle), and be of value for women with irregular cycles or for emergency suppression of bleeding.

Conclusion

Women now have a wide range of options for the management of menorrhagia. A thorough assessment, diagnosis and discussion of the options for the individual woman should improve the quality of life for many women.

CLINICAL PRESENTATION: Changing menstrual cycle

Changes in the menstrual cycle may cause varying levels of concern for women. A common concern may be not knowing what to expect or what is regarded as 'normal'. This can lead to some women with a normal pattern consulting and to others ignoring a change that may be significant in the belief that it is 'just menopause'. It is essential to check for indications of possible underlying pathology (Box 14.12).

BOX 14.12 Considerations for referral to exclude underlying pathology for women with a bleeding problem

- After 40 years of age: increased bleeding (amount or duration)
- Abnormal bleeding (IMB, PCB, PMB)
- Ever on unopposed oestrogen
- Women with cancer risk factors

CLINICAL PRESENTATION: Menopausal symptoms

Many women pass through the menopause with minimal or no symptoms and the event has little impact on their lives. At the other end of the range are women who are so severely affected by the symptoms they experience that they are totally incapacitated. In between, a wide range of symptoms are experienced.[25] The perimenopause is the term given to the few years immediately preceding and after the last menstrual period. It is a time when symptoms may be experienced even though the woman is still menstruating.

For ease of description the symptoms experienced are often discussed in the following groups: vasomotor, genitourinary, psychological, sexual and musculoskeletal. Not all symptoms around this time are hormone-related; it is important to keep an open mind, particularly where there are multiple symptoms[26] (Box 14.13).

BOX 14.13 Principles of diagnosis applied to the multi-symptomatic woman around menopause

- Most likely: menopausal/stress/anxiety
- Not to be missed: depression/thyroid disease
- Life-threatening: cancer
- Pitfalls: attributing all symptoms to menopause
- Hidden message: sexual/relationship problem/abuse

Based on Murtagh's Principles of Diagnosis.[27]

Vasomotor symptoms

The classic symptoms are the vasomotor ones: hot flushes, palpitations and night sweats. If these occur during the night they may disturb sleep and lead to daytime tiredness. They may be experienced well before the menopause, often around the menses, when oestrogen levels are at their lowest.

Genitourinary symptoms

Oestrogen deficiency in the genitourinary tract can cause symptoms of urinary frequency, vaginal dryness and dyspareunia.

Psychological symptoms

These can often be the most distressing for women. They include irritability, emotional lability, anxiety, loss of memory and concentration, and depressed mood. The latter should be differentiated from true depression, which can occur at this time, although the incidence is no higher than at other times in a woman's life. Life stresses at this time may exacerbate these and other symptoms.

Sexuality

Changes in sexuality may occur that can be related to psychological effects or the physical changes of diminished oestrogen on the genital tissues, or may occur without either of these being present. The area is very complex and, as with all other symptoms, the context of the woman's life, past experiences and relationships need to be taken into account in discussions.[28] There is a positive relationship between previous sexual interest or the importance of sex and frequency of sexual activity in later middle life. Finally, cultural and societal notions of sexual attractiveness and attitudes concerning the expression of sexuality beyond the reproductive years have a significant influence on the maintenance of sexual activity in middle-aged and elderly women.

Other symptoms

Some women describe general muscle and joint aches around the time of menopause. An interesting but unexplained symptom is that of formication—the feeling of insects crawling under the skin. The experience of headaches is likewise poorly researched. Some women experience headaches for the first time around menopause, while in other women previously occurring headaches settle. Menstrual migraines, associated with the fall in oestrogens, are relieved with menopause and steady oestrogen levels.

Menopause

Menopause is defined as the last menstrual period in a woman's life and is therefore a retrospective diagnosis. The mean age at menopause is 51 years.[29] As women are now expected to live into their eighties, the postmenopausal period occupies one-third of a woman's life.

Menopause is a natural and universal event of the human female life cycle. The psychological impact of menopause is strongly influenced by the importance attached by a particular culture to procreation, fertility, ageing and female roles. In general, in those cultures where women receive rights at the time of menopause that are denied to them during the fertile period, menopausal symptoms are minimal. A culture where the society is youth-oriented and stereotypes of ageing women are largely negative does not provide a supportive environment for menopausal women. The individual experience is also affected by the other aspects of a woman's life[30] (Section 3).

Management of the woman in middle years[31]

Evaluation of symptoms

The issues may be simple or numerous and many may not be addressed unless an opportunity is given for discussion. Any areas that may be sensitive or embarrassing, such as sexual issues, psychosocial problems and incontinence, may not be revealed at the first visit. It may be helpful to suggest:

- Compiling a list of issues that are troubling her
- Maintaining a diary and arranging another visit
- Providing written information to read at home, and returning for discussion.

Health promotion

A consultation in the middle years presents an opportunity for reflection and planning for future health maintenance. Of all the lifestyle changes that could be made for any woman, regular exercise, weight reduction, stopping smoking, minimising alcohol intake and managing stress are those most likely to offer considerable benefits to health in older age (Section 17).

Medication

The ideological dispute as to whether menopause is a normal reproductive event or an endocrine deficiency disease requiring medical intervention continues. A practical approach is one that weighs up the short- and long-term consequences of oestrogen deficiency for and with the individual woman. Whether a woman chooses to begin HRT to alleviate symptoms depends on her own assessment of the degree of discomfort she is experiencing and the interference with her quality of life. Longer-term issues such as prevention of osteoporosis will also need to be considered (Box 14.14).

BOX 14.14 Individualising choices for management of menopause

- Every woman should be offered the choice of management for her individual problems.
- Decision making about management is between the woman and her doctor.
- Provide unbiased evidence-based information where this is available. Tell the woman where limited or no evidence currently exists.
- Balance individual risks and benefits of treatment options with every woman.
- Continuing care requires regular visits to reappraise the dynamic situation of changing symptoms, the development of medical conditions and appraisal of new research.

Vasomotor and urogenital symptoms have been shown to respond to oestrogen replacement.[32] Exogenous oestrogen (possibly in the form of oestrogen cream) alleviates atrophic vaginitis and associated dyspareunia, and increases vaginal lubrication. However, exogenous oestrogen does not increase sexual desire or libido. The role of testosterone is being evaluated. Regular sexual intercourse may be beneficial in maintaining the health of the vaginal mucosa. Psychological symptoms are more difficult to evaluate and assess for the individual woman. In this situation an individualised medication of effective treatment (IMET) could be undertaken.[33] Apart from possible hormone management, women may benefit from stress management and relaxation techniques.

Choices for treatment

For the woman with symptoms requesting treatment the choices are increasing.

Oral contraceptive pill

A woman still menstruating and with menopausal symptoms may find the low-dose 20 microgram OCP ideal. In addition to symptom relief, the OCP also can control bleeding problems and provide contraception. The usual contraindications apply and the question of how long to continue with the OCP needs to be considered (Section 12).

Hormone replacement therapy

If HRT is discussed it is important to defuse the misconception that once treatment starts it should be maintained lifelong. A commonsense approach that is acceptable to women is to review the situation annually. The woman should be advised that it is her choice to stop at any time, but that it would be helpful to discuss this with you first—not to persuade her to continue, but to understand and help with any concerns. Also it may be preferable to tailor the medication down gradually.

Hormone replacement therapy should consist of a continuous oestrogen therapy opposed by a progestogen in women for whom this is indicated (see below).[34] The same contraindications for oestrogen should be considered as for the OCP.

Oestrogen

There is a wide range of options for oestrogen delivery from daily pills, weekly or twice weekly patches, implants and skin gel and, in the future, a nasal spray. For the woman with urogenital symptoms not wanting or needing a systemic therapeutic dose, the vaginal creams, pessaries and rings are a useful option.

Progestogens

Women still menstruating should be prescribed progesterone for 12–14 days of the second half of the cycle (cyclical regimen) to prevent bleeding problems. In post-menopausal women the combined continuous regimen can be used. With this latter regimen—termed continuous combined treatment—bleeding may be experienced lightly but erratically during the first 3–6 months and then the woman should be amenorrhoeic. However, some women may choose to have a bleed each month (and use the cyclical regimen) and this remains their choice. A number of formulations are available and there may be individual sensitivity to these, necessitating a change of drug or regimen (Box 14.15).

BOX 14.15 Choices for women with intolerance to progestogen

- Low doses less often: regimens once every 3–12 months have been suggested but long-term data is not available on endometrial protection against increased risk of endometrial hyperplasia and cancer.
- No progestogen and check the endometrium annually (monitor with annual ultrasound and histological sampling).
- An alternative method of endometrial protection without systemic effects (Levonorgestrel intrauterine system; Section 12).
- An endometrial ablation: not ideal as complete removal of endometrium without regeneration cannot be guaranteed.
- A hysterectomy: major surgery. Consider if there are other indications (prolapse, urinary incontinence).

Route of administration

The woman's history and investigations are important as the metabolic effects are different between different forms of HRT. For example, the oral route of oestrogen and a non-androgenic progesterone would be preferred for a woman with cardiovascular risk factors and decreased high density lipoprotein. If the triglycerides are elevated then the transdermal route is the better choice. A low-dose transdermal oestrogen would be the most beneficial for a woman with a thrombogenic risk as this route does not affect the haemostatic parameters. The woman's choice of route is important for long-term adherence.

KEY POINT

Unopposed oestrogen can cause endometrial hyperplasia and endometrial cancer. Progesterone should always be included in an HRT regimen for a woman with a uterus, after endometrial ablation, a sub-total hysterectomy or post hysterectomy where the indication was extensive endometriosis.

Assessing hormone levels

Changes occur from the early forties, and hormone levels are not of value in predicting menopausal status (Section 4). Symptomatic women can be monitored on clinical response. However, women may notice symptoms from changes in the hormone levels even though these are in the normal physiological range (for reproductive years). This is particularly important for women choosing hormone implants—these should not be reimplanted without checking the oestrogen level, to avoid supra-physiological levels.

Androgen

There is no agreed clinical definition of androgen deficiency in women. A number of symptoms have been suggested to indicate possible androgen deficiency in women: diminished or loss of desire, reduced general well-being, lack of energy, depressed mood, diminished confidence or self-esteem. No specific level of circulating androgen has been shown to be associated with a particular symptom.[35] Whether an age-related response should be treated depends on the effect on the woman's life and her choice of management.

Several prospective studies of surgically menopausal women have demonstrated that the addition of testosterone to an oestrogen replacement regimen increased sexual desire, sexual arousal and the frequency of sexual fantasies compared with women treated with oestrogen alone. However, the role of androgens in the menopause is still at an early stage of knowledge and much work is still to be done. It is important to counsel women about possible side effects (hirsutism, voice changes) and to take care in prescribing for women with an obvious androgenic tendency by asking, for example, about acne and the frequency of body hair removal.

Alternative management

Many women are concerned about using HRT because of the possible side effects. This may lead them to seek alternative treatments. In recent years there has been a great deal written about these alternatives, in particular the phytoestrogens.[36] It is important to weigh up the evidence for these preparations in the same way that the HRT preparations are assessed.[37] More good quality research is required to confirm benefits and risks, and their place in the management options.

Problems with using hormones

Problems with using hormones fall into three main groups—adherence, side effects and risks—all of which overlap to some extent.

- *Adherence* to treatment can be a problem. It is essential to allow adequate time to discuss all issues important to the woman before prescribing any treatment.
- *Side effects* are a nuisance for the woman or give rise to concern about possible underlying disease. This will often lead to the woman stopping therapy of her own volition without discussion with her medical practitioner. The most frequent reasons given by women for stopping HRT include:
  - irregular bleeding
  - breast tenderness
  - 'PMS' symptoms
  - weight gain
  - concern about increased cancer risk
  - concern about possible as yet unknown side effects.

  These can be pre-empted in part by explaining the possible side effects in advance and suggesting that a return visit for further assessment and treatment adjustment would be appropriate if they should occur. Many women worry about weight gain using hormone treatment. However, there is no evidence that HRT causes increase in weight in addition to that normally gained at menopause. There is insufficient evidence to assess the effect of HRT on waist–hip ratio, fat mass or skin fold thickness at present.[38]

  Most of the 'nuisance' side effects (breast tenderness and 'PMS') can be managed with an alteration in the regimen. Concern about cancer and other side effects that still cause a woman to feel worried, even though appropriate explanation has been given, may be a reason to discontinue therapy.

Bleeding on HRT

This is one of the most common causes for lack of adherence to treatment and causes of concern for women. It can be related to oestrogen or progestogen therapy.

Hyperplasia

Unopposed oestrogen therapy at moderate or high doses is associated with increased rates of endometrial hyperplasia, endometrial cancer, irregular bleeding and subsequent non-adherence (Section 16).[39] Oral progesterone use decreases this risk and improves adherence to therapy. The decrease in risk is for both sequential (cyclical) and continuous treatment, although there is a suggestion that continuous treatment is more protective over a long duration. The duration of progesterone therapy is more important than the daily dose in protecting against endometrial cancer.

Atrophy

When there is either continuous or too much progesterone used, the endometrium becomes decidualised, thin, fragile and atrophic with focal areas of bleeding. The precise mechanism is still to be determined.

Checking the endometrial response with bleeding on HRT

Intermittent bleeding in a woman on a combined continuous regimen can be checked with transvaginal ultrasound. For a woman on sequential therapy, the time to check is at the end of an episode of bleeding. A uniform double endometrial thickness < 5 mm is less likely to have underlying pathology. A saline infusion sonohysterography is more reliable in excluding focal thickening, polyps or submucous fibroids. A woman with any of these changes or a persistent problem should be referred for further investigation and histological assessment.

Managing bleeding on HRT

Options may include decreasing the progesterone or increasing the oestrogen in a woman with persistent light bleeding and a thin endometrium. There are many preferred 'tricks' by individual clinicians for heavier bleeding, such as decreasing the oestrogen, increasing the progesterone or commencing the regimen with a lower dose of oestrogen. However, continuation of the same regimen often produces the same results over time. Some women who are stressed by spotting or light irregular bleeding may prefer a cyclical regimen with predictable bleeding even though the combined continuous therapy is more protective to the endometrium in the long term. The occasional woman continues to have problems after changing regimens. She may need to consider the alternatives (L-IUD, endometrial ablation, hysterectomy).

Risks of HRT

One of the main problems is explaining to women in meaningful terms what is meant by 'risk and benefit' or 'loss and gain' (Table 14.4) (Section 1).[40]

Thrombosis

Although there are concerns regarding an increased thrombotic risk with post-menopausal oestrogen use, the absolute risk in non-users is 1 in 10 000 women and this increases to 3.6 per 10 000 women in HRT users. The history should include any previous episodes, predisposing factors and genetic predisposition (Section 18).

Endometrial cancer

It became clear in the 1970s that the use of unopposed oestrogen was associated in a marked increase in the instance of endometrial cancer. Adding a progesten to the therapy for 10 to 12 days a month provides protection to the endometrium, and combined oestrogen–progesten regimens are now recommended as HRT for women in whom the uterus is intact.[39]

TABLE 14.4 Comparison of outcomes from the Women's Health Initiative and observational studies*[41]

Outcome after 5 years of combined hormone placement therapy	Relative risk (± CI) in systematic reviews of observational studies	Hazard ratio (± adjusted CI) in WHI study at 5.2 years[a]
Cancer		
Invasive breast	1.35 (1.21–1.49)[b] 1.53[c]	1.26 (0.83–1.92)
Endometrial	0.8 (0.6–1.2)	0.83 (0.29–2.32)
Colorectal	0.72 (0.53–0.96)	0.63 (0.32–1.24)
Total	—	1.03 (0.86–1.22)
Fractures		
Hip	0.06 (0.4–0.91)	0.66 (0.33–1.33)
Vertebral	0.67 (0.45–0.98)	0.66 (0.32–1.34)
Total	—	0.76 (0.63–0.92)
Cardiovascular disease		
Stroke	1.45 (1.10–1.92)	1.41 (0.86–2.31)
Thromboembolism	2.14 (1.64–2.81)	2.11 (1.26–3.55)
Coronary heart disease		1.29 (0.85–1.97)
• Observational studies	0.66 (0.53–0.84)	
• HERS[d] overall	0.99 (0.8–1.22)	
• HERS[d] mortality	1.24 (0.87–1.75)	
Total mortality	—	0.98 (0.70–1.37)

*Observational studies and randomised controlled trials cannot be directly compared but it is reassuring to see that the magnitude of effect is similar in this case.

[a] Combined oestrogen and progestogen regimens

[b] All regimens of hormone replacement therapy

[c] Oestrogen and progestogen regimen

[d] The Heart and Estrogen/Progestin Replacement Study (HERS) was a randomised placebo-controlled trial.

CI = Confidence Interval.

Ovarian cancer

Past studies have shown that oral contraceptives with 30 and 50 micrograms or more of oestrogen reduce the risk of ovarian cancer with an estimated risk reduction odds ratio of 0.5. However, it is not clear whether newer, lower-dose 20 microgram formulations or HRT offer similar protection.

Breast cancer

Considerable controversy has existed regarding the association between HRT and the incidence of breast cancer in postmenopausal women (Section 18). Generally the increased risk for breast cancer has been over-emphasised and has become a cause of fear among women. It needs to be put into perspective for the individual woman.

Long-term benefits

Mental health

Oestrogen has effects on brain function. However, there is little evidence that HRT or ERT has beneficial effects on the brain post menopause, or in women with dementia.[42,43] Dehydroepiandrosterone (DHEA) is promoted to improve cognitive function but there is no support from the current data available.[44]

Osteoporosis

The aspects of osteoporosis to be considered are prevention and treatment. Hormone replacement therapy has a preventative role in maintaining BMD. Knowing her BMD may be useful for a woman who is deciding whether to use or continue using HRT (Figure 14.1). In addition, other issues should be addressed, such as calcium intake, diet, balance and fall prevention (Section 17). Treatment of osteoporosis with reduction in the rate of fractures involves other medications (Figure 14.2).

FIGURE 14.1 Bone mineral density: indications, results, management

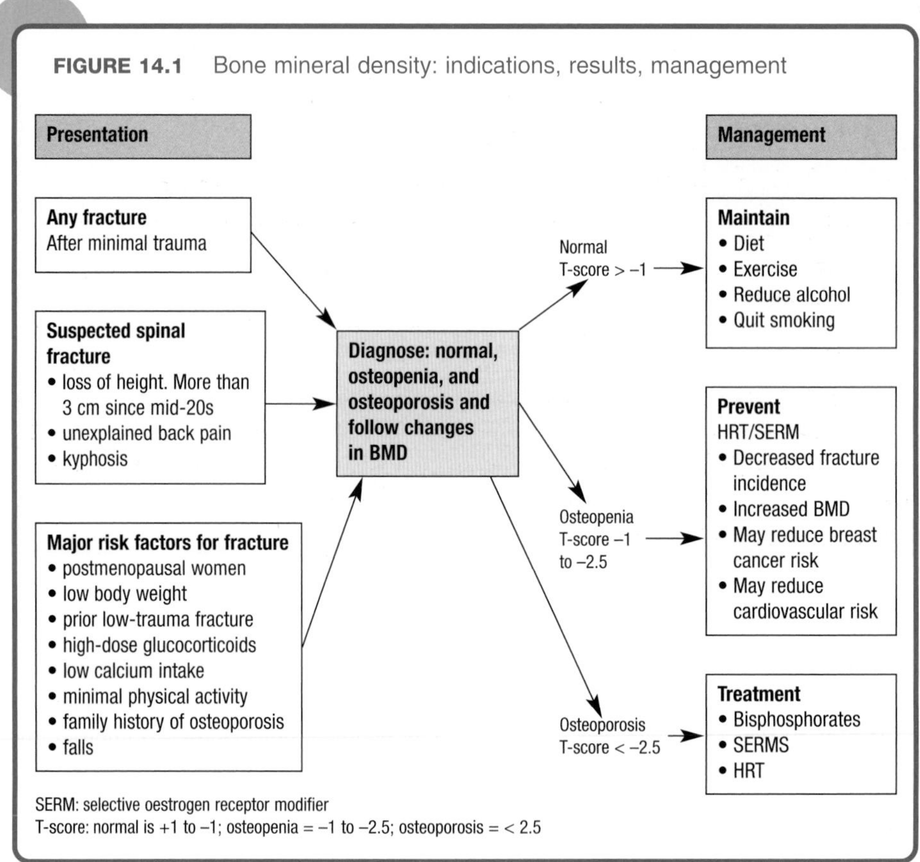

SERM: selective oestrogen receptor modifier
T-score: normal is +1 to –1; osteopenia = –1 to –2.5; osteoporosis = < 2.5

FIGURE 14.2 Development of osteoporosis over time

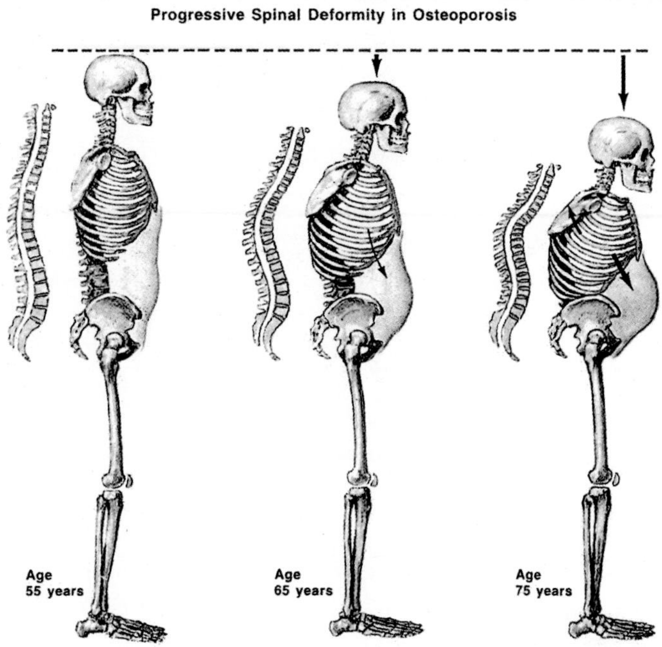

Continuing care

Once women are established on a hormone regimen that suits them, an annual review should be arranged. The situation is a dynamic one. The woman's beliefs, experiences and medical status may have changed. Also, there may be new treatment options and the woman may want to discuss these. New research may have elicited media coverage that may need to be put in perspective. The clinician needs to be aware of the various influences on the woman in the initial decision making and be prepared to reassess changes in these.

SECTION

15 Common complaints

Breast problems

Patterns of breast disease in Western women vary with age and social conditions. The factors responsible for these varying patterns are not fully understood but reproductive, other hormonal, dietary and breastfeeding factors are among those that may influence these patterns. These factors are themselves influenced by custom, culture and lifestyle within societal groups.

Breast problems vary significantly in incidence at different ages of women, and will affect the diagnostic process accordingly. The incidence of breast cancer increases in the late reproductive years and with increasing age. Variations in incidence with age are also seen with benign breast disorders. There are many consultations each year with clinicians in Australia for breast symptoms, with approximately 65 per cent of complaints due to the discovery of a breast lump. Other common presenting symptoms are breast pain and nipple discharge. With a lifetime risk of developing breast cancer of 1 in 11,[1] the possibility of symptoms indicating breast cancer is of concern to Australian women and their doctors. The majority (> 90 per cent) of these symptoms will not be due to breast cancer; however, it is critical to investigate any breast changes effectively in order to make the appropriate diagnosis and management plan. As disease presentation varies with the woman's age, so too does the effectiveness of the different imaging modalities. Keeping these differences in mind will assist in determining an appropriate diagnostic and management pathway for each woman.

CLINICAL PRESENTATIONS OF A BREAST PROBLEM

1. A problem found on self-examination or health professional examination: lump, thickening, nipple or skin changes
2. A symptomatic woman: pain, nipple discharge
3. A woman with a family history of breast disease
4. An asymptomatic woman undergoing breast screening (Section 14)

Further investigations

Multimodality diagnosis of breast disease has been refined into a highly sensitive and specific process. The principle that underpins the high degree of accuracy is the combining of diagnostic modalities such that the deficiencies of one modality are compensated for by the strengths of another. The modalities used are clinical examination, mammography, breast ultrasound and needle sampling. Each individually must be of the highest quality and their strengths and weaknesses understood to achieve the highest quality overall. Where the results of all investigations are congruent the diagnosis is more than 98 per cent probable. Different investigative modalities vary in their value for individual women and every case must be considered on an individual basis. Any discrepancy between tests requires further review and/or investigation following the approaches outlined below until a confident diagnosis is made.

- *Mammogram* (with additional work up views if necessary) (Figures 15.1 and 15.2)
- *Ultrasound*
- *Fine needle aspirate biopsy* (FNAB) generally uses a 20-gauge needle to obtain samples for cytological examination. It is used for confirmation of the impression gained from history and clinical and imaging examinations. Ultrasound or stereotactic guidance is used if the lesion is non-palpable. No local anaesthetic is required (Figure 15.3).
- *Core biopsy (CB):* as a histological examination is undertaken, this is more reliable than FNAB. Core biopsy uses a 12- or 14-gauge needle to remove tissue for examination (Figure 15.4). It can be performed with ultrasound or stereotactic guidance and requires local anaesthesia and a small skin incision.

CLINICAL PRESENTATION: A problem found on self-examination or examination by a health professional

During pregnancy and lactation

See Section 11.

In women aged > 55

See Section 16.

In women aged 35–55

(assuming menopause at approximately 50 years)

1 If doctor considers palpable area or sign to be discrete or otherwise significant:
   - Bilateral mammography is the imaging modality of first choice
   - If this is not diagnostic—perform bilateral breast ultrasound
   - Needle sampling indicated if solid or indeterminate lesion present: CB or FNAB
   - A surgical opinion or early clinical review in 1–3 months if pathology is not clarified by the above investigations.

2 If doctor considers palpable area to be not significant:
   - Review by doctor in 2–3 months or seek a second opinion. A change in the 'hormonal environment' may be helpful if indicated by the history (eg recently ceased COCP, restart on low-dose monophasic preparation if appropriate).

In all women, if the diagnosis is not conclusive one of the following two options must be taken, and the choice will vary with the index of suspicion:

- Diagnostic surgery
- Short-term review in 1–3 months with repeat needle sampling.

Breast cancer becomes increasingly common throughout this age group and every firm mass or other clinical change must be considered as a possible cancer. Investigation is therefore important whenever a persistent clinical change is noted in the breast. Failure to review or prolonged observation may create an unacceptable delay in diagnosis of sinister pathology.

FIGURE 15.1 Mammography being performed of the breast in the cranio-caudal (CC) position

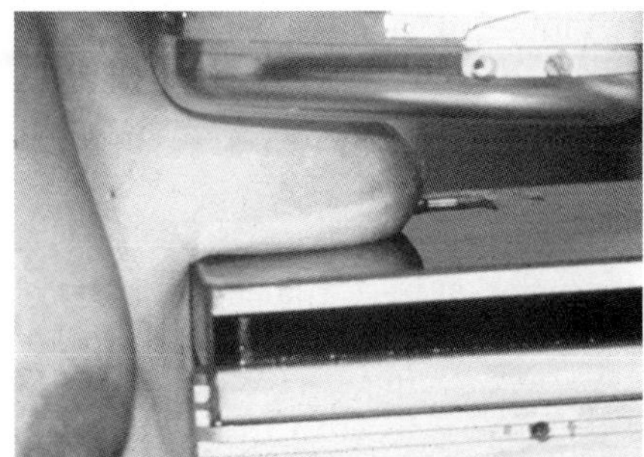

FIGURE 15.2 Mammography being performed of the breast in the medio-lateral oblique (MLO) position. The minimum mammographic examination includes bilateral MLO and CC views.

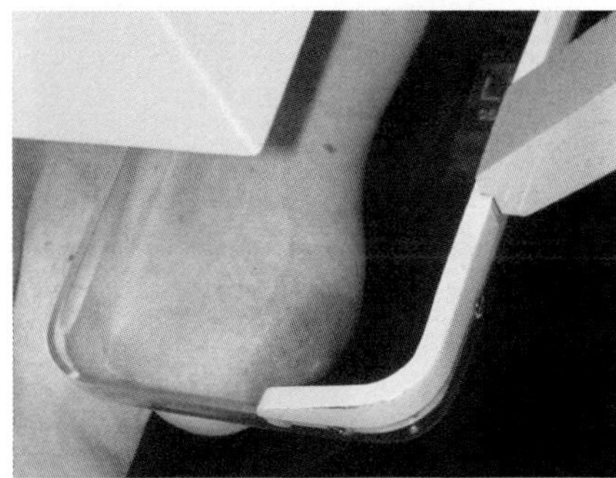

FIGURE 15.3 Fine needle biopsy being performed using ultrasound guidance

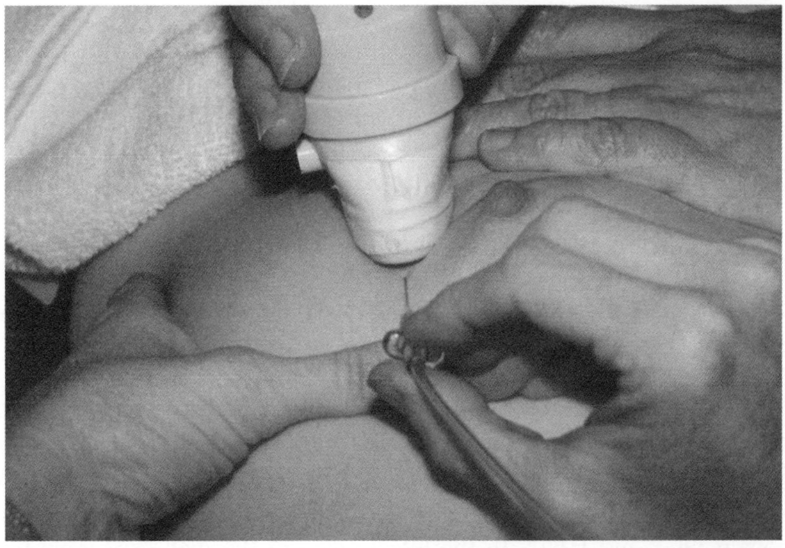

FIGURE 15.4 Core biopsy allows outpatient collection of a sample of tissue, which then undergoes a histological examination.

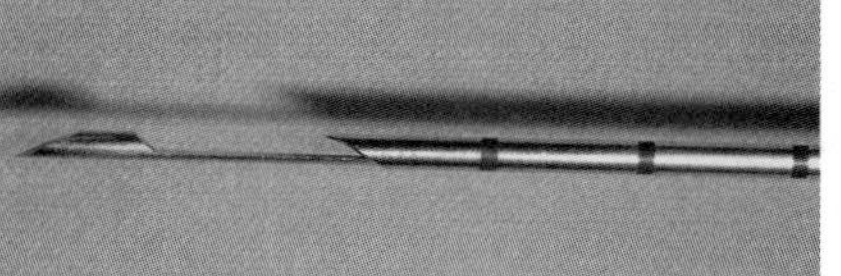

Commonly occurring conditions in this age group:

- Fibrocystic and benign breast change
- Periductal mastitis, duct papilloma and duct ectasia.
- Fibroadenoma (solitary or multiple)
- Mastalgia
- Breast cancer

Presentation by a woman with a breast symptom is an opportunity to assess any risk factors for breast cancer and provide advice to maximise the earliest detection of breast cancer (Table 15.1).

TABLE 15.1 Breast cancer risk factors[2]

Indicator	Low risk	High risk	Relative risk (RR)
Sex	Male	Female	150.0
Age	30–34 years	70–74 years	17.0
Age @ first child	< 20 years	> 30 years	2–3.5
Breastfeeding (m)	> 16 m	0	1.37
Parity	> 5	0	1.4
Age at bilateral oophorectomy	< 35 years	> 35 years	3.0
Age at menopause	< 45 years	> 55 years	2.0
Postmenopausal BMI	< 23	> 31	1.6
ERT	Never	Current	1.2
HRT	Never	Current	1.4
OCP usage	Never	Previous or current	1.07–1.2
FH Br Ca	No	Yes	2.6
BMD	Lowest quartile	Highest quartile	2.7–3.5
Serum E2	Lowest quartile	Highest quartile	1.8–5
Breast density on mammogram	Lowest quartile	Highest quartile	6.0

Benign breast change

In a normal menstrual cycle many women may have palpable thickenings or lumpiness in the breasts and fluctuating pain and tenderness, especially premenstrually. This frequently becomes worse in the later reproductive years (Figure 15.5). The symptomatology is associated with hormonal variations, both endogenous and exogenous (COCP and HRT). In the luteal phase of the menstrual cycle there is marked proliferation of the breast epithelium as well as an increase in mammary blood flow, partly explaining the premenstrual exacerbation of these symptoms. Examination will reveal 'tender lumpy breasts', usually occurring bilaterally and often more pronounced in the upper outer quadrants of the breasts. The onset of menses is usually associated with symptom relief; therefore, reviewing women at this time in their cycle is often helpful. These changes are common and do not represent a 'disease state'; hence the term 'benign breast changes' is used. Reassurance, after appropriate investigation, about the 'normality' of these symptoms is frequently all that is necessary. Commencing or changing to a low-dose, single-phase continuous COCP may alleviate symptoms for some women.

FIGURE 15.5 Incidence of normal breast lumpiness[3]

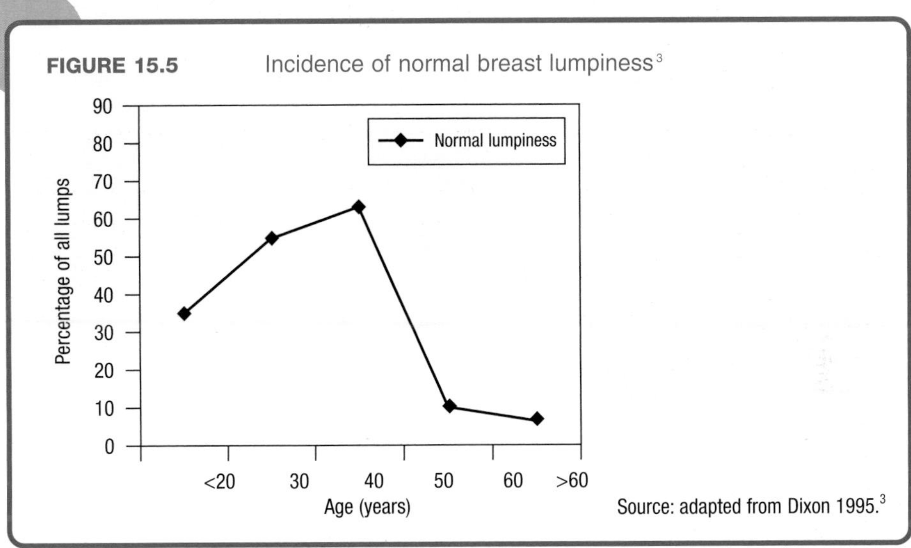

Source: adapted from Dixon 1995.[3]

Breast macrocysts

Macrocysts are most commonly found in women between the ages of 35 and 50 years (although the use of HRT can extend their incidence). They present as a lump or thickening, are often tender and may also increase suddenly in size. They may be single, multiple or recurring. Many cysts are also discovered on mammographic screening in an otherwise asymptomatic patient (Figure 15.6). Ultrasound examination confirms the diagnosis in almost all cases (Figure 15.7). If painful, or if the diagnosis is uncertain, they can easily be aspirated with ultrasound guidance, although they may later recur. Cytological examination of the aspirate should be undertaken if the fluid is blood-stained or if the lesion persists following attempted aspiration. The routine aspiration of typical cysts is not recommended in the absence of symptoms.

Traumatic or spontaneous rupture of a breast cyst with extravasation of the cyst fluid into the surrounding tissues can result in sudden onset of erythema and tenderness. There may or may not be a mass palpable. The differential diagnosis includes an inflammatory carcinoma. Previous history of cysts and the rapid resolution of symptoms will favour the diagnosis of cyst rupture; however, short-term follow-up ultrasound examination is recommended to ensure that there is no underlying pathology. Fibrocystic changes without associated proliferative activity on histology do not constitute a significant risk factor for breast cancer.

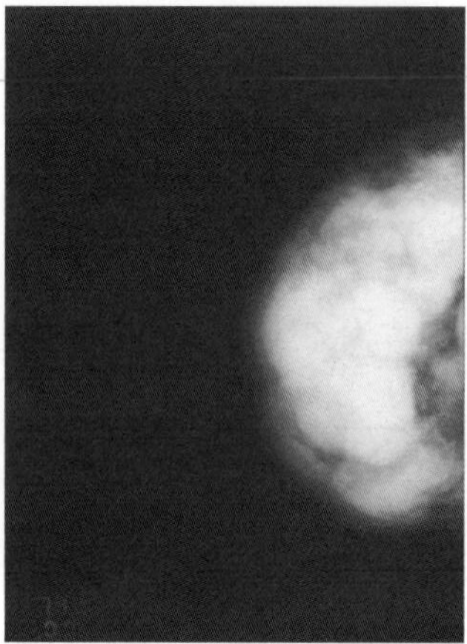

FIGURE 15.6 Mammogram (CC view) showing dense breast tissue containing multiple rounded densities

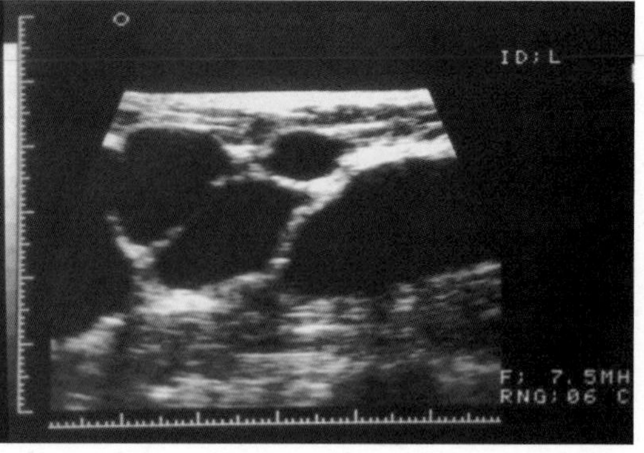

FIGURE 15.7 Ultrasound examination of the same woman clearly showing multiple well-defined anechoeic lesions (typical features of benign breast macrocysts)

Inflammatory changes

Periductal mastitis is most commonly seen in women in the mid reproductive years. There is active inflammation around non-dilated subareolar lactiferous ducts. Cigarette smoking appears to be an aetiological factor. Both anaerobic and aerobic organisms are involved. A woman may present with inflammation (with or without an associated mass) or with an established abscess. Pain is experienced centrally. There may also be nipple retraction and nipple discharge.

Duct ectasia largely affects women in the early postmenopausal age range, and is associated with dilatation and inflammation of the subareolar lactiferous ducts. There is frequently a characteristic appearance on mammography of 'cigar-shaped calcifications' in the subareolar region. Women may present with nipple discharge, nipple retraction (classically slit-like) or, occasionally, a palpable mass.

Fibroadenomata

These tumours are common in women in the early to middle reproductive years and will appear de novo. In as many as 30 per cent of cases they will be multiple and synchronous, and many women will have multiple asynchronous fibroadenomata during their lives. Fibroadenomas are composed of combinations of proliferating epithelial and stromal elements. Occasionally they may become very large, over 5 cm, in which case they are termed giant fibroadenoma. Fibroadenomata may or may not be visible on mammography, depending on the density of the surrounding parenchyma. They may or may not be palpable depending on their size and position within the breast. Careful and thorough ultrasound examination should always identify fibroadenomata, although they can be difficult to distinguish from a lobulated piece of fat or even a cancer. For this reason needle sampling either by fine needle aspiration or by core biopsy should be undertaken to confirm the diagnosis (Figure 15.8). The natural history of fibroadenomas suggests that fewer than 10 per cent increase in size and about one-third will decrease in size or disappear. Excision biopsy may be necessary if the nodule is increasing in size, if follow-up monitoring is difficult or if there is any uncertainty about the diagnosis.

FIGURE 15.8 Ultrasound showing a well-defined, lobulated, hypoechoic lesion. There is no shadowing posterior to the lesion and the horizontal axis is greater than the vertical axis. These features suggest the diagnosis of fibroadenoma. An FNAB is being performed to confirm this diagnosis (note the shadow of the biopsy needle in lesion).

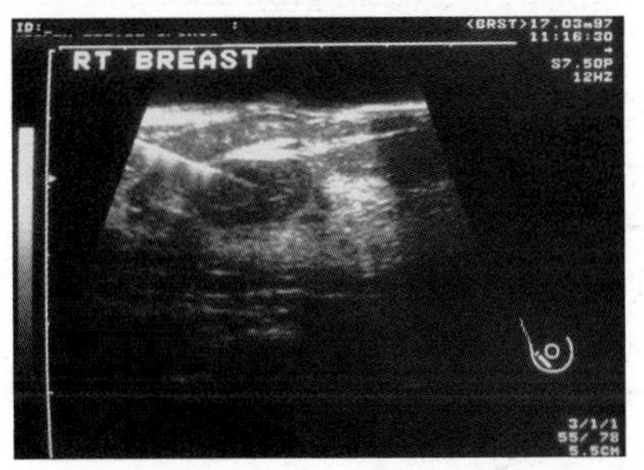

Cystosarcoma phyllodes tumour (phyllodes tumour)

Despite the name, most of these tumours (around 80 per cent) are benign. They are rare and found typically in women aged 30–50 years (slightly older age group than for fibroadenoma). The formation of leaf-like processes protruding into cystic spaces gives the tumour its name, and a characteristic 'cauliflower' appearance is often seen on ultrasound examination. The mass, with clinical characteristics similar to fibroadenoma, usually increases rapidly in size, and surgical excision is necessary to establish the diagnosis and to remove the enlarging mass. Although usually benign, careful evaluation by the pathologist of size, contour, stromal atypia and mitotic activity is essential to assess the behaviour of the tumour. Clinical and imaging follow-up for at least 2–3 years is indicated. For the malignant variety, most recurrences occur within two years of the diagnosis.

CLINICAL PRESENTATION: Women with breast symptoms

These women should be investigated as described in the previous section.

Breast pain

Mastalgia or breast pain is common, affecting more than 70 per cent of women at some time in their lives. Some of these women will seek medical attention for the relief of their symptoms, and many fear a sinister explanation for their pain and seek reassurance. Most breast pain is cyclical, although it can be non-cyclical and also can be generalised or localised. Non-cyclical pain should be differentiated on clinical examination from localised chest wall pain or referred pain.

Generalised (particularly if bilateral), cyclical breast pain is indicative of a normal physiological process. Women at any age can experience mastalgia but it is more common in premenopausal women. It is generally a chronic symptom, beginning during the reproductive years, frequently becoming more intense in the premenopausal years, with the majority resolving at menopause. The mechanism of breast pain is not well understood. The particular role of oestrogen, progestogen, prolactin and the gonadotrophins is unclear, with no clear differences in levels between those who complain of mastalgia and those without it. There is no association between total body water measurements and symptoms.

In order to reassure women that they do not have breast cancer, a history, clinical examination and appropriate investigations need to be undertaken.

Management

Reassurance after appropriate investigation will often improve symptoms. A daily pain chart can be helpful in tracking the frequency and severity of symptoms and monitoring response to any management strategies. Initial simple measures are often effective:

- Simple analgesics can be used on days of more severe pain.
- There appears to be a small increase in risk for cyclical mastalgia associated with smoking, high caffeine intake and perceived stress.[4] Lifestyle modifications addressing these factors, including relaxation, exercise, decreasing smoking and caffeine intake, and wearing a well-fitting bra while exercising, may be of benefit.
- Evening primrose oil (gamma linolenic acid) is effective. Daily doses of between 1000 and 3000 mg are usually required. It is well tolerated, although a few will experience bloating or nausea.[5] No benefit from vitamin A, B or E supplementation has been demonstrated in placebo-controlled trials.
- COCPs may either help or aggravate the symptom in different women. Similarly, HRT often initiates or exacerbates the symptoms. These problems can usually be overcome by time and adjustments in the regimen and dosage, with lower dose, single-phase combinations being most appropriate.

For the small group of patients with resistant severe breast pain and decreased quality of life, there are a number of agents that can be of benefit, although side effects can be troublesome.

- Danazol, an anti-gonadotrophin, binds to progesterone and androgen receptors in breast tissue. Androgenic side effects (menstrual irregularity, irritability, hirsuitism, acne and weight gain) occur in 20 per cent of women.
- Bromocriptine, a prolactin inhibitor, may also be effective. Postural hypotension, nausea and fatigue can be a problem.
- Tamoxifen, a selective oestrogen receptor modulater (SERM), is highly effective for breast pain. Side effects include hot flushes and vaginal dryness, as well as an increased incidence of vascular thrombotic disorders and endometrial cancer. Other SERMs may prove useful in the future.

Nipple discharge

Nipple discharge is a common complaint in women of reproductive age but is seldom caused by serious pathology. Despite this, it frequently raises concerns of breast cancer or pituitary tumour. History and physical examination will allow the selection of appropriate diagnostic investigations by dividing the possibilities into either ductal or endocrinological causes for the nipple discharge.

Ductal causes

All discharges not classified as galactorrhea fall into this category and may be due to benign or malignant causes (Table 15.2). The discharge may vary in colour,

TABLE 15.2 Ductal causes of nipple discharge

Pathology	Features
Benign	
Ductal ectasia	Discharge often green to black and multiductal. Subareolar dilatation of ducts associated with inflammation and fibrosis. May or may not be identified on imaging.
Fibrocystic breast changes	Serous, green or brown discharge, often multiductal, may be spontaneous or provoked. Dense nodular breast tissue with or without macrocysts. Some features may be seen on imaging.
Intraductal papilloma	Blood-stained, sometimes serous, uniductal discharge, which is often spontaneous and reproducible on palpation over affected duct. Papillomas are usually located within 1–2 cm of the areolar edge within the major ducts. Because of their association with proliferative lesions, women may be at slightly higher lifetime risk for breast cancer. Mammogram usually negative, sometimes an intraluminal lesion is seen on ultrasound. Galactography is sometimes helpful, although limitations include discomfort, invasiveness, and false positives for filling defects and doesn't obviate the need for surgery to make the diagnosis.
Malignant	
Intraductal cancer (DCIS)	Discharge usually serous or blood-stained and occurs unprovoked. May be marker of extensive DCIS requiring mastectomy to achieve adequate margins.
Invasive ductal cancer (papillary carcinoma)	May have associated palpable thickening and imaging signs.

Source: Adapted from Falkenberry 2002.[6]

with serous or blood-stained discharges more likely to be associated with sinister pathology. Apart from discharges associated with fibrocystic change and ductal ectasia, most will be unilateral and usually from a single duct orifice. History, physical examination, mammography and ultrasound are the diagnostic modalities used in evaluating a uni-ductal discharge. Galactography, where the duct orifice is cannulated and a small amount of water-soluble radio-contrast is introduced prior to coned mammography being performed, is sometimes of benefit but usually will not affect the need for surgery. Surgical duct excision is undertaken to establish the diagnosis in the case of single duct discharges and, for discharges that turn out to have a benign cause, is therapeutic. Undertaking cytology of the discharge generally is not useful because the absence of malignant cells does not exclude cancer, and a positive result cannot distinguish intraductal from invasive cancer.

Endocrinological causes

A relative or absolute increase in serum prolactin (secreted by the anterior pituitary gland) may result in galactorrhea. The discharge is milky in appearance, occurs from multiple ducts, and is most commonly bilateral. This is a normal end organ response to an inappropriate endocrine signal. Evaluation to define the specific aetiology of the galactorrhoea should be undertaken (Table 15.3; Section 13).

CLINICAL PRESENTATION: Women with a strong family history of cancer

The significance of family history in terms of assessing risk of developing breast cancer (Figure 15.9) ranges across a spectrum from 'normal risk' to 'very high' depending on the proportion of female relatives with the disease, the age of their diagnosis and whether they were first- or second-degree relatives. More than one first-degree relative with premenopausal cancer may be considered a rough threshold above which risk is high. Genetic counselling may be available for some of these women (Section 6). These women are fully aware that they are at increased risk and have often had negative experiences with breast cancer in their family members.

FIGURE 15.9 Mammogram (MLO view) showing a spiculated density which is tethered to the skin, causing distortion. These features are suggestive of malignancy and are easily seen, as fatty involution of the breast has occurred.

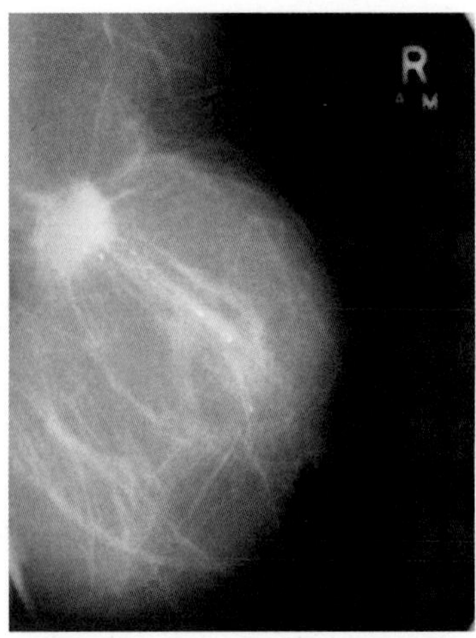

TABLE 15.3 Causes of increased prolactin release

Normal physiological conditions	Physical and emotional stress Eating (especially midday, high protein) Sleep Orgasm Exercise Late follicular and luteal phase of menstrual cycle Excessive breast stimulation Pregnancy/puerperium/nursing (up to 1 year after weaning)
Medications (via dopamine antagonism or stimulating pituitary lactotrophs)	Opiates Oral contraceptives Tricyclic antidepressants Methyldopa Metoclopramide Phenothiazine Cimetidine Calcium channel blockers Prochlorperazine Butyrophenones Amphetamines
Pituitary tumour	Pituitary adenoma (prolactinoma) also oligo- or amenorrhoea • Microadenoma (< 1 cm) most benign and remain stable or regress • Macroadenoma often associated with headache and bitemporal hemianopia Growth hormone producing pituitary lesions
Other	Hypothyroid (thyroid replacement results in resolution of hyperprolactinaemia as TSH normalises) Bronchogenic carcinoma and thoracic neoplasms Chronic renal failure Herpes zoster Hypernephroma

Source: Adapted from Falkenberry 2002.[6]

Investigations for diagnosis are no different from that of other women in their age group but a higher threshold of suspicion should be entertained at all times. To enhance early detection, mammographic screening is usually undertaken from an earlier age (10 years before the first degree relative was diagnosed, or 40 years of age, whichever is earlier) and at more frequent intervals (annually). There is some encouragement for regular ultrasound examinations for women in this high-risk category under the age of 35, but there is no population-based evidence of benefit on which to base such practices.

CLINICAL PRESENTATION: Asymptomatic women undergoing breast screening

See Section 14.

Pelvic floor disorders

The female pelvic floor is a remarkable structure representing a compromise between a number of different functions. It supports internal organs against gravity, has to guarantee urinary and faecal continence, allow evacuation of waste products and be elastic enough to permit birth. Anyone witnessing childbirth may wonder how normal function could possibly be resumed after such an event.

Pelvic floor dysfunction affects women about three times more commonly than men, resulting in pelvic organ prolapse, and urinary and faecal incontinence. Overall, up to half may suffer from such problems during the course of their lives, although many women don't actively seek help, despite the suffering caused by such symptoms. More than 10 per cent of women in the developed world will undergo surgery for pelvic floor disorders at least once in their lifetime. Pelvic floor dysfunction has significant effects on quality of life and important cost implications.

Anatomy and physiology

The female pelvic floor is a gutter-shaped structure, closing off the pelvis caudally and supporting the pelvic viscera. From above, it comprises endopelvic fascia, levator ani muscles, perineal membrane and external perineal muscles. It comprises three central openings: the urethra, the vagina and the anal canal (Figure 15.10). The former two are considered together and called 'urogenital hiatus'. The pelvic floor consists of:

- *Connective tissue:* the 'endopelvic fascia' above the levator muscle is a continuous sheet of connective tissue supporting uterus, bladder and urethra to the pelvic sidewall. The, pubocervical, transverse cervical (cardinal) and uterosacral ligaments are condensations of this fascia.
- *Muscle:* the 'pelvic floor muscle' or levator ani comprises the pubovisceral (pubococcygeus and puborectalis) and iliococcygeus muscles. The portion closest to the vagina can be palpated 3–4 cm above the hymen. The pubovisceral muscle is V-shaped and surrounds the urogenital hiatus and anal canal posteriorly, fusing with the vaginal wall and connecting the os pubis anteriorly with the vagina, perineal body, anal canal and coccyx.
- *Nerves:* the importance of the pudendal nerve is controversial but it seems clear that motor supply is via the sacral nerve roots S3 and S4 (see figures in Section 7).

FIGURE 15.10
Lateral view diagram of pelvic structures and 'pelvic floor muscles'

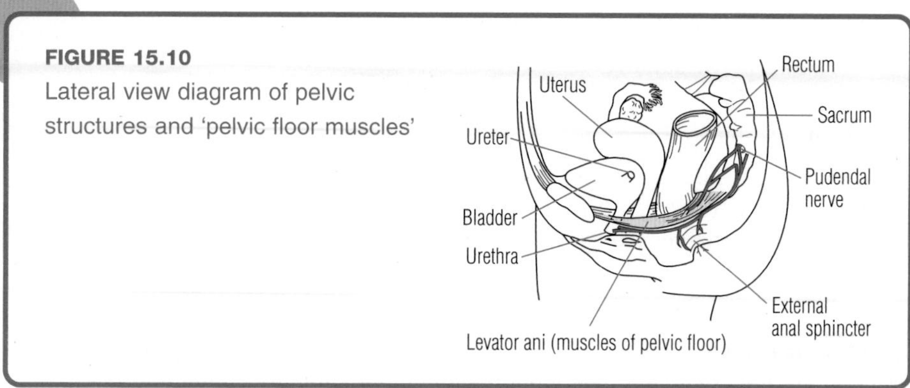

Aetiology of pelvic floor problems

Childbirth is important in the development of pelvic floor problems. However, nulliparous women can also be affected.

1 *Congenital factors* likely play a role in determining fascial strength, elasticity and resistance to trauma. Some women may have an inherently weak endopelvic fascia and therefore be at an increased risk of developing prolapse and stress incontinence.
2 *Acquired factors* play a major role.
   - *Childbirth:* stress incontinence and prolapse are associated with vaginal delivery, forceps or vacuum delivery, and possibly with birth weight and the length of the second stage of labour. It is unclear whether this association is due to fascial trauma or damage to muscle or nervous structures.
   - *Lifestyle:* obesity, chronic cough or constipation and such lifestyle factors as habitual lifting of heavy loads may also contribute, as do ageing and previous pelvic surgery.

Pelvic organ prolapse

CLINICAL PRESENTATION

Pelvic organ prolapse is the downwards displacement of urethra, bladder, uterus, small bowel and rectum, singly or in combination. Prolapse is generally more marked later in the day. Symptoms include:

- The feeling of a lump in the vagina, dragging sensation, low backache
- Bleeding and/or discharge from an ulceration.
- Voiding difficulty (see Table 15.4 on p. 546), which may occur with a large cystocele and urethral kinking
- Incomplete bowel emptying from a rectocele. Some women need to digitally replace the prolapse in order to defecate and micturate.

History

A number of risk factors and exacerbating factors should be covered in the history:

- Vaginal childbirth

- Operative delivery
- Previous pelvic surgery
- Obesity
- Constipation
- Chronic cough
- Smoking
- Connective tissue quality: history of hernia surgery or a family history of prolapse.

Clinical examination

Prolapse assessment is performed with the patient supine in lithotomy or the left lateral position, with a Sims speculum and after bladder (and if necessary bowel) emptying. Maximum descent of pelvic organs is observed during a strong valsalva manoeuvre. The vagina is divided into three compartments and the descent specified accordingly (Figure 15.11):

- Anterior compartment with urethra and bladder ('cystocele' or 'cysto-urethrocele')
- Central compartment with uterus or, if absent, the vaginal vault with small bowel ('uterine prolapse', or 'vault prolapse')
- Posterior compartment with small bowel and rectum/anal canal ('rectocele' and/or 'enterocele')

FIGURE 15.11 Varieties of uterovaginal prolapse

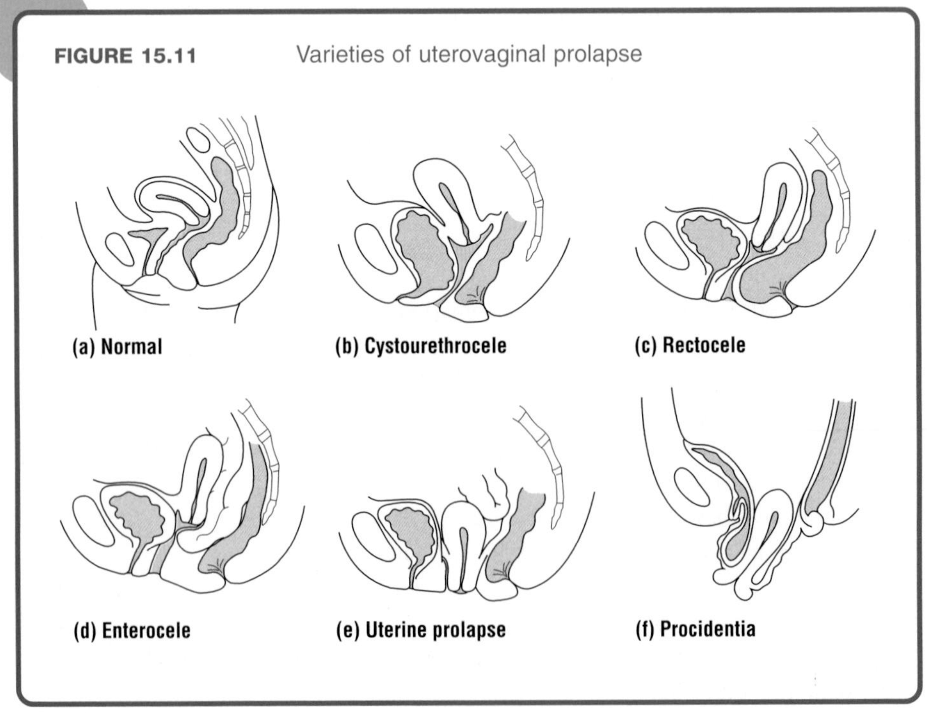

All those findings are graded:

- A first degree uterine prolapse descends to 1 cm above the hymen.
- A second degree uterine prolapse to within 1 cm below the hymen.
- A third degree further, until a fourth degree prolapse is reached with the organ completely outside the vagina (procidentia) (Figure 15.12).

FIGURE 15.12
Grades of uterovaginal prolapse

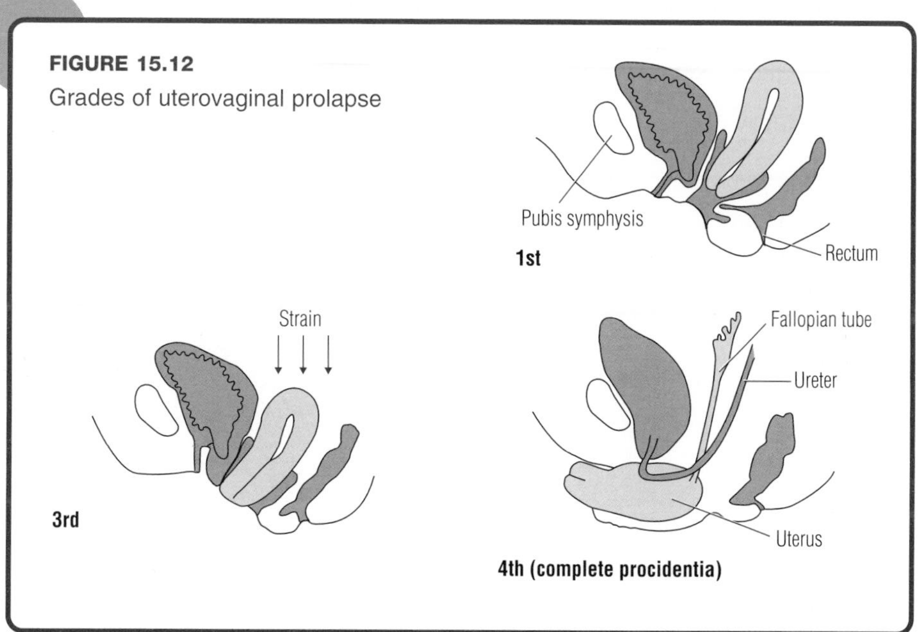

Differential diagnosis

Occasionally a cervical fibroid in vagina or introitus mimics prolapse; a vaginal (Gartner's) cyst or a large urethral diverticulum may do likewise.

Management

These conditions do not pose a threat to life but affect the quality of life. Treatment depends predominantly on symptoms and is influenced by the woman's medical fitness and her wish for further children. While enteroceles are true hernias, the hernial neck is so large that strangulation is not an issue. However, marked cystocele can result in urinary retention due to urethral kinking. Prolapse can also impair voiding, increasing the risk of urinary tract infections. Ulceration can lead to discharge and bleeding. Management comprises the following options:

- *Pelvic floor muscle exercises* or 'functional bracing' against increases in intra-abdominal pressure may reduce symptoms of prolapse.
- *Pessaries* are plastic rings, balls or more complex structures that are inserted vaginally to prevent descent of the pelvic organs. They have to be exchanged every 3–4 months. After menopause, local oestrogen is used to prevent ulceration.

- *Vaginal surgery:* the traditional mainstay of prolapse repair is anterior and posterior colporrhaphy often with vaginal hysterectomy. Colporrhaphy aims to repair defects in the fascia supporting anterior and posterior vaginal wall.
- *Abdominal surgery* is carried out in specialised units for recurrent prolapse. If vault prolapse occurs after hysterectomy, the vaginal apex may be sutured to the sacrospinous ligaments by dissecting the ischiorectal fossa until the ligament is reached (Figure 15.13, sacrocolpopexy).
- *Laparoscopic surgery* has recently been used for prolapse and incontinence procedures. Success rates seem to be similar to those of abdominal procedures.

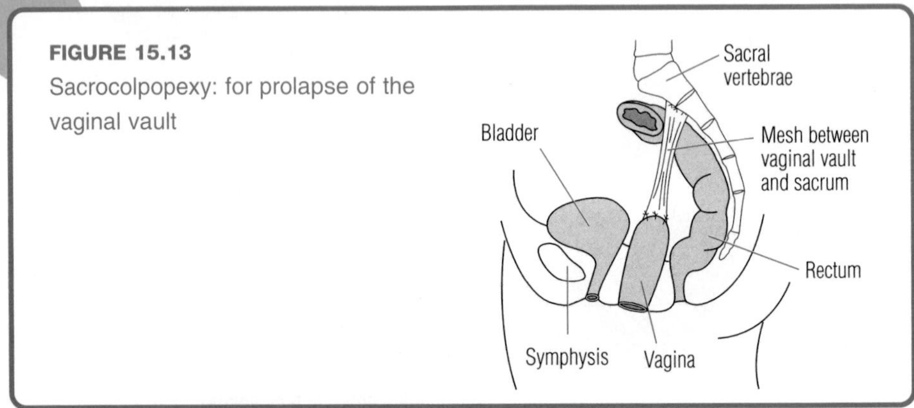

FIGURE 15.13
Sacrocolpopexy: for prolapse of the vaginal vault

Urinary incontinence

Urinary incontinence is a distressing condition with significant social implications. It is common, affecting 20 per cent of women aged over 40. Prevalence rises with age; urinary incontinence is not part of normal ageing, but age-related changes predispose to its occurrence (Section 17). Incontinence in women differs greatly between less developed and more developed countries.

Continence is maintained by several mechanisms which allow urethral pressure to exceed bladder pressure (Figures 15.14 and 15.15).

- *Bladder factors:* during bladder filling, bladder elasticity and cortical inhibition of the sacral reflex arc ensure that intravesical pressure changes very little.
- *Urethral factors:* urethral pressure is maintained by smooth and striated muscle, elastic tissue, blood vessel turgor in urethral wall and by mucosal folds of the lining.
- *Pressure transmission factors:* normally, bladder neck and proximal urethra are well supported intra-pelvic structures. When intra-abdominal pressure is raised (eg with coughing), this is transmitted to the proximal urethra as well as the bladder. This may be helped by active contraction of urethral striated muscle and levator complex. Thus the pressure gradient between urethra and bladder is maintained, and the patient stays continent.

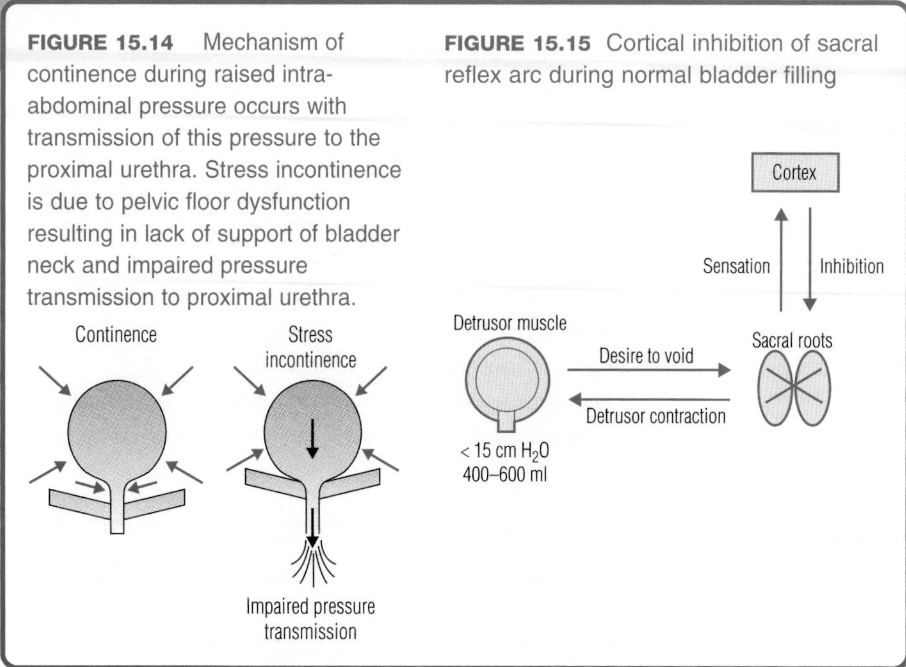

FIGURE 15.14 Mechanism of continence during raised intra-abdominal pressure occurs with transmission of this pressure to the proximal urethra. Stress incontinence is due to pelvic floor dysfunction resulting in lack of support of bladder neck and impaired pressure transmission to proximal urethra.

FIGURE 15.15 Cortical inhibition of sacral reflex arc during normal bladder filling

Classification of incontinence

The common and less common causes, pathophysiology and symptoms of incontinence are listed in Table 15.4.

History

This is generally more useful than examination. Combinations of symptoms (eg stress and urge incontinence) are common.

CLINICAL PRESENTATION

Urinary symptoms

- Involuntary leakage
- Urgency
- Frequency
- Urge incontinence
- Nocturia
- Nocturnal enuresis
- Situation during which leakage occurs
- Voiding dysfunction (hesitancy, poor stream, stop–start voiding),
- Dysuria
- Haematuria

Other symptoms

- Symptoms of prolapse
- Constipation

TABLE 15.4 Common and less common types of incontinence

Type of incontinence	Pathophysiology	Symptoms
Common		
Stress incontinence	Lack of bladder neck support and/or poor urethral closure	Involuntary leakage on effort, exertion, coughing and sneezing
Detrusor overactivity/ overactive bladder (Previously called detrusor instability/unstable bladder)	Failure of cortical inhibition of sacral reflex arc Idiopathic—anxiety, coffee intake and cold weather are said to influence symptoms Neurogenic (upper motor neuron lesion, ie multiple sclerosis, spinal trauma and cerebral vascular accidents) ? Urethral obstruction after surgery	Urgency: compelling desire to void, accompanied by fear of leakage and/or discomfort Frequency: > 7 voids during daytime hours Urge incontinence: involuntary loss of urine associated with a strong desire to void Nocturia: awoken at night one or more times to void Nocturnal enuresis: bedwetting
Less common		
Retention with overflow	Over-distension of bladder following surgery or delivery Urethral obstruction from a pelvic mass or faecal impaction Drugs or neurological disease	Dribble incontinence, symptoms of the overactive bladder and of voiding difficulty
Fistula	Less developed countries: prolonged obstructed labour and pressure necrosis of bladder base and vagina. More developed countries: pelvic surgical complications, radiation, advanced pelvic surgery.	Uncontrollable, continuous leakage

Effects

- Effect on quality of life, including protective clothing/pads worn

Past history

- Past urinary tract infections
- Symptoms of prolapse
- Previous treatment: conservative, pelvic or pelvic floor surgery
- Urinary complications of previous treatment (infection, retention of urine)
- Medical: neurological, cardiac, renal and endocrine abnormalities
- Childhood bedwetting as this is associated with later bladder overactivity

Drug history

- Benzodiazepines may cause confusion.
- Diuretics, lithium and caffeine may exacerbate urgency, frequency, nocturia and urge incontinence.
- Alpha-blockers such as prazosin may lead to stress incontinence.
- Antidepressants with their anticholinergic side effects can impair bladder emptying.
- Hormone replacement therapy is also relevant, as oestrogen deficiency, leading to atrophy of the urethra, may result in frequency, dysuria, urgency and voiding dysfunction.
- Smoking

Clinical examination

1 *General.* A limited general examination assessing overall health and mobility should be performed, since restricted mobility can precipitate incontinence if accompanied by urgency or inaccessible toilet facilities.

2 *Neurological.* A simplified neurological examination should be performed and the sensation in the sacral dermatomes (S2-S4) checked.

3 *Abdominal and pelvic* examinations are carried out to look for atrophic changes, prolapse and to exclude abdominal masses and retention. A clinical stress test (repeated coughs with or without valsalva manoeuvre) with a full bladder and, if necessary, in the standing position, demonstrates stress incontinence. Pelvic masses and faecal impaction should be excluded with a bimanual examination, and the pelvic floor assessed by the patient squeezing on the examiner's fingers.

Investigations

- Midstream urine is tested for glucose and protein, and cultured to exclude infection.
- A urinary diary records the timing of micturitions and voided volumes, incontinent episodes and the volume lost, pad usage and other information such as fluid intake.

History, examination and the above simple tests are the mainstay of investigation at a primary care level and allow the practitioner to make a presumptive diagnosis and start appropriate management.

Primary care management of stress incontinence

Stress incontinence is a common complaint among physically active women and may not require treatment. If treatment is requested by the patient, management options include:

- *Lifestyle intervention:* weight loss, caffeine reduction and avoidance of constipation
- *Adjust medication* if necessary (see above)

- *Pelvic floor muscle training* (PFMT): this is the mainstay of the conservative treatment of stress incontinence. After ensuring correct technique, a set of instructions is given. More important than the locally used protocol is the concept of using the levator when it is needed—that is, prior to coughing, heavy lifting etc. The success of PFMT is very dependent on the patient's motivation, and physiotherapists and nurse continence advisers have a very important role in this. Women have to continue with PFMT for at least 15–20 weeks to reach maximal effect. Up to 70 per cent can be expected to benefit.
- *Devices:* in particular those which support the bladder neck (Figure 15.16) are useful in selected patients, especially for 'exercise' induced stress incontinence. A wet tampon inserted prior to exercise may be enough to preserve continence in young active women.

FIGURE 15.16 Vaginal bladder neck supportive device (continence guard) for the treatment of stress incontinence

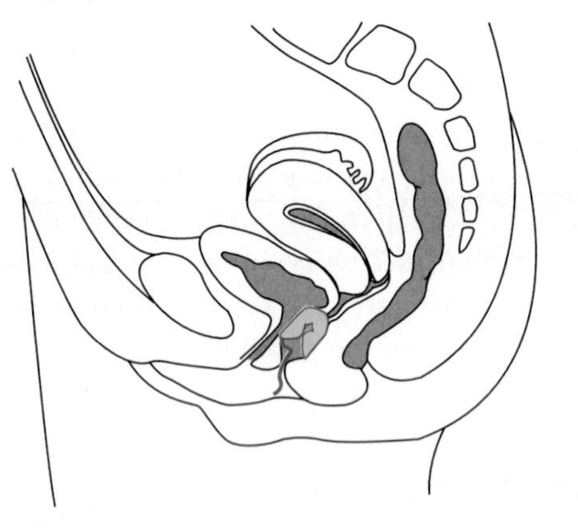

Primary care management of detrusor overactivity

All treatment of the overactive bladder is aimed at shifting the balance between factors favouring storage and those favouring leakage. This can be achieved in a number of ways:

- *Lifestyle intervention* aims at dietary modification to remove bladder irritants such as caffeine (tea, coffee, cola, chocolate).
- *Pelvic floor muscle training:* similar to stress incontinence, as pelvic floor muscle contractions can suppress uninhibited detrusor contractions.
- *Bladder retraining* uses urinary diaries to modify voiding habits. Times between voids are slowly increased, intake monitored (ideally 1.5–2 litres/day) and 'just in case' voiding discouraged. Behaviour modification is made possible either by mental distraction or by trying to suppress urgency. This is helped by a levator contraction until the urge subsides, but other tricks (sitting on the edge of a chair, crossing one's legs, curling one's toes) are also used.

- *Anticholinergics* are used to reduce the likelihood of an unstable contraction and to increase bladder volume. The most common drugs are imipramine (Tofranil), oxybutynin (Ditropan) and tolterodine (Detrusitol). All share anticholinergic side effects (dry mouth, palpitations, visual disturbances) and the possibility of urinary retention.
- *Vaginal oestrogens:* for postmenopausal women with oestrogen deficiency (atrophic vaginitis/ urethritis), vaginal oestrogens may improve frequency, urgency and recurrent UTIs and are recommended as a trial for three months, provided there is no contraindication.

Specialist management

Management by a gynaecologist, urologist or urogynaecologist is indicated for women with a complex history (recurrent incontinence, haematuria, recurrent infection, suspected fistula), voiding dysfunction, significant pelvic organ prolapse, and for women who are not significantly improved after a trial of conservative treatment.

The mainstay of specialist investigations is urodynamic testing. Cystometry, the measurement of bladder pressure in relation to volume changes, is used to diagnose detrusor overactivity (Figure 15.17). It is often combined with ultrasound or fluoroscopic imaging to diagnose 'urodynamic stress incontinence'—that is, urine leakage through the urethra in the absence of a detrusor contraction. Voiding function can also be assessed in detail.

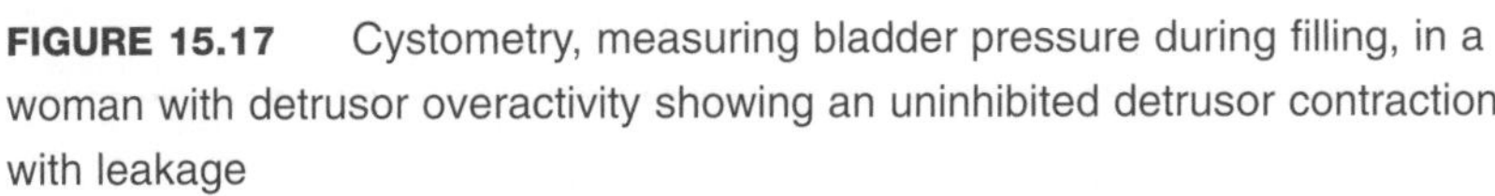

FIGURE 15.17 Cystometry, measuring bladder pressure during filling, in a woman with detrusor overactivity showing an uninhibited detrusor contraction with leakage

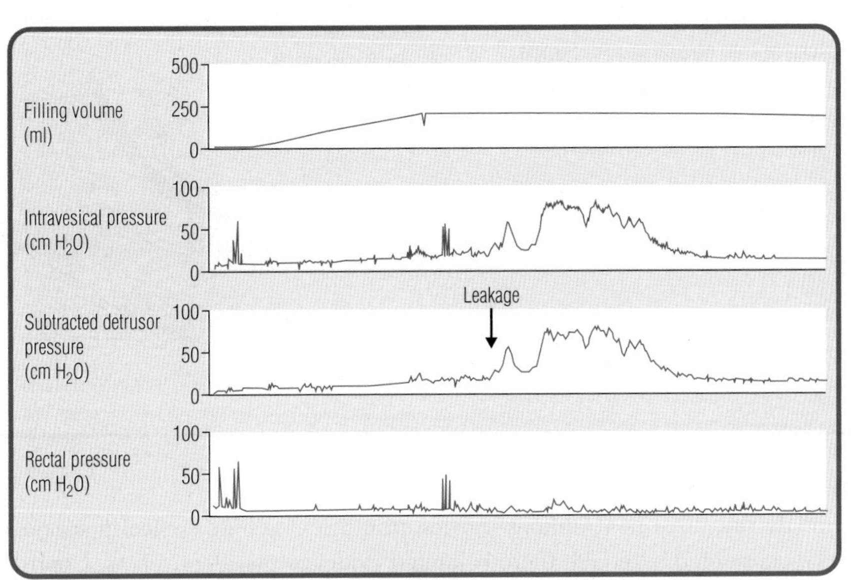

1 Urodynamic stress incontinence

Surgery aims to elevate a hypermobile bladder neck (to facilitate pressure transmission to the proximal urethra) or to compress the urethra, or both. Women with urodynamic stress incontinence should be counselled regarding the principles, types, success rates and complications of surgery to allow informed choice.

- *Anterior vaginal repair (colporrhaphy)* aims to support the bladder neck from below.
- *Colposuspension* elevates and immobilises the bladder neck by suspending the vaginal fornices to the iliopectineal ligament.
- *Slings:* fascial slings have mainly been used for recurrent stress incontinence. The advent of safe, simple synthetic slings such as the TVT (tension-free vaginal tape) has increased their popularity: they can be done as day cases. Success rates seem to be as high as for colposuspensions (Figure 15.18).
- *Injectables:* if the above procedures appear unsuitable, relief of stress incontinence can be achieved with the injection of collagen or other viscous fluids around the proximal urethra.

Retropubic operations give better results than vaginal repairs, with the first operation having the best chance of success. Colposuspension and sling procedures have a 70–85 per cent success rate and vaginal repairs and injectables an approximate 50 per cent success rate.

Complications of surgery include failure, voiding difficulty (5–10 per cent) and bladder overactivity (5–10 per cent).

FIGURE 15.18 Tension-free vaginal tape (TVT) sling for urodynamic stress incontinence—self-fixing prolene mesh sling supporting the mid-urethra

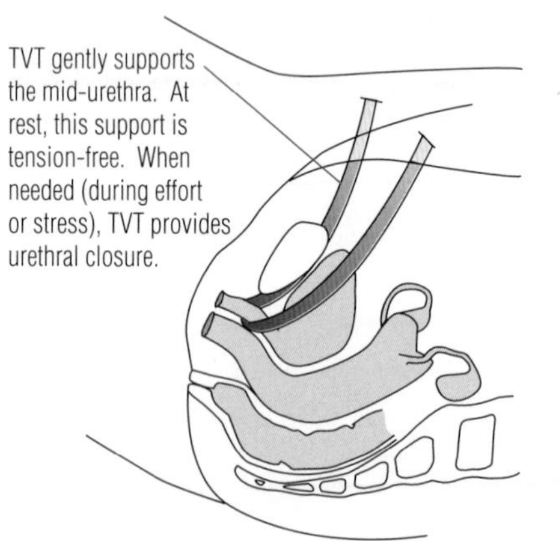

2 Overactive bladder

If primary care treatment options provide insufficient relief, surgical management may be considered, although there is limited evidence on effectiveness. Controlled overfilling of the bladder under anaesthetic, chemical denervation, sacral nerve stimulation via an implanted pacemaker and, for extremely disabling cases, bladder augmentation and urinary diversion, are offered mainly by urologists.

3 Voiding dysfunction

Voiding impairment is common, although often asymptomatic. If present, symptoms include hesitancy (slow start), poor stream, stop–start voiding, the feeling of incomplete emptying and/or the need to revoid. The history may reveal recurrent urinary tract infections. Any underlying cause should be identified and treated, such as a pelvic mass or significant prolapse such as a large cystocele with urethral kinking. Symptomatic treatment focuses on infection prevention (double voiding, urinary antiseptics, prophylactic antibiotics). If this is insufficient, then clean intermittent self-catheterisation is the best long-term option, and most women cope well with it.

CLINICAL PRESENTATION: Faecal incontinence

Problems with faecal incontinence can markedly impair quality of life and lead to people becoming housebound. Faecal incontinence is consistently reported to affect one per cent of the adult population living in the community and has been documented in seven per cent of healthy people over the age of 65 years. It is more common in women than men in a ratio of about 3:1. There is a frequent association with urinary incontinence and 26 per cent of people presenting to a urogynaecology clinic also complain of faecal incontinence.

Anatomy and physiology

The anal sphincter is about 3 cm in length and comprises external and internal sphincter and the overlying epithelium. The *internal sphincter* is under involuntary control, and is the main contributor to continence at rest. It only relaxes during evacuation and during sampling (momentary relaxation to detect rectal content). The *external sphincter* is thicker and made up of striated muscle, the upper third fusing with the puborectalis muscle. It is under voluntary control and is recruited when one needs extra assistance to ensure that rectal pressure does not exceed anal pressure when the rectum fills.

Aetiology of faecal incontinence

Many patients probably have a combination of varying degrees of both nerve and muscle damage.

- *Sphincter injury:* childbirth is often implicated in the development of faecal incontinence. In about 15 per cent of primiparous women the external anal sphincter is disrupted anteriorly by vaginal delivery. Sphincter injury may be part of a perineal tear but is often 'occult' with no disruption of the overlying epithelium.
- Denervation of the external anal sphincter has also been demonstrated in patients with incontinence. As the pelvic floor stretches during delivery the pudendal nerve and its branches may be damaged.

History

Symptoms of faecal incontinence may start soon after childbirth (one per cent of all deliveries) or occur in middle or later life. Symptoms may be of urgency or silent leakage.

- *Severity of faecal incontinence.* The frequency and amount of incontinence (use of pads) should be documented and whether this is to solid, liquid or gas. Enquiry should be made as to the effect of incontinence on the patient's quality of life and to the limitation on daily activities.
- *Obstetric history.* The risk of sphincter injury is greater with instrumental delivery (forceps), and increases with number of deliveries.
- *Other conditions.* A history of any previous anorectal surgery or problems, degenerative neurological disease, spinal cord injury or congenital abnormalities is important. In the work-up other anorectal or colonic pathology such as cancer or inflammatory bowel disease needs excluding.

Clinical examination

This involves inspection of the anus and perineum to note any scars, prolapse, haemorrhoids, fissures or fistulas. The perineum is often shortened with an external sphincter injury. The patient should be asked to valsalva to inspect for perineal descent and prolapse, and sensation of the perianal skin should be checked. Rectal examination may reveal a lax sphincter and the patient should be asked to squeeze to assess voluntary contraction.

Investigation

The most important investigation is *endoanal ultrasound* to examine the sphincter muscles for an anterior sphincter injury that could be repaired surgically (Figure 15.19). Anorectal physiology is often done to document anal pressures and pudendal nerve conduction.

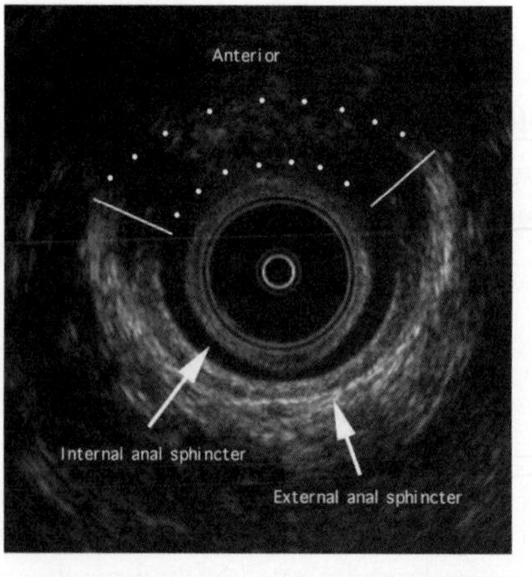

FIGURE 15.19 Endoanal ultrasound to assess integrity of anal muscles

Management

Conservative measures are tried first. This involves using loperamide to make a firmer stool that doesn't fragment and is easier for a weak sphincter to control. The majority of patients are greatly improved by achieving a state of relative constipation and some require the assistance of glycerine suppositories for regular evacuation. In addition to loperamide some recommend a low-residue diet as helpful, while others think a stool bulking agent is useful.

If conservative measures are unhelpful, *surgery* in the form of various pelvic floor operations can be used to tighten the sphincter. If there is an anterior sphincter injury demonstrated on ultrasound, this can be repaired with an 80 per cent success rate. Results with other procedures are poor and patients may need a permanent colostomy to restore continence.

Postmenopausal bleeding and discharge

This is a frequent presentation that may reflect the increased use of HRT, the early reporting by women and referral by the health practitioner for investigation.

CLINICAL PRESENTATION

Vaginal bleeding > six months after menopause.

The main aim is to exclude a malignancy. The risk of endometrial cancer increases with age and the number of risk factors present.

History

- Nature of bleeding: persistent, recurrent, or heavy bleeding is more suggestive of an endometrial carcinoma. Post-coital bleeding might suggest a cervical lesion. A watery discharge has been reported from carcinoma of the uterine tube.
- Risk factors for malignancy:
  - Early menarche (< 10 years)
  - Late menopause (> 55 years)
  - Nulliparity
  - Unopposed oestrogen therapy
  - Obesity
  - Diabetes
  - Hypertension
  - Liver disease
- Other symptoms:
  - Vaginal or vulval irritation
  - Bowel habit change
  - Abdominal discomfort, pain, swelling
  - Other vaginal discharge (Section 12)
- Local causes:
  - Use of a ring pessary

- Drug use:
  - Hormones
  - Herbal/OTC preparations
  - Warfarin/aspirin/NSAIDs
  - Pap test and mammography history

Examination

General: weight, blood pressure.
Pelvic: cervix and vagina for local causes. Bimanual for pelvic organs.

Investigations

See Box 15.1. Ultrasound of the pelvic organs can be valuable to check for ovarian tumours and endometrial pathology. It is dependent on the expertise of the operator. The 'cut-off' thickness of the endometrium in the postmenopausal woman not on oestrogen therapy, over which further investigation is indicated, has been suggested as < 5 mm. Uniformity of the endometrium is important as some lesions (polyps, cancer) may be focal.

Sampling of the endometrium is necessary to exclude hyperplasia or malignancy. However, the sensitivity of the different 'blind' sampling devices is variable and hysteroscopy and endometrial sampling is regarded as the 'gold standard' for diagnosis.

BOX 15.1 Investigations for postmenopausal bleeding

- Outpatient:
  - Transvaginal ultrasound
  - Sonohysteroscopy
  - Endometrial sampling
  - Hysteroscopy and directed endometrial biopsy
- Inpatient:
  - Hysteroscopy
  - Directed endometrial biopsy
  - Curettage

Differential diagnosis

This includes local and systemic causes (Table 15.5).

Management

The investigations are tailored to the individual woman after the history, examination and investigations have been taken into account.

TABLE 15.5 **Causes of postmenopausal bleeding**

General	Exogenous oestrogen	HRT, ginseng
	Endogenous oestrogen	Obesity (peripheral conversion of plasma androstenedione to estrone) Oestrogen-producing tumour
	Bleeding disorder	Warfarin, aspirin ingestion Diathesis
Non-genital tract	Bleeding from bowel, bladder or urethra	
	Bleeding due to a secondary cancer	Ovarian, colorectal, breast
Genital tract	Vulva	*Benign:* trauma, dermatitis, dystrophy *Malignant:* carcinoma
	Vagina	*Benign:* atrophic vaginitis, trauma, inflammation *Malignant:* carcinoma
	Cervix	*Benign:* polyps, atrophic changes, trauma, inflammation *Malignant:* carcinoma, adenocarcinoma
	Uterus	*Benign:* polyps, endometritis (HRT use) *Pre-malignant:* hyperplasia *Malignant:* adenocarcinoma
	Uterine tube	*Malignant:* carcinoma

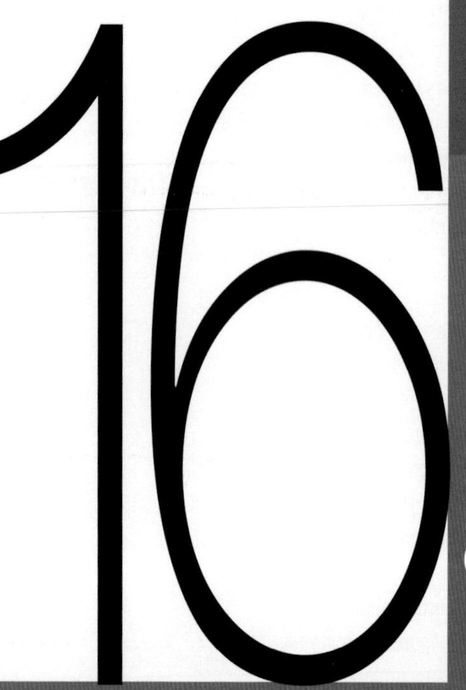

SECTION 16 Pre-cancer and cancer

Biology of cancer

Cancer arises because of genetic alterations which disrupt numerous cellular functions, thereby leading to an uncontrolled proliferation of one cell population. Cancers are characterised by their ability to metastasise and to invade surrounding tissues. The regulation of proliferation is a major determinant of the number of cells in a population. Alterations in genetic function may lead to stimulation of proliferation (oncogene) or loss of growth inhibition (tumour suppressor gene). Normal cells can undergo only a fixed number of cell divisions before the shortening of telomeres, the structures that cap each chromosome, arrests division. Malignant cells appear to be able to avoid this process by coding for telomerase, an enzyme that lengthens telomeres. Loss of growth inhibition can occur via two pathways—apoptosis (cell death) or senescence. Apoptosis is an active energy-dependent process that involves cleavage of DNA by endonucleases and proteases. Apoptosis may be triggered by a number of pathways but the most frequent is via the p53 tumour suppressor gene. The vast majority of cancer cell populations increase because of a decrease in apoptosis (tumour suppressor genes) as opposed to proliferation (oncogenes).

What causes genetic damage?

It is thought that all cancers arise from a series of genetic alterations, the origins of which are diverse and include exposure to carcinogens, inherited mutations or endogenous mutagenic processes. It is estimated that three to six alterations are required to fully transform a cell. In inherited cancers, several mutations may already be present at birth. The most common mutations responsible for hereditary cancer syndromes occur with tumour suppressor genes and DNA repair genes. There are only a few circumstances of oncogenes in germ line mutations being responsible for hereditary cancers.

Examples of tumour suppressor genes include PTEN, BRCA 1 and 2, p53, p16 and p27. Tumour suppressor genes usually involve a two-stage process of initiation of both copies of the gene. In most cases there is a mutation of one copy and deletion of a large segment of the other. Mutation of p53 is the most frequent genetic event described in human cancers. Approximately 20 per cent of endometrial carcinomas demonstrate p53 overexpression and mutation.[1] Many cancers have a 'missense' copy that is able to encode full-length proteins, but the produced proteins are unable to bind to receptor sites. The other important tumour suppressor gene in gynaecological malignancies is *PTEN/MMAC1*, located on chromosome 10q23, which is the genetic abnormality involved in hereditary non-polyposis colonic cancer (HNPCC) linked endometrial and ovarian cancer.[2] The *DCC* gene is another tumour-suppressor gene which is located on chromosome 18q. Expression is absent or decreased in 50 per cent of colorectal, pancreatic, breast and prostatic carcinomas.

Examples of oncogenes are Her-2/neu, EGF, K-ras and myc. Oncogenes produce peptide growth factors that bind to cell membrane receptors and then stimulate a cascade of events leading to nuclear changes and cell proliferation.

Invasion and metastasis

Normal tissue structure depends on cell-to-cell (cadherins) and cell-to-stroma (integrins) adhesion molecules. Cadherins are a superfamily of cell glycoproteins. Integrins are transmembrane adhesion receptors that bind to collagen, laminin, vitonectin and fibronectin. The genetic changes in cancer cells result in them gaining the ability to break down normal tissue structure by breaking the cell-to-cell and cell-to-stroma bonds via metalloproteases and thus obtain the capacity to invade tissue.

Solid cancers also need a new blood supply in order to grow. A solid tumour that is greater than 1 mm^3 has the ability to stimulate angiogenesis through proliferation of endothelial cells.

Premalignant change

Cervix

Cytology

Most cervical cancers are squamous cell carcinomas (85–90%), and only 10–15 per cent are glandular. The Pap test is the most successful screening tool for cervical pre-cancer. Pap testing is not designed to diagnose an invasive lesion or lesions of the endocervix. It is a screening test designed to detect pre-cancerous changes that may require further investigation. A false negative result may occur in the presence of an invasive cancer. This is most likely when the surface of the cervix becomes necrotic and produces an inflammatory exudate. It is vital therefore to always visualise the whole cervix; and anything that appears clinically suspicious, even in the presence of a normal Pap test, should be referred for biopsy.

Classification

The original Papanicolaou terminology has now been superseded by the Bethesda system (USA), which has several advantages. It has a specific statement about the adequacy of the Pap test and uses standardised terminology: normal, reactive changes, atypical squamous cells of uncertain significance (ASCUS), low-grade squamous intraepithelial lesion (LSIL), high-grade squamous intraepithelial lesion (HSIL) and malignancy. ASCUS suggests inflammatory or low-grade lesion. LSIL incorporates human papilloma virus, condyloma (warts) and cervical intraepithelial neoplasia (CIN) 1 (mild dysplasia in the old terminology). HSIL incorporates CIN 2 and 3 (moderate and severe dysplasia in the old terminology). In Australia, an additional category is used: 'inconclusive—possible high-grade abnormality', to indicate a lesion requiring immediate investigation.[3]

In the UK the term 'dyskaryosis' is used on Pap test reports. This is the cytological nuclear change associated with a histological diagnosis of CIN. The cytological report may include a prediction of histology (Table 16.1).

Glandular abnormalities can be detected by Pap test but may also represent abnormalities from higher up in the female reproductive system (cervix, endometrium, fallopian tubes and ovary). The standardised terms in the Bethesda system for glandular changes are atypical glandular cells of uncertain significance (AGCUS), adenocarcinoma in situ (ACIS) and adenocarcinoma. ACIS is defined as a replacement of endocervical glandular epithelium by cytologically malignant cells without evidence of stromal invasion. It is associated with HSIL in 50 per cent of cases.

TABLE 16.1 Papanicolaou, Bethesda and UK terminology of cytological and histological changes

Papanicolaou/UK	Bethesda	Cytological/histological appearance of the tissue
Atypia Inflammation	ASCUS	Atypia Inflammatory changes
Human papilloma virus (HPV) Predictive of CIN 1	LSIL	Characterised by the koilocyte, cells with perinuclear vacuolisation
'Borderline nuclear abnormalities' (BNA) introduced by British Society of Cervical Cytology (BSCC)	LSIL	BNA to be used when cellular changes differentiating benign atypia from early dyskaryosis are not clear cut.
Mild dyskaryosis Predictive of CIN 1	LSIL Inconclusive, possible HGIL	The lower third of the epithelium is undergoing dysplastic change with increased mitotic cells and loss of cellular polarity.
Moderate dyskaryosis Predictive of CIN 2	HSIL	The middle and lower third of the epithelium is undergoing dysplastic change with increased mitotic cells and loss of cellular polarity.
Severe dyskaryosis Predictive of CIN 3	HSIL	The full thickness of the epithelium is undergoing dysplastic change with increased mitotic cells and loss of cellular polarity.

CIN: cervical intraepithelial neoplasia, is a histological diagnosis.

Dyskaryosis is a cytological diagnosis.

ASCUS: atypical cells of undetermined significance; LSIL: low-grade squamous intraepithelial lesion; HSIL: high-grade squamous intraepithelial lesion.

CLINICAL PRESENTATION: Asymptomatic woman presents for Pap test screening

The main aim of Pap test screening is to detect women with significant degrees of pre-cancer, and to prevent progression to invasive cancer by removal or destruction of these changes. In the UK the mortality of cervical cancer was 15 per 100 000 population in 1986 and 8.9 per 100 000 in 1997 and continues to fall. The target of at least 80 per cent of women aged 20–64 having had a Pap test within five years has been exceeded since 1997.

A flaw in the Pap process is false negative results. These may occur because of:

- *Inadequate sampling.* Failure to visualise the whole cervix or sample the whole of the transformation zone and squamo-columnar junction (SCJ) with a full 360 degree sweep of the sampler. Where the SCJ is irregular and part or all of it lies outside the initial sweep, a second sample should be taken to ensure this zone is included. The presence of endocervical cells on the Pap test is a valid and convenient surrogate for sampling the SCJ[4] but should not be a substitute for adequate visualisation (Figure 16.1).
- *Poor sample obtained.* This may occur if:
  - The smear is too thick
  - There is blood or infection present
  - Too few cells are obtained (atrophy, drying effects, small lesion)
  - The Pap test consists almost solely of endocervical cells
  - The smear is poorly fixed.

  Improving the sample. In the postmenopausal woman the use of vaginal oestrogens nightly for 2–3 weeks before the Pap test is taken will improve the sample. If the cervix is dry or atrophic then dampening the spatula with normal saline will help cell recovery. Recommendations on types of samplers include the use of the extended-tip spatula for primary screening and investigation of women before and after treatment for cervical intra-epithelial neoplasia; the Ayre's spatula is the least effective device for cervical sampling.[4]
- *Liquid-based cytology* involves making a suspension of cells from the cervical samplers. This is used to produce a thin layer of cells on a slide and has the advantage of reducing the numbers of polymorphs and red blood cells, therefore making interpretation easier.
- *Incorrect laboratory processing*
- *Interpretative errors of the cell samples.*

Inflammation of the cervix is common. This may be due to acute or chronic inflammation or a repair process and should be able to be distinguished from neoplasia. Some infections can present in routine smears. These are *Trichomonas vaginalis*, candida, Actinomyces-like organisms, bacteria and herpes simplex cytopathic effects. A specific infection should be treated and the Pap smear test repeated.

False negative results may be minimised first by improving the sampling technique and second by automation allowing rapid re-screening of all negative smears. The development of laboratory standards in all developed countries minimises these problems.

Investigation of a Pap test change

Repeat Pap test

This is indicated at six months for an inadequate test or a low-grade change:

- After testing and treating for infection
- After treating with oestrogen in the postpartum and postmenopausal woman
- Using a sampler moistened with saline if the area is dry.

In the future HPV status may be used to refine referral for colposcopy.

FIGURE 16.1 The position of the squamocolumnar junction throughout life (a)–(d) Sagittal view (e)–(f) View through speculum

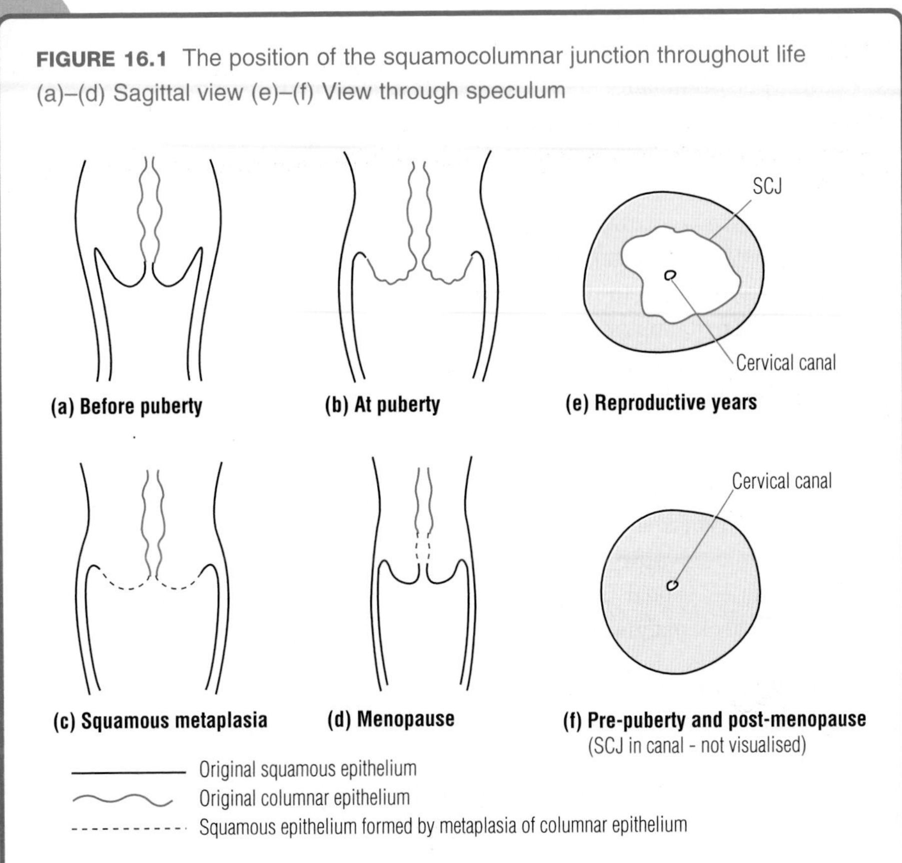

Colposcopy

Colposcopy is the system that allows both magnification and illumination of the cervix. The magnification range is usually between six- and forty-fold. The procedure involves exposure of the cervix and upper vagina with a bi-valve speculum and application of acetic acid (3% or 5%) that is left in situ for 5–10 seconds. The acetic acid will cause the columnar epithelium and abnormal epithelium to appear white (acetowhite) and is easily distinguishable from the normal pink squamous epithelium. Acetowhite epithelium is not diagnostic of CIN. It may also be found in association with HPV infection, immature squamous metaplasia, congenital transformation zone and regenerating epithelium. In general, the more intense the degree of change, the more extreme the cytological abnormality. The pattern and calibre of the sub-epithelial capillaries gives particular colposcopic appearances. These findings can be graded and may suggest the degree of abnormality. Markedly abnormal vessels are highly suggestive of early invasive disease but microinvasive lesions are frequently underdiagnosed.

Lugol's iodine may be used to outline atypical epithelium as this contains little or no glycogen and will therefore not take up the stain. Columnar epithelium also contains little or no glycogen and fails to take up the stain (Schiller's test).

Reasons to refer for colposcopy

- Women with HSIL on Pap test
- LSIL persistent after a repeat Pap test at 6 and 12 months. Between 20 and 40 per cent of women who have low-grade smear reports will have HSIL on biopsy. These lesions tend to be smaller than those presenting with high-grade cytological abnormalities on Pap test.
- Inconclusive—possible high-grade lesion on Pap test
- Abnormal/suspicious appearance of the cervix
- Abnormal bleeding or discharge as part of the investigation
- Persistent irritation or skin changes in the vulva or perineum
- Follow-up of any treatment of dysplasia and some cancers
- Post coital bleeding.

Biopsy

Diagnosis of cervical dysplasia usually requires a sample of tissue in the form of a punch biopsy. Where a high-grade lesion is reported on a Pap test, confirmed on colposcopy and an invasive lesion considered unlikely, then a punch biopsy may be omitted and an excisional method of treatment used (to obtain a final histological diagnosis and check margins of excision).

Human papilloma virus

The papilloma virus genus consists of many similar DNA viruses that are species-specific. At present over 80 human papilloma virus (HPV) genotypes and many sub-types have been identified. They all target and are confined to the epithelium, either the mucosal/genital or other cutaneous sites.

HPV infection may be:

- *clinical:* exophytic warts (HPV 2, 6, 11)
- *subclinical* (flat warts—only visualised after application of acetic acid. HPV 16, 18)
- *latent*.

The virus is transmitted during sexual intercourse and oral sex. The infection is often transient and causes mild, reversible cytological changes. In a minority of women the infection persists and results in cervical disease. The HPVs are described as 'low cancer risk' (HPV 2, 6, 11) or 'high cancer risk' (HPV 16, 18, 31, 33, 35, 45, 51, 52, 56). The latter is based on the detection of these types in most high-grade CIN and 95 per cent of cervical cancer,[5] their presence in cell lines derived from cervical cancer (eg HeLa), and their integration into the host genomic DNA in cervical cancers. HPV 16 accounts for 60–85 per cent of high-grade CIN and cervical cancer and HPV 18, 31, 33 and 35 for most of the remainder.

Correlation between histology and HPV status is not 100 per cent.

The progressive potential of CIN

Cervical intraepithelial neoplasm can progress to cervical cancer in some women. This is related to the grade (high-grade or low-grade), the size of the lesion and possibly other factors such as smoking. Invasive changes can be seen in association with all grades of change—not every woman passes through each change in turn and some invasive lesions can occur de novo or after an LGIL. Women who have been treated for CIN 3, compared to women without this change, have approximately a three-fold incidence of invasive carcinoma.

Treatment

Approximately eight per cent of cervical smears demonstrate some form of abnormality. However, the majority of patients only have minor cytological abnormalities and only a small percentage would develop cancer. Therefore, a balance needs to be made between treating all abnormalities and at the same time not missing any important changes. There is general agreement that high-grade lesions should be treated immediately, but that low-grade lesions may be observed over 6–12 months. This should take into account the chance of a woman defaulting from follow-up.

The whole transformation zone should be treated or excised. Cervical intraepithelial neoplasm can involve gland crypts, and so treatment to below the level of crypts (minimum 7 mm) is essential.

Main types of treatment:

- *Excisional methods*, where the sample is available for histological assessment—loop transformation zone (TZ) excision, loop biopsy, laser excision and cone biopsy. Large loop excision of the transformation zone appears to provide the most reliable specimens for histology.[6]
- *Destructive or ablative methods*, including cold (cryosurgery) or heat (laser ablation, electrodiathermy).

The evidence suggests that there is no obviously superior surgical technique for treating cervical intraepithelial neoplasia.[6] These procedures may be done under local analgesia (LA) or general anaesthesia. Hysterectomy is only used if there is another indication for the hysterectomy.

Complications

- Immediate: haemorrhage and pain
- Late complications:
  - Secondary haemorrhage (usually the result of a minor infection).
  - Pelvic infection and cervical stenosis.

Bleeding associated at the time of surgery under LA appears to be reduced by an injection of vasopressin into the cervix.[6] Cervical stenosis is more likely after large conisations, and affects 1–2 per cent of women managed by loop excision of the TZ. It is more likely in the postmenopausal woman. Stenosis may be asymptomatic or cause dysmenorrhea or, rarely, haematometra. Although a theoretical possibility, there is no data to confirm that local destructionary excision reduces fertility, or increases miscarriage, preterm labour or failure of the cervix to dilate in labour.

Follow-up

The arrangement for any investigation or procedure should also include an agreed method of communicating the results and making a future plan. Follow-up may include review at six months for cytology and possible colposcopy. The length of required follow-up by colposcopy is not known but most units will perform review colposcopy for up to 12 months depending upon the grade of the initial lesion.

Women who have had a hysterectomy and have never had any abnormal cytological changes in the cervix do not need follow-up Pap tests. However, continuing smears are required when:

- There has been treatment of CIN in the past.
- The hysterectomy has been as part of treatment of CIN.
- CIN is an incidental finding on the histology after hysterectomy.

Guidelines for follow-up have been developed in many countries and most countries are introducing national cervical screening databases that can be used to assist follow-up and recall in a mobile population.

Endometrial pre-cancer

Endometrial hyperplasia

These are classified as either having cellular atypia (endometrial intraepithelial neoplasia, EIN) or not having cellular atypia (endometrial hyperplasia, EH). The exact malignant potential of endometrial hyperplasia is controversial, with the presence or absence of cytological atypia being the most important indicator of malignant potential (Table 16.2). The amount of architectural abnormality appears to be irrelevant. The difference between EIN and invasive cancer is that in EIN there is no invasion into the underlying stroma.

TABLE 16.2 Risk of endometrial cancer with hyperplasia

Type of hyperplasia	Risk of progression to cancer
Hyperplasia without atypia (EH)	1–3%
Hyperplasia with atypia (EIN)	8–29%

CLINICAL PRESENTATION AND DIAGNOSIS

This is made on a histological sample of the endometrium taken as part of the investigation for heavy or abnormal bleeding, anovulation and infertility, or bleeding on oestrogen therapy.

Management

This depends on the fertility desired and menopausal status.

- In the peri- and postmenopausal woman, progestin therapy is effective at reversing endometrial hyperplasia without atypia. Daily continuous treatment should be given with a follow-up histological sample. If atypia is present, a hysterectomy is recommended.
- For the woman in reproductive years without atypia, either cyclical progestin or ovulation induction if a pregnancy is desired. If atypia is present then daily progestin is required and follow-up sampling of the endometrium.

Ovarian pre-cancer

Ovarian serosa is descended from coelomic epithelium that covers the nephrogenital ridge from where the ovary arises. Coelomic epithelium gives rise to both Müllerian and Wolffian ducts and therefore ovarian tumours can differentiate down either of these pathways. Ovarian tumours are classified as benign, low malignant potential (borderline) and carcinoma. There is no recognisable premalignant lesion of the ovary.

Vulvar pre-cancer

CLINICAL PRESENTATION

Persistent vulvar symptoms or a skin change.

A parallel preinvasive classification for vulval intraepithelial lesions is described essentially the same as for the cervix. The term *vulval intraepithelial neoplasia* (VIN) encompasses low-grade VIN 1 to high-grade VIN 2 and 3, which refer to squamous lesions. Vulval intraepithelial neoplasia has a similar histological profile to CIN but the malignant potential of VIN is low. It has been reported that progression to malignant disease of untreated VIN occurs in seven out of eight patients in eight years, whilst only four per cent of treated VIN progressed to cancer.

Management

Vulval intraepithelial neoplasia is frequently multifocal. It is evaluated with the colposcope and local biopsies taken for a histological diagnosis. Treatment is by local excision with regular annual follow-up once the lesion has been cleared.

Vaginal pre-cancer

This may be detected as part of a colposcopic follow-up for other genital tract pre-cancers. As with vulval premalignant conditions, there exists a vaginal intraepithelial neoplasia (VAIN) with mild dysplasia (VAIN I) through to severe dysplasia (VAIN III). Colposcopic evaluation, biopsy and local excision are indicated.

Gynaecological cancer: specific sites

Cervix

CLINICAL PRESENTATION

1 *Abnormal vaginal bleeding:* the most common symptom and in sexually active women this is manifested as postcoital bleeding (PCB).
2 *Vaginal discharge:* offensive in advanced tumours. Rarely the discharge may be the result of urine or faeces via the vagina, indicating a fistula.

Early diagnosis can be a challenge because of the asymptomatic nature of early disease, the significant false negative rate of Pap tests and because the origin of some tumours from inside the endocervical canal may make visualisation impossible.

Examination

Speculum examination should be performed and the *entire* cervix should be visualised. Digital vaginal/rectal examination is necessary to determine the extent of the disease and is usually performed under anaesthesia as a staging procedure.

Investigations (for diagnosis)

1 Histology. Biopsy of the tumour must be made to determine the cell type.
2 Pap tests are designed to predict the presence of preinvasive lesions and consequently have a false negative rate of up to 50 per cent in the presence of an invasive tumour.

Staging

This is clinical. According to International Federation of Gynaecology and Obstetrics (FIGO) staging rules the only other investigations allowable are CXR, IVP and examination under anaesthesia (EUA) with cystoscopy and/or proctoscopy. However, MRI has been used increasingly as a measure of tumour volume and size. Computerised tomography scanning has been used to determine the presence of enlarged pelvic lymph nodes and recently the use of PET scanning has been employed to determine whether metastases have occurred.

Metastases from cervical cancer

1 Direct (less than 1% to ovary; usually as per staging).
2 Lymphatic: sequentially up the nodal chain (bifurcation of internal/external iliac artery to para-aortic nodes)
3 Haematogenous—lung, liver, bones

Histology

Squamous lesions of the cervix

Squamous cell carcinoma involves invasion of cells into the underlying stroma with a desmoplastic response (stromal reaction). Diagnosis of cervical cancer usually requires a sample of tissue in the form of a biopsy. This sample may be small (a punch biopsy) or larger (obtained from a large loop excision of the transformation zone (LLETZ), laser cone or a cold knife cone biopsy of the cervix).

Glandular lesions of the cervix

Adenocarcoma in situ is defined as a replacement of endocervical glandular epithelium by cytologically malignant cells *without evidence of stromal invasion*. It is associated with HGSIL in 50 per cent of cases.

Adenocarcinoma can exhibit a variety of morphological patterns. The most common is the endocervical (mucinous) type.

Other tumours of the cervix

Numerous other types of tumours can develop as primary tumours of the cervix. These include sarcomas (derived from connective tissue elements in the cervix), melanoma, lymphoma or metastatic tumours (endometrium, vagina, ovary, bladder, bowel, colon, stomach and breast).

Epidemiology

Cervical cancer is the major cause of death from gynaecological cancers worldwide, with great variation in incidence dependent upon screening programs and cultural issues (eg Brazil 83/100 000, Israel 3/100 000, age-standardised mortality rates).

Early age of first intercourse appears to be important in the development of cervical cancer, probably due to adolescence being a period of heightened squamous metaplasia, with exposure to HPV virus increasing the likelihood of atypical transformation. Multiple sexual partners increase the risk of exposure to high-risk HPV serotypes. Both these factors suggest that safe sexual practices and the use of barrier contraception may reduce the risk of cervical cancer.

Human papilloma virus detection carries a minimum 10-fold increase in risk of cervical neoplasia, with over 90 per cent of CIN and 95 per cent of invasive cancers attributable to HPV infection. Smoking creates potentially mutagenic substances which are secreted in the cervical mucus and is an independent risk factor for cervical cancer. Long-term use of the OCP may lead to an increase in adenocarcinoma but this is far from proven. Immunosuppressed women (women with AIDS or a transplant) are far more likely to have progression of their CIN than women with normal immunology. Population studies have shown a declining mortality from cervical cancer due to cytological screening programs (Pap test). Case control studies have shown a risk reduction by a factor of 10 if a woman has a Pap test every three years.

Treatment

Treatment can be divided into either surgical or chemoradiation (concurrent chemotherapy and radiation) with the aim of selecting patients so that only one modality will be used for treatment. This is done to reduce the risk of complications that, generally speaking, increase if more than one form of treatment is required. It is felt that surgery has fewer ongoing complications than chemoradiation and, if possible, should be the mode of treatment even though the two carry the same chance of cure stage-for-stage.

The goal of radiation is to encompass the primary tumour, paracervical tissue and regional lymph nodes within the radiation field. If needed, the para-aortic nodes can be included.

Concurrent chemotherapy (cisplatin) and radiation has now become the standard of care for treatment of cervical cancer with an improvement in survival of approximately 25 per cent (National Cancer Institute 1999). The possible positive interaction occurs through inhibition of repair of radiation damage, cell synchronisation, recruitment of non-proliferating cells into cell cycle and reduction of the hypoxic fraction.

For stage IA1 the treatment is cone biopsy if fertility is required, or hysterectomy. For all other tumours up to 4 cm in size a radical hysterectomy and resection of pelvic lymph nodes is required.

Once the tumour is greater than 4 cm in size there is a 40 per cent chance of lymph node involvement and pelvic radiation is indicated. In an effort to reduce the increased morbidity of combined surgery and radiation, the primary treatment modality is chemoradiation for larger tumours.

Very occasionally, a woman will present with a vesicovaginal or rectovaginal fistula that can be treated by primary exenteration (removal of rectum, bladder and vagina) or radiation and diversion of the bowel or ureters (colostomy or ureterostomy).

Recurrence

If the initial disease extended into the parametrium or nodes were positive, then exenteration is not indicated. However, if the recurrence is central with no pelvic wall involvement, then pelvic exenteration is an option. Chemotherapy is used in some cases for palliation, with the drug of choice being cisplatin.

Prognosis

The five-year survival illustrates the importance of early diagnosis (see Staging, survival and spread, Table 16.3, p. 582). Poor prognostic features include positive lymph nodes, larger tumour size, depth of cervical stromal invasion, lymph/vascular space invasion, small cell carcinoma and close vaginal margins.

Endometrial cancer

CLINICAL PRESENTATION

Abnormal vaginal bleeding:

- Ninety per cent of women with endometrial cancer have abnormal vaginal bleeding, most commonly postmenopausal bleeding (PMB). It should be noted that of women presenting with PMB only 15 per cent will have endometrial cancer.
- Intermenstrual bleeding or heavy prolonged bleeding in the premenopausal woman should be treated with suspicion.

Examination

Routine vaginal examination: note the size and mobility of the uterus, cervical involvement and whether the adnexa appears normal.

Investigation

1 Endometrial biopsy in clinic setting: 10 per cent false negative rate
2 Hysteroscopy and curettage if:
   - Biopsy unsuccessful or shows hyperplasia
   - Ultrasound of the endometrium shows irregularity or increased endometrial thickness (5 mm or more) in a postmenopausal woman.

Staging

This is surgical. The pelvic and para-aortic nodes should be evaluated. There are no specific investigations other than a CXR which is used as part of the staging of the disease. Tumour volume is the most important prognostic factor for all tumours.

Histology

Adenocarcinoma

There are numerous morphological types named after the tissue most closely resembled by the tumour—endometrioid (uterine), serous papillary (tube), clear cell (renal) and mucinous (endocervix). Squamous cell carcinomas of the endometrium are rare.

Sarcoma

Uterine sarcomas are rare tumours arising from the mesoderm and account for about three per cent of uterine tumours. There are numerous classification systems but a simple version is to divide them into *pure* or *mixed*. Pure represents those tumours arising *only* from mesodermal elements such as leiomyosarcoma and endometrial stromal sarcomas. Mixed represents tumours arising from both mesodermal and epithelial elements, such as carcinosarcoma. The number of mitoses present per 10 high power fields is the best predictor of malignant behaviour.

Epidemiology

Endometrial cancer (EC) is the sixth most common cancer in women and interestingly the fourth most common cancer in women aged 25 to 59 years.[7] It has a cumulative risk to age 75 of 1.4 per cent, with 25 per cent of these women dying from endometrial cancer.

Type 1 endometrial cancer (typically endometrioid) is due to excess exposure to oestrogen. This can be due to either an increased circulating level of oestrogen or from normal levels unopposed by progesterone:

- Obesity (increased peripheral conversion of androstenedione)
- Diabetes via the actions of insulin-like growth factor 1, hyperinsulinaemia or increased oestrogen levels. This association may only hold true for obese diabetic women.
- Oestrogen-producing tumour
- Anovulatory cycles: polycystic ovarian syndrome
- Unopposed oestrogen used in hormone replacement therapy.

Type 2 endometrial cancer (serous papillary and clear cell) is not oestrogen driven and is possibly related to p53 abnormalities. These cancers carry a mortality of at least 50 per cent.

Women with a family history of hereditary non-polyposis colonic cancer (HNPCC) are at greater risk of developing EC before the age of 50, with studies showing lifetime risks of between 22 and 46 per cent in these cases. The OCP protects against EC through its strong progestogenic effects.

Treatment

There are few circumstances where primary treatment should not be surgical, where the aim is to remove all disease. The procedure of choice is total abdominal hysterectomy and bilateral salpingo-oophorectomy (BSO), with pelvic and para-aortic lymph nodes being removed in high-risk cases. In grossly obese women a vaginal hysterectomy may be performed and in some units a laparoscopic-assisted vaginal hysterectomy with BSO will be performed.

The following cases are deemed to be at high risk of lymphatic spread of the tumour and require pelvic and para-aortic lymph node dissection: grade 3 lesions, grade 2 tumours > 2 cm in size, clear cell carcinoma or serous papillary carcinoma, greater than 50 per cent myometrial invasion and/or cervical extension of the disease.

The presenting pathological grade or cell type from either an endometrial biopsy or dilatation and curettage is a *poor* predictor of the true pathological specimen obtained upon removal of the uterus. Therefore, intraoperative assessment of the uterus is used, with studies showing it has a high predictive value (> 90%) of the true and final pathology.[8]

It is uncommon for endometrial cancer to present as Stage IV (widespread metastases most likely to lung). Surgical treatment may still be appropriate to obtain local control of the disease and for palliation of symptoms (bleeding, foul discharge, fistula formation).

The role of radiation in endometrial cancer can be divided into five categories:

1 Adjuvant treatment after surgery to reduce pelvic recurrences (either external beam radiotherapy (EBRT) or brachytherapy—intravaginal) is given to deeply invasive tumours.
2 External beam radiation for women with proven positive lymph nodes.
3 Curative intent for patients not deemed suitable for surgery.
4 Curative intent for isolated vaginal/pelvic recurrence if not previously given radiation.
5 Palliation for metastatic disease.

Chemotherapy is not effective for endometrial cancer, nor has progesterone any role in adjuvant treatment.

Sarcomas are uncommon uterine mesodermal (non-epithelial) tumours that are treated primarily by surgical removal of the uterus. Adjuvant treatment may be useful in some cases, with commonly used modalities being irradiation to the pelvis and chemotherapeutic agents such as doxorubicin or ifosfamide.

Prognosis

Stage I has a 75 per cent five-year survival, which appears to be poor but it must be remembered that within this group there are some extremely high-risk cancers. Grading by architectural pattern and nuclear criteria are important prognostic factors and are related to other prognostic factors. In general, as the grade becomes more poorly differentiated there is a greater chance of deep myometrial invasion, extension to the endocervix and node involvement.[9]

Ovarian cancer

Epithelial ovarian cancer

CLINICAL PRESENTATIONS

Most women with epithelial ovarian cancer have no symptoms for long periods of time and this is the main reason for late presentation of this disease.

1 Vague and non-specific with abdominal bloating and changes in bowel function being common
2 In advanced cases, anorexia, weight loss, nausea, vomiting, abdominal distension from ascites and bowel obstruction may occur.

Examination

Routine abdominal and pelvic examination may demonstrate a pelvic mass (See Pelvic mass).

Investigations

The diagnosis of ovarian cancer requires an exploratory laparotomy to obtain tissue for histology and staging information about the spread of the disease. Some pre-operative tests may be useful.

1 CA-125 determination is non-specific for ovarian cancer.
   - *Post menopause:* an increased level and a pelvic mass in a postmenopausal woman is 90 per cent predictive of an ovarian cancer.
   - *Pre menopause:* endometriosis and fibroids may also be associated with a raised level.
2 A CXR may show a pleural effusion. This would then require a pleural tap to obtain cytology and, if positive, means stage IV disease is present and may change treatment.
3 CT scan may diagnose intrahepatic lesions or may be useful when there is no mass present with ascites in excluding other intra-abdominal causes of cancer.

Staging

Surgical staging should be performed because every subsequent treatment will be determined by the initial stage of the disease. In some series where careful staging was performed by gynaecological oncologists after an initial laparotomy, 30 per cent of the cancers were upstaged from stage 1 to stage 3.

Histology

These are usually serous, endometrioid or mucinous. About 10 per cent of ovarian serous tumours are low malignant potential and carry a good prognosis. However, serous carcinomas account for 75–80 per cent of all ovarian cancers and are bilateral in 60 per cent of cases.

Mucinous tumours of low malignant potential carry an excellent prognosis unless associated with a condition called pseudomyxoma peritonei, which occurs when pools of floating mucin are found free within the abdominal cavity. Mucinous carcinoma accounts for 10 per cent of all ovarian cancers. Endometrioid and clear cell tumours are less common, with the later carrying a poor prognosis.

Epidemiology

The incidence of ovarian epithelial cancer is influenced by country of origin, race and age. The highest are in industrialised countries (except Japan) with the lowest in non-industrialised countries (incidence varies from 14.9/100 000 population to 2.7/100 000 population).

Multiple factors have been mooted for the development of ovarian cancer, from environmental (radiation/talc) to rubella exposure, coffee, fat and vitamin consumption. More established relationships exist between number of children, oestrogen replacement, oral contraceptives, tubal ligation, hysterectomy, BRCA1 and 2 mutations and mismatch repair gene mutations and the development of ovarian cancer.

Continuous OCP use may reduce the risk of developing ovarian cancer by up to half. The safety of menopausal hormone replacement has been debated, with some epidemiological papers stating that there is an increase in risk. However, other studies have not shown this effect.

Several independent groups have reported that tubal ligation confers a protective effect (OR 0.72). Hysterectomy also confers a protective effect.

Genetic

About 5–10 per cent of all ovarian cancer will be due to a genetic predisposition, with the most common being due to BRCA1 (long arm chromosome 17) and BRCA2 (chromosome 13). Each offspring has a 50 per cent chance of inheritance but for unknown reasons it has variable penetrance, with some clusters causing ovarian cancer dominated families and others (more commonly) causing breast cancer dominated families. BRCA1 confers a risk of ovarian cancer of between 28 and 40 per cent (depending on penetrance and the population studied) of developing ovarian cancer by age 70. The BRCA2 risk is about 27 per cent.

Approximately three per cent of ovarian cancer is caused by mismatch repair gene mutations, commonly hMSH2 and hMLH1, on the short arm of chromosomes 2 and 3 respectively. These are associated with HNPCC but affected people can have renal and endometrial cancer in addition to colon and ovarian cancer.

Prophylactic oophorectomy may add 2.5 life years to the above groups but up to five per cent will develop primary peritoneal carcinomatosis. This is a disease very similar to ovarian carcinoma arising from the peritoneum. Prophylactic oophorectomy reduces the risk of breast cancer to a hazard ratio of 0.53. Laparoscopic prophylactic oophorectomy has a significant role to play in the management of these women.

Treatment

For early stage cancer (stage 1a & b), the staging laparotomy (TAH, BSO, collection of peritoneal washings and lymph node biopsies, omentectomy and careful inspection) may be all that is required for treatment. In women wanting fertility a unilateral salpingo-oophorectomy (USO) may be performed but requires careful follow-up.

Advanced stage disease requires 'debulking' surgery followed by chemotherapy. Debulking or cytoreductive surgery aims to eliminate the primary tumour and all of the metastatic disease in the abdomen. The rationale for this extensive surgery is three-fold—firstly to reduce the physiological effects of ascites and the intestinal masses and obstruction that may occur; secondly to improve tumour perfusion and increase growth fraction, which may help the effects of chemotherapy; and thirdly to improve the immunological function, as large tumours masses have been shown to be immunosuppressant.

All patients if medically fit will receive six cycles of chemotherapy consisting of carboplatin and paclitaxel as soon as possible after surgery.

Radiation therapy is not first-line treatment and has limited application to situations such as recurrent disease limited only to the pelvis. It can be given either as whole abdominal or pelvic field depending on the circumstances. Chemotherapy is generally favoured over radiotherapy.

Non-epithelial ovarian cancers

Germ cell tumours

CLINICAL PRESENTATION

In contrast to the relatively slow-growing epithelial tumours, germ cell tumours are rapidly expanding tumours.

1 Acute pelvic pain, which may be due to haemorrhage into the tumour or necrosis.
2 Bladder and bowel pressure symptoms
3 Menstrual irregularities.

Examination

Abdominal examination may reveal a mass or tenderness. Vaginal examination is inappropriate in premenarchal girls.

Investigations

1 Expert ultrasound examination: abdominal (and vaginal if appropriate).
2 Adnexal masses greater than 2 cm in size in *premenarchal* girls or complex masses in premenopausal women require surgical exploration for diagnosis.
3 Tumour markers in the form of AFP, HCG, LDH and PALP are useful in the evaluation of a pelvic mass in this population.
4 CT or MRI scan is useful to exclude retroperitoneal lymph nodes or liver metastases.
5 A karyotype should be obtained in all *premenarchal* girls as tumours often arise from dysgenetic gonads.

Treatment

Surgery is the mainstay of treatment, with the aim of completely removing the tumour if possible. It also provides invaluable data on the staging of the tumour and, in early dysgerminomas and immature teratomas where disease is confined to the ovary, is curative.

Chemotherapy is required in all other cases after surgical staging. Radiation, whilst effective in some instances, causes loss of fertility and is therefore not used as first-line treatment.

Other types of ovarian tumour

- *Germ cell tumours* of the ovary are thought to derive from the primordial germ cell and consequently can be a mixture of various cell lines. Seventy per cent of tumours in the first two decades of life are germ cell tumours, with only one-third of these being malignant. Mature teratomas (dermoid cysts) are the most common germ cell tumour, which has a very low chance of malignancy (approximately 1%). Macroscopically these tumours consist of mostly ectodermal elements such as hair, skin, sebaceous glands plus some endodermal elements such as bone and cartilage.
  The malignant germ cell tumours are dysgerminoma, endodermal sinus tumour, embryonal carcinoma and immature teratoma.
- *Sex cord stromal tumours* account for approximately eight per cent of all primary ovarian tumours and contain derivatives of embryonic gonads (granulosa and Sertoli cells) and ovarian stroma (theca, lutein and Leydig cells). Most are benign tumours with the exception of granulosa cell tumours (which are a low-grade malignancy) and Sertoli-Leydig cell tumours (well differentiated tumours have a good prognosis; poorly differentiated tumours have a poor prognosis).

Vulval cancer

CLINICAL PRESENTATION

1 Lump, ulceration or skin change on the vulva
2 Pruritus
3 Bleeding, pain, discharge or dysuria are less common.

Examination

Careful examination of the vulva, anus, vagina and cervix are required because five per cent of these cancers will be multifocal. Areas on the vulva causing symptoms that do not settle with treatment should have a biopsy to obtain a diagnosis.

Investigation

1 Biopsy of the area that includes the underlying tissues to obtain accurate results.
2 CT scan of the groin and pelvis is useful to determine the presence of enlarged nodes but has a significant false negative rate.
3 CXR is required for staging (Stage IV if positive).

Staging

Staging is surgical and spread to nodes can only confidently be excluded after surgical removal of the groin nodes. The role of sentinel node biopsy is still being evaluated.

Histology

Ninety per cent of vulval cancers are squamous cell carcinomas.

Epidemiology

Vulval cancer constitutes about four per cent of female genital tract malignancies. The common association between cervix, vaginal and vulval cancer suggests HPV and smoking as high risk. HPV DNA has been identified in 20–60 per cent of invasive cancers of the vulva. The HPV-positive group are usually younger, have greater tobacco use and have VIN present with the invasive part of the tumour.

In contrast, the disease in older women is unrelated to HPV but is more likely associated with lichen sclerosis. Of note is that up to 20 per cent of women with vulval malignancy have an invasive or pre-invasive lesion elsewhere in the genital tract but usually of the cervix.

Treatment

Management of vulval cancer should be broken into two parts.

Primary lesion

- *Small:* if small enough to be completely excised with a 1 cm clear margin without resorting to some sort of pelvic exenteration, then surgery is the choice of treatment. This is usually performed as a radical wide local excision, with the defect being closed primarily or with some type of flap. If an adequate margin is not obtained then local radiation is required.
- *Large:* if effective removal will require exenteration then pre-operative radiation with chemotherapy is now the primary mode of treatment. This is followed by wide excision of the tumour bed. If there are enlarged nodes (> 2 cm) on CT that may act as 'sanctuary sites' for the cancer, then these can be removed prior to irradiation.

Groin nodes

The groin nodes are removed through one or two separate incisions (left and/or right depending on the relationship between the primary cancer and the midline of the vulva). If the nodes contain two or fewer micrometastases then no further treatment is required.

Role of radiation

Radiation therapy may be used in the following circumstances:

1 Patients with inguinal node metastases, to reduce recurrence and improve survival.
2 Positive surgical margins or other high-risk features—positive pelvic nodes.
3 Used instead of exenterative surgery where the disease involves the anus or urethra.
4 Primary treatment for small tumours in the clitoral areas.
5 Treatment of vulval recurrences.

Increasingly, chemoradiation is being used in the treatment of vulval cancers, with the most active compounds being 5-FU and cisplatin.

Prognosis

The number of positive groin nodes is the single most important prognostic variable in the five-year survival (see Staging, survival and spread, Table 16.3).

Other vulval malignancies

Ten per cent of invasive cancers are adenocarcinoma. Other cancers of significance are melanomas, basal cell carcinoma, verrucous carcinoma and sarcomas.

Paget's disease of the vulva is an adenocarcinoma in situ of sweat glands with a small proportion having an underlying invasive adenocarcinoma (< 10%). It is difficult to treat because the macroscopic margins are usually involved with microscopic disease and recurrence is common.

Vaginal cancer

CLINICAL PRESENTATION

1 Painless bleeding or discharge from the vagina most likely presentation.
2 No symptoms: about 10 per cent of cases will be detected on Pap test alone.

Examination

Most lesions are on the upper one-third of the vagina and are usually exophytic. The tumour is easily missed on speculum examination of the vagina as it can lie under the bills. If there is no obvious tumour and there is an abnormal Pap test, careful colposcopic examination with Lugol's iodine is required.

Investigations

1 Multiple biopsies of the vaginal mucosa may be required to make a diagnosis and indeed excision of the upper vagina may be required for definitive diagnosis.
2 CXR.
3 Examination under anaesthesia with cystoscopy.
4 MRI and CT scanning are used in an attempt to determine the extent of disease and direct treatment but not for staging.

Histology

The most common cancer type is SCC, with adenocarcinoma comprising a much smaller proportion. The most widely known sarcoma is embryonal rhabdomyosarcoma, which grows from the vagina in young children and if possible is treated primarily with surgery.

Only 20 per cent of vaginal tumours are primary (arising from the vagina), with the rest being metastases from cervix, endometrium, colon, rectum, ovary, vulva and kidney.

Vagina: lymphatic drainage

The upper third is the same as the cervix; the middle third may crossover; the lower third is the same as the vulva.

Epidemiology

Vaginal cancer represents one per cent of malignancies of the female genital tract. Eighty per cent are metastatic from the cervix, endometrium, colon, ovary, vulva or renal. The aetiology is unknown but a similar aetiology to the cervix and vulva is suspected. Of interest is the concept of a multifocal carcinoma of the female genital tract involving cervix, vagina and vulva.

The true malignant potential of vaginal intraepithelial neoplasia (VAIN) is unknown, with studies showing five per cent of VAIN progressing to invasive cancer despite radiotherapy. Thirty per cent of primary vaginal cancer patients had a history of either CIN or cervical cancer leading to three possible causes for the disease in these cases:

- occult residual disease
- new primary disease
- radiation transformation in areas receiving sub-lethal doses.

Treatment

Due to the low frequency of the disease there is no consistent approach to vaginal cancer. A reasonable management is to treat surgically only those tumours that are Stage I confined to the upper vagina. Another role for surgery is in the young woman where transposition of ovaries can be performed prior to radiation. Pelvic exenteration may be appropriate for a central recurrence after treatment with radiation.

Chemoradiation is now the standard of care with data extrapolated from cervical cancer, and comprises a combination of brachytherapy and external beam radiation. The most commonly used chemotherapy is cisplatin and/or 5 FU.

Prognosis

The major predictors of poor outcome are large tumour volume/size, low vaginal lesions and lesions of the posterior wall (see Staging, survival and spread, Table 16.3).

Principles of treatment

Surgery

The role of surgery in gynaecological oncology is multifaceted and ranges from early diagnosis to palliation. Early diagnosis and prevention may be attained by the treatment of preinvasive lesions such as CIN and VIN. In women at high risk of developing ovarian cancer (HNPCC, BRCA) then prophylactic oophorectomy can substantially reduce risk.

Diagnosis and staging are required to optimise treatment. Diagnosis should always be a histological diagnosis and may be made by punch or excision biopsy. Fine needle aspiration (cytology) may be adequate for determining the extent of spread of disease but not for diagnostic purposes. With the exception of cervical and vaginal cancers, all cancers are surgically staged. Staging and diagnosis requires cooperation between the pathologist, cytologist and gynaecological oncologist.

Surgery can be used for primary treatment with the aim of clearing gross and microscopic disease with minimal removal of normal tissues. In cases such as Stage Ia2 to Ib2 cervix cancer, Stage I vaginal cancer and Stage I to III vulval cancer, the surgical procedure is based on removal of the primary disease site and the regional lymph nodes with the intent to cure without the need for adjuvant treatments.

Surgery is also combined with other modalities (chemo, hormonal, radiation) for treatment. Ovarian cancer relies on debulking surgery (removing all macroscopic disease) with adjuvant chemotherapy.

Occasionally, surgery can be used as salvage treatment in cases such as recurrent cervical, vulval, vaginal and endometrial cancers. In such cases, exenteration followed by reconstructive procedures may be curative.

Reconstructive surgery, particularly for vulval cancers, in the form of grafts, rotation and advancement flaps is important in attempting to normalise the visual damage created by treatment.

Occasionally, metastatic tumours will be resected—this is usually for symptom control but in some instances may prolong survival.

Palliative surgery may be required for symptom control, eg small bowel diversion/ bypass procedures or interrupting sensory nerve transmissions. There is a balance between the provision of relief of symptoms and the detrimental effects of the surgical procedure, which should always be discussed with the patient. Sometimes the relief of one symptom, such as placement of a ureteric stent, may be replaced by a more difficult symptom to treat (nerve root infiltration by the tumour) due to the change in the natural history of the cancer.

Radiation oncology

Radiation oncology is a specialised field of medicine using ionising radiation alone or in combination with other modalities. Ionising radiation is defined as radiation that is able to knock bound electrons from their orbit. This has a direct and indirect effect on the cells' DNA. The direct effect is the electron striking the DNA moiety, causing damage. The indirect effect (more common for X-rays) causes the formation of a hydroxyl radical, which in turn produces the DNA damage.

The aim is to deliver a precisely measured dose of irradiation to a defined tumour volume (and field) with minimal damage to surrounding normal tissues. This is performed using the known extent of the tumour, the pathological cell type and the intent of treatment (cure or palliation). This leads to an optimal dose to be delivered and follow-up evaluation to examine the effects.

Radiation techniques

Radiation can be delivered by a variety of means:

- *Teletherapy*—delivered at a distance from the body (EBRT)
- *Brachytherapy*—source placed within or adjacent to cancer
- *Radioactive solutions*—placed into a cavity, eg peritoneum.

Effects of radiation

No correlation has been found between the incidence and severity of acute reactions and the same parameters for late effects. Factors enhancing the propensity to injury are general and nutritional condition, hygiene, infection, surgery and chemotherapy.

The main areas affected in gynaecology are skin, small and large intestine, bladder, ovaries, bone marrow, peripheral nerves and sometimes liver and kidney.

1 Acute—within the first six months:
   - Skin changes—dry and moist desquamation and ulceration
   - Intestinal reactions—watery diarrhoea, abdominal cramps, rectal discomfort and passage of blood and mucus
   - Bladder dysfunction—cystitis, spasm and haematuria
2 Late effects occurring after six months:
   - Skin changes—atrophy
   - Bladder—in more severe cases chronic cystitis, fibrosis, reduced bladder volume and vesicovaginal fistula may occur.
   - Ovarian function is susceptible to even scattered low-dose irradiation, with doses causing significant damage and higher doses inducing menopause and loss of fertility.
   - Vaginal stenosis is common.
   - Peripheral nerve damage, renal and liver damage are unusual in gynaecological treatments.

Chemotherapy

Tumour biology

There are three populations of cells in normal tissues: static, expanding and renewing. Static populations, represented by striated muscle, neurons and oocytes, rarely undergo cell division. Expanding populations, represented by liver parenchyma and vascular epithelium, proliferate only under times of stress. Renewing populations, represented by bone marrow, epidermis, GIT and spermatocytes, undergo continuous proliferation.

This can be used to explain some of the problems seen with toxicity of chemotherapy. Normal tissues with static populations are unlikely to suffer significant problems, while renewing populations with constant cell turnover are most sensitive to acute problems.

Tumour cell growth undergoes 'Gompertzian' growth, which means in the early phases of tumour life, growth is occurring at an exponential rate but as the tumour enlarges growth slows (that is, as mass increases so does the time taken to double its volume). Most chemotherapeutic agents act by disrupting critical DNA, RNA or protein synthesis and are therefore more likely to be effective on rapidly proliferating cells.

The use of chemotherapy is a balance of benefits versus risk of toxicity. In some germ cell tumours of the ovary, chemotherapy has been responsible for dramatic increases in survival, whilst in epithelial ovarian cancer there is a high response rate initially but only a modest improvement in survival. A third group of gynaecological cancers such as endometrial cancer has a moderate response rate but very little improvement for survival for the majority of patients.

Choice of regimens

Adjuvant chemotherapy refers to the initial use of chemotherapy after surgery and /or radiation therapy with intent to cure the cancer. It is used in situations where, after initial therapy, the relapse rate without adjuvant chemotherapy is high.

Concurrent chemoradiation refers to the use of chemotherapy as a way to sensitise the tumour to the effects of radiation. It is given concurrently with curative intent. This can increase the toxicity to bone marrow in particular.

Neoadjuvant chemotherapy refers to the use of chemotherapy in situations where the management of locally advanced tumours precludes curative surgery, or the morbidity of curative surgery can be significantly reduced if chemotherapy is given before surgery.

Salvage chemotherapy refers to states where disease has returned after initial treatment and the goal is palliation of symptoms rather than cure.

Toxicity

Chemotherapy regimens are universally toxic with a narrow therapeutic window. Toxicity is common and falls into following categories: bone marrow, GIT, skin and hair, neurotoxicity, genitourinary and hypersensitivity reactions.

Bone marrow

This is the most frequent dose-limiting toxicity encountered, generally occurring 7 to 10 days post treatment. White blood cells are most often affected, with the absolute neutrophil count the best predictor of dose tolerance and risk of infection. Febrile neutropenia (neutrophils < 500 and temperature over 38°C) is a life-threatening condition and needs immediate treatment with broad-spectrum antibiotics. Granulocyte-stimulating factor (G-CSF) may be of benefit in this situation. Thrombocytopenia occurs less commonly, later post treatment, and generally requires no active treatment unless bleeding occurs. Moderate degrees of anaemia are common and contribute to fatigue, with blood transfusions used for treatment in severe cases. Erythropoietin is a safe but expensive alternative. Dose modifications are made cycle to cycle depending on the degree of bone marrow toxicity.

Gastrointestinal toxicity

Most chemotherapy agents cause some degree of nausea, vomiting and anorexia. Prophylactic treatment reduces these problems and increases the acceptance of the treatment. Most regimens include a 5-HT antagonist with dexamethasone. Anticipatory nausea and vomiting can also be a significant problem. Diarrhoea, oral mucositis, oesophagitis and gastroenteritis can also occur.

Skin and hair

Although almost always reversible, scalp alopecia is an emotionally taxing side effect of chemotherapy. In gynaecological cancers the most common cause is the use of paclitaxel; however, alopecia occurs with many other chemotherapeutic agents. There is no effective treatment. Skin problems include hypersensitivity and allergic reactions, hand foot syndrome and local extravasation necrosis.

Neurotoxicity

Peripheral neurotoxicity manifested by decreased proprioception and fine motor tasks, loss of vibratory sense, high-frequency hearing loss and deep tendon reflexes is common with the use of cisplatin and paclitaxel. It can progress after therapy has ceased and may resolve slowly, but sometimes it can be irreversible. It is related to the cumulative dose and dose intensity, and while there is no effective treatment, switching to carboplatin avoids many of these problems.

Renal toxicity

The main culprit is cisplatin even though only small proportions are cleared through the kidney. Maintaining good hydration and attention to urinary output during and after treatment is required. Switching to carboplatin virtually eliminates the problem.

Hypersensitivity reactions

Paclitaxel is a natural product with poor solubility and is formulated in cremephor, the compound associated with mast cell degradation and clinical hypersensitivity reactions. These can be managed with prophylactic antihistamines/steroids followed by rechallenge at a lower rate.

There are many different follow-up protocols. There is no evidence that intensive follow-up improves outcomes, however, psychological support may improve quality of life (see Women and cancer).

Staging, survival and spread

Staging

This is a method of assessing the spread of the cancer. It is used to direct management, evaluate modes of treatment and estimate outcome. Tumour volume is the most important prognostic factor for all tumours (Table 16.3).

Pattern of spread

1 Direct to surrounding tissues
2 Lymphatic
3 Haematogenous

TABLE 16.3 Staging of and survival after gynaecological cancer

Cancer		Staging	Five-year survival
Cervical	I	Confined to cervix	
		A1 ≤ 3 mm depth and ≤ 7 mm lateral	A > 95%
		A2 > 3 mm ≤ 5 mm depth of invasion and ≤ 7 mm lateral	B 80%
		B1 > 7 mm ≤ 40 mm	
		B2 > 40 mm	
	II	Stage IIa—extension to upper $^2/_3$ of vagina	
		Stage IIb – extension to parametrium but not to pelvic walls	66%
	III	Stage IIIa—extension to lower $^1/_3$ of vagina	
		Stage IIIb—extension to pelvic sidewall or radiological evidence of hydronephrosis	35%
	IV	Stage IVa—extension posteriorly or anteriorly to bladder or rectum	20%
		Stage IVb—distant spread	
Endometrial (surgical)	I	Confined to uterus	
		a endometrium only	75%
		b inner $^1/_2$ myometrium	
		c outer $^1/_2$ myometrium	
	II	Spread to cervix	
		a endocervical glands only	60%
		b cervical stroma	
	III	Mixture of tumour outside of uterus	
		a serosa, adnexa, or positive cytology	30%
		b vaginal metastasis	
		c retroperitoneal node metastasis	
	IV	a bladder/bowel involvement	
		b distant metastasis	10%
Ovarian (surgical)	I	Confined to ovary	
		a one ovary	
		b both ovaries	
		c tumour or surface of ovary/ies, rupture, ascites or positive washings	
	II	Still within pelvis	
		a to uterus/tubes	
		b other pelvic structures	
	III	Outside pelvis but within abdominal cavity	
		a microscopic seeding of peritoneum	
		b < 2 cm implants on peritoneum	
		c > 2 cm implants or spread to retroperitoneal nodes	
	IV	Stage IV––distant metastases	
		Parenchyma of liver, pleural effusion with positive cytology	

TABLE 16.3 continued

Cancer		Staging	Five-year survival
Vulva	I	Confined to vulva and < 2 cm in size	
		a invasion ≤ 1 mm deep	90%
		b invasion > 1 mm deep	
	II	Confined to vulva/perineum > 2 cm in size	75%
	III	Two distinct groups:	
		• any spread to vagina/urethra/anus	50%
		• spread to unilateral lymph nodes	
	IV	a Two groups:	
		• upper vagina (urethra/anal mucosa)	20%
		• bilateral lymph node involvement	
		b Distant metastases	
Vagina	I	Confined to vagina	70%
	II	Into paravaginal tissues	50%
	III	To pelvic side wall	30%
	IV	a bladder/rectal invasion	20%
		b distant metastases	

The development of breast cancer

In the last few decades there has been an increasing awareness among women of the importance of early detection of breast cancer. As a consequence of this, and particularly the contribution made by mammographic screening programs, the average size of detected breast cancers has decreased, as has the incidence of lymph node involvement at the time of initial treatment (Table 16.4).

Breast cancer death rates have been falling in Australia, the UK and the USA since the early 1990s. Improvements in adjuvant (systemic) treatment together with earlier detection by mammographic screening are thought to have contributed to this decline.

TABLE 16.4 Effect of breast screening on stage at which cancer is detected

Tumour size/node involvement	Screen detected	All cancers
< 15 mm	60.3%	42.7%
Node positive	22.5%	30.0%
1–3 nodes positive	18.7%	23.4%
> 3 nodes positive	8.4%	14.2%

Source: AIHW 2001.[10]

The use of breast-conserving surgery has increased substantially in the last two decades as a consequence of the evidence that a mastectomy confers no benefit in survival and also as a result of the detection of smaller primary tumours which are more amenable to breast-conserving treatment.

The development of a breast carcinoma probably involves a series of transformations which begins with proliferation of the epithelial cells that line the milk ducts (ductal hyperplasia). The next step is a change in the appearance of the epithelial cells, described as atypical ductal hyperplasia, which may progress to a *non-invasive malignancy*—ductal carcinoma in situ (DCIS). Ductal carcinoma in situ is a proliferative condition in which malignant cells are confined within the basement membrane of the ducts. When these malignant cells breach the basement membrane and extend into the surrounding tissues, this is described as *invasive* ductal carcinoma (IDC). Lobular carcinoma in situ (LCIS) follows a similar process but in spite of the name, LCIS is no longer classed as a malignant process. However, evidence shows that, as with DCIS, women with LCIS have an increased risk for the subsequent development of invasive cancer (about 15 per cent within 15 years).

Ductal carcinoma in situ is a non-invasive malignant process that appears to arise from the epithelium of the breast ducts. Of the various histological types, some show the feature known as 'comedo necrosis' with the formation of microscopic deposits of calcium in the affected ducts.

These microcalcifications are easily detected on mammography so that most cases of DCIS are now detected on routine screening mammography (Figure 16.2). In some cases with more extensive disease, the changes in the breast may develop into a palpable mass or thickening. Atypical ductal hyperplasia is sometimes associated with mammographic calcification and in these circumstances it is usually excised to exclude the possibility of adjacent DCIS.

Ductal carcinoma in situ

Since DCIS is a disease confined within the ducts, it has no ability to spread to the regional lymph nodes or to metastasise elsewhere, but spread along the ducts will occasionally produce a change in the nipple known as Paget's disease.

Although DCIS is a non-invasive malignancy with no resultant mortality, it is likely that it is a stage in the sequential development of many invasive breast cancers. If left alone, DCIS may eventually transform into invasive carcinoma, and women who have had DCIS treated have a substantial increase in risk of subsequent invasive carcinoma (Table 16.5). For all these reasons, it is usually recommended that when DCIS is identified, it should be completely excised (Figure 16.3). Where the process is extensive, this may require a mastectomy. Paradoxically, small invasive cancers can be treated conservatively more easily than extensive intra-duct (in situ) disease, and this may be difficult for a woman to understand.

Adjuvant radiation treatment is also used in some cases of DCIS, particularly high-grade lesions or those with close surgical margins. Evidence shows that in such cases, radiotherapy can reduce the risk of local recurrence (as in the case of invasive cancer). In fact, following treatment of DCIS almost half the recurrences are invasive rather than in situ: this subset of invasive cancers is also reduced by adjuvant radiation treatment. Although tamoxifen has been trialled as adjuvant therapy for DCIS, the evidence suggests that any benefit is small.

TABLE 16.5 Risk of invasive breast cancer after treatment for DCIS

Year since diagnosis	SIR	(95% CI)
< 1	8.0	(1.6–23.3)
1–4	6.5	(2.6–13.3)
≥ 5	11.7	(5.6–21.5)

n=186
13/19 (68%) were ipsilateral
SIR: standardised incidence ratio (ie in DCIS cases versus normal population)
Source: adapted from Franceschi et al 1998.[11]

FIGURE 16.2 Mammogram showing extensive malignant calcification due to ductal carcinoma in situ (craniocaudal view)

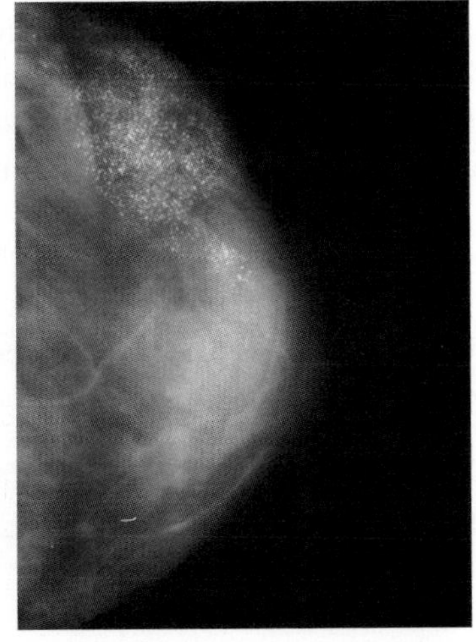

FIGURE 16.3 Operative specimen mammogram showing tiny focus of ductal carcinoma in situ (calcification) excised after guidewire localisation

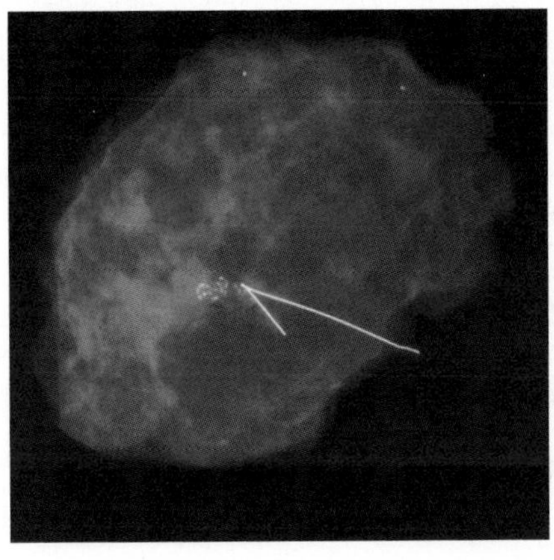

Lobular carcinoma in situ

Lobular carcinoma in situ (LCIS), in spite of its name, is a benign proliferative change which begins in the acini of the terminal duct—lobular unit. Although in some cases LCIS may extend into the ducts, it is essentially a change in the lobules and it is no longer regarded as a malignant condition. Lobular carcinoma in situ is usually diagnosed by chance in the course of a breast biopsy for another purpose, for example in tissue removed at the time of a breast reduction. Lobular carcinoma in situ itself causes no symptoms and is not usually identifiable on mammography.

The atypical hyperplasias

The atypical hyperplasias occur in both the ducts (atypical ductal hyperplasia, ADH) and the lobules (atypical lobular hyperplasia, ALH). Again, these are non-malignant processes but they may indicate the first step in a progression which is eventually expressed as invasive malignancy.

The significance of the breast pre-cancer lesion

Lobular carcinoma in situ, ADH and to a lesser extent ALH, are associated with an increased risk of subsequent invasive malignancy, and so women who have these conditions diagnosed should enter a surveillance program with regular (usually annual) mammography.

Breast cancer management

Historically, breast cancer was detected when a woman discovered a lump or other breast change (Box 16.1). Although some breast cancers are still discovered as a breast lump by the woman or her doctor, an increasing proportion of primary breast cancers are now detected by mammographic screening (in Australia, approximately 50 per cent of breast cancers are screen-detected). The quality of the mammogram and the experience of the reader are key elements in the detection of early breast cancer. In optimal conditions, it is not unusual to detect primary cancers of 6–7 mm in size.

Examination

It is useful to document clinical findings describing the position of a lump either according to the breast quadrant (eg right or left upper outer quadrant, RUOQ or

BOX 16.1 Clinical presentation of breast cancer

- Asymptomatic:
  - Abnormality detected on mammographic screen
- Symptomatic:
  - Breast lump or thickening
  - Nipple distortion/ulceration
  - Pain—localised and non-cyclical
  - Nipple discharge—serous or bloody
  - Skin changes—distortion, oedema, tethering
  - Pathological lymph node

LUOQ) or as a clock face with the nipple as the center of the clock (eg 3 o'clock position), and also the distance from the nipple. The size of the lump should be recorded (in two dimensions for larger lesions), in addition to any associated features.

Investigations for a diagnosis of breast cancer

When a lesion is detected on a screening mammogram, further investigation usually includes ultrasound examination and fine needle aspiration or core biopsy of the abnormality (Box 16.2). Cytological examination of a fine needle aspirate has a high diagnostic accuracy but core biopsy provides a precise histological diagnosis. For this reason there has been a drift away from cytology towards core biopsy in recent years.

The aim of these investigations is to provide a preoperative diagnosis so that the initial and subsequent treatment can be discussed in detail with the woman prior to surgical treatment. In cases where there remains doubt about the diagnosis after thorough investigation, an open surgical biopsy may be necessary to establish the diagnosis.

BOX 16.2 Investigations used in the diagnosis of breast cancer

- Mammography—primary diagnostic tool. Limited benefit in women < 30 years and in women with breast prostheses.
- Breast ultrasound—additional imaging investigation after clinical or mammographic abnormality detected. Also, first imaging choice for women < 30 years.
- Fine needle aspiration cytology
- Core biopsy
- Vacuum assisted core biopsy
- Large core biopsy (ABBI)

  (Core biopsy, vacuum assisted core biopsy and large core biopsy: under local anaesthetic for histological diagnosis)
- MRI—rarely, because of high cost, limited availability, technical demands and non-specificity of some findings. Useful in assessing integrity of breast prosthesis.

Pathology

In almost 90 per cent of cases, carcinoma of the breast arises in the lactiferous ducts and is therefore described as *ductal carcinoma*. In the remainder of cases, the disease arises in the glandular acini and has a characteristic histological pattern identified as *lobular carcinoma* (Box 16.3).

As an epithelial malignancy, breast cancer behaves in much the same way as other invasive cancers. In some cases, at an early stage, it may show extension into blood vessels or lymphatics of the breast and spread to the regional lymph nodes, usually of the axilla and internal mammary group. Irrespective of the position of the tumour in the breast, the majority of lymph node metastases appear in the axillary nodes. In the case of breast cancer, distant metastases appear most frequently in bone (typically the axial skeleton), liver and lungs.

BOX 16.3 **Classification of breast cancer**

Invasive cancer (90%)

- Potential for local and distant metastatic spread
  - Invasive ductal carcinoma (not otherwise specified, 75%)
    - Medullary carcinoma (5%)
    - Mucinous (colloid) carcinoma (5%)
    - Tubular carcinoma (3%)
  - Invasive lobular carcinoma (10%)
  - Other forms (2%)
    - Papillary carcinoma
    - Adenoid cystic carcinoma
    - Inflammatory carcinoma

In situ cancer (10%)

- Metastatic disease should not occur unless unrecognised invasive cancer is present.
  - Ductal carcinoma in situ
  - Paget's disease of the nipple

Prognostic factors

The prognosis of primary breast cancer is determined principally by three factors: tumour size, tumour grade and nodal status. Of these, lymph node status is the most powerful predictor and the risk of recurrence (and death from breast cancer), is directly related to the *number* of nodes involved at the time of initial surgery. The larger the tumour at the time of diagnosis, the greater the risk of metastatic disease, and of the three conventional histological grades, Grade III has the highest risk of subsequent metastatic disease. Each of these (size, grade and nodal status) is an independent prognostic variable, so the effect of each variable adds to the overall prognosis.

Epidemiology

Like many other malignancies, breast cancer is an age-related disease, with a higher incidence among women in their later years. From an annual incidence of 2 per 100 000 among women aged 20–29, the incidence of breast cancer rises steadily to approximately 300 per 100 000 among women in their eighties. Many earlier studies showed a transient fall in incidence among Western women in the early menopausal years but more recent data shows a biased increase in incidence among women in their fifties, due to the implementation of mammographic screening programs.

Risk factors

The cause of breast cancer is assigned to mutations in the relevant genes. In any individual, a concurrence of genetic errors, including loss of DNA repair/tumour suppressor genes, may be required to initiate the malignant process. In a small proportion of cases, an inherited mutation may determine the development of a cancer (see Familial/genetic factors). Other factors that influence the risk of breast cancer are summarised in Table 15.1.

Of the external influences, the use of combined HRT in postmenopausal women is associated with a small increase in risk of breast cancer. The magnitude of this risk is similar, year by year, to the effect of a late menopause.[12] A randomised controlled trial conducted in women with a mean age of 63 years suggests that HRT may exert this effect by stimulating the growth of pre-existing tumours.[13] There is no biological basis for the assumption that HRT causes breast cancer, nor is there evidence to show any increase in mortality from breast cancer in women who use HRT.[14]

The majority of studies show no increase in the risk of dying from breast cancer among women who use HRT. This suggests that any effect of adjuvant oestrogen in relation to breast cancer may be to accelerate the growth of established tumours rather than to initiate the process of carcinogenesis.

Other variables such as diet, alcohol consumption and smoking have been implicated. The long-term use of hormonal contraceptives does not appear to increase the risk of breast cancer in later years.[15]

Familial/genetic factors

Identifiable genetic mutations account for less than 10 per cent of the incidence of breast cancer. In families affected by an inherited mutation, there is a high incidence of breast cancer among male and female members, often occurring at an early age.

The best known familial mutation is on the BRCA-1 gene. More than 100 mutations have been identified. A woman who carries a BRCA-1 mutation has a lifetime risk of breast cancer of almost 80 per cent and half of breast cancers in these families occur before the age of fifty. Genetic testing can identify mutations of BRCA-1 and other relevant genes (BRCA-2, ataxia telangiectasia gene, p53 etc). When a BRCA-1 mutation is identified, management options include intensive surveillance (annual mammography with or without ultrasound), tamoxifen for breast cancer prevention or prophylactic mastectomy.

Management

The decisions and treatment planning for breast cancer are always made after detailed discussion with the woman, involving a full explanation of the treatment options, benefits and hazards.

The primary tumour

The first principle of treatment for invasive breast cancer is complete excision of the primary tumour. This can be achieved either by a complete local excision (CLE) of the tumour or by a total mastectomy. In either case, if this can be done before the cancer has begun to metastasise (as in the case of small tumours), the treatment is curative. Where there is a likelihood that metastatic disease has already occurred, no treatment is likely to be curative but appropriate surgery will at least minimise the risk of local recurrence of the cancer in the breast or chest wall.

In planning surgical treatment, tumour size, tumour position and breast size are all taken into consideration. As a rough guide, breast-conserving surgery (CLE with axillary sampling) is used for tumours 3 cm or less in size; larger tumours are treated more safely with mastectomy. Signs that indicate extension of the disease into the nipple or overlying skin, or the recurrence of cancer in a breast already treated conservatively, are additional indications for mastectomy.

Conservative therapy versus mastectomy

Australian data from 1995 reveals that for the primary surgical management of early breast cancer, 53 per cent of women underwent breast-conserving surgery, compared to 47 per cent undergoing mastectomy. In the case of advanced disease, 32 per cent had conservative surgery against 68 per cent undergoing mastectomy.

Over time there has been a decrease in the proportion of mastectomies being performed and a corresponding increase in the proportion of lumpectomies with or without axillary clearance. This is in line with the expected shift towards more conservative surgical management, with the evidence that conservative management has an equally good long-term outcome compared with mastectomy. Although there is a higher risk of local recurrence after breast-conserving surgery, the risk of distant metastases and contralateral tumours is identical to that for mastectomy (Table 16.6).

TABLE 16.6 Comparison of local recurrence rates twenty years after breast conservation versus mastectomy

	Mastectomy	Quad + XRT*
Local recurrence	8 (2.3%)	29 (8.2%)
Distant metastases	83 (23.8%)	81 (23.0%)
Contralateral tumour	31 (8.9%)	29 (8.2%)
N	349	352

*Quadrantectomy and radiation therapy
Source: adapted from Salvadori et al, 1999.[16]

Lymph node excision

In addition to excision of the primary tumour, surgical treatment for invasive cancers usually includes sampling of the axillary lymph nodes to determine whether metastasis to these nodes has already occurred. The condition of the axillary nodes is the most powerful predictor of prognosis in breast cancer and the probability of recurrence and survival is related directly to the number of lymph nodes that contain metastases (Table 16.7).

Sampling of the axillary nodes nowadays is usually confined to level 1 or level 2 depending on the perceived probability of lymph node involvement. This less radical excision of lymph nodes is intended to reduce the risk of arm lymphoedema, which can occur after axillary dissection.

However, even more conservative methods of lymph node sampling are now employed in some centres using the 'sentinel node' technique. The sentinel node is

TABLE 16.7 Recurrence (treatment failure) according to number of axillary nodes involved

Nodal status	Treatment failure
Negative	13%
1–3 positive	39%
4+ positive	69%

the primary draining node which serves the part of the breast containing the tumour. Two techniques are available to identify the sentinel node at the time of surgery. In one of these, a radionucleide tracer is injected around the tumour a few hours prior to surgery and passage into the axillary or other (eg internal mammary) nodes is identified with a gamma probe during the surgical procedure. Lymphoscintigraphy can be used before surgery to provide a 'map' of the lymphatic drainage of the primary tumour. In another technique, a patent blue dye is injected around the tumour at the commencement of the surgical procedure. Passage of the dye identifies the relevant lymph channels and the sentinel nodes as they take up the tracer colour. This use of these two methods in combination gives the greatest probability of success in identifying sentinel nodes.

Numerous studies have shown that there is a high correlation between sentinel node histology and axillary node metastases as determined by more extensive lymph node sampling. The sentinel node should be examined with multiple sections, preferably using immuno-histochemical stains. If lymph node metastases are identified, the addition of systemic therapy to any local treatment should be considered.

It is recognised that in the assessment of axillary lymph nodes, the standard procedure for examining the nodes with a single section is insufficient to identify small metastases. Several studies have shown that multiple sections through apparently 'normal' lymph nodes will reveal very small 'occult' metastases, particularly when these sections are examined with immuno-histochemical stains. These studies also show that the presence of these micrometastases does have an adverse effect on disease-free survival and overall survival.

Adjuvant therapy

Radiotherapy

The risk of local recurrence after breast-conserving surgery can be substantially reduced by the use of adjuvant radiotherapy. Without radiation treatment the probability of local recurrence after CLE may reach 50 per cent within 10 years: radiation treatment can reduce this to nearly 10 per cent. Studies have not yet revealed a subset of women with breast cancer in whom radiation treatment can be omitted safely. Even in the case of small primary tumours with clear margins, radiotherapy reduces the risk of local recurrence (Table 16.8). However, there is some evidence that the risk of local recurrence after complete excision of small, low-grade tumours in older women is so low that radiotherapy may not confer any useful benefit in these cases.

TABLE 16.8 Effect of radiation treatment in reducing local recurrence after breast-conserving surgery (four studies)

Study	Local recurrence	
	CLE	CLE + XRT
NSABP B-06 (< 40 mm/12 years)	36.8%	10.9%
Ontario (< 40 mm/7.6 years)	35.2%	11.3%
Uppsala-Orebro (≤ 20 mm/10 years)	24.0%	8.5%
Milan III (≤ 20 mm/10 years)	22.0%	5.9%

Radiation treatment is usually confined to the breast (excluding the regional nodes) and is delivered with external beam therapy. Some centres use implantation/brachytherapy. The advantage of this technique is that the radiation can be given in a very short period of time compared with the six or seven weeks required for a series of small fractional doses. Typically, a dose of 50 to 55 Gy is delivered to the entire breast with the possible addition of a boost of up to 10 Gy to the tumour site. Treatment usually begins three to four weeks after the initial surgery but where systemic therapy is planned, the radiation may be deferred for six months.

Systemic therapy

Systemic adjuvant therapy includes all forms of cytotoxic chemotherapy and/or hormonal manipulation used in conjunction with local therapy for early breast cancer. The aim of adjuvant therapy is to treat residual micrometastatic disease, to reduce the risk of tumour recurrence and ultimately improve survival. There is strong evidence of benefit from published overviews of randomised trials which demonstrate the effectiveness of adjuvant systemic therapies.[17,18] The potential benefits of systemic adjuvant therapy depend on the prognosis without adjuvant treatment. Benefits of adjuvant systemic therapy are expressed as proportional reductions in the risk of disease recurrence and risk of death from breast cancer with treatment. Thus the higher the risk of disease recurrence the greater the potential benefits from adjuvant therapy. Systemic therapy should be considered in all women at moderate to high risk of recurrence after local therapy. This includes women with involved lymph nodes and also many women with node-negative breast cancer, with the exception of small tumours associated with a very low risk of recurrence. The decision regarding suitability for adjuvant therapy should also incorporate the age, general health and personal preferences of the woman.

Tamoxifen

Tamoxifen, a selective oestrogen receptor modulator (SERM), has been shown to improve disease-free and overall survival in women of all age groups with hormone receptor positive tumours (Table 16.9). The recommended duration of tamoxifen is five years. No clear benefit has been found in patients with hormone receptor-negative tumours. Tamoxifen has also been shown to reduce the incidence of contralateral breast cancer by approximately half.

The most common side effects of tamoxifen from the anti-oestrogenic effects include hot flushes and vaginal dryness; the oestrogenic effects may cause increased vaginal discharge and also positive effects on bone.

Importantly, tamoxifen is associated with a 2.5-fold increased incidence of endometrial cancer, and abnormal bleeding should be investigated promptly. Ultrasound results are not reliable as tamoxifen gives rise to oedema in the myometrium that may mimic thickened endometrium; histological sampling is required to diagnose any underlying cause of uterine bleeding. Statistically, this is a small absolute risk, equal to one case per thousand treated women per year and the tumours are of low malignant potential and treatable. Other rare side effects include an increased incidence of stroke, pulmonary embolism, deep venous thrombosis and ocular toxicity.

Ovarian ablation

Ovarian ablation has also been shown to be an effective adjuvant treatment for premenopausal women with hormone receptor positive breast cancer.[17] This can be achieved by removing the ovaries surgically, irradiating them or suppressing their function using luteinising hormone releasing hormone (LHRH) analogues such as goserelin. This treatment is associated with premature menopause and its associated complications. Additional benefit can be obtained by adding tamoxifen.

Multi-agent chemotherapy

Multi-agent chemotherapy reduces the risk of recurrence and death for women with early breast cancer.[18] Adjuvant chemotherapy appears to be more effective in women less than 50 years of age, with less but still significant benefit seen in older women. Similar proportional benefits are seen in women with node-negative and node-positive breast cancer (Table 16.10). Evidence shows that moderately prolonged (several months) combination chemotherapy is more effective than single-agent therapy and treatment lasting less than one month.

The chemotherapy regimen which has been studied most extensively consists of a combination of three drugs: cyclophosphamide, methotrexate and 5-fluorouracil (CMF). Chemotherapy regimens using anthracyclines including doxorubicin or epirubicin have been examined in more recent trials. The most recent overview showed that anthracycline-containing chemotherapy regimens were associated with slightly superior results when compared to CMF for both recurrence-free survival and overall survival.[18]

Nausea, vomiting, tiredness and alopecia are the most frequent side effects associated with cytotoxic chemotherapy. Less common short-term side effects include mucositis, diarrhoea, febrile neutropenia, infection, anaemia, conjunctivitis, chemical cystitis and haemorrhage. Longer-term side effects include premature menopause, impairment of sexual function, possible problems with impaired concentration and with memory and, rarely, therapy-induced leukaemia. Congestive cardiac failure is an uncommon side effect associated with higher cumulative doses of anthracyclines. It may be exacerbated by radiation therapy, particularly to the left chest.

TABLE 16.9 Absolute benefit in terms of percentage risk reduction in 10-year overall survival with tamoxifen[18]

Lymph node status	10-year survival: No tamoxifen	10-year survival: With tamoxifen	Absolute benefit
Negative	73.3%	78.9%	5.6%
Positive	50.5%	61.4%	10.9%

TABLE 16.10 Absolute benefit in terms of percentage risk reduction in 10-year overall survival with multi-agent chemotherapy at 10 years[17]

Age	Lymph node status	10-year survival: No chemotherapy	10-year survival: With chemotherapy	Absolute benefit
< 50 years	Negative	71.9%	77.6%	5.7%
	Positive	41.4%	53.8%	12.4%
50–69 years	Negative	64.8%	71.2%	6.4%
	Positive	46.3%	48.6%	2.3%

Newer agents under evaluation

Aromatase inhibitors that reduce the amount of oestrogen produced at extra-ovarian sites in postmenopausal women may provide a ‘second line’ treatment for metastatic disease in hormone-receptor-positive tumours after initial treatment with tamoxifen.

Taxanes have anti-tumour activity in advanced breast cancer. They cause little nausea or emesis but are myleosuppressive.

HER2-neu receptor-blocking agents have potential to block tumour cell growth.

All women should be fully informed about all available treatment options. For most women, the benefits of adjuvant therapy as measured by the reduction in risk of breast cancer recurrence will significantly outweigh the risk of side effects.

Outcomes/prognosis

There has been a shift towards more conservative surgical management as no controlled trials have shown that there is any improvement in survival of breast cancer among women treated with mastectomy, compared with those treated by breast conservation. The risk of local recurrence within the breast after breast-conserving surgery is related to the size of the tumour, the margin of surgical clearance around the tumour and the presence or absence of vascular and/or lymphatic permeation.

An average measure of the risk of local recurrence (in the breast) is about one or two per cent per year. After mastectomy, the *lifetime* risk of local recurrence is approximately one per cent.

Follow-up

Depending on the length of the disease-free interval, a clinical review is undertaken on a 3–6 monthly basis. Mammographic examination is performed annually; however, an initial baseline mammogram of the affected breast may be taken at six months after local excision.

Metastatic work-up (including bone scan, chest X-ray and liver scan) may be undertaken at the time of diagnosis if there is concern about the possibility of distant disease. Subsequent investigations are undertaken if indicated by symptom development.

Emerging issues

Other tests for breast cancer

There are no reliable serum markers for breast cancer although carcinoembryonic antigen (CEA) and CA15-3 are elevated in about 20 per cent of women with advanced metastatic disease. At present, MRI is of uncertain value in the diagnosis of primary breast cancer. Thermography, a crude imaging method based on the heat emitted from blood flow in a malignant tumour is of no value in the early detection of breast cancer.

Women and cancer

The diagnosis of cancer represents a major crisis in the life of any person. For women diagnosed with breast or gynaecological cancer, concerns about threat to life are often compounded by the profound impact on the sense of self, body image and sexual adjustment, and changes in hormonal status and reproductive capacity. The diagnosis challenges the woman's view of the world, and consequently there are often profound changes in her hopes and expectations for herself and her family.

Grief and loss

Grief is implicit in the diagnosis of cancer. However, the particular meaning of the cancer depends on the woman's age and past experiences, her personality style, her social obligations and roles. For the woman whose own mother has died from breast cancer, the diagnosis may mean a death sentence, while for another it may provide the impetus to make major changes such as in relationships or work. There is mourning for the loss of innocence, for the life before cancer, and for relationships untarnished by the threat of recurrence.

Making treatment choices

For women with breast cancer, it is increasingly common for the woman to be offered a choice between mastectomy and breast-conserving surgery, and there is evidence that women offered a choice may be less depressed.[19] Not every woman is comfortable making a choice, and each woman should be asked for her preference about decision making. It is also important not to make presumptions, for example that an older woman 'doesn't mind' losing her breast. Similarly a young woman may feel that mastectomy is a reasonable price to pay to survive the disease.

Body image and sexuality

The damaging impact of mastectomy on body image has long been known, and in general, body image is better preserved in women who have breast-conserving surgery.[20] Treatment of gynaecological malignancy has a direct impact on body image and sexuality, often compounded by a change in hormonal status and imposition of infertility. Pelvic exenteration or radical vulvectomy has a profound impact on body image and self-esteem.[21] However, coping with this may be made more difficult by shame and guilt, especially if the woman has delayed seeking treatment. It is important for health professionals to ask about body image concerns, as women may be reticent about expressing them lest they are seen as ungrateful.

Concerns about family

A pervasive theme for women with cancer is concern about the impact of their disease on the partner and children. There is evidence that the partners of women with breast cancer have high levels of distress, sometimes exceeding that of the woman herself.[23] This merits attention in its own right, and also because lack of support from a partner undermines the coping of the woman.[22] Parents may be reluctant to discuss the cancer with children, in the belief that this will protect them from distress. Such avoidance in fact compounds the distress of children who perceive that something is happening, with parental silence confirming their fear that it is too terrible to discuss. Young children in particular need reassurance that they will be safe, and that the family will hold together.[23] Adolescent daughters appear particularly vulnerable when a mother has cancer.[24] This may relate in part to issues of emerging sexuality and body image, and the tendency of mothers to rely on their daughters for emotional support, exacerbated by increasing domestic responsibilities which often isolate the daughter from friends and supportive social networks.

Depression and anxiety

Grief and sadness are normal responses to loss (Section 3). However, when distress is severe and persistent, and interferes with social and occupational functioning, a diagnosis of depression or anxiety should be considered. Factors associated with increased risk of psychological problems include:

- Younger age
- Being single, widowed or divorced
- Having children younger than 21 years of age
- Economic adversity
- Perceived poor social support
- Poor marital or family functioning

- History of psychiatric illness
- Cumulative stressful life events
- Past history of alcohol or other substance abuse.[25]

In addition, women who have advanced disease, higher disease burden or pain are more vulnerable to becoming depressed. Treatment of depression or anxiety usually involves a combination of pharmacotherapy, supportive and cognitive techniques (Section 3), with specific focus on the meaning of the cancer for the particular woman.

Advanced disease

When confronted with advanced disease, people change the criteria by which they evaluate their lives.[26] Relationships and emotional connections assume greater importance, but for many women the opportunity to talk about fundamental issues of living and dying is militated against by social pressure to 'be positive' or 'keep on fighting'. These admonitions are more often founded in a desire to reduce the distress of the listener than that of the woman, although this is rarely spoken. Some women feel profoundly isolated, as friends become avoidant in order to reduce their shame that they just do not know what to say. Health professionals will often be avoidant too, fearful of not knowing what to say, or of making things worse. Perhaps more basically, many health professionals still equate death with failure, and find disease progression too threatening at a personal level. A fundamental aspect of the care of the woman with advanced cancer must be providing an atmosphere in which she can discuss the awfulness of her predicament, without fear of being rejected or abandoned.

Interventions to promote well-being

Effective communication skills are at the heart of optimal care of the woman with cancer. In addition, health professionals can optimise the adjustment of the woman with cancer by providing appropriate, detailed information, and encouraging her to talk about her feelings and concerns.[26] Identification of risk factors offers the opportunity for preventative interventions to reduce psychological disorder, or to identify and treat this early, as there is evidence that the emotional adjustment of the woman affects the functioning of the whole family.[27]

Part 5
Older years

SECTION 17

Ageing and its problems

Normal ageing

Demography of ageing

Since 1900, life expectancy at birth in the Western world has increased steadily; in 1996 it was approximately 82 years for women and 76 for men in Australia, 80 for women and 75 for men in the UK, and 80 for women and 74 for men in the USA. Consequently there are more older women than older men, and women live more of their lives as older people than men do. Increases in life expectancy have been accompanied by a continuing decline in the mortality rate, particularly among those aged 80–99 (an age group mainly comprising females), mostly because of declining death rates for specific diseases such as cardiovascular disease. Table 17.1 shows the proportion of people aged 65 and over in Australia, the UK and the USA in 2000 and the projected increase by 2050. The greatest increase for both men and women will be in the age group 85 and over. It is within this age group, however, that the difference in numbers between older men and women is expected to be greatest (Table 17.1).

It is also important to recognise that ageing is a global phenomenon. By 2050 the number of older people is expected to increase from approximately 600 million now to almost two billion.[1]

While life expectancy in some 'developing' countries may not be as high as in the Western world, in part because of wars, famine and lack of essential health care, in

TABLE 17.1 UN population figures 2000 and projected for 2050 for Australia, the UK and the USA

	2000	2050
Australia		
Total population	19 135 000	26 472 000
65+	12.3%	22.45%
85+	1.28%	4.25%
Males: % of 85+	30.33%	33.84%
Females: % of 85+	69.67%	66.16%
United Kingdom		
Total population	59 415 000	58 931 000 (Note: ↓)
65+	15.75%	27.31%
85+	1.96%	5.91%
Males: % of 85+	26.95%	34.73%
Females: % of 85+	73.05%	65.27%
United States		
Total population	283 230 000	397 061 000
65+	12.3%	21.09%
85+	1.51%	4.4%
Males: % of 85+	28%	34.08%
Females: % of 85+	72%	65.92%

absolute numbers there are more older people in 'developing' than in 'developed' countries—by 2050, 80 per cent of the world's older people (ie 60+) will be in developing countries.

Physiology of ageing

A definition of ageing is the 'progressive, generalised impairment of function resulting in loss of adaptive responses to stress (eg homeostatic mechanisms) and increasing risk of age-related disease…'.[2] The overall effect of these changes is that the older we get the more likely we are to die. But mortality rates rise throughout life from puberty and the rate is uniform; ageing therefore begins around puberty. However, there are certain older-age-related changes that are recognised in terms of the function of different organs. For instance, in terms of intellectual function, neuropsychological testing does show slowing of central processing time and acquisition of new information as well as the decline of what is called 'fluid intelligence'. Slight memory loss is common with ageing, but not usually sufficient to cause problems with daily functioning. There are people with subjective complaints and objective evidence of memory impairment, with normal physical and mental functioning. This condition is called mild cognitive impairment (MCI)[3] and people with MCI have an increased risk of developing dementia. Similarly, in terms of eyesight, there is a decline with age in ability to accommodate for near objects in early ageing (presbyopia) and a proportion of older people will require corrective lenses.

True ageing changes can be divided into intrinsic processes, meaning those that occur independent of environmental conditions, and extrinsic processes, those that are influenced strongly by environmental conditions. Two examples of age-related physiology leading to 'disease': older people exposed to low ambient temperatures during the winter months may develop hypothermia; older people may be more prone to heat strokes in the summer.

Tissues in the body vary in their degree of renewability—for instance, teeth that grow following loss of baby teeth are present until they fall out, break, are extracted or are knocked out. Other organs such as the liver and bone marrow have considerable regenerative/repair capacity. Organs such as the heart are intermediate between the non-regenerative and regenerative ones.

It is important to understand that age and ill-health are not synonymous terms. Most older people are healthy and active, and participate in the community. In the Australian Bureau of Statistics (ABS) 1995 National Health Survey, 64 per cent of older Australians rated their health as good, very good or excellent, and older people actually have higher ratings for emotional and mental health than younger people. A 1994 telephone survey of 12 793 adults, using the SF-36 Health Survey, found that:

> *For physical functioning, role limitations due to physical problems, bodily pain and general health, scores decreased as age group increased. Conversely, scores for role limitations due to emotional problems and mental health increased with age and were highest for both men and women in those over 65.*[4]

In the 1995 Australian National Health Survey, people aged over 75 scored the highest in terms of their mental health. Even those with chronic illness generally maintain satisfaction with life by adjusting their expectations and daily routines. However, many biomedical and other factors can affect the health, well-being and independence of older people. This section is concerned with the biomedical factors (Boxes 17.1 and 17.2).

BOX 17.1 Common disorders experienced by older women

- Postural hypotension
- Systolic hypertension
- Falls
- Osteoporosis
- Arthritis
- Ageing skin
- Urinary tract infection/incontinence
- Diabetes mellitus
- Depression

BOX 17.2 Additional disorders of increasing age and frailty

- Renal impairment
- Cerebrovascular accidents
- Paget's disease
- Parkinson's disease
- Cancer
- Dementia
- Hypothermia
- Heat stroke
- Malnutrition

Cardiovascular disease (including coronary heart disease and stroke) is the most common cause of death and disability in older people in Australia, the UK and USA, along with cancer. 'In 1983, approximately 30% of all cancer deaths occurred in people aged 75 years and over … by 1996 this proportion had increased to around 40%'.[5]

Breast cancer has increasing age as the greatest risk factor, yet 'screening mammography is underutilised among older women who are more likely to benefit from this',[6] with many doctors saying that they do not routinely do a breast examination on every woman over the age of 50 years.[7]

Presentation of ill health in old age

It is common for older patients to have up to six or seven separate pathological conditions. All of these conditions interact and the situation may be further exacerbated by the contribution of polypharmacy. Because old age impairs homeostatic mechanisms, even minor perturbations may have a dramatic effect on an elderly person's equilibrium. Often the illness presentation is very atypical. For example, myocardial infarction may not have the 'textbook' presentation—the patient may present with shortness of breath or collapse. Thyrotoxicosis may present with weight loss rather than with the classical symptoms of tremor, diarrhoea or exophthalmus. Tremor in an older person is more likely to be a senile or physiological tremor. Similarly, clinical signs may be different; it is common in older people for pneumonia to present with delirium, rather than with fever, cough and productive sputum.

Elderly patients with acute illnesses frequently present with functional disability—immobility, instability, incontinence, intellectual impairment—any of which may have iatrogenic causes. These are termed the 'Giants of Geriatrics' and they cause disability, loss of independence and institutionalisation. None of these giants is caused by old age. They are the result of pathology. These conditions must be very carefully sought and, as far as possible, remedied. Rehabilitation from day one is a fundamental principle of geriatric medicine, as is a multidisciplinary team approach involving most health professionals. If the conditions cannot be remedied, their effects can be ameliorated, thus restoring functional capacity to the patient and restoring independence.

All these conditions lead to loss of independence and institutionalisation.

KEY POINT

The five I's *not* caused by old age:
- **Immobility**
- **Instability**
- **Incontinence**
- **Intellectual impairment**
- **Iatrogenic illness.**

Immobility

Immobility is usually considered as a restriction in everyday activity. The prevalence of more severe immobility rises with increasing age.

Causes of immobility in old age

The causes of immobility in old age may be physical, mental and/or social.

- *Physical barriers* include:
  - Joint problems, especially osteoarthritis in women
  - Neurological deficit: impaired balance, stroke, Parkinson's disease
  - Sensory deprivation: deafness, impaired vision, impaired proprioception
  - Cardiovascular and respiratory disease
  - Previous falls and fear of further falls.
- *Mental barriers* include:
  - Reduced expectations of an 'active' life
  - Loss of adaptability and creativity
  - Introversion with reduced social contact
  - Anxiety and fear of going out (or of allowing others in)

- *Social barriers* include:
  - Retirement: with dangers of reduced income and social contact
  - Living alone: an endemic problem in ageing women
  - Insufficient outside interests or activities
  - Urgency incontinence: need to get to the toilet quickly and fear of social embarrassment.

Consequences of immobility

Immobility can lead to a variety of 'losses':

- Loss of choice: for example, being able to get to where they want/do what they want
- Loss of capability: for example, getting to the toilet in time/answering the door
- Loss of social responsiveness
- Loss of independence.

An older person's world may thus contract, eventually to what geriatricians sometimes call a 'triangular' existence—from bed to chair to commode.

Prevention of immobility

Prevention begins in middle age and involves maintenance of physical fitness and adequate diagnosis/treatment of minor ailments before they become major.

Assessing a patient with impaired mobility

It is important to fully assess impaired mobility, in order to be able to correct or ameliorate medical problems and offer assistance for mental and social issues. A useful approach is outlined here.

History

- When did she last go out of the house unaccompanied? (eg to use public transport, cross a busy street, go to the shops)
- Why did she stop going out? Was it because of pain? Breathlessness? Fear—of what?
- What difficulties are experienced with stairs, walking, getting on and off the chair, toilet or bed?
- What aids are used?

Examination

General pattern of movement, gait speed, step length, symmetry; transfer efficiency, style; range of movements of joint; muscle strength, tone, coordination; proprioception; vision.

Differential diagnoses

- What is the causal condition?
- What are the contributory conditions?

Outcome

- What is the treatment?
- What is the prognosis?

Management

Management depends on the correct diagnosis. For example, postural hypotension and giddiness may be alleviated by readjusting or stopping the offending drug. Osteoarthritis will respond to physiotherapy and analgesia; levodopa may alleviate the rigidity of Parkinson's disease.

Instability/falls

There is an increasing incidence of falls with age. Approximately 30 per cent of people over 65 experience at least one fall per year. Falls are the leading cause of injury and accidental death in older women. Of even greater burden, however, are the femoral neck fractures following falls and the resulting episodes of hospitalisation. In 1997–98, hospital separations per 100 000 population due to falls among people aged 65 years and over was 2184.[8] Many of these admissions result in long hospital stays and the need for (although not necessarily the receipt of) extensive rehabilitation. Although only five per cent of falls result in fractures and five per cent in soft tissue injuries, the remaining 90 per cent may result in loss of confidence.

Medications have been implicated in falls, particularly among older people in residential care. Older people taking three or four medications are at increased risk of falls.[9] Those most often associated with falls are tricyclic antidepressants, antipsychotics, diuretics and benzodiazepines. There is a small but consistent association between psychotropic drugs and falls.[9]

The causes of falls are numerous (Box 17.3) and there may be more than one factor operating.

Management

It is essential to take a good history, particularly with regard to loss of consciousness, position or activity at the time of the fall, and specific symptoms such as chest pain. It is also important to know how long the patient was on the floor. Full examination with particular reference to lying and standing blood pressure, any neurological disorders, vision and gait should be performed. Investigation is guided by history and examination. All identifiable causes such as polypharmacy or untreated Parkinson's disease should be managed. Rehabilitation and the multidisciplinary approach will not only restore confidence but also increase stability and ensure safety if falls occur. A home visit is mandatory when patients present with recurrent falls, to identify/modify environmental risks and increase patient safety.

In addition, it is important to assess four things:

- The injuries from this fall
- The reason for the fall
- Preventing further falls
- Preventing injury from future falls, which will be inevitable (hip protectors, home modification, treating osteoporosis and vitamin D deficiency).

In the UK falls prevention is part of the recommendations of the National Service Framework for Older People and current practices can be reviewed against this framework.[10,11]

BOX 17.3 Causes of falls in older women

- Impaired balance due to ageing
- Environmental factors, such as lack of grab rails, uneven floor surfaces
- Neurological and visual factors:
  - Confusion (acute and chronic)
  - Cerebrovascular disease:
    - Parkinsonism
    - Epilepsy
    - Visual impairment
    - Vertigo
    - Normal pressure hydrocephalus
- Cardiovascular issues:
  - Postural hypotension
  - Arrthythmias
  - Aortic stenosis
  - Other causes of syncope – micturition, cough
  - Vasovagal
  - Carotid sinus syndrome
- Locomotor
- Arthritis
  - Muscle weakness
  - Foot problems
  - Footwear
- Drugs (see above)

Arthritis

Osteoarthritis is a major cause of disability, particularly in the ageing population, and has both social and economic consequences.[12] The disease is more prevalent in women who suffer a particular economic burden.[13]

Osteoporosis

The definition of osteoporosis from the National Osteoporosis Foundation, Australia, is 'a progressive systemic skeletal disease characterised by low bone mass and micro-architectural deterioration of bone tissue, with a consequent increase in bone fragility and susceptibility to fracture' (Figures 17.1, 17.2). In terms of bone mineral density (BMD) the definition by the World Health Organization is a BMD of more than 2.5 standard deviations below the mean of a young adult population. Radiographic

FIGURE 17.1 Normal bone

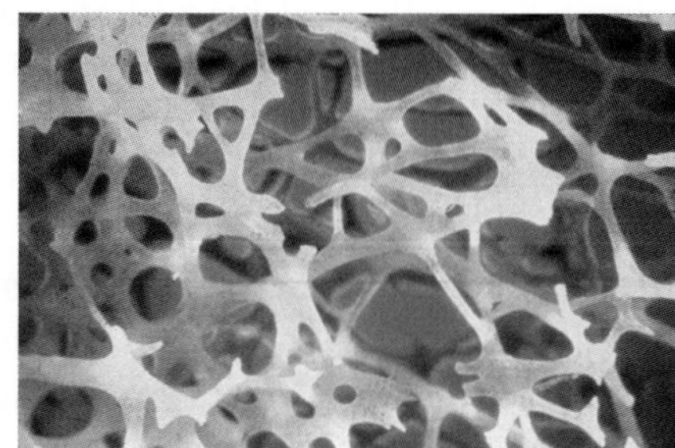

FIGURE 17.2 Osteoporotic bone with loss of architecture

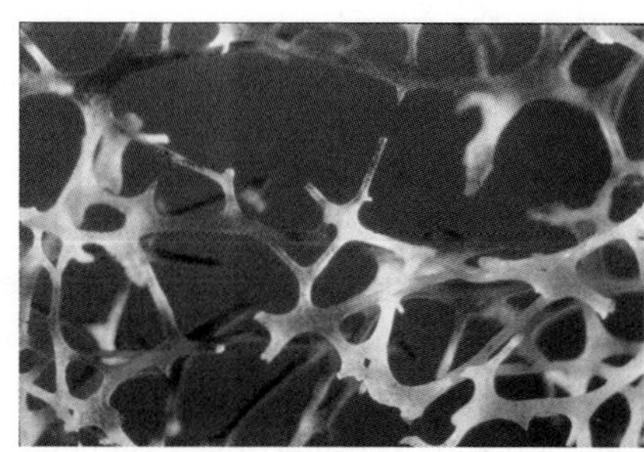

evidence is insensitive, bone loss only becoming apparent after a decrease in bone mass by 30–50 per cent. Bone mineral density is an intermediate outcome rather than a clinical outcome. However, the estimation of BMD allows detection of osteoporosis at a stage when a preventative intervention could be offered.

In the elderly almost all fractures are linked to osteoporosis. The most common fractures that present clinically are those of the proximal femur, the distal forearm and the vertebrae. Many vertebral fractures will heal and cause minimal problems; however, others will result in deformity, chronic pain, disability and the need for supportive or institutional care. While bone mineral density is important, the risk of falling will obviously be essential to whether or not a limb is fractured.

Bone loss prevention can be achieved by a number of agents (Table 17.2). Many elderly women may be vitamin D deficient (even in Australia) as they may be mostly

TABLE 17.2 Treatment options to maintain bone mineral density post menopause

BMD	Treatment options	Follow-up
Normal	Consider HRT for other reasons	Repeat BMD 3–5 years
–1 to –2.5	ERT	After 5–10 years (according to choice and symptoms) change to: a raloxifene b bisphosphonates
> –2.5 No fracture on X-ray	ERT Bisphosphonates Raloxifene + Ca + vitamin D (if deficient)	Repeat BMD every 2nd year to ensure adequate therapy
> –2.5 Fracture on X-ray	Bisphosphonates Raloxifene + Ca + vitamin D (if deficient)	Repeat BMD every 2nd year to ensure adequate therapy

ERT: oestrogen replacement therapy; Ca: calcium.

housebound. Research is focused on developing the ideal selective oestrogen receptor modulator (SERM). This would be an agent with all the beneficial effects of oestrogen (positive effects on bone, cardiovascular system and the brain; negative effects on the breast, uterus and clotting system). Currently available SERMs are clomiphene, tamoxifen and raloxifene; these have different uses, actions and side effect profiles.

Incontinence

It is important to consider incontinence (Section 15) in relation to older women because, for many older women, conditions such as incontinence and prolapse of the uterus may contribute significantly to restriction of activity, with resultant isolation, depression and eventually institutionalisation.

Urinary incontinence

Causes of urinary incontinence in older women may include:

- Urinary tract infection
- Stress incontinence. Pelvic floor muscle weakness may be due to atrophic urethritis which is often associated with pruritis vulvae and frequency of micturition. In older women this may be compounded by oestrogen deficiency, leading to atrophic vaginitis.
- Constipation, causing bladder outlet obstruction or reducing bladder capacity, which in turn may cause urinary retention. Frequent straining at stools may lead to neuromyopathy of the pelvic muscles.
- Polyuria, often caused by drug-induced diuresis, poorly controlled diabetes, hypercalcaemia, renal failure and excessive fluid intake. This may also result from mobilisation of peripheral oedema.
- Loss of awareness of bladder filling (eg in dementia).
- Unstable bladder—common in patients with global cerebral disease (eg dementia, cerebrovascular disease).

Assessment/investigations

History

Includes drug history.

Examination

- *Vaginal examination*—for stress leakage, vaginal wall and uterine prolapse, and atrophic vaginitis which is associated with atrophic urethritis.
- *Rectal examination*—assess all patients for the presence of faecal impaction.

Investigations

- MSU/urine cytology—cystoscopy may be indicated if haematuria is present without urinary infection.
- Incontinence chart—keep record initially for 48 hours. Record fluid intake (aim for 1500–2000 ml/day) and urine output at each voiding (gives indication of bladder capacity), episodes of urinary and faecal incontinence.

- Residential volume assessment ≥ ultrasound or 'in and out' catheter.
- Urodynamic assessment—in most elderly patients it is possible to diagnose the cause of incontinence from the history and examination findings. Urodynamic assessment is indicated when there is difficulty making precise diagnosis, when treatment has not been successful or when surgical treatment is being considered.
- Pelvic floor muscle assessment.

Treatment of urinary incontinence

- Review medication. Stop the offending drug(s) if possible or use an alternative drug. When diuretic therapy is required, a short-acting diuretic with a predictable effect should be used.
- Urinary tract infection—antibiotic medication as indicated from urine culture and sensitivity results.
- Stress incontinence—individual exercise program (Section 15).
- Bladder neck repair—indicated for older patients with stress incontinence who do not respond to the above treatment and are fit for an anaesthetic.
- Uterine and vaginal wall prolapse. This can be treated surgically if the woman is medically fit for an anaesthetic. If she is at high risk for problems from anaesthesia, a vaginal ring pessary can be used. This can often give good symptomatic relief.
- Constipation—use laxatives or enemas.
- Urge incontinence/unstable bladder—toileting: bladder drill or timed voiding to empty the bladder before the onset of urgency and/or bladder contraction. The usual interval between micturition is two hours. Restrict fluid intake after 6.00 pm if nocturnal incontinence persists.
- Environmental adjustment—useful aids include a commode placed beside the bed or chair for patients with nocturia and with limited mobility; raised toilet seat; frame around toilet; modifications to clothes (eg velcro fastenings).
- Anticholinergic drugs (eg oxybutynin, 3 mg bd to 5 mg tds) to increase bladder capacity and reduce the distending volume at which urgency occurs.
- Oestrogen for atrophic vaginitis—traditionally given in the form of pessaries or vaginal cream. Older women may have difficulty with traditional medications (for instance, vaginal application may be difficult if the woman has arthritis), and may require an alternative route.

Faecal incontinence

Causes of faecal incontinence include:

- Anorectal incontinence (idiopathic faecal incontinence)
- Colorectal disease
- Diarrhoea
- Faecal impaction

- Neurological (including dementia and unconsciousness)
- Immobility.

In the elderly the aetiology is usually multifactorial, with the most common cause being faecal impaction, which may include massive faecal loading with soft or even liquid stool. Immobile patients tend to be slow to respond to the 'call to stool'. They are therefore liable to incontinence when they are given a laxative, especially with potent preparations. This should always be remembered when older patients are being prepared for a barium enema, colonoscopy or surgery.

Treatment of faecal incontinence

The preferred treatment is to empty the rectum from below by administering an enema each day until the faecal mass is cleared. Occasionally this is ineffective, usually because the enema is not retained and in these patients the best result may be achieved with a micro-enema or suppository. Some patients will require manual evacuation, especially if they are impacted with very hard faeces.

Many elderly impacted patients have a continuing tendency to constipation even after their impaction has been cleared. The next step is preventing the recurrence of constipation. High fibre intake is not advisable as it has been shown to be associated with colonic faecal loading in immobile elderly patients. An alternative approach is to use a laxative, the choice of which must be guided by the character of the stool and the patient's ability to defecate. However, laxatives are not always successful for older patients and many patients require regular emptying of the bowel from below, using either enemas or suppositories.

Faecal incontinence should be seen as a curable and preventable problem. It must not be accepted as inevitable.

Intellectual/cognitive impairment

Intellectual/cognitive impairment implies a global disturbance of brain function:

- Memory—especially registration and recall of recent events
- Orientation—time, place, person
- Attention—increased distractibility
- Perception—increased misinterpretations, illusions, hallucinations
- Logical thought—muddled thinking and speech.

Impairment includes delirium (acute confusional state) and dementia (chronic confusional state). Cognitive impairment is a syndrome, not a diagnosis. Full assessment to determine the diagnosis and cause is essential.

Assessing a patient with suspected cognitive impairment

- Interview with the patient and/or carers/relatives
- Formal mental status test[14] (Box 17.4)
- Examination of patient/diagnostic tests

Is cognitive impairment present?

Suspicion will be aroused by:

- Memory/orientation problems: eg repeating questions, forgetting familiar names, getting lost in familiar surroundings
- Social problems: eg neglect of appearance, nutrition or hygiene, withdrawal from social surroundings
- Behavioural problems: eg wandering, leaving the stove on, irresponsible use of money

Other problems may include poor compliance with medication, incontinence, and stress to carers (potential for abuse).

Interviewing the patient

- Observe grooming, mood, behaviour.
- Is the patient easily distracted or drowsy?
- Does behaviour fluctuate from minute to minute?
- Normal social conversation provides the most information:
  - Avoid questions with yes/no answers
  - Leave formal mental testing to the end
  - Note language use (exclude aphasia)
  - Note evasiveness in answering questions (eg 'Do you think your memory is all right for your age'?)

Formal mental status testing

There are a number of instruments available to conduct formal testing. One of the most widely used is Folstein's Mini Mental State Examination (MMSE). This is a brief, objective screening test for cognitive impairment. It was not intended as a diagnostic test and its sensitivity as a screening test is poor, but it is a good measure of changes over time. The MMSE does not assess frontal lobe function and requires the subject to have good eyesight, intact speech, literacy and fluency in English.[15] An amended scoring chart has recently been produced to take account of age and education levels but other tests may be more appropriate (eg the six-step capacity assessment instrument, Box 17.4). Subtle memory loss in educated people can be detected with a word task list.[16]

Physical examination

A comprehensive physical examination, including full neurological examination, should be conducted. Diagnostic tests should include routine haematology and biochemistry (because they might indicate underlying infection, dehydration, metabolic abnormality, etc, which could be the causative or contributing factor) in addition to any targeted investigations (eg chest X-ray for suspected pneumonia or CT of brain for subdural haematoma).

Common causes of cognitive impairment

Dementia

Dementia is an age-related disorder. Because the population is ageing, the number of sufferers will double in 20 years.[17] The most common causes of dementia in older

BOX 17.4 The six-step capacity assessment process[18]

This process starts with the 'assumption of capacity'—a fundamental legal principle and looks for evidence of incapacity. If there is no evidence of incapacity, then capacity is assumed to be present—although an error may sometimes occur, this will err on the side of autonomy, not beneficence.

Step 1 Ensure a valid 'trigger to assess' is present. It requires events that put either the individual being assessed, or others, at risk. It also calls the person's capacity into question.

Step 2 Engage those being assessed—inform the person of the capacity assessment process; obtain assent if possible (cannot ask for informed consent to the assessment of capacity).

Step 3 Gather information—from the person being assessed and additional collateral information if available. In relation to health care this would include:

- The medical condition
- The proposed treatments
- Available alternatives
- Foreseeable consequences of treatments and/or alternatives (including the consequences of not having treatment)
- Exploring personal values/beliefs that might affect choices.

Step 4 Ensure opportunity to learn needed information has been provided – ignorance does not equal incapacity. Barriers to communication include language, culture, and/or education.

Step 5 Assess capacity, using a decisional aid such as a structured interview that can be scored.

Step 6 Act on results of assessment. If lack of capacity is found, arrange for a substitute decision-maker (eg someone with enduring power of attorney). If capacity is confirmed the person may still require assistance to deal with the fact that they have had a challenge to their personhood. Others have tried to show that they lack capacity. This latter issue is often overlooked.

Note: a diagnosis of incapacity may actually be a response to a structural problem, such as no community supports, or be related to side effects of medication.

people are Alzheimer's disease and vascular dementia. Alzheimer's disease typically has a slow onset, steady progression, parietal and frontal features following early memory impairment and often a family history. In vascular dementia there are history and clinical examination features of vascular disease both in the brain and systemically. Dementia with lewy body disease is increasingly being diagnosed; the main features of this disorder are rapid onset, fluctuating confusion, visual hallucinations, extrapyramidal signs and sensitivity to phenothiazines.

It is rarely possible to cure or arrest the causal factors of the dementia. However, it is important to consider what the likely exacerbating factors are. What brought the patient to present today? For example, occult infections, inadvertent medication side effects, worsening behaviour causing carer stress.

Management of dementia[19]

- Explain the diagnosis to the carer and where appropriate to the patient
- Identify and treat intercurrent medical illness early
- Correct sensory impairment
- Minimise medications
- Consider safety to drive
- Care for the carer: the Alzheimer's Association/Society are carers' groups which provide information and peer support. Advise about support services such as day care and respite care. Where necessary, nursing home placement should be sought.
- Consider cholinesterase drugs to treat Alzheimer's and lewy body dementia.
- Psychosocial strategies:
  - Simplify communication without patronising
  - Companionship
  - Predictable routine
  - Reality orientation etc
  - Advise regarding advance care planning, living wills, etc.

Delirium

Any systemic illness can produce delirium in an elderly person. Consider:

- Occult infection
- Metabolic disturbance
- Drug toxicity. Sedatives and any drug with anticholinergic activities such as Parkinsonian drugs can produce delirium.

Table 17.3 illustrates the distinguishing features of dementia and delirium, but in clinical practice the boundary line is often blurred. Pre-existing cognitive impairment or dementia is associated with an increased risk of delirium. Outcome studies of delirium suggest that it may be substantially less transient than was previously believed and that only a minority of patients fully recovers to their previous level of cognitive function after an episode of delirium.[20]

TABLE 17.3 Distinction between dementia and delirium[21]

	Dementia	**Delirium**
Onset	Insidious	Acute
Decline	Relatively slow	Rapid
Consciousness level	Alert	Clouding of consciousness
Sensory perceptions	No hypersensitivity	Hypersensitivity
Visual hallucinations	Less common	More common
Stability	Fairly stable	Fluctuating mental state

Depression

Depession is one of the few 'reversible' causes of cognitive impairment. Depression is not always easy to diagnose and mild depression is frequently missed, so other features to support the diagnosis should be sought (Section 3).

Loss and grief in older age can trigger a depressive episode. In addition to losses such as loss of body image, loss of role as mother and possibly loss of a career, older women are more likely than older men to face the loss of a spouse. It is important that older women receive counselling and support for these losses, and that they not be seen as just a 'normal' part of ageing (Section 3).

Other major issues for older women

Drugs

Older people use a disproportionate share of prescribed drugs (40 per cent of prescriptions in 1996 were for people aged 65 and over, who constitute 12 per cent of the population)[22] partly because many older patients suffer from multiple diseases and require increasing numbers of drugs, although frequent review should occur in order to avoid unnecessary polypharmacy.

The handling of drugs by the individual (pharmocokinetics) as well as the responsiveness of the body systems to drugs (pharmacodynamics) is altered with ageing and disease. Increasing problems with compliance are seen with increasing numbers of medications and complex dosing regimens, resulting in drug-related adverse events occurring with increasing frequency. Most of the adverse reactions are preventable, with proper knowledge and adequate thinking (Section 1).

Impaired vision/hearing

In the 1995 ABS survey, vision and hearing problems were almost as prevalent as arthritis among older Australians.

Activity and nutrition

Physical activity and balanced nutrition have been shown to offer some protection against a number of diseases and physical conditions affecting older people, including coronary heart disease, stroke, diabetes, femoral neck fractures and mental disorders,[23] in addition to arthritis and depression. Inadequate nutritional intake is a major problem for older people, especially those who live alone, and dental problems, including ill-fitting dentures, can exacerbate this.

Sexuality

Stereotypes about ageing and sexuality may negatively influence how older people both think and act sexually and can lead to gross errors in the clinical management of the sexual concerns of older people. Disfigurement, such as mastectomy, may make older women feel doubly devalued. There is increasing evidence that not only can older people continue to enjoy sexual activity to the end of their lives but that people aged 65 and older are often having as much sex, and in some cases more sex, than people aged 18 to 26,[24] particularly if they have 'an interested and interesting partner'.

Death and dying

Also see Section 3.

Advance care planning

When working with older patients an important aspect of care is to introduce the concept of advance care planning while the patient is still healthy. Depending on the legislative options in a specific area, advance care planning options may include the use of written instructions for a future time when the patient has lost capacity (an advance health directive or living will) and/or the appointment of a proxy or agent to make decisions at such a time (under an enduring power of attorney).

Palliative care/pain management

It is important that terminally ill patients be given adequate information about available palliative care services, and that they also be reassured about the issue of pain management. There is some fear in the community (including among doctors and other health professionals) that adequate pain relief is euthanasia. This is absolutely not the case and it is very important that patients, their families/carers and the treating medical team all understand this.

Skills required when dealing with older patients

1 The clinical competence to *communicate* optimally with patients, particularly those with impaired hearing, speech or cognition and the social/ethical competence to treat older people with respect, including the use of appropriate language.
2 The clinical competence to *physically examine* elderly patients, including confused or dysphasic patients and the social/ethical competence to be sensitive to embarrassment, to ensure privacy for the examination, to explain what is going to be done and to seek the older person's permission before touching them.
3 The *problem-solving* skills to analyse and address the *multiple pathologies* that characterise medical problems in old age.
4 A sound knowledge base to appreciate that care of the elderly requires a sound foundation in good clinical medicine and to understand that the gains to be achieved from treatment of elderly people do not diminish with increasing age of patient—in fact, the opposite may apply.
5 Flexibility, to allow for the longer consultation time required.

The future

All developed countries have an ageing population. Appropriate medicalisation of old age can improve the health of the ageing.[25] Caring for the older person, in and out of hospital, should also focus on their functional state.[26] The National Service Framework for Older People in Britain and the Adding Life to Years report from Scotland has made recommendations to meet the needs of this ageing population to maintain their health and quality of life.[27]

Part 6
Women and illness

SECTION 18

Surgical, medical and research issues for women

Surgery

The decision to undertake a surgical procedure needs to weigh up the risks and benefits for the individual (Box 18.1). Many procedures are now undertaken as day case surgery and even for women admitted to hospital the length of stay is often short. It is essential that women be fully informed and medically assessed before any procedure, that community resources be established to support early discharge, and that good communication be maintained between general practitioners, community services and the hospital.

BOX 18.1 Risks/complications of gynaecological surgery

- Immediate:
  - Anaesthetic complications
  - Haemorrhage
  - Infection: pelvic abscess
  - Thrombosis
  - Specific complications related to the procedure
- Long-term:
  - Damage to organs
  - Anaemia
  - Thrombotic effects: oedema, vascular insufficiency

Pre-operative assessment

Pre-operative assessment is undertaken to detect any particular additional risk a woman may have and instigate management where possible to minimise this risk. Most hospitals would ask the woman to complete an assessment form and any items on this can be further clarified by the medical and nursing staff. The history and examination will identify specific problems and indicate specific investigations for further clarification. It is important that the investigations be undertaken for a reason that will benefit the patient (Section 1). In addition to current medications, it is important to remember that many women take over-the-counter drugs and herbal products which they may not perceive as 'medications'. This is particularly important where these may affect the coagulation system (eg aspirin, NSAIDs).

Informed consent

It is important that a woman have sufficient information to consent to an operative procedure (Section 1). This includes all the common complications in general and specific to the procedure, including the chance of a failed procedure—particularly relevant for sterilisation procedures. Unless the procedure is an emergency, the woman should be given written information and a copy of the consent form to take home and consider before signing the consent form.

Risks from surgical procedures

Emergency surgery

An emergency procedure is associated with greater hazards than one that is planned. Intraoperative and postoperative considerations can affect the outcome and there may be special considerations for women (Box 18.2).

BOX 18.2 Operative considerations

- Intraoperative care:
  - Anaesthesia: LA, GA, regional
  - Sutures: absorbable : nonabsorbable
  - Indwelling urinary catheter (IDC)
  - Drains into peritoneal cavity and abdominal wall
  - Protection of personnel: needlestick injuries, eye protection
- Postoperative care:
  - Analgesia
  - Intravenous fluids
  - Oral intake
  - Physiotherapy
  - Ambulation
  - DVT prophylaxis
- Special considerations:
  - Pregnancy and postpartum (hypercoagulable state: section 9)
  - Oestrogen preparations:
    - Thrombosis and OCP increases RR × 3–4
    - Thrombosis and HRT RR × 3–4
      (associated with a 10-fold higher absolute risk because of older age)[1]
    - Thrombosis increases with age, obesity and smoking.

Venous thrombosis

This major health problem has an annual incidence of 160 per 100 000 for deep venous thrombosis (DVT), 20 per 100 000 for symptomatic non-fatal pulmonary embolus (PE) and 50 per 100 000 for fatal autopsy detected pulmonary embolism. Deep vein thrombosis can lead to chronic venous insufficiency and this is the underlying condition leading to 25 per cent of venous ulcers.[2] In addition it causes cellulitis, chronic oedema and decreased quality of life.

Prevention of thromboembolism

In low-risk surgical patients (short operations for a woman < 40 years with no additional risk factors) without thromboprophylaxis the estimated risk of DVT in the calf is 2 per cent, a clinical PE is 0.2 per cent and a fatal PE is 0.002 per cent.[3]

Some procedures pose a higher risk to the patient than others (Box 18.3). The rate of embolism following gynaecological surgery without prophylaxis has been reported as an average of 16 per cent and fatal PE as 0.4 per cent.[3] However, a number of prophylactic measures can be taken to prevent these deaths (Box 18.4). The rates of PE in prospective studies of gynaecological surgery patients demonstrated a 75 per cent risk reduction with thromboprophylaxis.[3] Women taking oestrogen hormone or who are pregnant have an increased risk of thrombosis, and it is recommended that hormone preparations cease 4–6 weeks before major surgery.

BOX 18.3 Risk of deep vein thrombosis without prophylaxis in different patient groups/situations[2]

- General medicine (17%)
- Gynaecological surgery (14–22%)
- General surgery (25%)
- Hip fracture (45%)
- Elective hip replacement (51%)
- Stroke (56%).

BOX 18.4 Prophylactic measures for preventing deep vein thrombosis

- Hydration
- Ambulation
- Graduated compression stockings
- Intermittent pneumatic compression (IPC)
- Calf stimulator
- Drug treatment (timing, anaesthetic and surgical considerations):
  - Heparin
  - Warfarin
  - Dextran
- Combination treatments

Specific risks for obstetric and gynaecological surgery

There may be risks associated with a particular procedure. For most obstetric and gynaecological procedures, operating in the pelvic area involves close contact with both the ureter and bladder, and so a knowledge of the anatomical relationship to the ureter and pelvic blood vessels is essential (Figure 18.1). There is increased risk to these structures in the presence of malignant disease, inflammatory conditions (PID or endometriosis), adhesions, or where there is distortion of the normal anatomy from tumours, such as cervical fibroids.

FIGURE 18.1 Anatomical relationship of the pelvic area to the ureter and pelvic blood vessels

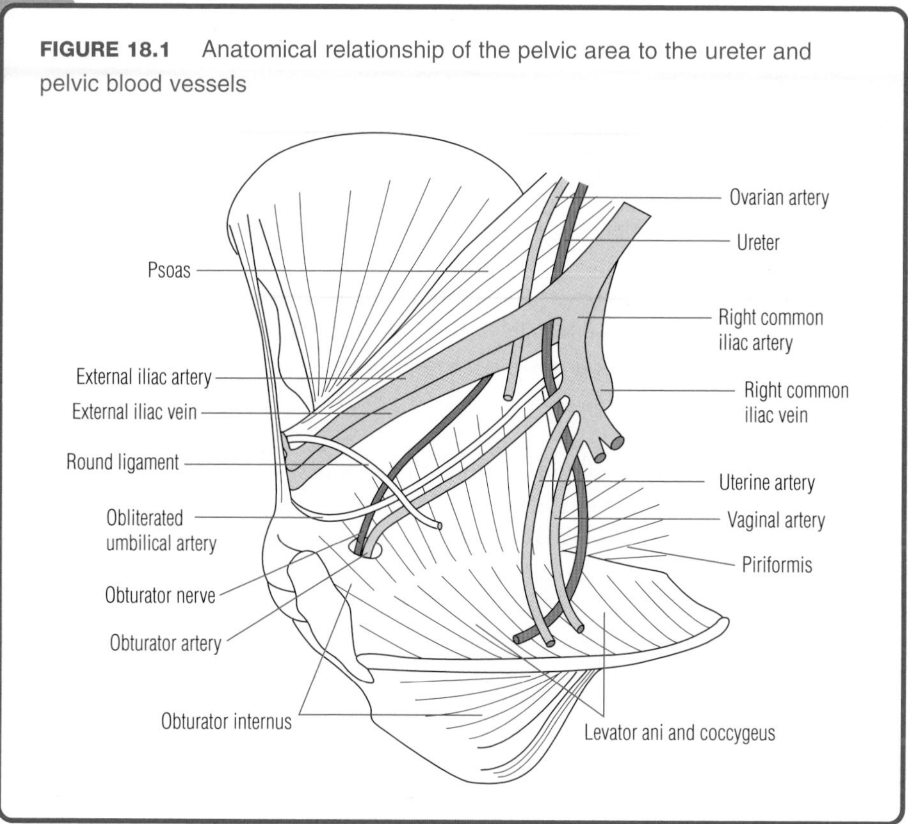

Common procedures

See also the summary list provided in Table 18.1 at the end of this section.

Hysteroscopy

Hysteroscopy is a procedure used for both diagnosis and treatment.

Endometrial ablative treatments for dysfunctional uterine bleeding

These can be performed via the hysteroscope and include endometrial ablation by diathermy or laser, or transcervical resection of the endometrium (TCRE). The ablation may also be achieved by microwave and other newer techniques. The current studies to compare these approaches are limited by the number of participants, length of follow-up and comparison with the alternatives. The advantages to women are shorter hospital stays, less severe and less frequent complications, and more rapid return to everyday activities.[4]

Long-term considerations of endometrial ablation

It is possible for some endometrium to regenerate after any of these techniques designed to ablate the endometrium. Consideration should be given for any women subsequently taking HRT (even though she has amenorrhoea) to use combined treatment (with progesterone to protect the 'endometrium' together with oestrogen). Also it should be kept in mind that the risk and difficulty in diagnosing a future endometrial cancer in the presence of intrauterine adhesions has not been determined.

The success rates, complications, outcome and cost comparisons with hysterectomy favour hysteroscopic methods. But the long-term data comparing both methods is not yet complete. Approximately 3–13 per cent of heavy menstrual bleeding is not improved at one year after an endometrial ablative procedure and 10–18 per cent of women will require re-treatment or a subsequent hysterectomy. The risks are low at 4.4 per cent and include uterine perforation, haemorrhage and fluid overload. Pregnancy after these techniques is rare but has been reported.

Laparoscopy

Laparoscopy is a procedure commonly used to investigate pelvic pain, infertility and ectopic pregnancy. It is also used as a procedure to treat these conditions and perform procedures such as sterilisation. The technique involves insertion of a Veress needle and insufflation of the abdominal cavity with carbon dioxide. A larger (2–5 mm diameter) instrument is then introduced through which a telescope is passed and a picture obtained on a TV screen. Complications are uncommon but include damage to any intra-abdominal structure (eg bowel, blood vessels) that may be contacted during 'blind' entry into the abdominal cavity.

Hysterectomy

The chance of a woman undergoing hysterectomy varies around the world and the decision-making process to reach this endpoint involves many factors (Box 18.5). Hysterectomy, in whatever geographical location, by whatever surgical route and by whichever surgeon, has an associated morbidity (infection 2%; haemorrhage 0.5% injury to bowel, ureter or bladder) and mortality (6–11 per 10 000).

The procedure can be through the abdomen or the vagina. Vaginal hysterectomy has a quicker recovery for the woman. It is not advised where the uterus is equivalent to or > 14 week pregnancy, or where malignancy is a possibility.

BOX 18.5 Factors influencing decision to undertake a hysterectomy

- Symptoms
- Clinical signs
- Presence of pathology
- Woman's:
  - wishes
  - knowledge
  - experience
- Medical practitioner's:
  - characteristics
  - preferences
  - skills and experience
- Available technologies
- Woman's socio-economic status
- Local economic issues
- Health policy guidelines
- Medical insurance category

Consideration should be given by any woman over the age of 45 years, who is having a hysterectomy, as to whether or not she wishes to have the ovaries removed (Box 18.6). If the woman is premenopausal, HRT would also need to be discussed.

BOX 18.6 Removal of ovaries at hysterectomy:[5] points for discussion

- Benign disease of ovary:
  - x 2 risk of further benign disease[6]
- Residual ovary syndrome—chronic pelvic pain:
  - More likely in women with pre-existing pelvic pain
- Endometriosis:
  - Further surgery for pelvic pain with ovary in situ reported[7,8]
- Premenstrual syndrome:
  - Symptoms continue with ovaries in situ
- Ovarian cancer:
  - Not common
  - Difficult to detect at an early stage
  - Lifetime risk is 2% with no family history of the disease
  - 7–18% of women developed ovarian cancer who had undergone a procedure where oophorectomy could have been done.[9]

Caesarean section

The incidence of caesarean sections has been increasing in developed countries in recent years and has been the subject of much debate. Caesarean section may be undertaken as an elective procedure or as an emergency (Section 14). The incision into the uterus is made into the lower segment. This is that part of the uterus that lies between the attachment of the peritoneum of the uterovesical pouch superiorly and the histological internal os inferiorly (Figure 18.2). This area has less muscle, more connective tissue, is thinner than the upper uterine segment, and there is less blood loss at operation and easier repair. In the last few weeks of pregnancy and/or at the onset of labour this area thins progressively as the thick muscle of the upper segment pulls on the cervix (Section 7). The majority of caesarean sections are carried out under regional anaesthesia (epidural or spinal anaesthetic). This is safer for the mother, who then has intact airway reflexes and the chance of inhalation of regurgitated acidic gastric contents and the development of a chemical pneumonia (Mendelson's syndrome) is reduced. It also has the advantage that the woman can be involved in the birth and have her partner or a support person with her in the operating theatre. Regional anaesthetic also has an advantage for the fetus, who avoids respiratory depression from general anaesthesia. An epidural can be used to provide postoperative pain relief. Complications are rare but may include transient hypotension and dural tap (in 1%), which may be followed by headache.

A decision-to-delivery interval of 30 minutes for an emergency caesarean section has been suggested but as a universal standard this may be unrealistic[10] and not of proven benefit.[11] Antibiotic prophylaxis has been shown to reduce the risk of endometritis by two-thirds to three-quarters.[12]

FIGURE 18.2 The lower uterine segment in late pregnancy

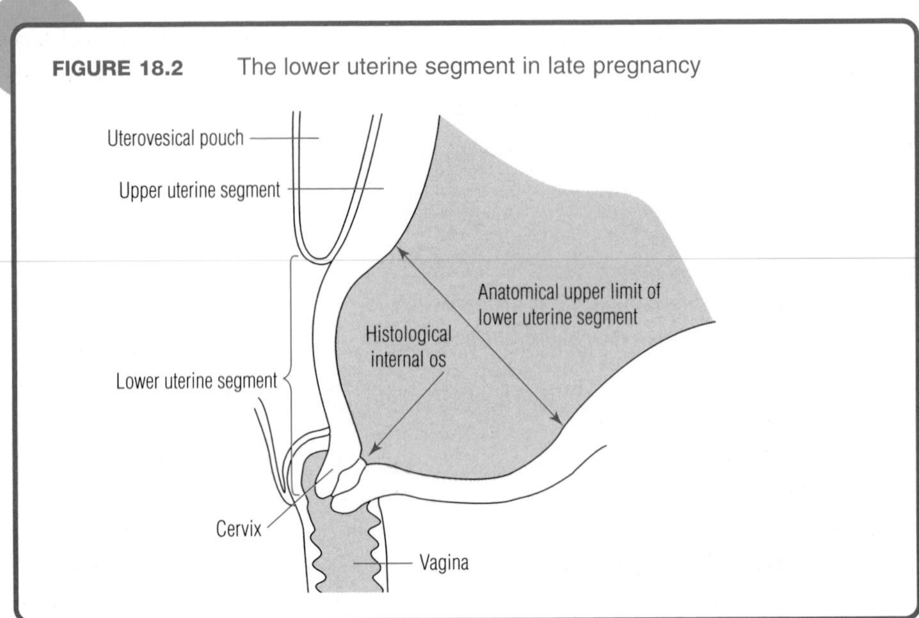

Postoperative care

A minimum of daily visits to the patient while in hospital is essential. Routine observations include charts to record the temperature, fluid balance and medication. Monitor the recovery process: be alert for early signs of complications (Box 18.1), provide information and answer the patient's questions. The details of each visit and any instructions to the patient or staff should be clearly recorded and signed in the patient's notes.

Adverse events

Everyone wants to avoid an adverse outcome during hospitalisation. Nevertheless, medical treatment is associated with risks; complications and errors can occur and can involve any member of staff. A medical error should be defined in terms of failed processes that are clearly linked to an adverse health outcome. Adverse outcomes include events that are the result of a complication, medical error or negligence. In one large study, 3.7 per cent of patients were identified with disabling injuries after treatment.[13] Drug complications were the most common adverse event (19%), followed by wound infection (14%) and technical complications (13%). Forty-eight per cent of adverse events were associated with an operation. Errors were identified in 58 per cent of the adverse events and nearly half of these were attributed to negligence: diagnostic mishaps (75%), non-invasive therapeutic mishaps—'errors of omission' (75%), and events in the emergency room (70%).

Adverse patient events can be detected, and their frequency reduced, using multiple detection methods and clinical improvement strategies as part of an integrated clinical risk management program. Efforts to reduce errors should be proportional to their impact on outcomes (preventable morbidity, mortality, and patient satisfaction) and the cost of preventing them.[14] Most types of adverse events occur too infrequently to be characterised at a hospital level and require large-scale (preferably national) collections of incidents and events.[15]

Medical problems

The concept of considering sex and gender differences in medicine (apart from reproductive issues) is a relatively recent idea. Latest research indicates that some problems are more serious, more common, or have different interventions and outcomes, in women than in men.

At present we do not know the answer to many questions about diseases in women. The questions should nevertheless be asked and the possibility that there are differences in the same disease occurring in men and women, even for common conditions, should be considered by any treating clinician or health professional.

There are numerous examples of differences in disease between genders; however, this knowledge is at an early stage and we need to keep asking questions. Those listed in Box 18.7 are a few examples; these will change over time as more information becomes available.

Some of these conditions have been covered in this text: for example, eating disorders, breast disease and urinary incontinence. Others may be less obvious; for

BOX 18.7 Possible gender differences in disease

- Do socio-economic determinants of disease affect men and women differently? (eg access to care)
- Does the degree of power and control over one's life affect health? (eg abuse, decision making about management options)
- Are the presenting symptoms the same? (eg chest pain and cardiovascular disease, appendicitis in pregnancy)
- Does the disease occur more commonly in women? (eg autoimmune disease, rheumatoid arthritis, irritable bowel syndrome)
- Is the aetiology the same? (eg substance abuse)
- Are there different risk factors? (eg osteoporosis, lung cancer)
- Are the findings the same? (eg depression)
- Does the disease have a different significance? (eg periodontal disease may be associated with preterm delivery, women with HIV have different outcomes)
- Does the disease behave differently? (eg higher rates of cardiovascular disease in diabetic women)
- Are the investigations appropriate for a particular symptom? (eg abdominal pain)
- Is a condition affected by the hormone differences? Does a disease behave differently during the menstrual cycle, in pregnancy, while taking the OCP? (eg epilepsy)

example, heart disease is the most common cause of death in both genders but in women this may have an atypical presentation; women's lipid profiles change after menopause (increase in LDL and decrease in HDL), and outcomes from treatment may not be the same.

Research

It is also important to reflect on the research on which the management is based. Have women participated in the research—or have the research outcomes simply been extrapolated from the data on men (Box 18.8)?

In many instances it may be appropriate to apply the same results, in others perhaps not. Students and clinicians working in the area of women's health should remain alert and questioning if there is to be further progress in improving knowledge about women in health and disease.

BOX 18.8 Questions to consider in the analysis of research evidence

- Is there gender bias in the study hypothesis?
- Has there been appropriate inclusion or exclusion of women in the study?
- Does the analysis include a breakdown of the results by sex?
- Can the findings from studies that exclude particular groups, such as women, children or a particular race or cultural group, be generalised and applied to those groups?

Source: adapted from Phillips 2002.[16]

TABLE 18.1 A summary of common gynaecological and obstetric operations

Name of operation	Procedure	Useful notes	Indications
Bartholin's marsupialisation	The dilated duct from Bartholin's gland is opened and the edges stitched to surrounding tissue	If infected, a small ribbon gauze pack is left in situ for 24 hours. Defect heals over several days	
Caesarean section	LSCS: lower segment of uterus incised. Upper segment may be used for delivery of premature fetus, hysterotomy, anterior placenta praevia	See above	Elective or emergency

TABLE 18.1 continued

Name of operation	Procedure	Useful notes	Indications
Cervical suture	CI manifested by opening of cervix, prolapse and rupture of membranes and loss of pregnancy < 24 weeks	Suture removed towards end of pregnancy or if labour ensues	Cervical incompetence (CI)
Cone biopsy	Cone-shaped cervical tissue removed by Fischer/LLETZ biopsy, laser, scalpel	Tailored to remove diseased tissue but to maintain the integrity of the internal cervical os in women desiring future pregnancies—damage to this causes cervical incompetence	*Diagnostic:* adenocarcinoma cervix, microinvasive or invasive squamous carcinoma cervix *Therapeutic:* CIN in endocervical canal
Cystoscopy	Passage of a rigid or flexible telescope through the urethra into the bladder	Prior to and on completion of an incontinence procedure Staging of a gynaecological cancer Suspected damage to bladder during surgery Assessment of bladder neck, suspected abnormality Infective history or haematuria	Bladder infection
D & C (dilatation and curettage)	Cervix gradually dilated and uterine lining (endometrium) removed	Uterine perforation (more likely if uterine wall is soft: pregnancy or malignancy) is a complication	*Diagnostic:* abnormal bleeding *Pregnancy complications:* abortion, hydatidiform mole
Evacuation of retained products of conception (ERPC)	Under GA	Pregnant uterine wall soft and more likely to be perforated	Incomplete: miscarriage, termination of pregnancy, removal of placenta
Examination under anaesthesia	Undertaken where discomfort for the woman can be avoided. Also for assessing medical condition.	Forms part of assessment for staging gynaecological cancer and exploring uterine cavity after a post-partum haemorrhage	

(continued overleaf)

TABLE 18.1 continued

Name of operation	Procedure	Useful notes	Indications
1 Abdominal hysterectomy	1 Removal of uterus and cervix	Removal of both ovaries in the pre-menopausal woman requires discussion on HRT	Bleeding problems, pelvic pain, cancer of endometrium, cervix, ovary
2 + bilateral salpingo-oophorectomy (BSO)	2 + Removal of both tubes and ovaries	Subtotal: suggested benefits on bowel, bladder and sexual function. Less likelihood	*Oophorectomy:* endometriosis; PID; ovarian cysts (after accident, torsion, or
3 Subtotal hysterectomy	3 Removal of the body of the uterus with conservation of the cervix	of damage to bladder and ureters. Woman require to continue with Pap tests	rupture); cancer *Salpingectomy:* ectopic pregnancy; PID; cancer
4 Vaginal hysterectomy (± BSO)	Uterus and cervix removed via vagina. No abdominal scar	May be combined with bladder or posterior vaginal wall repair	Bleeding problems Prolapse Bladder repair
5 Laparosopically assisted vaginal hysterectomy	Upper pedicles divided via laparoscope. Uterus removed via vagina	Combination of laparoscopy and vaginal hysterectomy	Useful where minimal uterine descent
6 Radical hysterectomy eg Wertheim's	Total abdominal hysterectomy, BSO, upper vagina, and pelvic lymph nodes removed	Risk of damage to bowel, ureters and bladder	Cancer of cervix
Hysteroscopy	Small-diameter rigid or flexible telescope is passed through the cervix to inspect the uterine cavity.	Complications: perforation of uterus, fluid overload, pelvic inflammatory disease (if infection present)	Abnormal bleeding Suspected uterine malformation Suspected Asherman's syndrome
Hysterotomy	Upper segment incision into uterus to remove POC before 24 weeks		Termination of pregnancy
Laparoscopy	To investigate abdominal symptoms or masses or for sterilisation (dividing or sealing the uterine tubes)	Discomfort under ribs, shoulders and neck for 24 hours (from CO_2 gas in abdominal cavity). 2–3 × 1 cm abdominal scars	*Diagnostic:* acute and chronic abdominal pain, infertility *Procedural:* sterilisation; ovarian cysts; ectopic pregnancy *Endometriosis:* staging and ablative treatment

TABLE 18.1 continued

Name of operation	Procedure	Useful notes	Indications
LLETZ/LEEP/Loop biopsy	A heated wire loop to remove cervical tissue. Area to be removed often outlined with acetic acid or iodine	Usually minimal blood loss	Cervical intraepithelial neoplasia (CIN)
Manchester repair	Cervix amputated and lateral uterine ligaments shortened. Used for uterovaginal prolapse preserving the uterus	Often performed with anterior and posterior vaginal repair	Prolapse, retaining the uterus
Manual removal of placenta	Under general (GA) or regional anaesthesia	Maintain contraction of uterus at end of procedure by bimanual compression and intravenous syntocinon	Retained placenta
Marshall Marchetti, sling operation, Burch colposuspension	Elevating and fixing bladder neck to pubic symphysis or nearby tissue	Bladder catheterisation for 3–7 days post operation	Stress incontinence
Myomectomy	Fibroids shelled out of uterine muscle wall and defects repaired	Postoperative morbidity similar to abdominal hysterectomy	Fibroids, conserving the uterus
Ovarian cystectomy	Cyst shelled out of ovary and remaining ovarian tissue repaired and conserved	Ovary retains normal function	Benign ovarian cysts, conserving the ovary
Salpingostomy	Opening but conserving uterine tube		Ectopic pregnancy, PID, conserving uterine tube
Vaginal repair: anterior, posterior		Newer procedures: involving tape inserted via vagina or suprapubically (Section 15)	Cystocele; cystourethrocele Rectocele; enterocele; perineal body laxity
Ventrosuspension	Round ligaments between upper uterine angles and pelvic side walls are shortened. This lifts the uterus out of the pouch of Douglas	Useful if pathology (endometriosis or PID) in pouch of Douglas. Prevents dyspareunia by lifting ovaries away from pouch of Douglas	Retroverted uterus; endometriosis and PID (to prevent the uterus adhering to pouch of Douglas)
Vulvectomy: simple/radical	Current approach for less extensive surgery to minimise morbidity and disfigurement		Cancer; pre-cancer

References

(Coch Rev: Cochrane Review. In: The Cochrane Library, Oxford: Update Software, 2002.)

1 The health professional role

1 O'Flynn N, Rymer J. Women's attitudes to the sex of medical students in a gynaecology clinic: cross sectional survey. BMJ 2002;325(7366):683–4.

2 Wensing M, Jung HP, Mainz J, Olesen F, Grol R. A systematic review of the literature on patient priorities in general practice care. Part 1: Description of the research domain. Soc Sci Med 1998;47(10):1573–88.

3 Coulter A. Patients' views of the good doctor. BMJ 2002;325(7366):668–9.

4 Dean B, Barber N, Schachter M. What is a prescribing error? Q Health Care 2000;9(4):232–7.

5 Mechanic D. How should hamsters run? Some observations about sufficient patient time in primary care. BMJ 2001;323(7307):266–8.

6 Freeman G, Horder JP, Howie JG, Hungin P, Hill AP, Shah NC et al. Evolving general practice consultation in Britain: issues of length and context. BMJ 2002;324(7342):880–2.

7 Maguire P, Pitceathly C. Key communication skills and how to acquire them. BMJ 2002; 325(7366):697–700.

8 Stewart M. Effective physician–patient communication and health outcomes: a review. Can Med Assoc J 1995;152(9):1423–33.

9 Lewin SA, Skea ZC, Entwistle V, Zwarenstein M, Dick J. Interventions for providers to promote a patient-centred approach in clinical consultations. Coch Rev.

10 Ferriman A. Patients need to be more involved in care decisions. BMJ 2001;323(7303):10.

11 Gask L, Usherwood T. ABC of psychological medicine. The consultation. BMJ 2002; 324(7353):1567–9.

12 Edwards A, Elwyn G, Mulley A. Explaining risks: turning numerical data into meaningful pictures. BMJ 2002;324(7341):827–30.

13 Holmes-Rovner M, Llewellyn-Thomas H, Entwistle V, Coulter A, O'Connor A, Rover DR. Patient choice modules for summaries of clinical effectiveness: a proposal. BMJ 2001; 322(7287):664–7.

14 Levinson W, Roter DL, Mullooly JP, Dull VT, Frankel RM. Physician–patient communication. The relationship with malpractice claims among primary care physicians and surgeons. JAMA 1997;277(7):553–9.

15 O'Connor AM, Rostom A, Fiset V, Tetroe J, Entwistle V, Llewellyn-Thomas H et al. Decision aids for patients facing health treatment or screening decisions: systematic review. BMJ 1999; 319(7212):731–4.

16 Deyo RA. A key medical decision maker: the patient. BMJ 2001;323(7311):466–7.

17 Murtagh J. General practice. 4th edn. North Ryde, Australia: McGraw Hill, 1999.

18 Harris DM, Guten S. Health-protective behavior: an exploratory study. J Health Soc Behav 1979;20(1):17–29.

19 McGuire TM, Vernon J. Queensland Medication Helpline Annual Report 2000–2001. Mater Pharmacy Services, Health Services, South Brisbane, 1 October 2001.

20 MacLennan AH, Wilson DH, Taylor AW. Prevalence and cost of alternative medicines in Australia. Lancet 1996;347(9001):569–73.

21 Eisenberg DM, Davis RB, Ettner SL, Appel S, Wilkey W, Van Rompay M et al. Trends in alternative medicine use in the United States, 1990–1997: results of a follow-up national survey. JAMA 1998;280(18):1569–75.

22 Thomas KJ, Nicholl JP, Coleman P. Use and expenditure on complementary medicine in England: a population-based survey. Complement Ther Med 2001;9(1):2–11.

23 Astin JA. Why patients use alternative medicine: results of a national study. JAMA 1998;279(19):1548–53.

24 Harris RZ, Benet LZ, Schwartz JB. Gender effects in pharmacokinetics and pharmacodynamics. Drugs 1995;50(2):222–39.

25 Tanaka E. Gender-related differences in pharmacokinetics and their clinical significance. J Clin Pharm Ther 1999;24(5):339–46.

26 Meibohm B, Beierle I, Derendorf H. How important are gender differences in pharmacokinetics? Clin-Pharmacokinet 2002;41(5):329–42.
27 Yukawa E, Honda T, Ohdo S, Higuchi S, Aoyama T. Population-based investigation of relative clearance of digoxin in Japanese patients by multiple trough screen analysis: an update. J Clin Pharmacol 1997;37(2):92–100.
28 Schuetz EG, Furuya KN, Schuetz JD. Interindividual variation in expression of P-glycoprotein in normal human liver and secondary hepatic neoplasms. J Pharmacol Exp Ther 1995; 275(2):1011–18.
29 Guengerich FP. Inhibition of oral contraceptive steroid-metabolizing enzymes by steroids and drugs. Am J Obstet Gynecol 1990;163(6 Pt 2):2159–63.
30 Yonkers KA, Kando JC, Cole JO, Blumenthal S. Gender differences in pharmacokinetics and pharmacodynamics of psychotropic medication. Am J Psychiatry 1992;149(5):587–95.
31 Australian Drug Evaluation Committee. Prescribing medicines in pregnancy. 4th edn. Canberra: Therapeutic Goods Administration, 1999.
32 Jewell D. Nausea and vomiting in early pregnancy. Clin Evid 2002;7:1279–81.
33 Briggs GG, Freeman RK, Yaffe SJ. Drugs in pregnancy and lactation. A reference guide to fetal and neonatal risk. 6th edn. Baltimore: Williams & Wilkins, 2002.
34 Kennedy D. Drugs in pregnancy. Medicine Today 2002;3(2):26–34.
35 Last JM. A dictionary of epidemiology. 4th edn. New York: Oxford University Press, 2001.
36 Cervical Cancer Prevention Taskforce. Screening for the prevention of cervical cancer. Canberra: Department of Health, Housing and Community Services, 1991.
37 Rembold CM. Number needed to screen: development of a statistic for disease screening. BMJ 1998;317(7154):307–12.
38 Muir Gray JA. Evidence-based health care: how to make health policy and management decisions. 2nd edn. London: Churchill Livingstone, 2001.
39 Barratt AL, Les Irwig M, Glasziou PP, Salkeld GP, Houssami N. Benefits, harms and costs of screening mammography in women 70 years and over: a systematic review. Med J Aust 2002;176(6):266–71.
40 Dickinson JA. Cervical screening: time to change the policy. Med J Aust 2002;176(11): 547–50.
41 Leung GM, Lam TH, Hedley AJ. Screening mammography re-evaluated. Lancet 2000; 355(9205):750–1.
42 Dickinson JA, Wun YT, Wong SL. Modelling death rates for carriers of hepatitis B. Epidemiol Infect 2002;128(1):83–92.
43 Hirst G, Ward J, Del Mar CB. Screening for prostate cancer: the case against. Med J Aust 1996;164(5):285–8.
44 Dent TH, Sadler M. From guidance to practice. Why NICE is not enough. BMJ 2002; 324(7341):842–5.
45 Silagy C, Haines A. Evidence-based practice in primary care. London: BMJ Books, 2002.
46 Sackett DL, Straus SE, Richardson WS, Rosenberg W. Haynes RB. Evidence-based medicine. 2nd edn. Edinburgh: Churchill Livingstone, 2000.
47 Chang CL, Donaghy M, Poulter N. Migraine and stroke in young women: case-control study. The World Health Organisation Collaborative Study of Cardiovascular Disease and Steroid Hormone Contraception. BMJ 1999;318(7175):13–18.
48 Tzourio C, Tehindrazanarivelo A, Iglesias S, Alperovitch A, Chedru F, d'Anglejan-Chatillon J et al. Case-control study of migraine and risk of ischaemic stroke in young women. BMJ 1995;310(6983):830–3.
49 Henrich JB, Horwitz RI. The contributions of individual factors to thromboembolic stroke. J Gen Intern Med. 1989;4(3):195–201.
50 WHO Collaborative Study of Cardiovascular Disease and Steroid Hormone Contraception. Ischaemic stroke and combined oral contraceptives: results of an international, multicentre, case-control study. Lancet 1996;348(9026):498–505.
51 WHO Collaborative Study of Cardiovascular Disease and Steroid Hormone Contraception. Haemorrhagic stroke, overall stroke risk, and combined oral contraceptives: results of an international, multicentre, case-control study. Lancet 1996;348(9026):505–10.
52 Del Mar CB, Glasziou PP. Ways of using evidence-based medicine in general practice. Med J Aust 2001;174(7):347–50.

53 Brassey J, Elwyn G, Price C, Kinnersley P. Just in time information for clinicians: a questionnaire evaluation of the ATTRACT project. BMJ 2001;322(7285):529–30.
54 Del Mar CB, Silagy CA, Glasziou PP, Weller D, Spinks AB, Bernath V et al. Feasibility of an evidence-based literature search service for general practitioners. Med J Aust 2001; 175(3):134–7.
55 Muir Gray JA. Where's the chief knowledge officer? BMJ 1998;317(7162):832.

2 Women and health

1 Charles N. Gender Divisions and Social Change. Hemel Hempstead: Harvester Wheatsheaf, 1993.
2 Doyal L, ed. Women and Health Services: an agenda for change. Buckingham: Open University Press, 1998.
3 Fee E, Krieger N. Women's health, politics and power: essays on sex/gender, medicine and public health. Amityville NY: Baywood Publishing Co, 1994.
4 Kitts J, Roberts J. The health gap: beyond pregnancy and reproduction. Ottawa: IDRC, 1996.
5 Stein J. Empowerment and women's health. London: Zed Books, 1997.
6 Carroll S. The which? guide to men's health. London: Consumers' Association, 1994.
7 Harrison J, Chin J, Ficarrotto T. Warning: masculinity may be dangerous to your health. In: Kimmel M, Messner M, eds, Men's lives. New York: Macmillan, 1992.
8 Huggins A, Lamb B. Social Perspectives on Men's Health in Australia. Melbourne: Maclennan and Petty, 1998.
9 Sabo D, Gordon D. Men's health and illness: Gender, power and the body. London: Sage, 1995.
10 Oakley A. Sex, Gender and Society. London: Temple Smith, 1972.
11 Birke L. Feminism and biology. Brighton: Wheatsheaf, 1986.
12 Wizemann S, Pardue ML. Exploring the biological contribution to human health: does sex matter? Washington DC: National Academy Press, 2001.
13 Kraemer S. The fragile male. BMJ 2000;321(7276):1609–12.
14 Doyal L. What makes women sick: gender and the political economy of health. London: Tavistock, 1995.
15 Sargent C, Brettell C, eds. Gender and health: an international perspective. New Jersey: Prentice-Hall, 1996.
16 Papenek H. To each less than she needs, from each more than she can do: allocations, entitlements and values. In: Tinker I, ed. Persistent inequalities: women and world development. New York: Oxford University Press, 1990.
17 United Nations Development Programme Human Development Report. New York: UNDP, 1995.
18 World Health Organization. Gender and health: technical document. Geneva: WHO, 1998.
19 Allottey P. Travelling with excess baggage: health problems of refugee women in Western Australia. Women & Health 1998;28(1):63–81.
20 Markovic M, Manderson L. Nowhere is as at home: adjustment strategies of recent immigrant women from the former Yugoslav Republics in South East Queensland. J Sociology 2000; 36(3):315–28.
21 Busfield J. Men, women and madness: understanding gender and mental disorder. London: Macmillan, 1996.
22 Desjarlais R, Eisenberg L, Good B, Kleinman A. World mental health: problems and priorities. Oxford: Oxford University Press, 1995.
23 Payne S. Hit and miss: the success and failure of psychiatric services for women. In: Doyal L, ed. Women and health services: an agenda for change. Buckingham: Open University Press, 1998.
24 Australian Institute of Health and Welfare. Mental Health of Australians. Canberra: AIHW and AGPS, 1998.
25 Brown P, Brown W. Leisure: all work and no play does Jill no good. Australian Parks and Leisure Health 2001;4(4)38–9.
26 Lee C. Family care giving: a gender-based analysis of women's experiences. In: Payne S, Ellis Hill C, eds. Chronic and terminal illness: new perspectives on caring and carers. New York: Oxford University Press, 2001.
27 Schofield H, Bloch S, Nankervis J, Murphy B, Singh B, Herrman H. Health and wellbeing of women family carers: a comparative study with a generic focus. ANZ J Public Health 1999;(6):585–9.

28 Lee C and Porteous J. Experiences of family care-giving among middle aged Australian women. Feminism & Psychology 2002;12(1)79–96.

29 Australian Bureau of Statistics Year Book Australia 1998 (special article: violence against women). Canberra: AGPS; 1998.

30 Mirrlees-Black C. Domestic violence: findings from a new British Crime Survey self-reporting questionnaire. Home Office Research Studies no 192. London: Home Office, 1998.

31 Webster J, Sweett S, Stoltz TA. Domestic violence in pregnancy: a prevalence study. Med J Aust 1994;161(8):466–70.

32 Arber S. Health, ageing and older women. In: Doyal L, ed. Women and health services: an agenda for change. Buckingham: Open University Press, 1998.

33 World Health Organization. Women, ageing and health: controlling health across the lifespan. Geneva: WHO, 1996.

34 Drever F, Whitehead M, eds. Health inequalities: decennial supplement. Series DS: 15. London: Stationery Office, 1997.

35 Office for National Statistics. Living in Britain: results from the 1995 General Household Survey. London: Stationery Office, 1997.

36 Australian Bureau of Statistics. Australian social trends 1999. Canberra: AGPS, 1999.

37 Smaje C. Health, 'Race' and ethnicity: making sense of the evidence. London: King's Fund Institute, 1995.

38 Fenton S, Sadiq A. The sorrow in my heart: sixteen Asian women speak about depression. London: Commission for Racial Equality, 1995.

39 Australian Bureau of Statistics. National Aboriginal and Torres Strait Islander Survey. Canberra: AGPS, 1994.

40 Kildea S, Bowen F. Reproductive health, infertility and sexually transmitted infections in Indigenous women in a remote community in the Northern Territory. Aust NZ J Public Health 1994;24(4):382–6.

41 Kennir B. Family planning clinic cuts: a survey of NHS family planning clinics in Greater London. London: Family Planning Association, 1990.

42 Black K, Fisher J, Groves S. Public hospital pregnancy termination services: are we meeting demand? Aust NZ J Public Health 1999;(5):525–7.

43 Taylor R, Mamoon H, Morell S, Wain G. Cervical screening by socio-economic status in Australia. Aust NZ J Public Health 2001;(3):256–6.

44 Wain G, Morrell S, Taylor R, Mamoon H, Bodkin N. Variation in cervical cancer screening by region, socio-economic, migrant and indigenous status in women in New South Wales. Aust NZ J Obstet Gynaecol 2001;(3):320–5.

45 Young A, Dobson A, Byles J. Determinants of general practitioner use among women in Australia. Soc Sci Med 2001;53(12):1641–51.

46 Roberts H. The patient patients: women and their doctors. London: Pandora Press, 1985.

47 Graham H, Oakley A. Competing ideologies of reproduction: medical and maternal perspectives on pregnancy. In Roberts H, ed. Women, health and reproduction. London: Routledge & Kegan Paul, 1981.

48 Todd A. Intimate adversaries: cultural conflict between doctors and women patients. Philadelphia PA: University of Pennsylvania Press, 1989.

49 White E. Black women's health book: speaking for ourselves. Seattle: Seal Press, 1990.

50 Young A, Byles J, Dobson A. Women's satisfaction with general practice consultations. Med J Aust 1998;(168):386–9.

51 Tsianakas V, Liamputtong P. What women from an Islamic background in Australia say about care in pregnancy and pre-natal testing. Midwifery 2002;18(1):25–34.

52 Jirojwong S, Manderson L. Beliefs and behaviours about Pap and breast self-examination among Thai immigrant women in Brisbane, Australia. Women Health 2001;33(3/4): 47–66.

53 Holmes H, Purdy C. Feminist perspectives in medical ethics. Bloomington: Indiana University Press, 1992.

54 Sherwin, S. No longer patient: feminist ethics and health care. Philadelphia: Temple University Press, 1992.

55 Tong R. Feminist approaches to bioethics: theoretical reflections and practical applications. Boulder CO: Westview Press, 1997.

56 Mirza T, Kovacs G, McDonald P. The use of reproductive health services by young women in Australia. Aust NZ J Obstet Gynaecol 1998;(3):336–8.
57 Mintzes B, ed. A question of control: women's perspectives on the development and use of contraceptive technology. Amsterdam: Women and Pharmaceuticals Project, Health Action International and WEMOS, 1992.
58 Broom D. By women, for women: the continuing appeal of women's health centres. Women Health 1998;28(1):5–22.
59 Redberg RF. Coronary artery disease in women: understanding the diagnostic and management pitfalls. Medscape Women's Health 1998;3(5):1.
60 Sharp I. Gender issues in the prevention and treatment of coronary heart disease. In: Doyal L, ed. Women and health services: an agenda for change, Buckingham: Open University Press, 1998.
61 Foster S, Mallik M. A comparative study of differences in the referral behaviour patterns of men and women who have experienced cardiac-related chest pain. Intensive & Critical Care Nursing 1998;14(4):192–202.
62 Tobin JN, Wassertheil-Smoller S, Wexler JP, Steingart RM, Budner N, Lense L et al. Sex bias in considering coronary bypass surgery. Ann Intern Med 1997;107(1):19–25.
63 Travin M, Johnson L. Assessment of coronary artery disease in women. Curr Opin Cardiol 64 1997;12(6):587–94.
64 Petticrew M, McKee, M, Jones J. Coronary artery surgery: are women discriminated against? BMJ 1993;306(6886):1164–6.
65 Heller R, Powell H, O'Connell R, D'Este K, Lim L. Trends in the hospital management of unstable angina. J Epidem Comm Health; 2000;55(7):483–6.
66 Semmens J, Norman P, Lawrence-Brown M, Holman C. Influence of gender on outcome from ruptured abdominal aneurysm. Brit J Surg 2000;87(2)191–4.
67 LaRosa J, Pinn V. Gender bias in biomedical research. J Amer Med Women's Assoc 1993; 48(5):145–51.
68 Doyal L. Gender equity in health: debates and dilemmas. Soc Sci Med 2000;51(6):931–9.
69 Draper H. Consent in childbirth. In: Frith L, ed. Ethics and midwifery: issues in contemporary practice. Oxford: Butterworth-Heinemann, 1996.
70 Crosthwaite J. Gender and bioethics. In: Kuhse H, Singer P, eds. A companion to bioethics. Oxford: Blackwell, 2001.
71 Dresser R. Wanted: single, white male for medical research. Hastings Cent Rep 1992; 22(1):24–9.
72 Fisher S. In the patient's best interest: women and the politics of medical decisions. New Brunswick, NJ: Rutgers University Press, 1986.
73 Coney S. The unfortunate experiment: the full story behind the inquiry into cervical cancer treatment. Auckland, New Zealand: Penguin Books, 1988.
74 Sherwin S. No longer patient. Philadelphia: Temple University Press, 1992.
75 Mason JK, McCall Smith RA, Laurie, GT. Law, Medical ethics, 5th edn. London: Reed Elsevier (UK), 1999.
76 Warren M, Kuhse H, Singer P, eds. A companion to bioethics. Oxford: Blackwell Publishers Ltd, 2001.
77 Marquis D. Why abortion is immoral. J Philosophy 1989;86(4):183–202.
78 Purdy L. Assisted reproduction. In: Kuhse H, Singer P, eds. A companion to bioethics. Oxford: Blackwell, 2001.
79 Tong R. In: Donchin A, Purdy LM, eds. Embodying bioethics: recent feminist advances. Maryland, US: Rowman and Littlefield, 1999.
80 Steinbock B. Mother–fetus conflict. In: Kuhse H, Singer P, eds. A companion to bioethics. Oxford: Blackwell, 2001.
81 Rogers WA. Is menopause a disease and should we treat it? In: Donchin A, Purdy LM, eds. Embodying bioethics: recent feminist advances. Maryland, US: Rowman and Littlefield, 1999.
82 Gotzsche PC, Olsen O. Is screening for breast cancer with mammography justifiable? Lancet 2000;355(9198):129–34.
83 Inhorn MC, Whittle KL. Feminism meets the 'new' epidemiologies: toward an appraisal of antifeminist biases in epidemiological research on women's health. Soc Sci Med 2001; 53(5):553–67.

84 Rogers WA. Does evidence-based medicine discriminate against women? (in press).
85 Bryson L, Warner-Smith P. Choice of GP: who do young rural women prefer? Aust J Rural Health 1998;6(3):144–9.
86 Najman J. Class inequalities in health and lifestyle. In: Waddell C, Peterson AR, eds. Just health: inequality in illness care and prevention: South Melbourne: Churchill Livingstone, 1994.
87 Khoury P. Aboriginal health as a social product. In: Germov J, ed. Second opinion: an introduction to health sociology. Oxford: Oxford University Press, 1998;57–73.
88 Hunter E. Aboriginal health and history. Melbourne: Cambridge University Press, 1993.
89 Shannon C. Social and cultural differences affect medical treatment. Aust Fam Physician 1994;23(1):33–5.
90 Hill P. Aboriginal culture and the doctor–patient relationship. Aust Fam Physician 1994; 23(1):29–32.
91 Nassar N, Sullivan EA. Australia's mothers and babies 1999. AIHW Cat. No. PER 19. Sydney: AIHW National Perinatal Statistics Unit (Perinatal Statistics Series No. 11), 2001.
92 Day P, Sullivan EA, Lancaster P. Indigenous mothers and their babies Australia 1994–1996. AIHW Cat. No. PER 9. Sydney: Australian Institute of Health and Welfare National Perinatal Statistics Unit (Perinatal Statistics Series No 8), 1999.
93 Kirk M, Hoban E, Dunne A, Manderson L. Carriers and appropriate service delivery systems for cervical cancer screening in Indigenous communities in Queensland. Queensland Health, University of Queensland Press, 1999.
94 Manderson L, Reid JC. What's culture got to do with it? In: Waddell C, Petersen AR, eds. Just health: inequalities in illness care and prevention. South Melbourne: Churchill Livingstone, 1994.
95 Ferguson B. Concepts, Models and theories for immigrant health care. In: Ferguson B, Browne E, eds. Health care and immigrants: a guide for helping professions. Artarmon, NSW: MacLennan & Petty, 1991.
96 Allotey P. Travelling with 'excess baggage': health problems of refugee women in Western Australia. In: Manderson L, ed. Australian women's health: innovations in social science and community research. New York: Haworth Press, 1998.
97 Stevens PE. Structural and interpersonal impact of heterosexual assumptions on lesbian health care clients. Nursing Research 1995;44(1):25–30.
98 Lehmann JB, Lehmann CU, Kelly PJ. Development and health care needs of lesbians. J Women's Health 1998;7(3):379–87.
99 McNair RP, Anderson S, Mitchell A. Addressing health inequalities in Victorian lesbian, gay, bisexual and transgender communities. Health Promotion J Aust 2001;11(4):305–11.
100 Trippet SE. Lesbians' mental health concerns. Health Care Women Int 1994; 15(4):317–23.
101 Welch S, Collings SC, Howden-Chapman P. Lesbians in New Zealand: their mental health and satisfaction with mental health services. Aust NZ J Psychiatry 2000;34(2):256–63.
102 Remafedi G. Sexual orientation and youth suicide. JAMA 1999;282(13):1291–2.
103 Scherzer T. Domestic violence in lesbian relationships: findings of the lesbian relationships research project. In: Ponticelli CM, ed. Gateways to improving lesbian health and health care. New York: Haworth Press, 1998.
104 Victorian Gay and Lesbian Rights Lobby. Everyday experiments. Report of a survey into same-sex domestic partnerships in Victoria, 2001. Website: http://home.vicnet.net.au/~vglrl.
105 Mikhailovich K, Martin S, Lawton S. Lesbian and gay parents: their experiences of children's health care in Australia. Int J Sexuality Gender Studies 2001;6(3):181–91.
106 Gill CJ. The last sisters: health issues of women with disabilities. In: Ruzek SB, Olesen VL, Clarke AE, eds. Women's health: complexities and differences. Columbus: Ohio State University Press, 1996;96–111.
107 Larson M, Schatz M. HIV prevention strategies with homeless street youth. In Moore MK, Frost ML. AIDS education: reaching diverse populations. Praeger: Westport, Connecticut, 1996;115–32.
108 Hartley R. The social costs of youth homelessness. In: Sykes, H. ed. Youth homelessness: courage and hope. Melbourne: Melbourne University Press, 1993;100–20.
109 Van der Ploeg J, Scholte E. Homeless youth. Chapter 4, Biographical and psychological factors. London: Sage, 1994; 34–43.
110 Chamberlain C, Mackenzie D. Youth homelessness: early intervention and prevention. Chapter 11, National policy challenge. Sydney: ACEE, 1998; 165–88.

111 Easteal PW. Women and crime: imprisonment issues. No. 35, Trends and issues in crime and criminal justice. Canberra: Australian Institute of Criminology, 1992.
112 Caddle D, Crisp D. Mothers in prison. Research Findings No 38, Home Office Research and Statistics Directorate. London: Home Office, 1997.
113 Brockett L, Murray A. Thai sex workers in Sydney. In: Perkins R. et al, eds. Sex Work and Sex Workers in Australia. Sydney: UNSW Press, 1994.
114 Watts C, Zimmerman C. Violence against women: global scope and magnitude. Lancet 2002; 359(9313):1232–7.
115 Graham H, Der G. Patterns and predictors of tobacco consumption among women. Health Educ Res 1999;14(5):611–18.
116 Siahpush M, Borland R, Scollo M. Prevalence and socio-economic correlates of smoking among lone mothers in Australia. Aust NZ J Public Health 2002;26(2):132–5.
117 Abel EL, Hannigan JH. Maternal risk factors in fetal alcohol syndrome: provocative and permissive influences. Neurotoxicol & Teratol 1995;17(4):445–62.
118 Fagerstrom K. The epidemiology of smoking: health consequences and benefits of cessation. Drugs 2002;62(Suppl 2):1–9.
119 Unwin E, Codde J. Trends and patterns of drug-caused mortality in Australia and Western Australia. Aust NZ J Public health 1999;23(4):352–6.
120 McKenna C. UK has highest reduction in deaths from lung and breast cancer. BMJ 2002; 325(7355):63A.
121 Stellman SD, Garfindel L. Proportions of cancer deaths attributable to cigarette smoking in women. Women Health 1989;15(2):19–28.
122 Loewen GM, Romano CF. Lung cancer in women. J Psychoactive Drugs 1989;21(3):319–21.
123 Coker AL, Bond SM, Williams A, Gerasimova T, Pirisi L. Active and passive smoking, high-risk human papillomaviruses and cervical neoplasia. Cancer Detect Prev 2002;26(2):121–8.
124 Hughes EG, Brennan BG. Does cigarette smoking impair natural or assisted fecundity? Fertil Steril 1996;66(5):679–89.
125 Kleinman JC, Pierre MB, Madans JM, Land GH, Schramm WF. The effects of maternal smoking on fetal and infant mortality. Am J Epidemiol 1998;127(2):274–82
126 Gulmezoglu M, de Onis M, Villar J. Effectiveness of interventions to prevent or treat impaired fetal growth. Obstet Gynecol Surv 1997;52(2):139–49.
127 Zhou FM, Liang Y, Dani JA. Endogenous cholinergic activity regulates dopamine release in the striatum. Nat Neurosci 2001;4(12):1224–9.
128 Tomkins DM, Sellers EM. Addiction and the brain: the role of the neurotransmitters in the cause and treatment of drug dependence. CMAJ 2001;164(6):817–21.
129 Silagy C, Lancaster T, Stread L, Mant D, Fowler G. Nicotine replacement therapy for smoking cessation. Coch Rev.
130 Peters MJ, Morgan LC. The pharmacotherapy of smoking cessation. MJA 2002;176(10):486–90.
131 Westmaas JL, Wild TC, Ferrence R. Effects of gender in social control of smoking cessation. Health Psychol 2002;21(4):368–76.
132 Williamson DF, Madans J, Anda RF, Kleinman JC, Giovino GA, Byers T. Smoking cessation and severity of weight gain in a national cohort. N Engl J Med 1991;342(11):739–45.
133 Heatherton TF, Kozlowski LT, Frecker RC, Fagerstrom KO. The Fagerstrom Test for Nicotine Dependence: a revision of the Fagerstrom Tolerance Questionnaire. Br J Addiction 1991; 86(9):1119–27.
134 Mallin R. Smoking cessation: integration of behavioral and drug therapies. Am Fam Physician 2002;65(6):1107–14.
135 Fiore MC, Bailey WC, Cohen SJ, Dorfman SF, Goldstein MG, Gritz ER et al. Treating tobacco use and dependence. Clinical Practice Guideline. Rockville, MD: US Department of Health and Human Services. Public Health Service, June 2002.
136 Institute of Alcohol Studies, 'UK Consumption'. Website: www.eurocare.org/profiles/uk/ukconsumption.htm.
137 Ferner RE, Chambers J. Alcohol intake: measure for measure. BMJ 2001;323(7327):1439–40.
138 Bien TH, Miller WR, Tonigan JS. Brief interventions for alcohol problems: a review. Addiction. 1993;88(3):315–35.
139 Bradley KA, Boyd-Wickizer J, Powell SH, Burman ML. Alcohol screening questionnaires in women; a critical review. JAMA 1998;280(2):166–71.

140 Prytkowicz A. Female alcoholism: impacts on women and children. In: M Galanter, ed. Currents in alcoholism: recent advances in research and treatment, Vol 3. New York: Grune & Stratton, 1980;429–34.

141 Leimone P, Harousseau H, Borteyru JP, Menuet JC. Children of alcoholic parents—observed anomalies: discussion of 127 cases. Ther Drug Monit 2003(1968);25(2):132–6.

142 Jones KL, Smith DW, Ullelan C, Steissguth P. Pattern of malformation in offspring of chronic alcoholic mothers. Lancet 1973;1(7815):1267–71.

143 Spohr HL, Steinhausen HC, eds. Alcohol, pregnancy and the developing child. Cambridge: Cambridge University Press, 1996.

144 Kaminski M, Franc M, Lebouvier M, du Mazaubrun C, Rumeau-Rouquette C. Moderate alcohol use and pregnancy outcome. Neurobehav Toxicol Teratol 1981;3(2):173–81.

145 Lelong N, Kaminski M, Chwalow J, Bean K, Subtil D. Attitudes and behaviour of pregnant women and health professionals towards alcohol and tobacco consumption. Patient Educ Couns 1995;25(1):39–49.

146 West JR, Goodlett CR, Bonthius DJ, Hamre KM, Marcussen BL. Cell population depletion associated with fetal alcohol brain damage: mechanisms of BAC-dependent cell loss. Alcohol Clin Exp Res 1990;14(6):813–18.

147 Lee MJ. Marihuana and tobacco use in pregnancy. Obstet Gynecol Clin North Am 1998; 25(1):65–83.

148 Rey JM, Tennant CC. Cannabis and mental health. BMJ 2002;325(7374):1183–4.

149 Laegried L, Hagberg G, Lundberg A. Neurodevelopment in late infancy after prenatal exposure to benzodiazepines—a prospective study. Neuropediatrics 1992;23(2):60–7.

150 National Teratology Information Service (NTIS). Br J Clin Pharmacol 1998;45(2):184.

151 Rizk B, Atterbury JL, Groome LJ. Reproductive risks of cocaine. Hum Reprod Update 1996;2(1):43–55.

152 Ward RM Difficulties in the study of adverse fetal and neonatal effects of drug therapy during pregnancy. Semin Perinatol 2001;25(3):191–5.

153 Brown WJ, Dobson AJ, Mishra G. What is a healthy weight for middle aged women? Int J Obes Relat Metab Disord 1998;22(6):520–8.

154 Dasgupta S, Hazra SC. The utility of waist circumference in assessment of obesity. Indian J Public Health 1999;43(4):32–5.

155 Dobbelsteyn CJ, Joffres MR, MacLean DR, Flowerdew G. A comparative evaluation of waist circumference, waist-to-hip ratio and body mass index as indicators of cardiovascular risk factors. The Canadian Heart Health Surveys. Int J Obes Rel Metab Disord 2001;25(5): 652–61.

156 Seidell JC, Perusse L, Despres JP, Bouchard C. Waist and hip circumferences have independent and opposite effects on cardiovascular disease risk factors. The Quebec Family Study. Am J Clin Nutr 2001;74(3):315–21.

157 Nowson CA, Margerison C. Vitamin D intake and vitamin D status of Australians. Med J Aust 2002;177(3):149–52.

158 Diamond TH, Levy S, Smith A, Day P. High bone turnover in Muslim women with vitamin D deficiency. Med J Aust 2002;177(3):139–42.

159 Pasco JA, Sanders KM, Henry MJ, Nicholson GC, Seeman E, Kotowicz MA. Calcium intakes among Australian women: Geelong Osteoporosis Study. Aust NZ J Med 2000;30(1):21–7.

160 Abrams SA. Calcium turnover and nutrition through the life cycle. Proc Nutr Soc 2001; 60(2):283–9.

161 Fletcher RH, Fairfield KM. Vitamins for chronic disease prevention in adults: clinical applications. JAMA 2002;287(23):3127–9.

162 Willett WC. Dietary fat plays a major role in obesity: no. Obes Rev 2002;3(2):59–68.

163 Dunstan DW, Zimmet PZ, Welborn TA, Cameron AJ, Shaw J, de Courten M et al. The Australian Diabetes, Obesity and Lifestyle Study (AusDiab)—methods and response rates. Diabetes Res Clin Pract 2002;57(2):119–29.

164 Wilson BD, Wilson NC, Russell DG. Obesity and body fat distribution in the New Zealand population. NZ Med J 2001;113(1128):127–30.

165 United Kingdom Parliament, Select Committee on Public Accounts Ninth Report, Tackling obesity in England. Website: www.publications.parliament.uk/pa/cm200102/cmselect/cmpubacc/421/42103.htm.

166 Mokdad AH, Serdula MK, Dietz WH, Bowman BA, Marks JS, Koplan JP. The spread of the obesity epidemic in the United States 1991–1998. JAMA 1999;282(16):1519–22.
167 Chinn S, Rona RJ. Prevalence and trends in overweight and obesity in three cross sectional studies of British children, 1974–94. BMJ 2001;322(7277):24–6.
168 Cole TJ, Belllizzi MC, Flegal KM, Dietz WH. Establishing a standard definition for child overweight and obesity worldwide: international survey. BMJ 2000;320(7244):1240–3.
169 Wang Y. Cross-national comparison of childhood obesity: the epidemic and the relationship between obesity and socioeconomic status. Int J Epidemiol 2001;30(5):1129–36.
170 Sorensen TI, Echwald SM. Obesity genes. BMJ 2001;322(7287):630–1.
171 Lahti-Koski M, Pietinen P, Heliovaara M, Vartiainen E. Associations of body mass index and obesity with physical activity, food choices, alcohol intake and smoking in the 1982–1997 FINRISK Studies. Am J Clin Nutr 2002;75(5):809–17.
172 Gillman MW, Rifas-Shiman SL, Camargo CA Jr, Berkey CS, Frazier AL, Rockett HR, Field AE, Colditz GA. Risk of overweight among adolescents who were breastfed as infants. JAMA 2001;285(19):2461–7.
173 von-Kries R, Koletzko B, Sauerwald T, von Mutius E. Does breast-feeding protect against childhood obesity? Adv Exp Med Biol 2000;478:29–39.
174 Castracane VD, Henson MC. When did Leptin become a reproductive hormone? Sem Reprod Med 2002;20(2):89–92,08–11.
175 Heymsfield SB, Greenberg AS, Fujioka K, Dixon RM, Kushner R, Hunt T et al. Recombinant leptin for weight loss in obese and lean adults: a randomized, controlled, dose-escalation trial. JAMA 1999;282(16):1568–75.
176 National Institutes of Health. Clinical guidelines on the identification, evaluation, and treatment of overweight and obesity in adults: the Evidence report. Bethesda, MD: US Department of Health and Human Services, 1998.
177 Nightingale AL, Lawrenson RA, Simpson EL, Williamd TJ, MacRae KD, Farmer RD. The effects of age, body mass index, smoking and general health on the risk of venous thromboembolism in users of combined oral contraceptives. Eur J Contracept Reprod Health Care 2000;5(4):265–74.
178 American Institute for Cancer Research/World Cancer Research Fund. Food, nutrition and the prevention of cancer: a global perspective. Washington DC: American Institute for Cancer Research, 1997.
179 Sebire NJ, Jolly M, Harris JP, Wadsworth J, Joffe M, Beard RW et al. Maternal obesity and pregnancy outcome: a study of 287,213 pregnancies in London. Int J Obes Relat Metab Disord 2001;25(8):1175–82.
180 Reasner CA II. Promising new approaches. Diabetes Obes Metab (Suppl) 1999;1:S41–8.
181 Ogden J, Bandara I, Cohen H et al General practitioners' and patients' models of obesity: whose problem is it? Patient Educ Couns 2001;44(3):227–33.
182 Pirozzo S, Summerbell C, Cameron C, Glasziou P. Advice on low-fat diets for obesity. Coch Rev.
183 Brownell KD, Kramer FM. Behavioural management of obesity. Med Clin North Am 1989; 73(1):185–201.
184 Dobson R. Obesity drug approved as problem grows across the world. BMJ 2001; 323(7319):955.
185 Ballinger A, Peikin SR. Orlistat: its current status as an anti-obesity drug. Eur J Pharmacol 2001;440(2–3):109–17.
186 Foxcroft DR, Milne R. Orlistat for the treatment of obesity: rapid review and cost-effectiveness model. Obes Rev 2000;1(2):121–6.
187 Livingston E. Obesity and its surgical management. Am J Surg 2002;184(2):103.
188 Wadden TA, Brownell KD, Foster GD. Obesity: responding to the global epidemic. J Consult Clin Psychol 2002;70(3):510–25.
189 Maiese DR. Healthy people 2010—leading health indicators for women. Women's Health Issues 2002;12(4):155–64.
190 Miles A, Rapoport L, Wardle J, Afuape T, Duman M. Using the mass-media to target obesity: an analysis of the characteristics and reported behaviour change of participants in the BBC's 'Fighting Fat, Fighting Fit' campaign. Health Educ Res 2001;16(3):357–72.
191 Sarwer DB, Wadden TA. The treatment of obesity: what's new, what's recommended. J Women's Health Gend Based Med 1999;8(4):483–93.

192 Campbell K, Waters E, O'Meara S, Summerbell C. Interventions for preventing obesity in childhood. A systematic review. Obes Rev 2001;2(3):149–57.
193 Despres JP. Drug treatment for obesity. We need more studies in men at higher risk of coronary events. BMJ 2001;322(7299):1379–80.
194 Arterburn D, Noel PH. Extracts from 'Clinical Evidence'. Obesity. BMJ 2001;322(7299): 1406–9.
195 Lenskyj, H. Women, sport and physical activity: selected research themes. Canada: Sport Information Resources Centre, 1994.
196 Bauman A. Owen N, Rushworth RL. Recent trends and socio-demographic determinants of exercise participation in Australia. Community Health Stud 1990;14(1):19–26.
197 Martinez-Gonzalez MA, Varo JJ, Santos JL, De Irala J, Gibney M, Kearney J et al. Prevalence of physical activity during leisure time in the European Union. Med Sci Sport Exerc 2001; 33(7):1142–6.
198 Eyler AE, Wilcox S, Matson-Koffman D, Evenson KR, Sanderson B, Thompson J et al. Correlates of physical activity among women from diverse racial/ethnic groups. J Women's Health Gend Based Med 2002;11(3):239–53.
199 Steinbeck KS. The importance of physical activity in the prevention of overweight and obesity in childhood: a review and an opinion. Obes Rev 2001;2(2):117–30.
200 Hootman JM, Macera CA, Ainsworth BE, Addy CL, Martin M, Blair SN. Epidemiology of musculoskeletal injuries among sedentary and physically active adults. Med Sci Sport Exerc 2002;34(5):838–44.
201 Bruce DG, Devine A, Prince RL. Recreational physical activity levels in healthy older women: the importance of fear of falling. J Am Geriatr Soc 2002;50(1):84–9.
202 Brown WJ, Miller YD. Too wet to exercise: leaking urine as a barrier to physical activity in women. J Sci Med Sport 2001;4(4):373–8.
203 Eyler AA, Brownson RC, King AC, Brown D, Donatelle RJ, Heath G. Physical activity and women in the United States: an overview of health benefits, prevalence, and intervention opportunities. Women Health 1997; 26(3):27–49.
204 Humpel N, Owen N, Leslie E. Environmental factors associated with adults' participation in physical activity. A review. Am J Prev Med 2002;22(3):188–99.
205 Carnegie MA, Bauman A, Marshall AL, Mohsin M, Westley-Wise V, Booth ML. Perceptions of the physical environment, stage of change for physical activity, and walking among Australian adults. Res Q Exerc Sport 2002;73(2):146–55.
206 Ball K, Bauman A, Leslie E, Owen N. Perceived environmental aesthetics and convenience and company are associated with walking for exercise among Australian adults. Prev Med 2001; 33(5):434–40.
207 Brown WJ, Mishra G, Lee C, Bauman A. leisure time physical activity in Australian women: relationship with well being and symptoms. Res Q Exerc Sport 2000;71(3):206–16.
208 Powell, KE, Thompson PD, Caspersen CJ, Kendrick JS. Physical activity and the incidence of coronary heart disease. Ann Rev Public Health 1987;8:281–7.
209 Blair SN, Kampert JB. Influences of cardiorespiratory fitness and other precursors on cardiovascular disease and all-cause mortality in men and women. JAMA 1996;276(3):205–10.
210 Hagberg JM, Park JJ. The role of exercise training in the treatment of hypertension: an update. Sports Med 2000;30(3):193–206.
211 Durstine JL, Grandjean PW, Davis PG, Ferguson MA, Alderson NL, DuBose KD. Blood lipid and lipoprotein adaptations to exercise: a quantitative analysis. Sports Med 2001;31(15): 1033–62.
212 Ryan AS, Pratley RE, Elahi D, Goldberg AP. Changes in plasma leptin and insulin action with resistive training in postmenopausal women. Int J Obes Relat Metab Disord 2000;24(1):27–32.
213 Thune I, Furberg AS. Physical activity and cancer risk: dose-response and cancer, all sites and site-specific. Med Sci Sport Exerc 2001;33(6)(Suppl):S530–50.
214 Nilsen TI, Vatten LJ. Prospective study of colorectal cancer risk and physical activity, diabetes, blood glucose and BMI: exploring the hyperinsulinaemia hypothesis. Br J Cancer 2001; 84(3):417–22.
215 Gilliland FD, Li YF, Baumgartner K, Crumley D, Samet JM. Physical activity and breast cancer risk in hispanic and non-hispanic white women. Am J Epidemiol 2001;154(5):442–50.
216 Drake, DA. A longitudinal study of physical activity and breast cancer prediction. Cancer Nurs 2001;24(5):371–7.

217 Vuori IM. Dose-response of physical activity and low back pain, osteoarthritis, and osteoporosis. Med Sci Sport Exerc 2001;33(6)(Suppl):S551–86,609–10.
218 Janz K. Physical activity and bone development during childhood and adolescence. Implications for the prevention of osteoporosis. Minerva Pediatr 2002;54(2):93–104.
219 Day L, Fildes B, Gordon I, Fitzharris M, Flamer H, Lord S. Randomised factorial trial of falls prevention among older people living in their own homes. BMJ 2002;325(7356):128.
220 Department of Health. Physical activity and health outcomes: a review of the Chief Medical Officer. London: Department of Health, in press.
221 McCabe, Ricciardelli. Presentation at The Body Culture Conference: Melbourne, July 1999.
222 Paxton, Durkin. Presentation at The Body Culture Conference: Melbourne, July 1999.
223 Lamb CS, Jackson L, Cassidy P, Priest DJ. Body figure preferences of men and women: a comparison of two generations, Sex Roles 1993;28(5/6):345–58.
224 Wardle J, Bindra R, Fairclough B, Westcombe A. Culture and body image: body perception and weight concern in young Asian and Caucasian British women. J Comm Applied Social Psychology 1993;3(3):173–81.
225 Huon GF, Morris SE, Brown LE. Difference between male and female preferences for female body size, Australian Psychologist 1990;25:314–17.
226 Tiggemann M, Pennington B. The development of gender differences in body-size dissatisfaction, Australian Psychologist 1990;25:306–13.
227 Bush HM, Williams RG, Lean ME, Anderson AS. Body image and weight consciousness among South Asian, Italian and general population women in Britain. Appetite 2001;37(3):207–15.
228 Truby H, Paxton SJ. Development of the Children's Body Image Scale. Brit J Clin Psychol 2002;41(Pt 2):185–203.
229 Davis K. Reshaping the female body: the dilemma of cosmetic surgery. New York: Routledge, 1995.
230 Victorian Gay and Lesbian Rights Lobby: Enough is enough. A report on discrimination and abuse experienced by lesbians, gay men, bisexuals and transgender people in Victoria. Website: http://home.vicnet.net.au/~vglrl.
231 Cass VC. Homosexual identity formation: a theoretical model. J Homosex 1979;4(3):219–35.
232 Kinsey AC, Pomeroy WB, Martin CE, Gebhard PH. Sexual behaviour in the human female. Philadelphia: WB Saunders, 1953.
233 Bancroft J. Human sexuality and its problems. Edinburgh: Churchill Livingstone, 1998.
234 Aaron DJ, Markovic N, Danielson ME, Hannold JA, Janosky JE, Schmidt NJ. Behavioral risk factors for disease and preventive health practices among lesbians. Am J Public Health 2001;91(6):972–5.
235 Laumann EO, Paik A, Rosen RC. Sexual dysfunction in the United States: prevalence and predictors. JAMA 1999;281(6):537–44.
236 Deeks A. Sexual desire. Menopause and its psychological impact. Aust Family Physician 2002;31(5):433–9.
237 Ross MW, Channon-Little LD, Rosser BRS. Sexual Health Concerns. Interviewing and History Taking for Health Practitioners, 2nd Edn. MacLennan and Petty 2001;121.

3 Behavioural and mental health issues

1 Watts C, Zimmerman C. Violence against women: global scope and magnitude. Lancet 2002;359(9313):1232–7.
2 Campbell JC. Health consequences of intimate partner violence. Lancet 2002;359(9314): 1331–6.
3 Sassetti MR. Domestic violence. Prim Care 1993;20(2):289–305.
4 Australian Public Health Association. Domestic violence: Australian Public Health Association, 1990.
5 World Health Organization. WHO multi-country study on women's health and domestic violence progress report. Geneva: WHO/WHD, 2001.
6 McLennan W. Women's Safety Survey: Australian Bureau of Statistics, Canberra, Australia, 1996.
7 Finkelhor D. The international epidemiology of child sexual abuse. Child Abuse Negl 1994; 18(5):409–17.
8 Roberts G, O'Toole BI, Lawrence JM, Raphael B. Domestic violence victims in a hospital emergency department. Med J Aust 1993;159(5):307–10.
9 Webster J, Sweett S, Stolz T. Domestic violence in pregnancy. A prevalence study. Med J Aust 1994;161(8):466–70.

10 Hegarty K, Hindmarsh ED, Gilles MT. Domestic violence in Australia: definition, prevalence and nature of presentation in clinical practice. Med J Aust 2000;173(7):363–7.
11 McCauley J, Kern DE, Kolodner K, Dill L, Schroeder AF, De Chant HK et al. The 'battering syndrome': prevalence and clinical characteristics of domestic violence in primary care internal medicine practices. Ann Intern Med 1995;123(10):737–46.
12 Richardson J, Coid J, Petruckevitch A, Chung WS, Moorey S, Feder G. Identifying domestic violence: cross sectional study in primary care. BMJ 2002;324(7322):274.
13 Bradley F, Smith M, Long J, O'Dowd T. Reported frequency of domestic violence: cross sectional survey of women attending general practice. BMJ 2002;324(7322):271.
14 Eisenstat S, Bancroft L. Domestic violence. N Engl J Med 1999;341(12):886–92.
15 Hegarty KL, Taft AJ. Overcoming the barriers to disclosure and inquiry of partner abuse for women attending general practice. Aust NZ J Public Health 2001;25(5):433–7.
16 World Health Organization. Violence against women information package, July 1997.
17 Scott D, Walker L, Gilmore K. Breaking the silence: a guide to supporting adult victims/survivors of sexual assault. Melbourne: CASA House, 1995.
18 Heenan M, McKelvie H. Rape law reform evaluation project. Report No. 2. Melbourne: Department of Justice, 1997.
19 Welborn A, Adult sexual assault. Centre for Learning and Teaching Support. Churchill: Victoria: Monash University, Gippsland Campus, 2002.
20 FBI—Uniform Crime Reports. Crime in the United States. Washington DC: Government Printing Office,1988.
21 Wundersitz J. Rape and sexual assault: some statistics. Reproduced from conference papers, Preventing Adult Rape and Sexual Assault, Adelaide, 1997;17–24.
22 Dunn SF, Gilchrist VJ. Sexual assault. Prim Care 1993;20(2):359–73.
23 Burgess AW, Holstrom LL. Rape trauma syndrome. Am J Psychiatry 1974;131(9):981–6.
24 Briere J Conference proceedings. Satellite symposium in sexual assault. Perth: May 2002.
25 Gebhard PH. Sex offenders, an analysis of types. New York: Harper and Row, 1965.
26 Abel GG, Osborn C. The paraphilias: the extent and nature of sexually deviant and criminal behaviour. Psych Clin N Am 1992;15(3):675.
27 James M, ed. Paedophilia: Australian Institute of Criminology Trends and Issues in Crime and Criminal Justice. Series number 57. Canberra: Australian Institute of Criminology.
28 Davis GE, Leitenberg H. Adolescent sex offenders. Psychol Bull 1987;101(3):417–27.
29 Pathe M. Sex offenders. In: Adult sexual assault, Centre for Learning and Teaching Support. Monash University, Gippsland Campus: Churchill, Victoria, 2002.
30 Polaschek DLL, Ward T. The implicit theories of potential rapists: What our questionnaires tell us. Aggression & Violent Behaviour 2002;7:385–406.
31 Welborn A. The forensic examination: no more hushed whispers. Obstet Gynecol 2001; 3(4):246–50.
32 Kolodny R, Masters W, Johnson V. Textbook of sexual medicine. Boston: Little, Brown and Co, 1979;437.
33 Wellborn A. Adult sexual assault. Victoria: Monash University, 2000; Wells D. Forensic medicine: issues in causation. In: Freckleton I, Mendelson D, eds. Causation in law and medicine. England: Dartmouth Publishing, 2002.
34 Rosenfield S. Labelling mental illness: the effects of received services and perceived stigma on life satisfaction. Amer Soc Rev 1997;62:660–72.
35 Lyons D, McLoughlin DM. Recent advances: psychiatry. BMJ 2001;323(7323):1228–31.
36 Crisp AH, Gelder MG, Rix S, Meltzer HI, Rowlands OJ. Stigmatisation of people with mental illnesses. Br J Psychiatry 2000;177:4–7.
37 World Health Organization, The World Health Report 2001 (www.who.int/whr).
38 Mazza D, Dennerstein L, Garamszegi CV, Dudley EC. The physical, sexual and emotional violence history of middle-aged women: a community-based prevalence study. Med J Aust 2001;175(4):199–201.
39 Hall LA, Sachs B, Rayens MK, Lutenbacher M. Childhood physical and sexual abuse: their relationship with depressive symptoms in adulthood. Image J Nurs Sch 1993;25(4): 317–23.
40 Moeller TP, Bachmann GA, Moeller JR. The combined effects of physical, sexual, and emotional abuse during childhood: long-term health consequences for women. Child Abuse Neglect 1993;17(5):623–40.

41 Carlson LE, Sherwin BB. Higher levels of plasma estradiol and testosterone in health elderly men compared with age-matched women may protect aspects of explicit memory. Menopause 2000;7(3):168–77.

42 Grodstein F, Chen J, Pollen DA, Altert MS, Wilson RS, Folstein MF et al. Postmenopausal hormone therapy and cognitive function in healthy older women. J Am Geriatr Soc 2000; 48(7):746–52.

43 Burt VK, Hendrick VC. Women's mental health. Washington DC: American Psychiatric Press, 1997.

44 DeLongis A, Coyne JC, Dakof G, Folkman S, Lazarus RS. Relationship of daily hassles, uplifts, and major life events to health status. Health Psychology 1982;1:119–36.

45 Murray CJL, Lopez AD, eds. The global burden of disease and injury series. Volume 1: A comprehensive assessment of mortality and disability from diseases, injuries and risk factors in 1990 and projected to 2020. Cambridge, The Harvard School of Public Health, on behalf of the World Health Organization and the World Bank: Harvard University Press, 1996.

46 Wilhelm K, Parker G, Hadzi–Pavlovic D. Fifteen years on: evolving ideas in researching sex differences in depression. Psychol Med 1997;27(4):875–83.

47 Paykel E. Depression in women Br J Psychiatry 1991;158(Suppl 10):22–9.

48 Davidson JRT, Meltzer–Brody SE. The underrecognition and undertreatment of depression: What is the breadth and depth of the problem? J Clin Psych 1999:60(Suppl 7):4–9.

49 Alvidrez J, Azocar F. Self-recognition of depression in public care women's clinic patients. J Women's Health Gend Based Med 1999:8(8):1063–71.

50 Diagnostic and statistical manual of mental disorders, 4th edn. DSM–IV. Washington DC: American Psychiatric Association, 1994.

51 Gitlin MJ, Pasnau RO. Psychiatric syndromes linked to reproductive function in women: a review of current knowledge. Am J Psych 1989:146(11):1413–22.

52 Belle D. Poverty and women's mental health. Am Psychol 1990:45(3):385–9.

53 Pillow DR, Zautra AJ, Sandler I. Major life events and minor stressors: identifying mediational links in the stress process. J Pers Soc Psychol 1996;70(2):381–94.

54 Weiss EL, Longhurst JG, Mazure CM. Childhood sexual abuse as a risk factor for depression in women: psychosocial and neurobiological correlates. Am J Psych 1999;156(6):816–28.

55 Roberts GL, Lawrence JM, Williams GM, Raphael B. The impact of domestic violence on women's mental health. Aust NZ J Public Health 1998:22(7):56–61.

56 Yee JL, Schulz R. Gender differences in psychiatric morbidity among family caregivers: a review and analysis. Gerontologist 2000: 40(2):147–64.

57 Boyle FM, Vance JC, Najman JM, Thearle MJ. The mental health impact of stillbirth, neonatal death or SIDS: prevalence and patterns of distress among mothers. Soc Sci Med 1996: 43(8):1273–82.

58 Kissane DW, Clarke DM, Ikin J, Bloch S, Smith GC, Vitetta L et al. Psychological morbidity and quality of life in Australian women with early-stage breast cancer: a cross-sectional survey. Med J Aust 1998;169(4):192–6.

59 Brady KT, Randall CL. Gender differences in substance use disorders. Psych Clin N Am 1999;22(2):241–52.

60 Blum LN, Nielsen NH, Riggs JA for the Council on Scientific Affairs, American Medical Association. Alcoholism and alcohol abuse among women: report of the council on scientific affairs. Journal of Women's Health 1998;7(7):861–71.

61 Schaffer A, Levitt AJ, Bagby RM, Kennedy SH, Levitan RD, Joffe RT. Suicidal ideation in major depression: sex differences and impact of comorbid anxiety. Can J Psych 2000;45(9):822–6.

62 DeRubeis RJ, Gelfand LA, Tang TZ, Simons AD. Medication versus cognitive behavior therapy for severely depressed outpatients: mega-analysis of four randomized comparisons Am J Psych 1999:156(7):1007–13.

63 Kennedy SH, Lam RW, Cohen NL, Ravindran AV. CANMAT Depression Work Group. Clinical Guidelines for the treatment of depressive disorders. IV. Medications and other biological treatments. Can J Psychiatry 2001;46(Suppl 1):S38–58.

64 Altshuler LL, Cohen LS, Moline ML, Kahn DA, Carpenter D, Dochery JP. Expert consensus panel for depression in women. The expert consensus guideline series. Treatment of depression in women. Postgrad Med 2001;Mar:1–107.

65 Dubovsky SL, Giese A. Selected issues in the pharmacologic treatment of women with psychiatric disorders. J Practical Psychiatry Behavioral Health 1997;3:275–84.

66 Spigset O, Martensson B. Fortnightly review. Drug treatment of depression. BMJ 1999; 318(7192):1188–91.
67 Malhi GS, Mitchell PB, Caterson I. 'Why getting fat, Doc?' Weight gain and psychotropic medications. Aust NZ J Psychiatry 2001;35(3):315–21.
68 Hippisley–Cox J, Fielding K, Pringle M. Depression as a risk factor for ischaemic heart disease in men: population-based case-control study. BMJ 1998;316(7146):1714–19.
69 Michelson D, Stratakis C, Hill L, Reynolds J, Galliven E, Chrousos G, Gold P. Bone mineral density in women with depression. N Engl J Med 1996;335(16):1176–81.
70 Hammen C. Children of depressed parents. The stress context. In: Wolchik SA, Sandler IN, eds. Handbook of children's coping, linking theory and intervention. Chap 5. New York: Plenum Press, 1997.
71 Angst J. Fortnightly review. A regular review of the long-term follow up of depression. BMJ 1997;315(7116):1143–6.
72 Mueller TI, Leon AC, Keller MB, Solomon DA, Endicott J, Coryell W et al. Recurrence after recovery from major depressive disorder during 15 years of observational follow-up. Am J Psychiatry 1999;156(7):1000–6.
73 Andrews G. Should depression be managed as a chronic disease? BMJ 2001;322(7283):419–21.
74 Wittchen HU, Hoyer J. Generalized anxiety disorder: nature and course J Clin Psych 2001; 62(Suppl 11):15–19.
75 Howell HB, Brawman–Mintzer O, Monnier J, Yonkers KA. Generalized anxiety disorder in women. Psychiatr Clin North Am 2001:24(1):65–78.
76 Hettema JM, Neale MC, Kendler KS. A review and meta-analysis of the genetic epidemiology of anxiety disorders. Am J Psych 2001;158(10):1568–78.
77 Sansone RA, Sansone LA, Righter EL. Panic disorder: The ultimate anxiety. J Women's Health 1998;7(8):983–9.
78 Gale C, Oakley-Browne M. Anxiety disorder. BMJ 2000;321(7270):1204–7.
79 Work Group or Panic Disorder. American Psychiatric Association. Practice guideline for the treatment of patients with panic disorder. Am J Psychiatry 1998;155(Suppl 5):1–34.
80 Tjemsland L, Soreide JA, Malt UF. Traumatic distress symptoms in early breast cancer I. Acute response to diagnosis. Psycho-Oncology 1996;5(1):1–8.
81 Green BL, Rowland JH, Krupnick JL, Epstein SA, Stockton P, Stern NM et al. Prevalence of post-traumatic stress disorder in women with breast cancer. Psychosomatics 1998;39(2):102–11.
82 Lin J, Thompson DS. Treating premenstrual dysphoric disorder using serotonin agents. J Women's Health Gend Based Med 2001;10(8):745–50.
83 Yonkers KA. The association between premenstrual dysphoric disorder and other mood disorders. J Clin Psychiatry 1997;58(15):19–25.
84 Steiner M, Streiner DL, Steinberg S, Steward D, Carter D, Berger C et al. The measurement of premenstrual mood symptoms. J Affect Disord 1999;53(3):269–73.
85 Kessel B. Premenstrual syndrome. Advances in diagnosis and treatment. Obstet Gynecol Clin North Am 2000;27(3):625–39.
86 Parry BL. The role of central serotonergic dysfunction in the aetiology of premenstrual dysphoric disorder: therapeutic implications. CNS Drugs 2001;15(4):277–85.
87 Dimmock PW, Wyatt KM, Jones PW, O'Brien PM. Efficacy of selective serotonin-reuptake inhibitors in premenstrual syndrome: a systematic review. Lancet 2000;356(9236):1131–6.
88 Steiner M, Born L. Diagnosis and treatment of premenstrual dysphoric disorder: an update. Int Clin Psychopharmacol 2000;15(Suppl 3):S5–17.
89 Kowalenko N, Barnett B, Fowler C, Matthey S. The perinatal period: early interventions for mental health. Volume 4. In: R Kosky, A O'Hanlon, G Martin & C Davis, series eds. Clinical approaches to early intervention in child and adolescent mental health. Adelaide: The Australian Early Intervention Network for Mental Health in Young People, 2000.
90 Cox JL, Holden JM, Sagovsky R. Detection of postnatal depression: development of the 10-item Edinburgh Postnatal Depression Scale. Brit J Psychiatry 1987;150:782–6.
91 Evans J, Heron J, Francomb H, Oke S, Golding J. Cohort study of depressed mood during pregnancy and after childbirth. BMJ 2001;323(7307):257–60.
92 O'Connor TG, Heron J, Golding J, Beveridge M, Glover V. Maternal antenatal anxiety and children's behavioural/emotional problems at 4 years. Report from the Avon Longitudinal Study of Parents and Children. Brit J Psychiatry 2002;180:502–8.

93 Murray L, Cooper PJ, eds. Postpartum depression and child development. New York: Guilford Press,1997.
94 Barnett B, Fowler C. Caring for the family's future. Sydney: Norman Swan Medical Communications,1995.
95 MacLennan A, Wilson D, Taylor A. The self-reported prevalence of postnatal depression. Aust NZ J Obstet Gynaecol 1996;36(3):313.
96 Hoffbrand S, Howard L, Crawley H. Antidepressant treatment for post-natal depression. Coch Rev.
97 National Health and Medical Research Council. Information paper: Postnatal depression. A systematic review of published scientific literature to 1999. Commonwealth of Australia: NHMRC, 2001.
98 Shakespeare J. Evaluation of screening for postnatal depression against the NSC handbook criteria. National Screening Committee paper 2001. www.nelh.nhs.uk/screening/adult_pps/postnatal_depression.html.
99 Appleby L, Warner R, Whitton A, Faragher B. A controlled study of fluoxetine and cognitive-behavioural counselling in the treatment of postnatal depression. BMJ 1997;314(7085):932–6.
100 Buist A. Psychotropic medication in pregnancy. Obstet Gynaecol 2001;3:259–61.
101 Motherisk, www.motherisk.org.
102 Gerson LW, Jarjoura D, McCord G. Factors related to impaired mental health in urban elderly. Res Aging 1987;9(3):356–71.
103 Gray GR, Ventis DG, Hayslip B Jr. Socio-cognitive skills as a determinant of life satisfaction in aged persons. Int J Aging Hum Dev 1992;35(3):205–18.
104 Murray JA. Loss as a universal concept: a review of the literature to identify common aspects of loss in diverse situations. J Loss Trauma 2001;6(3):219–41.
105 Klass D, Silverman PR, Nickman SL. Continuing bonds: New understandings of grief. Philadelphia: Taylor and Francis, 1996.
106 Teel CS. Chronic sorrow: Analysis of the concept. J Adv Nurs 1991;16(11):1311–19.
107 Brown GW, Harris TO, Hepworth C. Loss, humiliation and entrapment among women developing depression: a patient and non-patient comparison. Psychol Med 1995;25(1):7–18.
108 Clark D, Between hope and acceptance: the medicalisation of dying. BMJ 2002;324(7342): 905–7.
109 Mitchell G, Currow D. Chemotherapy and radiotherapy. When to call it quits. Aust Fam Physician 2002;31(2):129–33.
110 van Lommel P, van Wees R, Meyers V, Elfferich I. Near-death experience in survivors of cardiac arrest: a prospective study in the Netherlands. Lancet 2001;358(9298):2039–45.
111 Writing Group. Therapeutic guidelines: Palliative care. Melbourne: Therapeutic Guidelines, 2001.

4 Hormones and early development

1 Witschi E. Gonad development and function. Rec Progr Horm Res 1951;6:1–23.
2 Erickson GF. The ovary: basic principles and concepts. In: Felig P, Baxter JD, Broadus AE, Frohman, LA, eds. Endocrinology and metabolism, 3rd edn. New York: McGraw-Hill, 1995; 973–1015.
3 Soules MR, Bremner WJ. The menopause and climacteric: endocrinologic basis and associated symptomatology. J Am Geriatr Soc 1982;30:547–61.
4 Wray S, Grant P, Gainer H. Evidence that cells expressing luteinizing hormone-releasing hormone mRNA in the mouse are derived from the progenitor cells in the olfactory placode. Proc Natl Acad Sci USA 1989;86(20):8132–6.
5 Rasmussen DD, Liu JH, Swartz WH, Tueros VS, Yen SS. Human fetal hypothalamic GnRH neurosecretion: dopaminergic regulation in vitro. Clin Endocrinol (Oxf). 1986;25(2):127–32.
6 Anderson DC. Sex-hormone-binding globulin. Clin Endocrinol (Oxf) 1974;3(1):69–96.
7 Teixeira J, Maheswaran S, Donahoe PK. Mullerian inhibiting substance: an instructive developmental hormone with diagnostic and possible therapeutic applications. Endocr Rev 2001; 22(5):657–74.
8 Reyes FI, Winter JS, Faiman C. Gonadotrophin–gonadal interrelationships in the fetus. Prog Clin Biol Res 1976;10:83–106.
9 Faiman C, Winter JS, Reyes FI. Patterns of gonadotrophins and gonadal steroids throughout life. Clin Obstet Gynaecol 1976;3(3):467–83.

10 Krantz KE, Atkinson JP. Pediatric and adolescent gynecology. I Fundamental considerations. Gross anatomy. Ann NY Acad Sci 1967;142(3):551–75.
11 Stanhope R, Adams J, Jacobs HS, Brook CG. Ovarian ultrasound assessment in normal children, idiopathic precocious puberty, and during low dose pulsatile gonadotrophin releasing hormone treatment of hypogonadotrophic hypogonadism. Arch Dis Child 1985;60(2): 116–9.
12 Salardi S, Orsini LF, Cacciari E, Bovicelli L, Tasson P, Reggiani A. Pelvic ultrasonography in premenarcheal girls: relation to puberty and sex hormone concentrations. Arch Dis Child 1985; 60(2):120–5.
13 Richter TA, Terasawa E. Neural mechanisms underlying the pubertal increase in LHRH release in the rhesus monkey. Trends Endocrinol Metab 2001;12(8):353–9.
14 Marshall WA, Tanner JM. Variation in pattern of pubertal changes in girls. Arch Dis Child 1969;44(235):291–303.
15 Rifkind AB, Kulin HE, Rayford PL, Cargille CM, Ross GT. 24-Hour urinary luteinizing hormone (LW) and follicle stimulating hormone (FSH) excretion in normal children. J Clin Endocrinol Metab 1970:31(5):517–25.
16 Treloar AE, Boynton RE, Behn BG, Brown BW. Variation of the human menstrual cycle through reproductive life. Int J Fertil 1970;12(1):77–126.
17 Knobil E. The neuroendocrine control of the menstrual cycle. Recent Prog Horm Res 1980;36:53–88.
18 Groome NP, Illingworth PJ, O'Brien M, Pai R, Rodger FE, Mather JP, McNeilly AS. Measurement of dimeric inhibin B throughout the human menstrual cycle. J Clin Endocrinol Metab 1996;81(4):1401–5.
19 Groome NP, Illingworth PJ, O'Brien M, Cooke I, Ganesan TS, Baird DT, McNeilly AS. Detection of dimeric inhibin throughout the human menstrual cycle by two-site enzyme immunoassay. Clin Endocrinol (Oxf). 1994;40(6):717–23.
20 Schwartz D, Mayaux MJ. Female fecundity as a function of age: results of artificial insemination in 2193 nulliparous women with azoospermic husbands. N Engl J Med 1982;306(7):404–6.
21 Lee SJ, Lenton EA, Sexton L, Cooke ID. The effect of age on the cyclical patterns of plasma LH, FSH, oestradiol and progesterone in women with regular menstrual cycles. Hum Reprod 1988;3(7):851–5.
22 Burger HG, Igarashi M. Inhibin: definition and nomenclature, including related substances. Mol Endocrinol 1988;2(4):391–2.
23 Aubert MJ, Grumbach MM, Kaplan SL. The ontogenesis of human fetal hormones. III Prolactin. J Clin Invest 1975;56(1):155–64.
24 Plymate SR, Jones RE, Matej LA, Friedl KE. Regulation of sex hormone binding globulin (SHBG) production in Hep G2 cells by insulin. Steroids 1988;52(4):339–40.
25 Dewis P, Petsos P, Newman M, Anderson DC. The treatment of hirsutism with a combination of desogestrel and ethinyl oestradiol. Clin Endocrinol (Oxf) 1985;22(1):29–36.
26 Treloar AE. Menstrual cyclicity and the pre-menopause. Maturitas 1981 Dec;3(3/4):249–64.
27 McKinlay SM, Brambilla DJ, Posner JG. The normal menstrual transition. Maturitas 1992;14(2):103–15.
28 Dennerstein L, Smith AM, Morse C, Burger H, Green A, Hopper J, Ryan M. Menopausal symptoms in Australian women. Med J Aust 1993;159(4):232–6.
29 Klein NA, Illingworth PJ, Groome NP, McNeilly AS, Battaglia DE, Soules MR. Decreased inhibin B secretion is associated with the monotropic FSH rise in older, ovulatory women: a study of serum and follicular fluid levels of dimeric inhibin A and B in spontaneous menstrual cycles. J Clin Endocrinol Metab 1996;81(7):2742–5.
30 Burger HG, Dudley E, Mamers P, Groome N, Robertson DM. Early follicular phase serum FSH as a function of age: the roles of inhibin B, inhibin A and oestradiol. Climacteric 2000;3(1):17–24.
31 Trevoux R, De Brux J, Castanier M, Nahoul K, Soule JP, Scholler R. Endometrium and plasma hormone profile in the peri-menopause and post-menopause. Maturitas 1986;8(4):309–26.
32 Orentreich N, Brind JL, Rizer RL, Vogelman JH. Age changes and sex differences in serum dehydroepiandrosterone sulfate concentrations throughout adulthood. J Clin Endocrinol Metab 1984;59(3):551–5.
33 Burger HG, Dudley EC, Cui J, Dennerstein, Hopper JL. A prospective longitudinal study of serum testosterone, dehydroepiandrosterone sulphate, and sex hormone-binding globulin levels through the menopause transition. J Clin Endocrinol Metab 2000;85(8):2832–938.

34 Abraham GE. Ovarian and adrenal contribution to peripheral androgens during the menstrual cycle. J Clin Endocrinol Metab 1974;39(2):340–6.
35 Judd HL, Judd GE, Lucas WE, Yen SS. Endocrine function of the postmenopausal ovary: concentration of androgens and estrogens in ovarian and peripheral vein blood. J Clin Endocrinol Metab 1974;39(6):1020–4.
36 Vierhapper H, Nowotny P, Waldhausl W. Determination of testosterone production rates in men and women using stable isotope/dilution and mass spectrometry. J Clin Endocrinol Metab 1997;82(5):1492–6.
37 Miller KK, Sesmilo G, Schiller A, Schoenfeld D, Burton S, Klibanski A. Androgen deficiency in women with hypopituitarism. J Clin Endocrinol Metab 2001;86(2):561–7.
38 Couzinet B, Meduri G, Lecce MG, Young J, Brailly S, Loosfelt H et al. The postmenopausal ovary is not a major androgen-producing gland. J Clin Endocrinol Metab 2001;86(10):5060–6.
39 Hughes LA. Normal sexual differentiation. In: Dramusic V, Ratnam SS, eds. Clinical approach to paediatric and adolescent gynaecology. Singapore: Oxford University Press, 1998;2.
40 Sizonenko PC. Development of the ovary and growth and pubertal development. In: Dramusic V, Ratnam SS, eds. Clinical approach to paediatric and adolescent gynaecology. Singapore: Oxford University Press, 1998;11–13.
41 Simpson JL. Genetics of sexual differentiation. In: Carpenter SEK, Rock JA, eds. Pediatric and adolescent gynecology. New York: Raven Press, 1992;6.
42 Shulman LP, Elias S. Developmental abnormalities of the female reproductive tract: pathogenesis and nosology. Adolesc Pediatr Gynecol 1998;1:231.
43 ACOG Committee on Adolescent Health Care. ACOG Committee Opinion No. 274. July 2002. Non-surgical diagnosis and management of vaginal agenesis. Obstet Gynaecol 2002;100(1):213–16.
44 Farkas A, Chertin B. Feminizing genitoplasty in patients with 46XX congenital adrenal hyperplasia. J Pediatr Endocrinol Metab 2001;14(6):713–22.
45 Sutphen R, Galan-Gomez E, Kousseff BG. Clitoromegaly in neurofibromatosis. Am J Med Genet 1995;55(3):325–30.
46 Reiner WG. Assignment of sex in neonates with ambiguous genitalia. Curr Opin Pediatr 1999;11(4):363–5.
47 Taha SA. Male pseudohermaphroditism: factors determining the gender of rearing in Saudi Arabia. Urology 1994;43(3):370–4.
48 Lee PA, Witchel S. Precocious Puberty. In: Dramusic V, Ratnam SS, eds. Clinical approach to paediatric and adolescent gynaecology. Singapore: Oxford University Press, 1998;106–7.
49 Simpson JL. Genetics of sexual differentiation. In: Carpenter SEK, Rock JA, eds. Pediatric and adolescent gynecology. New York: Raven Press,1992;1–37.
50 Speroff L, Glass RH, Kase NG. Clinical gynecologic endocrinology and infertility. Baltimore: Lippincott Williams & Wilkins, 1999;349–52.
51 Yordam N, Alikasifoglu A, Kandemir N, Caglar M, Balci S. True hermaphroditism: clinical features, genetic variants and gonadal histology. J Pediatr Endocrinol Metab 2001;14(4):421–7.
52 Saenger P. Turner's syndrome. In: Dramusic V, Ratnam SS, eds. Clinical approach to paediatric and adolescent gynaecology. Singapore: Oxford University Press, 1998;127–39.

5 The female child and adolescent

1 Sizonenko PC. Development of the ovary and growth and pubertal development. In: Dramusic V, Ratnam SS, eds. Clinical approach to paediatric and adolescent gynaecology. Singapore: Oxford University Press, 1998;12–13,18–19.
2 Lee P, Kulin HE, Guo SS. Age of puberty among girls and the diagnosis of precocious puberty. Pediatrics 2001;107(6):1493.
3 Cook, AS. Normal growth and development of the genitalia in infancy and childhood. In: Dramusic V, Ratnam SS, eds. Clinical approach to paediatric and adolescent gynaecology. Singapore: Oxford University Press, 1998;45.
4 Jordan EE. Tips, tricks and tests for the gynecologic exam of young females. In: Goldfarb AF, ed. Clinical problems in pediatric and adolescent gynaecology. New York: Chapman & Hall, 1996;3–18.
5 Hammerschlag MR, Alpert S, Rosner I, Thurston P, Semine D, McComb D et al. Microbiology of the vagina in children: normal and potentially pathogenic organisms. Pediatrics 1978; 62(1):57–62.
6 Paradise JE, Campos JM, Friedman HM, Frishmuth G. Vulvovaginitis in premenarchal girls: clinical features and diagnostic evaluation. Pediatrics 1982;70(2):193–8.

7 Wilson MD. Vaginal discharge and vaginal bleeding in childhood. In: Carpenter SEK, Rock JA, eds. Pediatric and adolescent gynecology. New York: Raven Press, 1992;142.
8 Bacon J. Pediatric vulvovaginitis. In: Goldfarb AF, ed. Clinical problems in pediatric and adolescent gynecology. New York: Chapman & Hall, 1996;19–32.
9 Sanci L, Young D. Engaging the adolescent patient. Aust Family Physician 1995; 24(11):2027–31.
10 Rey JM, Sawyer MG, Clark JJ, Baghurst PA. Depression among Australian adolescents. Med J Aust 2001;175(1):19–23.
11 Moon L, Meyer P, Grau J. Australia's young people—their health and wellbeing. Canberra: Australian Institute of Health and Welfare, Cat. No.PHE-19, 1999.
12 Australian Institute of Health and Welfare. The Health and Welfare of Australia's Aboriginal and Torres Strait Islander Peoples 2001. Australian Bureau of Statistics 2001;4704.0.
13 Mathers C, Vos T, Stevenson C. The burden of disease and injury in Australia. Summary report. Canberra: Australian Institute of Health and Welfare, Cat. No.PHE18, 1999.
14 Hawkins JD, Catalano RF, Miller JY. Risk and protective factors for alcohol and other drug problems in adolescence and early adulthood: implications for substance abuse prevention. Psychol Bull 1992;112(1):64–105.
15 Tanner JM. Trends: earlier menarche in London, Oslo, Copenhagen, the Netherlands and Hungary. Nature 1973;243(5402):95–6.
16 Wyshak G. Secular changes in age at menarche in a sample of US women. Ann Hum Biol 1983;10(1):75–7.
17 Hetherington EM, Kelly J. For better or for worse: divorce reconsidered. New York: Norton & Co, 2002.
18 Mann DR, Plant TM. Leptin and pubertal development. Semin Reprod Med 2002; 20(2):93–102.
19 Simon D. Puberty in chronically diseased patients. Horm Res 2002;57(Suppl 2):53–6.
20 Marshall WA, Tanner JM. Variations in the pattern of pubertal changes in girls. Arch Dis Child 1969;44(235):291–303.
21 Zacharias L, Wurtman RJ, Schatzoff M. Sexual maturation in contemporary American girls. Am J Obstet Gynecol 1997;108(5):833–46.
22 Meyer F, Moisan J, Marcoux D, Bouchard C. Dietary and physical determinants of menarche. Epidemiology 1990;1(5):377–81.
23 Apta D, Butzow TL, Laughlin GA, Yen SS. Gonadotrophin-releasing hormone pulse generator activity during pubertal transition in girls: pulsatile and diurnal patterns of circulating gonadotrophins. J Clin Endocrinol Metab 1993;76(4):940–9.
24 Wyatt KM, Dimmock PW, O'Brien PMS, Walker TJ. A new method to determine total menstrual blood loss. Fertil Steril 2001; 76(1):125–31.
25 Edmonds DK. Dysfunctional uterine bleeding in adolescence. Bailleres Best Pract Res Clin Obstet Gynecol 1999;13(2):239–49.
26 Quinlivan JA, Petersen RW, Gurrin LC. High prevalence of Chlamydia and Pap smear abnormalities in pregnant adolescents warrants routine screening. Aust NZ J Obstet Gynaecol 1998;38(3):254–7.
27 Australian Institute of Health and Welfare. Cervical screening in Australia 1997–98. Cat No 9. Canberra: Australian Institute of Health and Welfare (Cancer Series No 14); 2000.
28 Mitchell H, Medley G. Age and time trends in the prevalence of cervical intraepithelial neoplasia on Papanicolaou smear tests, 1970-1988. Med J Aust 1990;152(5):252–5.
29 Moerman ML. Growth of the birth canal in adolescent girls. Am J Obstet Gynecol 1982; 143(5):528–32.
30 Rees JM. Overview: nutrition for pregnant and childbearing adolescents. Ann NY Acad Sci 1997;817:241–5.
31 Frisancho AR. Reduction of birth weight among infants born to adolescents: maternal-fetal growth competition. Ann NY Acad Sci 1997;817:272–80.
32 Fraser AM, Brockert JE, Ward RH. Association of young maternal age with adverse reproductive outcomes. N Engl J Med 1995;332(17):1113–17.
33 Smith GC, Pell JP. Teenage pregnancy and the risk of adverse perinatal outcomes associated with first and second births: population based retrospective cohort study. BMJ 2001; 323(7311):476.
34 Allen Guttmacher Institute. Sex and America's teenagers. New York: AGI, 1994.

35 Nassar N, O'Sullivan EA 2001. Australia's mothers and babies, AIHW Cat No. PER 19. Sydney: AIHW National Perinatal Statistics Unit (Perinatal Statistics Series No 11); 1999.
36 Australian Bureau of Statistics. Births Australia. Cat. No. 3301.0 Canberra: AGPS, 1999.
37 Kmietowicz Z. US and UK are top in teenage pregnancy rates. BMJ 2002;324(7350):1354.
38 Wellings K, Kane R. Trends in teenage pregnancy in England and Wales: how can we explain them? J R Soc Med. 1999;92(6):277–82.
39 Smith T. Influence of socioeconomic factors on attaining targets for reducing teenage pregnancies. BMJ 1993;306(6887):1232-5.
40 Mawer C. Preventing teenage pregnancies: supporting teenage mothers. BMJ 1999; 318(7200):1713–14.
41 Van der Klis KA, Westenberg L, Chan A, Dekker G, Keane RJ. Teenage pregnancy: trends characteristics and outcomes in South Australia and Australia. Aust NZ J Public Health 2002;26(2):125–31.
42 Grunseit A, Kippax S, Aggleton P, Baldo M, Slutkin G. Sexuality education and young people's sexual behaviour: a review of studies. J Adolesc Res 1997;12(4):421–53.
43 DiCenso A, Guyatt G, Willan A, Griffith L. Interventions to reduce unintended pregnancies among adolescents: systematic review of randomised controlled trials. BMJ 2002; 324(7351):1426–32.
44 Education Department of South Australia. Supportive learning environment. Pregnant girls and teenage mothers, the educational implications. Education of Girls' Unit, Education Department of South Australia; 1991.
45 Rindfuss RR, St John C, Bumpass LL. Education and timing of motherhood: disentangling causation. J Marriage Family 1984;46(4):981–8.
46 Furstenberg FF, Brooks-Gunn J, Morgan SP. Adolescent mothers in later life. Cambridge: Cambridge University Press, 1987.
47 Quinlivan JA, Petersen RW, Gurrin LC. Adolescent pregnancy—psychopathology missed. Aust NZ J Psychiatry 1999;33(6):864–8.
48 Miller BC, Moore KA. Adolescent sexual behaviour, pregnancy, and parenting: research through the 1980s. J Marriage Family 1990;52(4):1025–44.
49 Quinlivan JA, Quinlivan JA, Evans SF. A prospective cohort study of the impact of domestic violence on young teenage pregnancy outcomes. J Pediatr Adolesc Gynecol 2001;14(1):17–23.
50 Secretary Department of Health and Community Services v JWB and SMB. Marion's Case. CLR 1991;218.
51 Gillick v West Norfolk. AHA, AC 1986;112.
52 Section 92E Crimes Act 1990 (ACT); section 129 Criminal Code (NT); sections 66A, C and D Crimes Act 1900 (NSW); section 215 Criminal Code (QLD); section 49 Criminal Law Consolidation Act 1935 (SA); section 124 Criminal Code (TAS); section 45 Crimes Act 1958 (VIC); section 320 Criminal Code (WA).

6 Pre-pregnancy and antenatal care

1 Kline J, Stein Z, Susser M. Conception to birth. New York: Oxford University Press, 1989; 259–94.
2 Lian ZH, Zack MM, Erickson JD. Paternal age and the occurrence of birth defects. Am J Hum Genet 1986;39(5):648–60.
3 Malaspina D, Harlap S, Fennig S, Heiman D, Nahon D, Feldman D, Susser E. Advancing paternal age and the risk of schizophrenia. Arch Gen Psychiatry 2001;58(4):361–7.
4 Stein Z, Susser M. The risks of having children later in life. Social advantage may make up for biological disadvantage. BMJ 2000;320(7251):1681–2.
5 Mathews F, Yudkin P, Neil A. Influence of maternal nutrition on outcome of pregnancy: prospective cohort study. BMJ 1999;319(7206):339–43.
6 Nolla-Salas J, Bosch J, Gasser I, Vinas L, de Simon M, Almela M et al. Perinatal listeriosis: a population-based multicenter study in Barcelona, Spain (1990–1996). Am J Perinatol 1998;15(8):461–7.
7 Lumley J, Watson L, Watson M, Bower C. Periconceptional supplementation with folate and/or multivitamins for preventing neural tube defects. Coch Rev.
8 George L, Mills JL, Johansson AL, Nordmark A, Olander B, Granath F et al. Plasma folate levels and risk of spontaneous abortion. JAMA 2002;288(15):1867–73.

9 Roizen NJ, Patteson D. Down's syndrome. Lancet 2003;361(9365):1281–9.
10 Perlow JH. Education about folic acid: the ob-gyn's role in preventing neural tube defects. Contemp Obstet Gynecol 1999;44(3):39–53.
11 Platt MJ, Stanisstreet M, Casson IF, Howard CV, Walkinshaw S, Pennycook S et al. St Vincent's Declaration 10 years on: outcomes of diabetic pregnancies. Diabetes Med 2002; 19(3):216–20.
12 Morrell MJ Epilepsy in women: the science of why it is special. Neurology 1999;53(4 Suppl 1):S42–8.
13 Madden V. Women with epilepsy are not getting pregnancy advice. BMJ 1999;318(7195):1374.
14 Phillips E. Toxoplasmosis. Can Fam Physician 1998;44:1823–5.
15 Neilsen JP. Symphysis–fundal height measurement in pregnancy. Coch Rev.
16 Villar J, Carroli G, Khan-Neelofur D, Piaggio G, Gulmezoglu M. Patterns of routine antenatal care for low risk pregnancy. Coch Rev.
17 Jewell D, Sharp D, Sanders J, Peters TJ. A randomised controlled trial of flexibility in routine antenatal care. Brit J Obstet Gynaecol 2001;107(10):1241–7.
18 Kroner C, Turnbull D, Wilkinson C. Antenatal day care unit versus hospital admission for women with complicated pregnancy. Coch Rev.
19 McFadyen A, Gledhill J, Whitlow B, Economides D. First trimester ultrasound screening. BMJ 1998;317(7160):694–5.
20 Cuervo LG, Mahomed K. Treatments for iron deficiency anaemia in pregnancy. Coch Rev.
21 Best JM, O'Shea S, Tipples G, Davies N, Al-Khusaiby SM, Krause A et al. Interpretation of rubella serology in pregnancy: pitfalls and problems. BMJ 2002;325(7356):147–8.
22 Report to the National Screening Committee. Antenatal syphilis screening in the UK: a systematic review and national options appraisal with recommendations. London: Public Health Laboratory Service, 1998.
23 Ades AE, Sculpher MJ, Gibb DM, Gupta R, Ratcliffe J. Cost effectiveness analysis of antenatal HIV screening in United Kingdom. BMJ 1999;319(7219):1230–4.
24 Smaill F. Antibiotics for asymptomatic bacteriuria in pregnancy. Coch Rev.
25 Whitlow BJ, Economides DL. Screening for fetal anomalies in the first trimester. Progress in Obstetrics and Gynaecology, Vol. 14. Ed. J Studd. London: Churchill Livingstone, 2000.
26 Neilson JP. Ultrasound for fetal assessment in early pregnancy. Coch Rev.
27 Wellesley D, Boyle T, Barber J, Howe DT. Retrospective audit of different antenatal screening policies for Down's syndrome in eight district general hospitals in one health region. BMJ 2002;235(7354):15.
28 Northern Regional Survey Steering Group. Fetal abnormality: an audit of its recognition and management. Arch Dis Child 1992;67(7 Spec No):770–4.
29 Crowley P. Interventions for preventing or improving the outcome of delivery at or beyond term. Coch Rev.
30 Chamberlain G, Wraight A, Crowley P. Homebirths. Carnforth: Parthenon, 1997.
31 Bastian H, Keirse MJ, Lancaster PA. Perinatal death associated with planned home birth in Australia: population based study. BMJ 1998;317(7155):384–8.
32 Olsen O, Jewell MD. Home versus hospital birth. Coch Rev.
33 Hodnett ED. Home-like versus conventional institutional settings for birth. Coch Rev.
34 Gazmararian J, Lazorick S, Spitz AM, Ballard TJ, Saltzman LE, Marks JS. Prevalence of violence against pregnant women. JAMA 1996;275(24):1915–20.
35 Campbell JC. Health consequences of intimate partner violence. Lancet 2002;359(9314):1331–6.
36 Murphy CC, Schei B, Myhr TL, Du Mont J. Abuse: a risk factor for low birth weight? A systematic review and meta-analysis. CMAJ 2001;164(11):1567–72.
37 World Health Organisation. Female genital mutilation: report of a WHO technical working group. Geneva: WHO/FRH/WHD, 1996.
38 Gagnon AJ. Individual or group antenatal education for childbirth/parenthood. Coch Rev.
39 MacEvilly M, Buggy D. Back pain and pregnancy: a review. Pain 1996;64(3):405–14.
40 Ostgaard HC, Zetherstrom G, Roos-Hansson E. Back pain in relation to pregnancy: a 6-year follow-up. Spine 1997;22(4):2945–50.
41 Albert H, Godskesen M, Westergaard J. Prognosis in four syndromes of pregnancy-related pelvic pain. Acta Obstet Gynecol Scand 2001;80(6):505–10.
42 Kramer MS. Aerobic exercise for women during pregnancy. Coch Rev.

43 Young GL, Jewell D. Interventions for leg cramps in pregnancy. Coch Rev.
44 Young GL, Jewell D. Creams for preventing stretch marks in pregnancy. Coch Rev.

7 Labour and childbirth

1 Howell EA, Gardiner B, Concato J. Do women prefer female obstetricians? Obstet Gynecol 2002;99(6):1031–5.
2 Waldenstrom U, Brown S, McLachlan H, Forster D, Brennecke S. Does team midwife care increase satisfaction with antenatal, intrapartum, and postpartum care? A randomized controlled trial. Birth 2000;27(3):156–67.
3 Shields N, Turnbull D, Reid M, Holmes A, McGinley M, Smith LN. Satisfaction with midwife-managed care in different time periods: a randomised controlled trial of 1299 women. Midwifery 1998;14(2):85–93.
4 Hundley VA, Milne JM, Glazener CM, Mollison J. Satisfaction and the three C's: continuity, choice and control. Women's views from a randomised controlled trial of midwife-led care. Br J Obstet Gynaecol 1997;104(11):1273–80.
5 Waldenstrom U. Continuity of carer and satisfaction. Midwifery 1998 Dec;14(4):207–13.
6 Brown S, Lumley J. Satisfaction with care in labor and birth: a survey of 790 Australian women. Birth 1994;21(1):4–13.
7 Changing Childbirth. Report of the Expert Maternity Group. London: HMSO, 1994.
8 Thomas C, Curtis P. Having a baby: some disabled women's reproductive experiences. Midwifery 1997;13(4):202–9.
9 Small R, Rice PL, Yelland J, Lumley J. Mothers in a new country: the role of culture and communication in Vietnamese, Turkish and Filipino women's experiences of giving birth in Australia. Women Health 1999;28(3):77–101.
10 Hanzon L, Hodnett E. Labour assessment program to delay admission to labour wards. Coch Rev.
11 Albers LL. The duration of labor in healthy women. J Perinatol 1999;19(2):114–19.
12 World Health Organization Maternal and Safe Motherhood Programme. WHO partograph in management of labour. Lancet 1994;343(8910):1399–404.
13 Fraser WD, Turcot L, Krauss I, Brisson-Carrol G. Amniotomy for shortening spontaneous labour. Coch Rev.
14 Prendiville WJ, Harding JE, Elbourne DR, Stirrat GM. The Bristol third stage trial: 'active' versus 'physiological' management of third stage of labour. BMJ 1988;297(6659):1295–300.
15 Prendiville W, Elbourne D, McDonald S. Active versus expectant management in the third stage of labour. Coch Rev.
16 McDonald SJ, Prendiville WJ, Blair E. Randomised controlled trial of oxytocin alone versus oxytocin and ergometrine in active management of third stage of labour. BMJ 1993;307(6913): 1167–71.
17 Carroli G, Bergel E. Umbilical vein injection for management of retained placenta. Coch Rev.
18 Thornton JG, Lilford RJ. Active management of labour: current knowledge and research issues. BMJ 1994;309(6951):366–9.
19 Thaker SB, Stroup D, Chang M. Continuous electronic heart rate monitoring for fetal assessment during labour. Coch Rev.
20 Cuervo LG, Rodriguez MN, Delgado MB. Enemas during labour. Coch Rev. Basevi V, Lavender T. Routine perineal shaving on admission in labour. Coch Rev.
21 Hodnett ED. Caregiver support for women during childbirth. Coch Rev.
22 Gupta JK, Nikodem VC. Position for women during the second stage of labour. Coch Rev.
23 Nikodem VC. Immersion in water in pregnancy, labour and birth. Coch Rev.
24 Williams FL, Du V, Florey C, Mires GJ, Ogston SA. Episiotomy and perineal tears in low-risk UK primigravidae. J Pub Health Med 1998;20(4):422–7.
25 Carroli G, Belizan J. Episiotomy for vaginal birth. Coch Rev.
26 Kettle C, Johanson RB. Continuous versus interrupted sutures for perineal repair. Coch Rev.

8 The newborn infant and postnatal care

1 Ballard JL, Khoury JC, Wedig K, Wang L, Eilers-Walsman BL, Lipp R. New Ballard Score, expanded to include extremely premature infants. J Pediatr 1991;119(3):417–23.
2 Dubowitz LM, Dubowitz V, Goldberg C. Clinical assessment of gestational age in the newborn infant. J Pediatr 1970;77(1):1–10.

3 Glazener CM, Abdalla M, Stroud P, Naji S, Templeton A, Russell IT. Postnatal maternal morbidity: extent, causes, prevention and treatment. Br J Obstet Gynaecol 1995;102(4):282–7.
4 Gunn J, Lumley J, Chondros P, Young D. Does an early postnatal check-up improve maternal health: results from a randomised trial in Australian general practice. Br J Obstet Gynaecol 1998;105(9):991–7.
5 Hytten F. The clinical physiology of the puerperium. London: Farrand Press, 1995.
6 McCalman J. Sex and suffering: Women's Health and a Women's Hospital. Melbourne University Press, 1999.
7 Brubaker L. Postpartum urinary incontinence. BMJ 2002;324(7348):1227–8.
8 Marchant S, Alexander J, Garcia J, Ashurst H, Alderdice F, Keene J. A survey of women's experiences of vaginal loss from 24 hours to three months after childbirth (the BLiPP study). Midwifery 1999;15(2):72–81.
9 Glazener C. Sexual function after childbirth: woman's experiences, persistent morbidity and lack of professional recognition. Br J Obstet Gynaecol 1997;104(3):330–5.
10 Brown S, Lumley J. Maternal health after childbirth: results of an Australian population-based survey. Br J Obstet Gynaecol 1998;105(2):156–61.
11 Byrd JE, Hyde JS, DeLamater JD, Plant EA. Sexuality during pregnancy and the year postpartum. J Fam Pract 1998;47(4):305–8.
12 Barrett G, Pendry E, Peacock J, Victor C, Thakar R, Manyonda I. Women's sexual health after childbirth. Br J Obstet Gynaecol 2000;107(2):186–95.
13 McNeilly AS. Neuroendocrine changes and fertility in breast-feeding women. Prog Brain Res 2001;133:207–14.
14 McNeilly AS, Glasier AF, Howie PW, Houston MJ, Cook A, Boyle H. Fertility after childbirth: pregnancy associated with breast feeding. Clin Endocrinol (Oxf) 1983;19(2):167–73.
15 Gross BA, Burger H. WHO Task Force on methods for the natural regulation of fertility. Breastfeeding patterns and return to fertility in Australian women. Aust NZ J Obstet Gynaecol 2002;42(2):148–54.
16 Brown S, Lumley J, Small R, Astbury J. Missing Voices: The experience of motherhood. Oxford University Press, Melbourne 1995.
17 McVeigh CA. An Australian study of functional status after childbirth. Midwifery 1997;13(4): 172–8.
18 Brown S, Lumley J. Physical health problems after childbirth and maternal depression at six to seven months postpartum. Br J Obstet Gynaecol 2000;107(10):1194–201.
19 Gunn J, Lumley J, Young D. Visits to medical practitioners in the first six months of life. J Paed Child Health 1996;32(2):162–6.
20 Gunn J, Brown S, Small R, Lumley J. Guidelines for assessing postnatal problems: evidence-based guidelines. Melbourne: Department of General Practice, University of Melbourne, 1999.
21 Bick DE, MacArthur C, Knowles H, Winter H. Postnatal care: evidence and guidelines for management. London: Churchill Livingstone, 2002.
22 MacArthur C, Bick DE, Keighley MR. Faecal incontinence after childbirth. Brit J Obstet Gynaecol 1997;104(1):46–50.
23 MacArthur C, Winter HR, Bick DE, Knowles H, Lilford R, Henderson C. Effects of redesigned community postnatal care on women's health 4 months after birth: a cluster randomised controlled trial. Lancet 2002; 359(9304):378–85.
24 Dowswell T, Piercy J, Hirst J, Hewison J, Lilford R. Short postnatal hospital stay: implications for women and service providers. J Pub Health Med 1997;19(2):132–6.
25 Brown S, Lumley J. Reasons to stay, reasons to go: results of an Australian population-based survey. Birth 1997;24(3):148–58.
26 Gunn J, Lumley J, Chondros P, Young D. Does an early postnatal check-up improve maternal health: results from a randomised trial in Australian general practice. Br J Obstet Gynaecol 1998;105(9):991–7.
27 Brown S, Small R, Faber B, Krastev A, Davies P. Early postnatal discharge from hospital for healthy mothers and term infants. Coch Rev.
28 Bick DE, MacArthur C. Attendance, content and relevance of the six week postnatal examination. Midwifery 1995;11(2):69–73.
29 Thompson JF, Roberts CL, Currie M, Ellwood DA. Prevalence and persistence of health problems after childbirth: associations with parity and method of birth. Birth. 2002;29(2):83–94.

30 Donath S, Amir L. Rates of breastfeeding in Australia by State and socio-economic status: evidence from the 1995 National Health Survey. J Paediatr Child Health 2000;36(2):164–8.

31 Hamlyn B, Brooker S, Oleinikova K, Wands S. Infant feeding 2000. London: Stationery Office, 2002.

32 RACGP Breastfeeding Position Statement, 2000; http://www.racgp.org.au.

33 Scott JA, Binns CW. Factors associated with the initiation and duration of breastfeeding: a review of the literature. Aust J Nutr Diet 1998;55(2):51–61.

34 McIntyre E, Hiller JE, Turnbull D. Determinants of infant feeding practices in a low socio-economic area: identifying environmental barriers to breastfeeding. Aust NZ J Public Health 1999;23(2):207–9.

35 Renfrew MJ, Woolridge MW, Ross McGill H. Enabling women to breastfeed. A review of practices which promote or inhibit breastfeeding—with evidence-based guidance for practice. London: Stationery Office, 2000.

36 Lawrence RA, Lawrence RM. Breastfeeding: a guide for the medical profession. 5th edn. St Louis: Mosby, 1999.

37 Riordan J, Auerbach KG. Breastfeeding and human lactation. Boston: Jones and Bartlett, 1993.

38 Protecting, promoting and supporting breastfeeding: the special role of maternity services. A joint WHO/UNICEF statement. Geneva: World Health Organization,1989.

9 Pregnancy problems

1 World Health Organization. Classification of Diseases. 10th edn. Geneva: WHO, 1992.

2 National Health and Medical Research Centre. Report on Maternal Deaths in Australia, 1994–96. Canberra: NHMRC, 2001.

3 Lipitz S, Achiron R, Zalel Y, Mendelson E, Tepperberg M, Gamzu R. Outcome of pregnancies with vertical transmission of primary cytomegalovirus infection. Obstet Gynecol 2002;100(3): 428–33.

4 Lazzarotto T, Varani S, Gabrielli L, Spezzacatena P, Landini MP. New advances in the diagnosis of congenital cytomegalovirus infection. Intervirology 1999;42(5/6):390–7.

5 Adler SP. Cytomegalovirus and pregnancy. Curr Opin Obstet Gynecol 1992;4(5):670–5.

6 Raynor BD. Cytomegalovirus in pregnancy. Semin Perinatol 1993;17(6):394–402.

7 Trincado DE, Rawlinson WD. Congenital and perinatal infection with cytomegalovirus. J Paediatr Child Health 2001;37(2):187–92.

8 Jones JL, Lopez A, Wilson M, Schulkin J, Gibbs R. Congenital toxoplasmosis: a review. Obstet Gynecol Surv 2001;56(5):296–305.

9 Beazley DM, Egerman RS. Toxoplasmosis. Semin Perinatol 1998;22(4):332–8.

10 Wallon M, Liou C, Garner P, Peyron F. Congenital toxoplasmosis: systematic review of evidence of efficacy of treatment in pregnancy. BMJ 1999;318(7197):1511–4.

11 Dufour P, de Bievre P, Vinatier D, Tordjeman N, Da Lage B, Vanhove J et al. Varicella and pregnancy. Eur J Obstet Gynecol Reprod Biol 1996;66(2):119–23.

12 Koren G. Varicella virus vaccine before pregnancy. Omortant breakthrough in protecting fetuses. Online: www.motherisk.com. October 2000.

13 Enders G, Miller E, Cradock–Watson J, Jolley I, Ridehalgh M. Consequences of varicella and herpes zoster in pregnancy: prospective study of 1739 cases. Lancet 1994;343(8912):950–1.

14 Harger JH, Adler SP, Koch WC, Harger GF. Prospective evaluation of 618 pregnant exposed to parvovirus B19: risks and symptoms. Obstet Gynecol 1998;91(3):413–20.

15 Miller E, Fairley CK, Cohen BJ, Seng C. Immediate and long term outcome of human parvovirus B19 infection in pregnancy. Br J Obstet Gynaecol 1998;105(12):1337–8.

16 Skjoldebrand-Sparre L, Tolfvenstam T, Papadogiannakis, Wahren B, Broliden K, Nyman M. Parvovirus B19 infection: association with third trimester intrauterine fetal death. Br J Obstet Gynaecol 2000;107(4):476–80.

17 Wong SF, Chan FY, Cincotta RB, Tilse M. Human parvovirus B19 infection in pregnancy: should screening be offered to the low risk population? Aust NZ J Obstet Gynaecol 2002; 42(4):347–51.

18 Mindel A, Taylor J, Tideman RL, Seifert C, Berry G, Wagner K et al. Neonatal herpes prevention: a minor public health problem in some communities. Sex Transm Infect 2000;76(4):287–91.

19 Eskild A, Jeansson S, Stray-Pedersen B, Jenum PA. Herpes simplex virus type-2 in pregnancy: no risk of fetal death: results from a nested case-control study within 35,940 women. Br J Obstet Gynaecol 2002;109(9):1030–5.

20 Brown ZA, Selke S, Zeh J, Kopelman J, Maslow A, Ashley RL et al. The acquisition of herpes simplex virus during pregnancy. N Engl J Med 1997;337(8):509–15.
21 Ugwumadu AH. Bacterial vaginosis in pregnancy. Curr Opin Obstet Gynecol 2002;14(2): 115–18.
22 Stephenson MD, Awartani KA, Robinson WP. Cytogenetic analysis of miscarriages from couples with recurrent miscarriage: a case-control study. Hum Reprod 2002 Feb;17(2):446–51.
23 Rai R, Regan L. Recurrent miscarriage. PACE 96/08. The Royal College of Obstetricians and Gynaecologists.
24 Li TC. Recurrent miscarriage: principles of management. Hum Reprod 1998;13(2):478–82.
25 Banerjee S, Aslam N, Woelfer B, Lawrence A, Elson J, Jurkovic D. Expectant management of early pregnancies of unknown location: a prospective evaluation of methods to predict spontaneous resolution of pregnancy, Br J Obstet Gynaecol 2001;108(2):158–63.
26 Luise C, Jermy K, Collons WP, Bourne TH/ Expectant management of incomplete, spontaneous first-trimester miscarriage: outcome according to initial ultrasound criteria and value of follow-up visits. Ultrasound Obstet Gynecol 2002;19(6):580–2.
27 Forna F, Gulmezoglu AM. Surgical procedures to evacuate incomplete abortion. Coch Rev.
28 Tham KF, Ratnan SS. The classification of gestational trophoblastic disease: a critical review. Int J Gynaecol Obstet 1998;60(Suppl):39–49.
29 Berkowitz RS, Im SS, Bernstein MR, Goldstein DP. Gestational trophoblastic disease. Subsequent pregnancy outcome, including repeat molar pregnancy. J Reprod Med 1998;43(1):81–6.
30 Waldenstrom U, Axelsson O, Nilsson S. Sonographic dating of pregnancies among women with menstrual irregularities. Acta Obstet Gynecol Scand 1991;70(1):17–20.
31 Selbing A. The pregnant population and a fetal crown-rump length screening program. Acta Obstet Gynecol Scand 1983;62(2):161–4.
32 Barker DJ, Winter PD, Osmond C, Margetts B, Simmonds SJ. Weight in infancy and death from ischaemic heart disease. Lancet 1989;2(8663):577–80.
33 Rouse DJ, Owen J, Goldenberg RL, Cliver SP. The effectiveness and costs of elective cesarean delivery for fetal macrosomia diagnosed by ultrasound. JAMA 1996;276(18):1480–6.
34 Neilson JP, Alfirevic Z. Doppler ultrasound for fetal assessment in high risk pregnancies. Coch Rev.
35 Robinson JN, Regan JA, Norwitz ER. The epidemiology of preterm labor. Semin Perinatol 2001;25(4):204–14.
36 Svigos JM. The fetal inflammatory response syndrome and cerebral palsy: yet another challenge and dilemma for the obstetrician. Aust N Z J Obstet Gynaecol 2001;41(2):170–6.
37 Papatsonis DN, Van-Geijn HP, Ader HJ, Lange FM, Bleker OP, Dekker GA. Nifedipine and ritodrine in the management of preterm labor: a randomized multicenter trial. Obstet Gynecol 1997;90(2):230–4.
38 Terzidou V, Bennett PR. Preterm labour. Curr Opin Obstet Gynecol 2002;14(2):105–13.
39 Kenyon S, Boulvain M, Neilson J. Antibiotics for preterm premature rupture of membranes. Cochrane Database Syst Rev 2001(4):CD001058.
40 Heath VC, Daskalakis G, Zagaliki A, Carvalho M, Nicolaides KH. Cervicovaginal fibronectin and cervical length at 23 weeks of gestation: relative risk of early preterm delivery. Br J Obstet Gynaecol 2000;107(10):1276–81.
41 Hague WM, North RA, Gallus AS, Walters BN, Orlikowski C, Burrows RF et al. A Working Group on behalf of the Obstetric Medicine Group of Australasia. Anticoagulation in pregnancy and the puerperium. Med J Aust 2001;175(5):258–63.
42 Scott F, Chan FY. Assessment of the clinical usefulness of the 'Queenan' chart versus the 'Liley' chart in predicting severity of rhesus isoimmunization. Prenat Diagn 1998;18(11):1143–8.
43 Wiley AW. Liquor amnii analysis in the management of the pregnancy complicated by rhesus sensitization. Am J Obstet Gynecol 1961;82:1359–70.
44 Tan KS, Thomson NC. Asthma in pregnancy. Am J Med 2000;109(9):727–33.
45 Hoffman L, Nolan C, Wilson JD, Oats JJ, Simmons D. Gestational diabetes mellitus—management guidelines. The Australasian Diabetes in Pregnancy Society. Med J Aust 1998;169(2):93–7.
46 Metzger BE, Coustan DR. Summary and recommendations of the Fourth International Workshop—Conference on Gestational Diabetes Mellitus. The Organizing Committee. Diabetes Care 1998;21(Suppl 2):B161–7.
47 American Diabetes Association. Gestational diabetes mellitus. (Position statement.) Diabetes Care 2002;25(1):S94–6.

48 American Diabetes Association. Pre-conception care of women with diabetes. (Position statement.) Diabetes Care 2002;25(1):S82–4.
49 Brown MA, Hague WM, Higgins J, Lowe S, McCowan L, Oats J et al. The detection, investigation and management of hypertension in pregnancy: executive summary. Aust NZ J Obstet Gynaecol 2000;40(2):133–8.

10 Induction of labour, assisted deliveries and postnatal problems

1 Hodnett E. Caregiver support for women during childbirth. Coch Rev.
2 Paterson-Brown S. Elective caesarean section—a woman's right to choose? Progr Obstet Gynaecol 2000;14:202–15.
3 Johanson R, Newburn M. Promoting normality in childbirth. BMJ 2001;323(7322):1142–3.
4 Paterson-Brown S. Should doctors perform an elective Caesarean section on request? Yes, as long as the woman is fully informed. BMJ 1998;317(7156):462–3.
5 McFarlane A. At last—maternity statistics for England. BMJ 1998;316(7131):566–7.
6 Royal College of Obstetricians and Gynaecologists, www.rcog.org.uk/guidelines/nscs–audit.pdf.
7 Clark SL, Koonings PP, Phelan JP. Placenta praevia/accreta and prior caesarean section. Obstet Gynecol 1985;66(1):89–92.
8 Sultan Ah. Anal incontinence after childbirth. Curr Opin Obstet Gynecol 1997;9(5):320–4.
9 Crowley P. Interventions for preventing or improving the outcome of delivery at or beyond term. Coch Rev.
10 Bishop EH. Pelvic scoring for elective induction. Obstet Gynecol 1964;24(2):266–8.
11 Hofmeyr GJ, Gulmezoglu AM. Vaginal misoprostol for cervical ripening and induction of labour. Coch Rev.
12 Nuutila M, Halmesmaki E, Hiilesmaa V, Ylikorkala O. Women's anticipation of and experiences with induction of labor. Acta Obstet Gynecol Scand 1999;78(8):704–9.
13 Lauzon L, Hodnett E. Labour assessment programs to delay admission to labour wards. Coch Rev.
14 Hofmeyr GJ. External cephalic version facilitation for breech presentation at term. Coch Rev.
15 Lau TK, Lo KW, Leung TY, Fok WY, Rogers MS. Outcome of labour after successful external cephalic version at term complicated by isolated transient fetal bradycardia. Br J Obstet Gynaecol. 2000;107(3):401–5.
16 Hannah ME, Hannah WJ, Hewson SA, Hodnett ED, Saigal S, Willan AR. Planned caesarean section versus planned vaginal birth for breech presentation at term: a randomised multicentre trial. Term Breech Trial Collaborative Group. Lancet 2000;356(9239):1375–83.
17 Hofmer GJ, Hannah ME. Planned Caesarean section for term breech delivery. Coch Rev.
18 Johanson RB, Menon BK. Vacuum extraction versus forceps for assisted vaginal delivery. Coch Rev.
19 James D. Caesarean section for fetal distress. BMJ 2001;322(7298):1316–17.
20 Glazenor CM, Abdulla M, Stroud P. et al. Postnatal maternal morbidity: extent, causes, prevention and treatment. Br J Obstet Gynaecol 1995;102(4):282–7.
21 Waterstone M, Bewley S, Wolfe C. Incidence and predictors of severe obstetric morbidity: case-control study. BMJ 2001;322(7294):1089–93; discussion 1093–4.
22 Ching-Chung L, Shuenn-Dhy C, Lin-Hong T. et al. Postpartum urinary retention: assessment of contributing factors and long term clinical impairment. Aust NZ J Obstet Gynaecol 2002; 42(4):365–8.
23 Kettle C, Johanson RB. Continuous versus interrupted sutures for perineal repair. Coch Rev.
24 Gorman WP, Davis KR, Donnelly R. ABC of arterial and venous disease. Swollen lower limb 1: General assessment and deep venous thrombosis. BMJ 2000;320(7247):1453–6.
25 Gates S, Brocklehurst P, Davis LJ. Prophylaxis for venous thromboembolic disease in pregnancy and the early postnatal period. Coch Rev.
26 Marchant S, Alexander J, Garcia J. Postnatal bleeding problems and general practice. Midwifery 2002;18(1):212–4.
27 MacLennan AH, Taylor AW, Wilson DH, Wilson D. The prevalence of pelvic floor disorders and their relationship to gender, age, parity and mode of delivery. Br J Obstet Gynaecol 2000;107(12):1460–70.
28 Brubaker L. Postpartum urinary incontinence. BMJ 2002;324(7348):1227–8.
29 Chiarelli P, Cockburn J. Promoting urinary continence in women after delivery: randomised controlled trial. BMJ 2002; 324(7348):1241.

30 Stamp G, Kruzins G, Crowther C. Perineal massage in labour and prevention of perineal trauma: randomised controlled trial. BMJ 2001;322(7297):1277–80.
31 Boyce P, Condon J. Psychological debriefing. Providing good clinical care means listening to women's concerns. BMJ 2001;322(7291):928.
32 Kenardy J. The current status of psychological debriefing. BMJ 2000;321(7268):1032–3.
33 Gamble JA, Creedy DK, Webster J, Moyle W. A review of the literature on debriefing or non-directive counselling to prevent postpartum emotional distress. Midwifery 2002;18(1): 72–9.
34 Livingstone VH. Problem-solving formula for failure to thrive in breast-fed infants. Can Fam Physician 1990;36:1541–5.

12 Sexual health

1 Rosenberg L, Palmer JR, Sands MI, Grimes D, Bergman U, Daling J et al. Modern oral contraceptives and cardiovascular disease Am J Obstet Gynecol 1997;177(3):707–15.
2 Larsson G, Milsom I, Linstedt G, Rybo G. The influence of a low-dose combined oral contraceptive on menstrual blood loss and iron status. Contraception 1992;46(4):327–34.
3 Rivera R, Yacobson I, Grimes D. The mechanism of action of hormonal contraceptives and intrauterine devices. Review. 1999;181(5 Pt 1):1263–9.
4 Collaborative Group on Hormonal Factors in Breast Cancer. Breast cancer and hormone contraceptives: collaborative reanalysis of individual data on 53 297 women with breast cancer and 100 239 women without breast cancer from 54 epidemiologcal studies. Lancet 1996; 347(9017):1713–27.
5 Anderson TJ, Battersby S, King RJ, McPherson K, Going JJ. Oral contraceptive use influences resting breast proliferation. Hum Pathol 1989;20(12):1139–44.
6 Clinical and Scientific Advisory Committee Interim Guidelines for doctors following the pill scare. Br J Fam Plann 1984;9:120–2.
7 Cundy T, Evans M, Roberts H, Wattie D, Ames R, Reid IR. Bone density in women receiving depot medroxyprogesterone acetate for contraception. BMJ 1991;303(6793):13–6.
8 Gbolade BA. Ellis S. Murby B. Kirkman R. Bone density in long term users of depot medroxyprogesterone acetate (DMPA). Brit J Obstet Gynaecol 1998;105(7):790–4.
9 Orr-Walker BJ, Evans MC, Ames RW, Clearwater JM, Cundy T, Reid IR. The effect of past use of the injectable contraceptive depot medroxyprogesterone acetate on bone mineral density in normal post-menopausal women. Clin Endocrinol 1998;49(5):615–18.
10 Peterson HB, Xia Z, Hughes JM, Wilcox LS, Tylor LR, Trussel J. The risk of pregnancy after tubal sterilization: Findings from the US Collaborative Review of Sterilization. Am J Obstet Gynecol 1996;174(4):1161–8; discussion 1168–70.
11 Boyle M. The experience of abortion in women's health: contemporary international perspectives. Ed. Ussher, JM. British Psychological Society Books, 2000.
12 Kaunitz AM, Rovira EZ, Grimes DA, Schultz KF. Abortions that fail. Obstet Gynecol 1985; 66:533–7.
13 The care of women requesting induced abortion. Evidence-based guideline No 7. RCOG Clinical Effectiveness Support Group. RCOG Press, 2000.
14 Ferriman A. Medical abortion still not available in most countries. BMJ 1999;319(7217):1091.
15 Zhang J, Thomas AG, Leybovich E. Vaginal douching and adverse health effects: a meta-analysis. Am J Public Health 1997;87(7):1201–11.
16 Howell MR, Quinn TC, Gaydos CA. Screening for *Chlamydia trachomatis* in asymptomatic women attending family planning clinics. A cost-effectiveness analysis of three stages. Ann Intern Med 1998;128(4):277–84.
17 Stokes T. Screening for *Chlamydia* in general practice: a literature review and summary of the evidence. J Public Health Med 1997;19(2):222–32.
18 Serlin M, Shafer MA, Tebb K, Gyamfi AA, Moncada J, Schachter J et al. What sexually transmitted disease screening method does the adolescent prefer? Adolescents' attitudes toward first-void urine, self-collected vaginal swab, and pelvic examination. Arch Pediatr Adolesc Med 2002;156(6):588–91.
19 Johnson RE, Newhall WJ, Papp JR, Knapp JS, Black CM, Gift TL et al. Screening tests to detect Chlamydia trachomatis and Neisseria gonorrhoeae infections—2002. Mortality & Morbidity Weekly Report. Vol 51, No. RR15; 2002;1–38.

20 Oakeshott P, Hay P, Hay S, Steinke F, Rink E, Kerry S. Association between bacterial vaginosis or chlamydial infection and miscarriage before 16 weeks' gestation: prospective community based cohort study. BMJ 2002;325(7376):1334.
21 Marrazzo JM, Handsfield HH, Whittington WL. Predicting chlamydial and gonococcal cervical infection: implications for management of cervicitis. Obstet Gynecol 2002; 100(3):579–84.
22 Hook EW III, Marra CM. Acquired syphilis in adults. N Engl J Med. 1992;326(16):1060–9.
23 Centers for Disease Control and Prevention. HIV/AIDS Surveillance Report 2001;13(2).
24 National Centre for HIV Epidemiology and Clinical Research. AIDS, hepatitis C and sexually transmissible infections. Annual Surveillance Report. Darlinghurst, Australia, 2000.
25 Johnson AM, Laga M. Heterosexual transmission of HIV. AIDS 1988;2(Suppl 1):S49–56.
26 Fleming PL, Ciesielski CA, Byers RH, Castro KG, Berkelman Rl. Gender differences in reported AIDS—indicative diagnoses. J Infect Dis 1993;168(1):61–7.
27 Homayoon Farzadegan H, Hoover DR, Astermborski J, Lyles CM et al. Sex differences in HIV1 viral load and progression to AIDS. Lancet 1998;352(9139):1510–14.
28 Sterling TR. Initial HIV 1 plasma RNA after seroconversion does not predict progression to AIDS in women. XIIIth International AIDS Conference, Durban B204, 2000.
29 Long EM, Martin HJL Jr, Kreiss JK, Rainwater SM, Lavreys L, Jackson DJ et al. Gender differences in HIV-I diversity at time of infection. Nat Med 2000;6(1):71–5.
30 Oliatitan A, Johnson MA. Cervical intraepithelial neoplasia in women with HIV. J Int Assoc Physicians AIDS Care 1997;3(5):15–18.
31 Maiman M. Management of cervical neoplasia in human immunodeficiency virus-infected women. J Natl Cancer Inst Monogr 1998;23:43–9.
32 Sun XW, Kuhn L, Ellerbrock TV, Chiasson MA, Bush TJ, Wright TC Jr. Human papillomavirus infection in women infected with the human immunodeficiency virus. N Engl J Med 1997; 337(19):1343–9.
33 Minkoff HL, Eisenberger-Matityahu D, Feldman J, Burk R, Clarke L. Prevalence and incidence of gynecologic disorders among women infected with human immunodeficiency virus. Am J Obstet Gynecol 1999;180(4):824–36.
34 Stephenson JM, Griffioen A. The effect of HIV diagnosis on reproductive experience. Study Group for the Medical Research Council Collaborative Study of Women with HIV. AIDS 1996;10(14):1683–7.
35 Carroll N, Goldstein RS, Wilson L, Mayer KH. Gynaecological Infections and sexual practices of Massachusetts lesbian and bisexual women. J Gay Lesbian Med Assoc 1997;1(1):15–23.
36 Diamant AL, Wold C, Spritzer K, Gelberg L. Health behaviours, health status and access to and use of health care: a population-based study of lesbian, bisexual and heterosexual women. Arch Fam Med 2000;9(10):1043–51.
37 Skinner WF, Otis MD. Drug and alcohol use among lesbian and gay people in a southern US sample: epidemiological, comparative, and methodological findings from the Triology Project. J Homosexuality 1996;30(3):59–92.
38 Marrazzo JM. Sexually transmitted infections in women who have sex with women: who cares? Sex Transm Infect 2000;76(5):330–2.
39 Booth C. Woman to woman: a guide to lesbian sexuality. Sydney: Simon & Schuster, 2002.
40 Johnson AM, Wadsworth J, Wellings K, Field J. Sexual attitudes and lifestyles. London: Blackwell, 1994.
41 Dunne MP, Bailey JM, Kirk KM, Martin NG. The subtlety of sex—atypicality. Arch Sex Behav 2000;29(6):549–65.
42 Purdie DM, Dunne MP, Boyle FM, Cook MD, Najman JM. Health and demographic characteristics of respondents in an Australian national sexuality survey: comparison with population norms. J Epidemiol Community Health 2002;56(10):748–53.
43 Laumann EO, Paik A, Rosen RC. Sexual dysfunction in the United States: prevalence and predictors. JAMA 1999;281(6):537–44.
44 Fleming JM. Prevalence of childhood sexual abuse in a community sample of Australian women. Med J Aust 1997;166(2):65–8.
45 Dunne MP, Purdie D, Cook M, Boyle FM, Najman JM. Is child sexual abuse declining? Evidence from a population-based survey of men and women in Australia. Child Abuse Negl 2003;27(2):141–52.

46 Jones LM, Finkelhor D, Kopiec K. Why is sexual abuse declining? A survey of state child protection administrators. Child Abuse Negl 2001;25(9):1139–58.
47 Fergusson D, Mullen P. Childhood sexual abuse: An evidence-based perspective. Thousand Oaks: Sage, 1999.
48 Tyler KA. Social and emotional outcomes of childhood sexual abuse: a review of recent research. Aggression & Violent Behavior 2002;7(6):567–89.
49 Nelson EC, Heath AC, Madden PA, Cooper ML, Dinwiddie SH, Bucholz KK et al. Association between self-reported childhood sexual abuse and adverse psychosocial outcomes: results from a twin study. Arch Gen Psychiatry 2002;59(2):139–45.

13 Common problems

1 National Breast Cancer Centre. Breast imaging: a guide for practice. Camperdown, NSW: NBCC, 2002.
2 Stephen EH, Chandra A. Updated projections of infertility in the United States: 1995–2025. Fertil Steril 1998;70(1):30.
3 Dunson DB, Colombo B, Baird DD. Changes with age in the level and duration of fertility in the menstrual cycle. Hum Reprod 2002;17(5):1399–403.
4 Grimes DA. Intrauterine device and upper genital tract infection. Lancet 2000; 356(9234):1031–9.
5 Jensen TK, Hjollund NH, Henriksen TB, Scheike T, Kolstad H, Giwercman A et al. Does moderate alcohol consumption affect fertility? Follow-up study among couples planning first pregnancy. BMJ 1998;317(7157):505–10.
6 Hakim RB, Gray RH, Zacur H. Alcohol and caffeine consumption and decreased fertility. Fertil Steril 1998;70(4):632–7.
7 Laurent SL, Thompson SJ, Addy C, Garrison CZ, Moore EE. An epidemiologic study of smoking and primary infertility in women. Fertil Steril 1992;57(3):565–72.
8 Akande V. Tubal pelvic damage: prediction and prognosis. Hum Reprod 2002;5(Suppl 1): S15–20.
9 Allingham-Hawkins DJ, Babul-Hirji R, Chitayat D, Holden JJ, Yang KT, Lee C et al. Fragile X is a significant risk factor for premature ovarian failure: The International Collaborative POF in Fragile X study—preliminary data. Am J Med Genet 1999;53(4):322–5.
10 The Initial Investigation and Management of the Infertile Couple: Evidence-based Clinical Guidelines No. 2. RCOG Press, 1998.
11 Watson AJ, Gupta JK, O'Donovan P, Dalton ME, Lilford RJ. The results of tubal surgery in the treatment of infertility in two non-specialist hospitals. Br J Obstet Gynaecol 1990;97(7):561.
12 Watson A, Vandekerekhove P, Lilford R. Techniques of pelvic surgery in infertility. Coch Rev, 2000.
13 Dhont M, De Sutter P, Ruyssinck G, Martens G, Bekaert A. Perinatal outcome of pregnancies after assisted reproduction: a case-control study. Am J Obstet Gynecol 1999;181(3):688–95.
14 Sutcliffe AG. Health risks in babies born after assisted reproduction. BMJ 2002;325(7356): 117–18.
15 Bonduelle M, Liebaers I, Deketelaere V, Derde MP, Camus M, Devroey P, Van Steirteghem A. Neonatal data on a cohort of 2889 infants born after ICSI (1991–1999) and of 2995 infants born after IVF (1983–1999). Hum Reprod 2002;17(3):671–94.
16 Venn A, Watson L, Bruinsma F, Giles G, Healy D. Risk of cancer after use of fertility drugs with in-vitro fertilisation. Lancet 1999;354(9190):1586–90.
17 Guzick DS, Sullivan MW, Adamson GD, Cedars MI, Falk RJ, Peterson EP, Steinkampf MP. Efficacy of treatment for unexplained infertility. Fertil Steril 1998;70(2):207–13.
18 Wang C, McDonald V, Leung A, Superlano L, Berman N, Hull L, Swerdloff RS. Effect of increased scrotal temperature on sperm production in normal men. Fertil Steril 1997; 68(2):334–9.
19 Cahill DJ, Wardle PG. Management of infertility. BMJ 2002;325(7354):28–32.
20 Silber SJ, Nagy Z, Liu J, Tournaye H, Lissens W, Ferec C et al. The use of epididymal and testicular spermatozoa for intracytoplasmic sperm injection: the genetic implications for male infertility. Hum Reprod 1995;10(8):2031–43.
21 Ferriman D, Gallwey JD. Clinical assessment of body hair growth in women. J Clin Endocrinol Metab 1961;21:1440–6.

22 Moncada E. Familial study of hirsutism. J Clin Endocrinol Metab 1970;31(5):556–64.
23 Moore J, Kennedy S. Causes of chronic pelvic pain. Baillière's Clinical Obstetrics & Gynaecology 2000;14(3):389–161.
24 Beard RW, Reginald PW, Wadsworth J. Clinical features of women with lower abdominal pain and pelvic congestion. Br J Obstet Gynaecol 1988;95(2):153–61.
25 Howard FM. The role of laparoscopy as a diagnostic tool in chronic pelvic pain. Baillière's Clinical Obstetrics & Gynaecology 2000;14(3):467–94.
26 Sampson JA. Perforating haemorrhagic (chocolate) cysts of the ovary. Their importance and especially their relation to pelvic adenomas of the endometrial type ('adenomyoma' of the uterus, rectovaginal septum, sigmoid etc). Arch Surg 1921;3:245–323.
27 Pellicer A, Albert C, Mercader A, Bonilla-Musoles F, Remohi J, Simon C. The follicular and endocrine environment in women with endometriosis: local and systemic cytokine production. Fertil Steril 1998;70(3):425–31.
28 Moen MH, Stockstad T. A long-term follow-up study of women with asymptomatic endometriosis diagnosed incidentaly at sterilization. Fertil Steril 2002; 78(4):773–6.
29 Cornillie FJ, Oosterlynck D, Lauweryns JM, Koninckx PR. Deeply infiltrating pelvic endometriosis: histology and clinical significance. Fertil Steril 1990;53(6):978–83.
30 Hughes EG, Fedorkow DM, Collins JA. A quantitative overview of controlled trials in endometriosis-associated infertility. Fertil Steril 1993;59(5):963–70.
31 Marcoux S, Maheux R, Berube S. Laparoscopic surgery in infertile women with minimal or mild endometriosis. Canadian Collaborative Group on Endometriosis. N Engl J Med 1997; 337(4):217–22.
32 Selak V, Farquhar C, Prentice A, Singla A. Danazol for pelvic pain associated with endometriosis. Coch Rev.
33 Proctor ML, Farquhar CM, Sinclair OJ, Johnson NP. Surgical interruption of pelvic nerve pathways for primary and secondary dysmenorrhoea. Coch Rev.
34 Benson CB, Chow JS, Chang-Lee W, Hill JA III, Doubilet PM. Outcome of pregnancies in women with uterine leiomyomas identified by sonography in the first trimester. J Clin Ultrasound 2001;29(5):261–4.
35 Pritts EA. Fibroids and infertility: a systematic review of the evidence. Obstet Gynecol Surv 2001;56(8):483–91.
36 Moorehead ME, Conard CJ. Uterine leiomyoma: a treatable condition. Ann NY Acad Sci 2001;984:121–9.
37 Farquhar C, Arroll B, Ekeroma A, Fentiman G, Lethaby A, Rademaker L et al. An evidence-based guideline for the management of uterine fibroids. Aust NZ J Obstet Gynaecol 2001; 41(2):125–40.
38 Walker WJ, Pelage JP, Sutton C. Fibroid embolization. Clin Radiol 2002;57(5):325–31.
39 Tanos V, Schenker JG. Ovarian cysts: a clinical dilemma. Gynecol Endocrinol 1994;8(1): 59–67.
40 Reimer T, Gerber B, Muller H, Jeschke U, Krause A, Friese K. Differential diagnosis of peri- and postmenopausal ovarian cysts. Maturitas 1999;31(2):123–32.
41 Ekerhovd E, Wienerroith H, Staudach A, Granberg S. Preoperative assessment of unilocular adnexal cysts by transvaginal ultrasonography: a comparison between ultrasonographic morphologic imaging and histopathologic diagnosis. Am J Obstet Gynecol 2001;184(2):48–54.
42 Ross J. Pelvic inflammatory disease. BMJ 2001;322(7287):658–9.
43 Adler MW. Complications of common genital infections. ABC of Sexually Transmitted Diseases. BMJ Publishing Group, 1998;17.
44 Peipert JF, Ness RB, Blume J, Soper DE, Holley R, Randall H et al, Pelvic Inflammatory Disease Evaluation and Clinical Health Study Investigators. Clinical predictors of endometritis in women with symptoms and signs of pelvic inflammatory disease. Am J Obstet Gynecol 2001;184(5):856–63; discussion 863–4.
45 Molander P, Sjoberg J, Paavonen J, Cacciatore B. Transvaginal power Doppler findings in laparoscopically proven acute pelvic inflammatory disease. Ultrasound Obstet Gynecol 2001; 17(3):233–8.
46 Ross JD. Outpatient antibiotics for pelvic inflammatory disease. BMJ 2001;322(7281):251–2.
47 Ross JD. European guideline for the management of pelvic inflammatory disease and perihepatitis. Int J STD AIDS 2001;12(Suppl 3):84–7.

48 Downing SJ, Tay JI, Maguiness SD et al. Effect of inflammatory mediators on the physiology of the human Fallopian tube. Hum Fertil 2002;5(2):54–60.
49 Nelson HD, Heland M. Screening for chlamydial infection. Am J Prev Med 2001;20(3): 95–107.
50 McMillan S. Chlamydia trachomatis in subfertile women undergoing uterine instrumentation: the clinician's role. Hum Reprod 2002;17(6):1433–6.
51 Zhang J, Thomas AG, Leybovich E. Vaginal douching and adverse health effects: a meta-analysis. Am J Public Health 1997;87(7):1201–11.

14 Health maintenance and disease prevention

1 Australian Institute of Health and Welfare, Australasian association of Cancer Registries and NHMRC National Breast Cancer Centre 1999. Breast cancer in Australian women 1982–1996. Canberra: AIHW (Cancer Series).
2 Holmberg L, Ekborn A, Calle E, Mokdad A, Byers T. Breast cancer mortality in relation to self-reported use of breast self-examination. A cohort study of 450,000 women. Breast Cancer Res Treat 1997;43(2):137–40.
3 UK Trial of Early Detection of Breast Cancer Group; sixteen year mortality from breast cancer in the UK Trial of Early Detection of Breast Cancer. Lancet 1999;353(9168):1909–14.
4 Kerlikowske K, Grady D, Rubin SM, Sandrock C, Ernster VL. Efficacy of screening mammography. A meta-analysis. JAMA 1995;273(2):149–54.
5 Kerlikowske K. Efficacy of screening mammography among women aged 40 to 49 years and 50 to 69 years: comparison of relative and absolute benefit. J Natl Cancer Inst Monogr 1997; 22:79–86.
6 Tabar L, Fagerberg G, Chen H, Duffy S, Smart C, Gad A, Smit R. Efficacy of breast cancer screening by age. New results from the Swedish Two-County Trial. Cancer 1995;75(10): 2507–17.
7 Barloon TJ, Young DC, Bergus G. The role of diagnostic imaging in women with breast implants. Am Fam Physician 1996;54(6):2029–36.
8 Gammon MD, John EM, Britton JA. Recreational and occupational physical activities and risk of breast cancer. J Natl Cancer Inst 1998;90(2):100–17.
9 Kushi LH, Sellers TA, Potter JD, Nelson CL, Munger RG, Kay SA. Dietary fat and postmenopausal breast cancer J Natl Cancer Inst 1992;84(14):1092–9.
10 Willet WC, Hunter DJ, Stampfer MJ, Colditz G, Manson JE, Spiegelman D et al. Dietary fat and fiber in relation to risk of breast cancer: An eight-year follow-up. JAMA 1992;268(15): 2037–44.
11 Feigelson HS, Jonas CR, Robertson AS, McCullough ML, Thun MJ, Calle EE. Alcohol, folate, methionine, and risk of incdient breast cancer in the American Cancer Society Cancer Prevention Study II Nutrition Cohort. Cancer Epidemiol Biomarkers Prev 2003;12(2): 161–4.
12 Cuzik J; International Breast Cancer Intervention Study. A brief review of the International Breast Cancer Intervention Study (IBIS), the other current breast cancer prevention trials, and proposals for future trials. Ann NY Acad Sci 2001; 949:123–33.
13 Hartmann LC, Schaid DJ, Woods JE, Crotty TP, Myers JL, Arnold PG et al. Efficacy of bilateral prophylactic mastectomy in women with a family history of breast cancer. N Engl J Med 1999;340(2):77–84.
14 Fraser IJ. Menorrhagia: a pragmatic approach to the understanding of causes and the need for investigation. Br J Obstet Gynaecol 1994;101(Suppl 11): 307.
15 Wyatt KM, Dimmock PW, Walker TJ, O'Brien PM. Determination of total menstrual blood loss. Fertil Steril 2001;76(1):125–31.
16 Janssen CA, Scholten PC, Heintz AP. Reconsidering menorrhagia in gynecological practice. Europ J Obstet Gynecol Reprod Biol 1998;78(1):69–72.
17 Working Party for Guidelines for the Management of Heavy Menstrual Bleeding. An evidence-based guideline for the management of heavy menstrual bleeding. NZ Med J 1999;112(1088): 174–7.
18 Naegle F, O'Connor H, Davies A, Badawy A, Mohammed H, Magos A. 2500 outpatient diagnostic hysteroscopies. Obstet Gynecol 1996;88(1):87–92.
19 P Sivyer. Pelvic ultrasound in women. World J Surg 2000;24(2):188–97.

20 Hurskainen R, Aalto AM, Teperi J, Grenman S, Kivela A, Kujansuu E et al. Psychosocial and other characteristics of women complaining of menorrhagia, with and without actual increased menstrual blood loss. Br J Obstet Gynaecol 2001;108(3):281–5.
21 Carlson KJ, Miller BA, Fowler FJ Jr. The Maine Women's Health Study: 1. Outcomes of hysterectomy. Obstet Gynecol 1994;83(4):556–65.
22 O'Connor VM. Heavy menstrual loss. Part 1. Is it really heavy loss? Medicine Today 2003;4(4):51–9. Part 2. Management options. Medicine Today 2003;4(5):45–55.
23 O'Flynn N, Britten N. Menorrhagia in general practice—disease or illness. Soc Sci Med 2000;50(5):651–61.
24 Lethaby A, Irvine G, Cameron I. Cyclical progestogens for heavy menstrual bleeding. Coch Rev. Iyer V, Farquhar C, Jepson R. Oral contraceptive pills for heavy menstrual bleeding. Coch Rev. Lethaby A, Augood C, Duckitt K. Nonsteroidal anti-inflammatory drugs for heavy menstrual bleeding. Coch Rev. Lethaby AE, Cooke I, Rees M. Progesterone/progestogen releasing intrauterine systems versus either placebo or any other medication for heavy menstrual bleeding. Coch Rev.
25 Avis NE, Crawford SL, MaKinley SM. Psychosocial, behavioural, and health factors related to menopause symptomatology. Women Health 1997;3(2):103–20.
26 O'Connor VM, Del Mar CB, Sheehan M, Siskind V, Fox-Young S, Cragg C. Do psycho-social factors contribute more to symptom reporting by middle aged women than hormonal status? Maturitas 1994;20(2/3):63–9.
27 Murtagh J. General practice. Sydney: McGraw-Hill,1998.
28 Dennerstein L, Lehert P, Burger H, Dudley E. Factors affecting sexual functioning of women in the mid-life years. Climacteric 1999;2(4):254–62.
29 Do KA, Treloar SA, Pandeya N et al. Predictive factors of age at menopause in a large Australian twin study. Hum Biol 1998;70(6):1073–91.
30 Dennerstein L, Lehert P, Burger H, Dudley E. Mood and the menopause transition. J Nerv Ment Dis 1999;187(11):685–91.
31 O'Connor VM. Menopause, Parts 1 and 2. Mod Med 2001, vol 1.
32 MacLennan A, Lester S, Moore V. Oral oestrogen replacement therapy versus placebo for hot flushes. Coch Rev.
33 Nikles CJ, Glasziou PP, Del Mar CB, Duggan CM, Mitchell G. N of 1 trials. Practical tools for medication management. Aust Fam Physician 2000;29(11):1108–12.
34 Khaw KT. Hormone replacement therapy again. Risk-benefit relation differs between populations and individuals. BMJ 1998;316(7148):1842–44.
35 Davis SR, Burger HG. Use of androgens in postmenopausal women. Curr Opin Obstet Gynecol 1997;9(3):177–80.
36 Eden J. Managing menopause—HRT or herbal. Mod Med Aust 1999; August: 32–5.
37 MacLennan AH. The four harms of harmless therapies. Climacteric 1999;2(2):73–4.
38 Norman RJ, Flight IHK, Rees MCP. Oestrogen and progestogen hormone replacement therapy for peri-menopausal and post-menopausal women: weight and body fat distribution. Coch Rev.
39 Lethaby A, Farquhar C, Sarkis A, Roberts H, Jepson R, Barlow D. Hormone replacement therapy in postmenopausal women: endometrial hyperplasia and irregular bleeding. Coch Rev.
40 Clinical Synthesis Panel on HRT. Hormone replacement therapy. Lancet 1999;354(9173):152–5.
41 MacLennan AH. Hormone replacement therapy: where to now? Australian Prescriber 2003;26(1):8–11.
42 Hogervorst E, Yaffe K, Richards M, Huppert F. Hormone replacement therapy for cognitive function in women with dementia. Coch Rev.
43 Hogervorst E, Yaffe K, Richards M, Huppert F. Hormone replacement therapy for cognitive function in postmenopausal women. Coch Rev.
44 Huppert FA, Van Niekerk JK. Dehydroepiandrosterone (DHEA) supplementation for cognitive function. Coch Rev.

15 Common complaints

1 Australian Institute of Health and Welfare, Australasian Association of Cancer Registries and NHMRC National Breast Cancer Centre. Breast cancer in Australian women 1982–1996 Canberra: AIHW (Cancer Series), 1999.
2 Clemons M, Goss P. Estrogen and the risk of breast cancer. N Engl J Med 2001;344(4):276–85.

3 Dixon JM, ed. ABC of Breast Diseases. London: BMJ Publishing, 1995;4.
4 Adler DN, South-Paul J, Adera T, Deuster PA. Cyclic mastalgia: prevalence and associated health and behavioral factors. J Psychosom Obstet Gynecol 2001;22(2):71–6.
5 Gateley CA, Miers M, Mansel RE, Hughes LE. Drug treatments for mastalgia: 17 years experience in the Cardiff Mastalgia Clinic. J R Soc Med 1992;85(1):12–5.
6 Falkenberry S. Nipple discharge. Obstet Gynecol Clin North Am 2002;29(1):21–9.

16 Pre-cancer and cancer

1 Kohler MF, Berchuck A, Davidoff AM, Humphrey PA, Dodge RK, Iglehart JD et al. Overexpression and mutation of p53 in endometrial carcinoma. Cancer Res 1992;52(6): 1622–7.
2 Risinger JI, Hayes AK, Berchuck A, Barrett JC. PTEN/MMAC1 mutations in endometrial cancers. Cancer Res 1997;57(21):4736–8.
3 National Pathology Accreditation Advisory Council. Requirements for gynaecological (cervical) cytology. Canberra: Australian Government Publishing Service, 1997.
4 Martin-Hirsch P, Lilford R, Jarvis G, Kitchener HC. Efficacy of cervical-smear collection devices: a systematic review and meta-analysis. Lancet 1999;354(9192):1763–70.
5 Syrjanen K, Parkkinen S, Mantyjarvi R, Vayrynen M, Syrjanen S, Holopainen H et al. Human papilloma virus (HPV) type as an important determinant of the natural history of HPV infections in uterine cervix. Eur J Epidemiol 1985;1(3):180–7.
6 Martin-Hirsch PL, Kitchener H. Interventions for preventing blood loss during the treatment of cervical intraepithelial neoplasia. Coch Rev.
7 Creasman WT. Endometrial cancer: incidence, prognostic factors, diagnosis and treatment. Semin Oncol 1997;24(1 Suppl 1):SI–140.
8 Quinlivan JA, Petersen RW, Nicklin JL. Accuracy of frozen section for the operative management of endometrial cancer. Br J Obst Gynaecol 2001;108(8):798–803.
9 Pecorelli S, Benedet JL, Creasman WT, Shepherd JH. On behalf of the 1994–97 FIGO Committee on Gynaecologic Oncology. FIGO staging of gynaecologic cancer. Int J Gynaecol Obstet 1998;64(1):5–10.
10 Breast cancer size and nodal status. Cancer monitoring no 2. Canberra National Breast Cancer Centre; Australasian Association of Cancer Registries; Breastscreen Australia; Department of Health and Aged Care; Australian Institute of Health and Welfare, October 2001.
11 Franceschi S, Levi F, LaVecchia C, Randimbison L, Te VC. Second cancers following in situ carcinoma of the breast. Int J Cancer 1998;77(3):392–5.
12 Beral V, Bull D, Doll R, Key T, Peto R, Reeves G. Collaborative Group on Hormonal Factors in Breast Cancer. Breast cancer and hormone replacement therapy: collaborative reanalysis of data from 51 epidemiological studies of 52 705 women with breast cancer and 108 411 women without breast cancer. Lancet 1997;350(9084):1047–59.
13 Roussow JE, Anderson GL, Prentice RL, LaCroix AZ, Kooperberg C, Stefantck ML et al. Risks and benefits of estrogen plus progestin in healthy post-menopausal women: principal results from the Women's Health Initiative randomized controlled trial. JAMA 2002;288(3): 321–33.
14 Cheek J, Lacy J, Toth-Fejel S, Morris K, Calhoun K, Pommier RF. The impact of hormone replacement therapy on the detection and stage of breast cancer. Arch Surg 2002;137(9): 1015–21, discussion 1019–21.
15 Marchbanks PA, McDonald JA, Wilson HG, Folger SG, Mandel MG, Daling JR et al. Oral contraceptives and the risk of breast cancer. N Engl J Med 2002;346(26):2025–32.
16 Salvadori B, Marubini E, Miceli R, Conti AR, Cusumano F, Andreola S et al. Reoperation for locally recurrent breast cancer in patients previously treated with conservative surgery. Br J Surg 1999;86(1):84–7.
17 Early Breast Cancer Trialists' Collaborative Group. Polychemotherapy for early breast cancer: an overview of the randomised trials. Lancet 1998;352(9132):930–42.
18 Early Breast Cancer Trialists' Collaborative Group. Tamoxifen for early breast cancer: an overview of the randomised trials. Lancet 1998;351(9114):1451–67.
19 Fallowfield LJ, Hall A, Maguire GP, Baum M, A'Hern RP. Psychological effects of being offered choice of surgery for breast cancer. BMJ 1994;309(6952):448.
20 Mock V. Body image in women treated for breast cancer. Nurs Res 1993;42(3):153–7.

21 Andersen BL, Golden-Kreutz DM. Sexual self-concept for the woman with cancer. Chapter 17 in Cancer and the Family, eds. Baider L, Cooper CL, De-Nour AK. Chichester: John Wiley & Sons, 1996;337–66.
22 Turner J. Children of mothers with advanced breast cancer: a review of needs and services. Cancer Forum 1998;22(3):191–5.
23 Northouse LL, Cracchiolo-Carraway A, Appel CP. Psychologic consequences of breast cancer on partner and family. Sem Oncol Nurs 1991;7(3):216–23.
24 Wellisch DK, Gritz ER, Schain W, Wang HJ, Siau J. Psychological functioning of daughters of breast cancer patients: Part II: Characterizing the distressed daughter of the breast cancer patient. Psychosomatics 1992;33(2):171–9.
25 National Health and Medical Research Council. Psychosocial Clinical Practice Guidelines: information, support and counselling for women with breast cancer. Canberra: Australian Government Publishing Service, 2000.
26 Devine EC, Westlake SK. The effects of psychoeducational care provided to adults with cancer: meta-analysis of 116 studies. Oncology Nursing Forum 1995;14(2):101–8.
27 Lewis F, Hammond MA. Psychosocial adjustment of the family to breast cancer: a longitudinal analysis. J Am Med Women's Assoc 1992;47(5):194–200.

17 Ageing and its problems

1 Anan K, UN Secretary-General, Address to 2nd UN World Assembly on Ageing, Madrid, Spain, 9 Apr 2002.
2 Davies I. Cellular mechanisms of ageing. In: Brocklehurst's textbook of geriatric medicine and gerontology, Edinburgh: Churchill Livingstone, 1998;51–83.
3 Hogan DB, McKeith I. Of MCI and dementia: Improving diagnosis and treatments. Neurology 2001;56(9):1131–2.
4 Watson EK, Firman DW, Baade PD, Ring I. Telephone administration of the SF-36 health survey: validation studies and population norms for adults in Queensland. Aust NZ J Pub Health 1996;20(4):1085–90.
5 Australian Institute of Health and Welfare. Australia's health 1998. Canberra: AIHW, 1998.
6 Scinto J, Gill TM, Grady JN, Holmboe ES. Screening mammography: is it suitably targeted to older women who are most likely to benefit? J Am Geriatr Soc 2001;49(8):110–14.
7 Haigney E, Morgan R, King D, Spencer B. Breast examination in older women; questionnaire survey of attitudes of patients and doctors. BMJ 1997;315(7115):1058–9.
8 Australian Institute of Health and Welfare. Australia's Health 2000. Canberra: AIHW, 2000.
9 Leipzig RM, Cumming RG, Tinnetti ME. Drugs and falls in older people: a systematic review and meta-analysis. Cardiac and analgesic drugs. J Am Geriatr Soc 1999;47:40–50.
10 National Service Framework for Older People, Department of Health, 2001, www.doh.uk/nsf/olderpeople.
11 Hughes M. Falls prevention among older adults. Is London ready for the NSF? Br J Commun Nurs 2002;7(7):352–8.
12 Brooks PM. Impact of osteoarthritis on individuals and society: how much disability? Social consequences and health economic implications. Curr Opin Rheumatol 2002;14(5):573–7.
13 Lapsley HM, March LM, Tribe KL, Cross MJ, Courtenay BG, Brooks PM. Living with rheumatoid arthritis: patient expenditures, health status, and social impact on patients. Ann Rheum Dis 2002;61(9):818–21.
14 Folstein MF, Folstein SE, McHugh PR. 'Mini-mental state': a practical method for grading the cognitive state of patients for the clinician. J Psychiatr Res 1975;12(3):189–98.
15 Burns A, Lawlor B, Craig S. Assessment scales in old age psychiatry. London: Martin Dunitz, 1999.
16 Small GW. What we need to know about age-related memory loss. BMJ 2002;324:1502–5.
17 Jorm AF, Henderson AS. The problem of dementia in Australia. 3rd edn. Canberra: AGPS, 1993.
18 Darzins P, Molloy W, Strang D. Who can decide? The six-step capacity assessment process. Adelaide: Memory Press Australia, 2000.
19 Doody RS, Stevens JC, Beck C, Dubinsky RM, Kaye JA, Gwyther L et al. Practice parameter: management of dementia (an evidence-based review). Report of the Quality Standards Subcommittee of the American Academy of Neurology. Neurology 2001;56(9):1154–66.

20 Levkoff SE, Evans DA, Liptzin B, Cleary PD, Lispitz LA, Wetle TT et al. Delirium: The occurrence and persistence of symptoms among elderly hospitalized patients. Arch Intern Med 1992;152(2):334–40.
21 Shah A, Ames D. Behavioural problems in patients with dementia. Mod Med Aust 1994; 37(5):67–72.
22 Nair B. Older people and medications: what is the right prescription? Aust Prescr 1999; 22:130–1.
23 Munro J, Brazier J, Davey R, Nicholl J. Physical activity for the over-65s: could it be a cost-effective exercise for the NHS? J Pub Health Med 1997;19(4):397–402.
24 Steinberg M, Donald K, Clark M, Tynan R. Towards successful ageing in the 21st century, Chapter 9. In Lupton GM, Najman JM eds. The sociology of health and illness. Macmillan Australia,1995;186–214.
25 Ebrahim S. The medicalisation of old age, BMJ 2002;324(7342):861–3.
26 Kurrle SE. Aged care medicine. Med J Aust 2002;176(1):4.
27 Expert Group on Healthcare of Older People. Adding life to years: report of the expert group on healthcare of older people. Glasgow: Scottish Executive, 2002.

18 Surgical, medical and research issues for women

1 Gorman WP, Davis KR, Donnelly R. Swollen lower limb—1: general assessment and deep venous thrombosis. BMJ 2000;320(7247):1453–56.
2 Adapted from: Prevention of venous thromboembolism. National Working Party on the Management and Prevention of Venous Thromboembolism. Best Practice Guidelines for Australia and New Zealand, 2nd edn, 2001. Health Education and Management International.
3 Geerts WH, Heit JA, Clagett GP, Pineo GF, Colwell CW, Anderson FA Jr et al. Prevention of venous thromboembolism. Chest 2001;119(Suppl 1):S132–75.
4 Lethaby A, Shepperd S, Cooke I, Farquhar C. Endometrial resection and ablation versus hysterectomy for heavy menstrual bleeding. Coch Rev.
5 Woodman N, Read MD. Oophorectomy at hysterectomy. In: Progress in Obstetrics and Gynaecology, Vol 14. Studd J. ed. Churchill Livingstone, 2000.
6 Plockinger B, Kolbl H. Development of ovarian pathology after hysterectomy without oophorectomy. J Am Coll Surg 1994;178(6):581–5.
7 Montgomery JC, Studd JW. Oestradiol and testosterone implants after hysterectomy for endometriosis. Contrib Gynecol Obstet 1987;16:241–6.
8 Reich H. Laparoscopic surgery for advanced endometriosis. In: The Yearbook of Obstetrics and Gynaecology, Vol 6. London: RCOG Press, 1998;377–93.
9 Schwartz PE. The role of prophylactic oophorectomy in the avoidance of ovarian cancer. Int J Gynaecol Obstet 1992;39(3):175–84.
10 Helmy WH, Jolaoso AS, Ifaturoti OO, Afify SA, Jones MH. The decision-to-delivery interval for emergency caesarean section: is 30 minutes a realistic target? Br J Obstet Gynaecol 2002;109(5):505–8.
11 MacKenzie IZ, Cooke I. What is a reasonable time from decision-to-delivery by caesarean section? Evidence from 415 deliveries. Br J Obstet Gynaecol 2002;109(5):498–504.
12 Smaill F, Hofmeyr GJ. Antibiotic prophylaxis for caesarean section. Coch Rev.
13 Leape LL, Brennan TA, Laird N, Lawthers AG, Localio AR, Bames BA et al. The nature of adverse events in hospitalzsed patients. Results of the Harvard Medical Practice Study II. N Engl J Med 1991:324(6):377–84.
14 Wolff AM, Bourke J, Campbell IA, Leembruggen DW. Detecting and reducing hospital adverse events: outcomes of the Wimmera clinical risk management program. Med J Aust 2001; 174(12):621–5.
15 Runciman WB, Edmonds MJ, Pradhan M. Setting priorities for patient safety. Qual Saf Health Care 2002;11(3):224–9.
16 Phillips SP. Evaluating women's health and gender. Am J Obstet Gynecol 2002;187 (Suppl 3):S22–4.

Abbreviations

A	androstenedione
ADEC	Australian Drug Evaluation Committee
ADHD	attention deficit/hyperactivity disorder
AFI	amniotic fluid index
AFP	alpha-fetoprotein
AIDS	acquired immune deficiency syndrome
ANC	antenatal clinic
APH	antepartum haemorrhage
ARM	artificial rupture of membranes
β-HCG	beta unit of HCG
BMD	bone mineral density
BMI	body mass index
BP	blood pressure
BPD	biparietal diameter
bpm	beats per minute
BSO	bilateral salpingo-oophorectomy
BV	bacterial vaginosis
Ca	cancer/calcium (according to context)
CAH	congenital adrenal hyperplasia
CHD	coronary heart disease
CIN	cervical intraepithelial neoplasia
CMV	cytomegalovirus
COC(P)	combined oral contraceptive (pill)
CPD	cephalopelvic disproportion
CTG	cardiotocogram/-graphy
CVP	central venous pressure
CVS	chorionic villus sampling
Cx	cervix
D&C	dilatation of cervix and curettage of uterus
DALY	daily adjusted life year
DCIS	ductal carcinoma in situ
DES	diethyl-stilboestrol
DHEA	dehydroepiandrosterone
DHEAS	dehydroepiandrosterone sulphate
DHT	dihydrotestosterone
DIC	disseminated intravascular coagulation
DMPA	depot medroxyprogesterone acetate
DUB	dysfunctional uterine bleeding
DVT	deep vein thrombosis
E_2	oestradiol
ECV	external cephalic version
EDD	expected date of delivery
EDS	Edinburgh depression scale
ERPC	evacuation of retained products of conception
EUA	examination under anaesthetic

FAE	fetal alcholol effect
FAS	fetal alcohol syndrome
FBC	full blood count
FGM	female genital mutilation
FISH	fluorescent in situ hybridisation test
FMP	final menstrual period
FNAB	fine needle aspiration biopsy
FSH	follicle-stimulating hormone
GA	general anaesthetic
GABA	G-aminobutyric acid
GBS	group B streptococci
GDM	gestational diabetes mellitus
GIFT	gamete intrafallopian transfer
GnRH	gonadotrophin-releasing hormone
GnRHa	gonadotrophin-releasing hormone analogue
GP	general practitioner or family physician (USA)
GSI	genuine stress incontinence
GTT	glucose tolerance test
Hb	haemoglobin
HBV	hepatitis B virus
HC	head circumference
HCG	human chorionic gonadotrophin
HCP	health care professional
HCV	hepatitis C virus
HDL	high-density lipoprotein
HELLP	haemolysis, elevated liver enzymes, low platelets
HIV	human immunodeficiency virus
HNPCC	hereditary non-polyposis colonic cancer
HPO	hypothalamic pituitary ovarian axis
HPV	human papilloma virus
HRT	hormone replacement therapy
HSIL	high-grade squamous intraepithelial lesion
HVS	high vaginal swab
HWY	hundred women years
IBS	irritable bowel syndrome
ICSI	intracytoplasmic sperm injection
IDC	invasive ductal carcinoma
IDDM	insulin-dependent diabetes mellitus
IgG	immunoglobulin G
IgM	immunoglobulin M
IMB	intermenstrual bleeding
IUCD	intrauterine contraceptive device
IUD	intrauterine death
IUGR	intrauterine growth retardation
IUS	intrauterine system
IVF	in vitro fertilisation
IVP	intravenous pyelogram

LA	local analgesia
LCIS	lobular carcinoma in situ
LDL	low-density lipoprotein
LFT	liver function test
LH	luteinising hormone
LIUS	levonorgestrel intrauterine system
LLETZ	large loop excision of the transformation zone
LMP	last menstrual period
lpm	litres per minute
LSCS	lower segment caesarean section
LSIL	low-grade squamous intraepithelial lesion
MSU	midstream specimen of urine
NEC	necrotising enterocolitis
NIDDM	non-insulin-dependent diabetes mellitus
NSAID	non-steroidal anti-inflammatory drug
NTD	neural tube defect
OA	occipitoanterior position
OCP	oral contraceptive pill
OHSS	ovarian hyperstimulation syndrome
OP	occipito-posterior position
OT	occipito-transverse position
OTC	over the counter
PCB	postcoital bleeding
PCOD	polycystic ovarian disease
PCOS	polycystic ovarian syndrome
PCR	polymerase chain reaction
PCT	postcoital test
PE	pulmonary embolism
PET	pre-eclampsia
PGA	pteroryl glutamic acid (folic acid)
PID	pelvic inflammatory disease
PMB	postmenopausal bleeding
PMDD	premenstrual dysphoric disorder
PMS	premenstrual syndrome
PND	postnatal depression
POC	products of conception
POP	progestogen-only pill
PPH	postpartum haemorrhage
PPP	postpartum psychosis
PPROM	preterm prelabour rupture of membranes
PRL	prolactin
PTL	preterm labour
RBS	random blood sugar (glucose)
RCT	randomised controlled trial
RDI	recommended daily intake
RDS	respiratory distress syndrome
Rh	Rhesus blood group

RIF	right iliac fossa
RNA	ribonucleic acid
ROP	retinopathy of prematurity
RPOC	retained products of conception
SCJ	squamo-columnar junction
SERM	selective oestrogen receptor modulator
SFD	small for dates
SGA	small for gestational age
SHBG	sex hormone binding globulin
SIDS	sudden infant death syndrome
SLE	systemic lupus erythematosus
SRM	spontaneous rupture of membranes
SRY	sex determining region of the Y chromosome
SSRI	selective serotonin reuptake inhibitor
STI	sexually transmitted infection
SVD	spontaneous vaginal delivery
TAH	total abdominal hysterectomy
TCA	tricyclic antidepressant
TDF	testicular determining factor
TFT	thyroid function test
TOP	termination of pregnancy
TORCH	viral screen for toxoplasma, cytomegalovirus and rubella
TVS	transvaginal ultrasound scan
TZ	transformation zone (of the cervix)
UDS	urodynamic studies
USS	ultrasound scan
UTI	urinary tract infection
VAIN	vaginal intraepithelial neoplasia
VBAC	vaginal bath after caesarean section
VIN	vulval intraepithelial neoplasia
/7	number of days
/12	number of months
/52	number of weeks
/40	number of weeks of pregnancy
6/28	notation of menstrual cycle; days of loss/length of cycle

Index